Handbook of Pharmacology & Physiology in Anesthetic Practice

SECOND EDITION

Handbook of Pharmacology & Physiology in Anesthetic Practice

SECOND EDITION

BY

ROBERT K. STOELTING, M.D.

Emeritus Professor and Chair, Department of Anesthesia Indiana University School of Medicine
Indianapolis, Indiana

SIMON C. HILLIER M.B., Ch.B; FRCA

Associate Professor, Department of Anesthesia
Indiana University School of Medicine
Indianapolis, Indiana

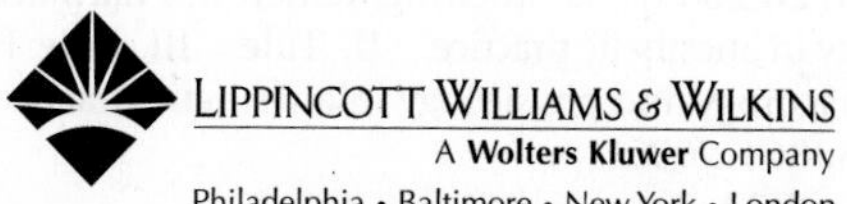

Acquisitions Editor: Brian Brown
Developmental Editor: Fran Murphy
Project Manager: Dave Murphy
Manufacturing Manager: Ben Rivera
Marketing Manager: Angela Panetta
Compositor: TechBooks
Printer: R. R. Donnelley

530 Walnut Street
Philadelphia, PA 19106 USA
LWW.com

Printed in China

Library of Congress Cataloging-in-Publication Data

Stoelting, Robert K.
Handbook of pharmacology & physiology in anesthetic practice / by Robert K. Stoelting. —2nd ed.
p. ; cm.
Companion v. to: Pharmacology and physiology in anesthetic practice / Robert K. Stoelting. 4th ed.
Includes bibliographical references and indexes.
ISBN 13: 978-0-7817-5785-0
ISBN 10: 0-7817-5785-1
1. Anesthetics—Physiological effect—Handbooks, manuals, etc.
[DNLM: 1. Anesthetics—pharmacology—Handbooks. 2. Anesthetics—pharmacology—Outlines. 3. Physiological Processes—Handbooks. 4. Physiological Processes—Outlines. QV 39 S872h 2005] I. Stoelting, Robert K. Pharmacology and physiology in anesthetic practice. II. Title. III. Title: Handbook of pharmacology and physiology in anesthetic practice.
RD82.2.S686 2005
615'.781—dc22

2005017549

RRS1109

10 9 8 7 6

To purchase additional copies of this book, call our customer service department at (800) 638-3030 or fax orders to (301) 824-7390. International customers should call (301) 714-2324.

Visit Lippincott Williams & Wilkins on the Internet: http://www.LWW.com. Lippincott Williams & Wilkins customer service representatives are available from 8:30 am to 6:00 pm, EST.

Contents

SECTION I: PHARMACOLOGY 1

Preface

The Handbook of Pharmacology and Physiology in Anesthetic Practice is intended to provide a rapid and accurate source of information relevant to the pharmacology of drugs encountered during anesthesia and the physiologic responses that impact the anesthetic experience. The handbook utilizes a format that follows the identical chapters and headings in the fourth edition of *Pharmacology and Physiology in Anesthetic Practice,* thus permitting the reader to refer to corresponding areas of the more detailed information in the textbook. As such, the intent of the handbook is to serve as a companion and to provide a practical cross-reference to *Pharmacology and Physiology in Anesthetic Practice* and its more in-depth discussion of drugs and physiology. The emphasis in the handbook is on presentation of information in a table format. This design provides rapid visibility of pertinent aspects of pharmacology and physiology that can be readily assessed at sites other than the individual's personal library.

The authors wish to thank Deanna Walker for her secretarial help in the preparation of the manuscript.

Robert K. Stoelting, M.D.
Simon C. Hillier, M.B., Ch.B., FRCA

Pharmacology

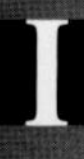

Pharmacokinetics and Pharmacodynamics of Injected and Inhaled Drugs

1

Pharmacokinetics is the quantitative study of the absorption, distribution, metabolism, and excretion of injected and inhaled drugs and their metabolites (Stoelting RK, Hillier SC. Pharamacokinetics and pharmacodynamics of injected and inhaled drugs. In: *Pharmacology and Physiology in Anesthetic Practice*, 4th ed. Philadelphia: Lippincott Williams & Wilkins, 2006:1–41). The selection and adjustment of drug dosage schedules and interpretation of measured plasma concentrations of drugs are facilitated by an understanding of pharmacokinetic principles. Pharmacodynamics is the study of the intrinsic sensitivity or responsiveness of receptors to a drug and the mechanisms by which these effects occur. The intrinsic sensitivity of receptors is determined by measuring the plasma concentrations of a drug required to evoke specific pharmacologic responses. The intrinsic sensitivity of receptors varies among patients. As a result, at similar plasma concentrations of a drug, some patients show a therapeutic response, others show no response, and in others, toxicity develops.

STEREOCHEMISTRY

Stereochemistry is the study of how molecules are structured in three dimensions. *Enantiomers* (substances of opposite shape) are pairs of molecules existing in two forms that are mirror images of one another (right- and left-hand) but that cannot be superimposed. A pair of enantiomers is distinguished by the direction in which, when dissolved in solution, they rotate in polarized light, either clockwise (dextrorotatory, d [+]) or counterclockwise (levorotatory, l [−]). When the two enantiomers are present in equal proportions (50:50), they are referred to as a *racemic mixture*. The most rapidly applicable and unambiguous convention for designating isomers is the sinister (S) and rectus (R) classification that specifies the absolute configuration in the name of the compound. Pharmacologically, not all enantiomers are created equal. Enantiomers can exhibit differences in absorption, distribution, clearance, potency, and toxicity (drug interactions). The administration of a racemic drug mixture may in fact pharmacologically represent two different drugs with distinct pharmacokinetic and pharmacodynamic properties.

Clinical Aspects of Chirality

More than one third of all synthetic drugs are *chiral* (thiopental, ketamine, inhaled anesthetics except sevoflurane, local anesthetics, neuromuscular-blocking drugs, opioids), although most of them are utilized clinically as racemic mixtures.

DESCRIPTION OF DRUG RESPONSE (TABLE 1-1)

PHARMACOLOGY OF INJECTED DRUGS

The pharmacokinetics of injected drugs usually is defined initially in healthy adults with a low fat-to-lean body ratio. Conversely, drugs are most likely to be administered to patients with chronic diseases (renal failure, cirrhosis of the liver, cardiac failure) at various extremes of age, hydration, and nutrition.

TABLE 1-1.
DESCRIPTION OF DRUG RESPONSE

Hyperactive (unusually low dose produces expected effect)
Hypersensitive (allergic, sensitized)
Hyporeactive (large does required to produce expected effect)
Tolerance (hyporeactivity that occurs with chronic exposure)
Cross-tolerance (develops between drugs of different classes that produce similar effects)
  Neuronal adaptation (cellular tolerance)
  Enzyme induction
  Depletion of neurotransmitters with sustained stimulation
Additive effect (second drug acting with first drug produces an effect equal to summation)
Synergistic effect (two drugs interact to produce an effect greater than either alone)
Antagonism (two drugs interact to produce an effect less than summation)
Agonist (drug activates receptors by binding to receptors)
Antagonist (drug binds to receptors without activating receptors)
  Competitive (increasing concentrations of the antagonist progressively inhibit the response to an unchanging concentration of agonist)
  Noncompetitive (even high concentrations of agonist cannot completely overcome the antagonism)

General anesthesia and surgery may alter the pharmacokinetics of injected drugs relative to the awake state because of alterations in renal blood flow, hepatic blood flow, and hepatic enzyme activity. Drug-induced changes in peripheral blood flow may further alter the perioperative distribution of injected anesthetics. The measured or calculated pharmacokinetic parameters of injected drugs include bioavailability, clearance, volume of distribution (Vd), elimination half-time, context-sensitive half-time, effect-site equilibration time, and recovery time. Context-sensitive half-time and effect-site equilibration time are more useful than elimination half-time in characterizing the clinical responses to drugs.

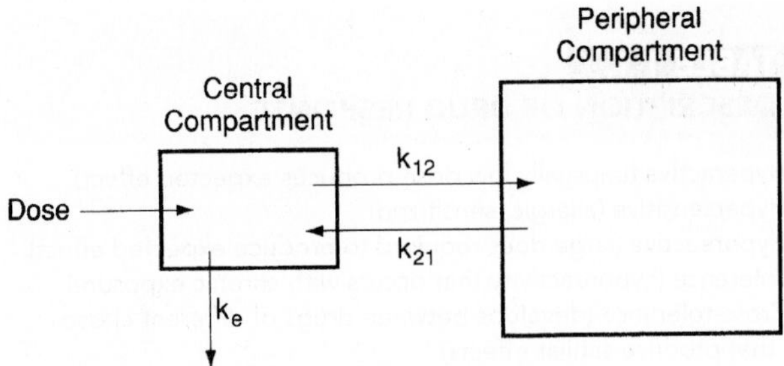

Figure 1-1. A two-compartment pharmacokinetic model as derived from a biexponential plasma decay curve (see Fig. 1-2). The rate constants that characterize the intercompartmental transfer of drugs are k12 and k21, and ke is the rate constant for overall drug elimination from the body. (From Stanski DR, Watkins WD. *Drug Disposition in Anesthesia*. New York: Grune & Stratton, 1982; with permission.)

Compartmental Models (Fig 1-1)

The central compartment includes intravascular fluid and highly perfused tissues (lungs, heart, brain, kidneys, liver) into which the uptake of drug is rapid. In adults, these highly perfused tissues receive almost 75% of the cardiac output but represent about 10% of the body mass. A large calculated volume for the peripheral compartment suggests extensive uptake of drug by those tissues that constitute the peripheral compartment.

Alternative Concepts in the Interpretation of Compartment Modeling

The traditional application of compartmental models to pharmacokinetics assumes that a drug is eliminated only from the central compartment. Atracurium and cisatracurium, however, are eliminated by pathways (Hoffman elimination, ester hydrolysis) that do not depend on the usual organs of clearance depicted by the central compartment. Elimination half-time, which provides a description of drug disposition in a single compartment model, may be of limited value in describing multicompartmental models.

Plasma Concentrsation Curves (Fig. 1-2)

The distribution phase of the plasma concentration curve begins immediately after the intravenous injection of a drug and reflects that drug's distribution from the circulation (central compartment) to peripheral tissues (peripheral compartments) (see Figs. 1-1 and 1-2). The elimination phase of the plasma concentration curve follows the initial distribution phase and is characterized by a more gradual decline in the drug's plasma

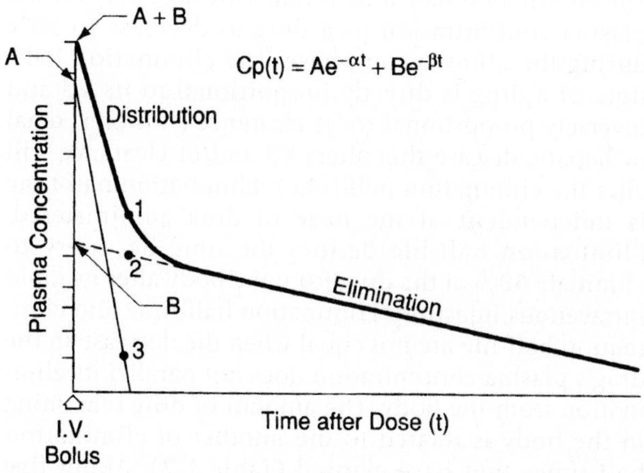

Figure 1-2. Schematic depiction of the decrease in plasma concentration of a drug with time after rapid intravenous injection into the central compartment (see Fig. 1-1). Two distinct phases (biexponential) that characterize this curve are designated the distribution (α) and elimination (β) phases. (From Stanski DR, Watkins WD. *Drug Disposition in Anesthesia*. New York: Grune & Stratton, 1982; with permission.)

concentration (see Fig. 1-2). This gradual decline reflects the drug's elimination from the circulation (central compartment) through renal and hepatic clearance mechanisms.

Alternative Concepts in Interpretation of Plasma Drug Concentration

The traditional concept that a drug's pharmacologic effect parallels its plasma (presumably receptor) concentration is not always valid (1 minute after the bolus administration of cisatracurium, the plasma concentration is already decreasing, whereas the pharmacologic effect is increasing).

Elimination Haslf-Time

The elimination half-time is that time necessary for the plasma concentration of a drug to decrease to 50% during the elimination phase. The elimination half-time of a drug is directly proportional to its Vd and inversely proportional to its clearance (however, renal or hepatic disease that alters Vd and/or clearance will alter the elimination half-time). Elimination half-time is independent of the dose of drug administered. Elimination half-life defines the time necessary to eliminate 50% of the drug from the body after its rapid intravenous injection. Elimination half-time and elimination half-life are not equal when the decrease in the drug's plasma concentration does not parallel its elimination from the body. The amount of drug remaining in the body is related to the number of elimination half-times that have elapsed (Table 1-2). About five elimination half-times are required for the nearly total (96.9%) elimination of drug from the body (drug accumulation is predictable if dosing intervals are less than this period). Drug accumulation continues until the rate of its elimination equals the rate of its administration.

TABLE 1-2.
RELATIONSHIP OF HALF-TIMES TO AMOUNT OF DRUG ELIMINATED

Number of Half-Times	Fraction of Initial Amount Remaining	Percent of Initial Amount Eliminated
0	1	0
1	1/2	50
2	1/4	75
3	1/8	87.5
4	1/16	93.8
5	1/32	96.9
6	1/64	98.4

Alternative Concepts in Interpretation of the Elimination Half-Time

Elimination half-time may be of little value in describing drug pharmacokinetics in multicompartmental models. Elimination half-times alone provide virtually no insight into the rate of decrease in the plasma concentration after the discontinuation of intravenous drug administration.

Context-Sensitive Half-Time

This value describes the time necessary for the plasma drug concentration to decrease by 50% (or any other percentage) after discontinuing a continuous infusion of a specific duration (Fig. 1-3). Context-sensitive half-time, in contrast to elimination half-time, considers the combined effects of distribution and metabolism as well as the duration of continuous intravenous administration on drug pharmacokinetics. Depending largely on the lipid solubility of the drug and the efficiency of its clearance mechanisms, the context-sensitive half-time increases in parallel with the duration of continuous intravenous administration (see Fig. 1-3). The context-sensitive half-time bears no constant relationship to the drug's elimination half-time.

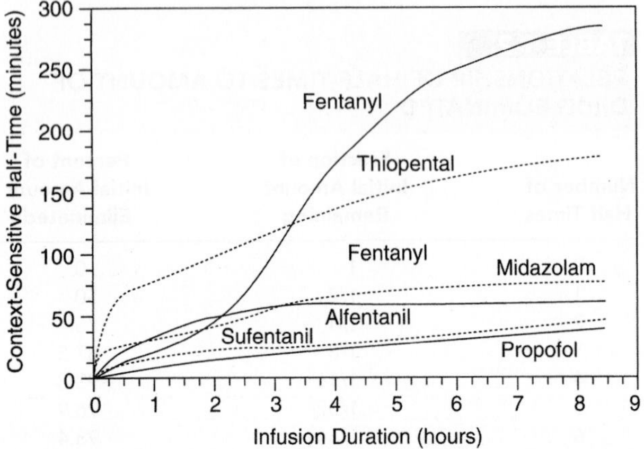

Figure 1-3. Context-sensitive half-times as a function of the duration of intravenous drug infusion for each of the computer-simulated pharmacokinetic models. (From Hughes MA, Glass PSA, Jacobs JR. Context-sensitive half-time in multicompartment pharmacokinetic models for intravenous anesthetic drugs. *Anesthesiology* 1992;76:334–341; with permission.)

Time to Recovery

The time to recovery depends on how far the plasma concentration of a drug must decrease to reach levels compatible with awakening (Fig. 1-4). The difference between the plasma concentration at the time that the continuous infusion of a drug is discontinued and the plasma concentration below which awakening can be expected is an important factor in determining time to recovery.

Effect-Site Equilibration

The delay between the intravenous administration of a drug and the onset of its clinical effect reflects the time necessary for the circulation to deliver the drug to its site of action (tissues such as the brain; measured as the time to produce a specific effect on the electroencephalo-

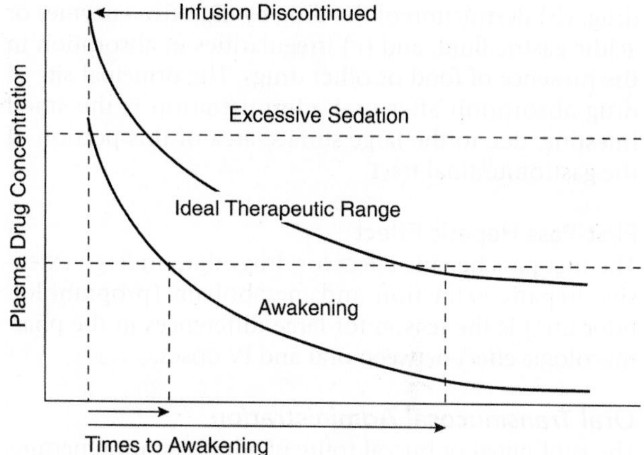

Figure 1-4. The time necessary for the plasma concentration of drug to decrease to a level associated with awakening depends on the plasma concentration present when the infusion of drug is discontinued.

gram). Drugs with a short effect-site equilibration time (remifentanil, alfentanil, thiopental, propofol) will produce a more rapid onset of pharmacologic effect compared with drugs that have a longer effect-site equilibration time (fentanyl, sufentanil, midazolam). The knowledge of effect-site equilibration time is important in determining dosing intervals, especially when titrating intravenous drugs to a given clinical effect.

Route of Administration and Systemic Absorption of Drugs

Systemic absorption, regardless of the route of drug administration, depends on the drug's solubility.

Oral Administration

The disadvantages of the oral route include (a) emesis caused by irritation of the gastrointestinal mucosa by the drug, (b) destruction of the drug by digestive enzymes or acidic gastric fluid, and (c) irregularities in absorption in the presence of food or other drugs. The principal site of drug absorption after oral administration is the small intestine, due to the large surface area of this portion of the gastrointestinal tract.

First-Pass Hepatic Effect

The first-pass hepatic effect for drugs that undergo extensive hepatic extraction and metabolism (propranolol, lidocaine) is the reason for large differences in the pharmacologic effect between oral and IV doses.

Oral Transmucosal Administration

The sublingual or buccal route of administration permits a rapid onset of drug effect, because it bypasses the liver and thus prevents the first-pass hepatic effect on the initial plasma concentration of drug.

Transdermal Administration

The transdermal administration of drugs provides sustained therapeutic plasma concentrations of the drug and decreases the likelihood of loss of therapeutic efficacy due to the peaks and valleys associated with conventional intermittent drug injections. The postauricular zone, because of its thin epidermal layer and somewhat higher temperature, is the only area that is sufficiently permeable for predictable and sustained absorption of scopolamine.

Rectal Administration

Drugs administered into the proximal rectum are absorbed into the superior hemorrhoidal veins and subsequently transported via the portal venous system to the liver, where they are exposed to metabolism (first-pass hepatic effect) before entering the systemic circulation.

Parenteral Administration

A parenteral route may be required to ensure the absorption of the active form of the drug, and it is the only acceptable route of administration in an unconscious or otherwise uncooperative patient.

Distribution of Drugs after Systemic Absorption

After the systemic absorption of a drug, the highly perfused tissues (heart, brain, kidneys, liver) receive a disproportionately large amount of the total dose (Table 1-3). As the plasma concentration of drug decreases below that in highly perfused tissues, the drug leaves these tissues to be redistributed to less well-perfused sites, such as skeletal muscles and fat (see Table 1-3). For example, awakening after a single dose of thiopental principally reflects a redistribution of the drug from the brain to less well-perfused tissue sites, such as skeletal muscles and fat, where thiopental is considered to be pharmacologically inactive. The capacity of tissues to accept a drug depends largely on the drug's solubility in the tissue and the mass of the tissue (Table 1-4).

Uptake into the Lungs

The pulmonary uptake of drugs may influence the peak arterial concentration of these drugs and serve as a reservoir to release the drug back into the systemic circulation.

TABLE 1-3.
BODY TISSUE COMPOSITION

	Body Mass (% of 70-kg adult)	Blood Flow (% of cardiac output)
Vessel-rich group	10	75
Muscle group	50	19
Fat group	20	6
Vessel-poor group	20	<1

TABLE 1-4.
RATE AND CAPACITY OF TISSUE UPTAKE OF DRUGS

Determinants of tissue uptake of drug
Blood flow
Concentration gradient
Blood-brain barrier
Physicochemical properties of drug
Ionization
Lipid solubility
Protein binding
Determinants of capacity of tissue to store drug
Solubility
Tissue mass
Binding to macromolecules
pH

Central Nervous System Distribution

The distribution of ionized water-soluble drugs to the central nervous system (CNS) from the circulation is restricted because of the limited permeability characteristics of brain capillaries, known as the *blood-brain barrier*. Cerebral blood flow is the only limitation to permeation of the CNS by nonionized lipid-soluble drugs. Acute head injury and arterial hypoxemia may be associated with a disruption of the blood-brain barrier.

Volume of Distribution

The Vd depicts the distribution characteristics of a drug in the body and is influenced by the physicochemical characteristics of the drug, including (a) lipid solubility, (b) binding to plasma proteins, and (c) molecular size. A lipid-soluble drug (thiopental, diazepam) that is highly concentrated in tissues, with a resulting low plasma concentration, will have a calculated Vd that exceeds total body water.

Ionization

Most drugs are weak acids or bases that are present in solutions as both ionized and nonionized molecules.

Characteristics of Ionized and Nonionized Molecules (Table 1-5)

Determinant of Degree of Ionization

When the pK and the pH values are identical, 50% of the drug exists in both the ionized and nonionized form. This is the degree of ionization.

Ion Trapping

A concentration difference of total drug can develop on two sides of any membrane that separates fluids having different pH values. The nonionized lipid-soluble fraction of drug equilibrates across the cell membranes, but the total concentration of drug is very different on each side of the membrane because of the impact of pH on the fraction of drug that exists in the ionized form.

TABLE 1-5.
CHARACTERISTICS OF NONIONIZED AND IONIZED DRUG MOLECULES

	Nonionized	Ionized
Pharmacologic effect	Active	Nonactive
Solubility	Lipids	Water
Cross lipid barriers (gastrointestinal tract, blood-brain barrier, placenta)	Yes	No
Renal excretion	No	Yes
Hepatic metabolism	Yes	No

Protein Binding

Most acidic drugs bind to albumin, whereas basic drugs select α-1-acid glycoprotein. Protein binding has an important effect on the distribution of drugs because only the free or unbound fraction is readily available to cross cell membranes. Alterations in protein binding are usually important only for those drugs that are highly protein bound, such as warfarin, propranolol, phenytoin, and diazepam.

Determinants of Protein Binding

The extent of protein binding parallels the lipid solubility of the drug. Statements about the percentage of protein binding of a drug are not meaningful unless the plasma concentration of the drug and availability of binding sites (plasma concentration of albumin) are also known. Renal failure may decrease the fraction of a drug bound to protein, even in the absence of changes in plasma concentrations of albumin or other proteins. Albumin concentrations tend to be lower in elderly patients, but the impact of this change is small compared with the effect of disease states that result in renal or hepatic dysfunction. Increases in the plasma concentration of α-1-acid glycoprotein occur in response to surgery, chronic pain, and acute myocardial infarction.

Clearance of Drugs From the Systemic Circulation

Clearance is the volume of plasma cleared of a drug through renal excretion and/or metabolism in the liver or other organs. Almost all drugs administered in the therapeutic dose ranges are cleared from the circulation at a rate proportional to the amount of drug present in the plasma (first-order kinetics). More drug is cleared from the plasma per unit time immediately following administration, when plasma concentrations are the highest (elimination rate is proportional to the concentration). Clearance is one of the most important pharmacokinetic variables to consider when defining a constant drug infusion regimen.

Hepatic Clearance

The hepatic clearance of a drug is the product of hepatic blood flow and the hepatic extraction ratio.

Biliary Excretion

Most of the metabolites of drugs produced in the liver are excreted in bile into the gastrointestinal tract.

Renal Clearance

Water-soluble compounds are excreted more efficiently by the kidneys than are compounds having high lipid solubility. Reabsorption is most prominent for lipid-soluble drugs that can easily cross the cell membranes of renal tubular epithelial cells to enter pericapillary fluid.

Metabolism of Drugs (Biotransformation)

Biotransformation converts pharmacologically active, lipid-soluble drugs into water-soluble and often pharmacologically inactive metabolites. Increased water solubility decreases the Vd for a drug and enhances its renal excretion and occasionally gastrointestinal elimination. A lipid-soluble parent drug is not likely to undergo extensive renal excretion because of the ease of reabsorption from the lumens of renal tubules into pericapillary fluid. Metabolism does not always lead to the production of pharmacologically inactive metabolites.

Rate of Metabolism

The metabolism rate is most often determined by the concentration of a drug at the site of metabolism and by the intrinsic rate of the metabolism process.

First-Order Kinetics

First-order kinetics describes metabolism of a constant fraction of available drug in a given period.

Zero-Order Kinetics

Zero-order kinetics occurs when the plasma concentration of a drug exceeds the capacity of metabolizing enzymes. As a result, the absolute amount of a drug eliminated per unit of time during zero-order kinetics is the same, regardless of the drug's plasma concentration.

Pathways of Metabolism

The metabolic pathways for drugs are (a) oxidation, (b) reduction, (c) hydrolysis, and (d) conjugation. Hepatic microsomal enzymes, which participate in the metabolism of many drugs, are located principally in hepatic smooth endoplasmic reticulum.

Phase I Enzymes

These enzymes include cytochrome P-450 enzymes, noncytochrome P-450 enzymes, and flavin-containing monooxygenase enzymes.

Cytochrome P-450 Enzymes

The enzymes of the cytochrome P-450 (CYP) system, a superfamily of membrane-bound heme proteins, catalyze the metabolism of endogenous compounds. P-450 3A4 is the most abundantly expressed P-450 isoform, comprising 20% to 60% of total P-450 activity. P-450 3A4/5 is considered to be responsible for metabolizing more than one half of all currently available drugs, including opioids (alfentanil, sufentanil, fentanyl), benzodiazepines, local anesthetics (lidocaine, ropivacaine), immunosuppressants (cyclosporine), and antihistamines (terfenadine).

Enzyme Induction

Enzyme induction is the increased enzyme activity produced by drugs or chemicals.

Noncytochrome P-450 Enzymes

Noncytochrome P-450 enzymes (esters or nonmicrosomal enzymes) catalyze those reactions responsible for the metabolism of drugs by conjugation, hydrolysis, and, to a lesser extent, oxidation and reduction. Noncytochrome P-450 enzymes, such as plasma cholinesterase and acetylating enzymes, do not, however, undergo enzyme induction. The activity of these enzymes is determined genetically, as emphasized by patients with atypical cholinesterase enzyme and individuals who are classified as being rapid or slow acetylators.

Flavin-Containing Monooxygenase Enzymes

Flavin-containing monooxygenase enzymes are nicotinamide adenine dinucleotide (NAD)-dependent microsomal enzymes that oxidize (phase I reactions) nitrogen, sulfur, and phosphorus-containing compounds.

Phase II Enzymes

Phase II enzymes include glucuronosyltrasferases, glutathione-S-transferases, *N*-acetyl-transferases, and sulfotransferases.

Glucuronosyltranserases

The glucuronosyltranserases are a family of hepatic microsomal enzymes that catalyze the covalent addition of glucuronic acid to a variety of endogenous and exogenous compounds, thus rendering them more water soluble. Glucuronides may be more or less pharmacologically active than their parent drugs. Glucuronidation is an important metabolic pathway for several drugs used during anesthesia. Propofol undergoes glucuronidation in the liver and kidneys. Opioids also undergo glucuronidation, as reflected by morphine-3-glucuronide and morphine-6-glucuronide. The glucuronide of 1-hydroxymidazolam is pharmacologically active and may contribute to prolonged midazolam effects in patients with renal insufficiency.

Glutathione-*S*-Transferase

Glutathione-S-transferase (GST) enzymes are primarily a defensive system for detoxification and protection against oxidative stress.

N-acetyl-transferase

N-acetyl-transferase (NAT) and resulting acetylation is a common phase II reaction for heterocyclic aromatic amines and arylamines hydrazines. Slow acetylators have a greater therapeutic response to drugs that are inactivated by NAT enzymes, and these individuals may be at greater risk for drug-induced side effects (isoniazid hepatotoxicity, hydralazine or procainamide lupuslike syndrome).

Oxidative Metabolism

Hepatic microsomal enzymes, including cytochrome P-450 enzymes, are crucial for the oxidation (hydroxylation, deamination, desulfuration, dealkylation, and dehalogenation) and resulting metabolism of many drugs. Epoxide intermediates present in the oxidative metabolism of drugs are capable of covalently binding with macromolecules and may be responsible for drug-induced organ toxicity, such as hepatic dysfunction.

Reductive Metabolism

Under conditions of low oxygen partial pressures, cytochrome P-450 enzymes transfer electrons directly to a substrate, such as halothane, rather than to oxygen.

Hydrolysis

Enzymes responsible for the hydrolysis of drugs (often an ester bond) do not involve the cytochrome P-450 enzyme system.

Conjugation with Glucuronic Acid Involves Cytochrome P-450 Enzymes

When conjugated to a lipid-soluble drug or metabolite, hydrophilic glucuronic acid renders the substance pharmacologically inactive and more water soluble. The resulting water-soluble glucuronide conjugates are unlikely to be reabsorbed into the systemic circulation and are thus preferentially excreted in bile and urine.

Dose–Response Curves

Dose–response curves depict the relationship between a dose of drug administered and the resulting pharmacologic effect (Fig. 1-5). A logarithmic transformation of dosage is frequently used, because it permits the display of a wide range of doses.

Potency

The potency of a drug is influenced by (a) absorption, (b) distribution, (c) metabolism, (d) excretion, and (e) affinity for the receptor. For clinical purposes, the potency of a drug makes little difference as long as the effective dose (ED50, ED90) of the drug can be administered conveniently. An increased affinity of a drug for its receptor moves the dose–response curve to the left.

Slope of the Dose–Response Curve

The slope of the curve is influenced by the number of receptors that must be occupied before a drug effect occurs. A steep dose–response curve is characteristic of neuromuscular blocking drugs and inhaled anesthetics (minimal alevolar concentration or MAC). When the

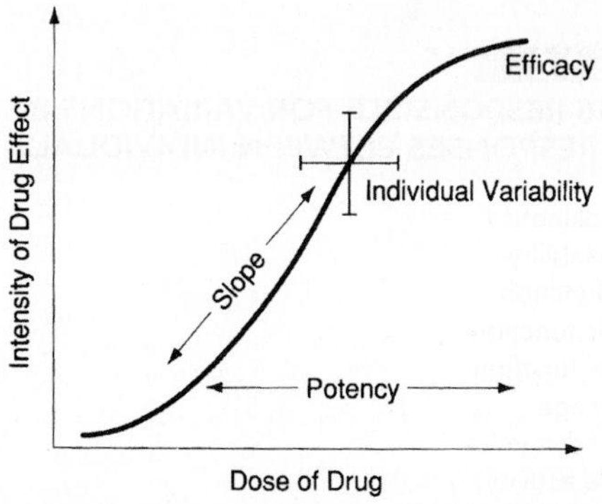

Figure 1-5. Dose–response curves are characterized by differences in potency, slope, efficacy, and individual responses.

dose–response curve is steep, the difference between a therapeutic and toxic concentration may be small (especially true for volatile anesthetics).

Efficacy

The efficacy of a drug is depicted by the plateau in dose–response curves. The side effects of a drug may limit dosage to below the concentration associated with its maximal desirable effect. Differences in efficacy are emphasized by the pharmacologic effects of opioids versus aspirin in relieving pain.

Individual Variability in Responses

The variability of response to a drug reflects the differences in pharmacokinetics and/or pharmacodynamics among patients (Table 1-6). This may account even for differences in pharmacologic effects of drugs in the same patient at different times. A five-fold range in the plasma concentrations of a drug may be required to achieve the same pharmacologic effect in different individuals. In clinical practice, the impact of interpatient variability may be masked by the administration of high doses of a drug (nondepolarizing neuromuscular-blocking drugs).

TABLE 1-6.
EVENTS RESPONSIBLE FOR VARIATIONS IN DRUG RESPONSES BETWEEN INDIVIDUALS

- Pharmacokinetics
  - Bioavailability
  - Renal function
  - Hepatic function
  - Cardiac function
  - Patient age
- Pharmacodynamics
  - Enzyme activity
  - Genetic differences
- Drug Interactions

Elderly Patients

Elderly patients who exhibit variations in drug response most likely reflect (a) decreased cardiac output, (b) enlarged fat content, (c) decreased plasma protein binding, and (d) decreased renal function. The net effect of these changes is an increased vulnerability of elderly patients to cumulative drug effects. Aging does not seem to be accompanied by changes in receptor responsiveness.

Enzyme Activity Alterations

Alterations in enzyme activity, as reflected by enzyme induction, may be responsible for variations in drug responses among individuals.

Genetic Disorders

Disorders that cause variations in drug responses among individuals are due, in part, to genetic differences that may also affect receptor sensitivity. Genetic variations in metabolic pathways (rapid versus slow acetylators) may have important clinical implications for drugs such as isoniazid and hydralazine. Examples of diseases that are unmasked by drugs include (a) atypical cholinesterase enzyme, revealed by prolonged neuromuscular blockade after administration of succinylcholine or mivacurium; (b) malignant hyperthermia, triggered by succinylcholine or volatile anesthetics; (c) glucose-6-phosphate dehydrogenase deficiency, in which certain drugs cause hemolysis; and (d) intermittent porphyria, in which barbiturates may evoke an acute attack.

Drug Interactions

Pharmacologic interactions occur when a drug alters the intensity of pharmacologic effects of another drug given concurrently. Drug interactions may reflect alterations in pharmacokinetics (increased metabolism of neuromuscular blocking drugs in patients receiving anticonvulsants chronically) or pharmacodynamics (decrease in volatile anesthetic requirements produced by opioids). The net result of a drug interaction may be the enhanced or diminished effects of one or both drugs, leading to desired or undesired effects. The potential for drug interactions in the perioperative period is great, considering the large number of drugs from different chemical classes that are likely to be part of anesthesia management.

PHARMACODYNAMICS OF INJECTED DRUGS

The most important mechanism by which drugs exert pharmacologic effects is by the interaction of the drug with a specific protein molecule (receptor) in the lipid bilayer of cell membranes (Fig. 1-6). A drug administered as an exogenous substance is an incidental "passenger" for these receptors. A drug–receptor interaction alters the function or conformation of a specific cellular component that initiates or prevents a series of changes that characterize the pharmacologic effects of the drug. The three classes of cell surface receptors, as defined by their signal transduction mechanisms, are categorized at G protein-coupled receptors, ligand-gated ion channels, and receptor-linked enzymes. *G protein-coupled receptors* constitute the largest family of cell surface receptors, and they mediate the cellular responses to diverse extracellular signals including hormones, neurotransmitters, and local mediators. A hallmark of signal transduction by G protein-coupled receptors is their ability to amplify extracellular signals.

Excitable Transmembrane Proteins

Voltage-Sensitive Ion Channels

Voltage-sensitive ion channels open and close in response to changes in voltage across cell membranes; these are represented by the classic sodium, chloride, potassium, and calcium ion channels. At normal resting membrane potentials (usually −60 to −80 mV), these channels remain closed. When cell membranes are depo-

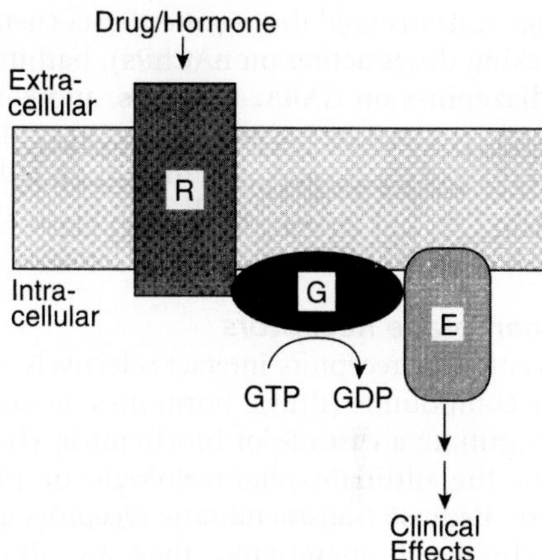

Figure 1-6. Transmembrane receptors (R) are located in the cell membrane and bind drugs or hormones on the extracellular surface. Agonist-bound receptors then interact with guanine nucleotide proteins (G proteins). With the energy provided by the hydrolysis of guanine triphosphate (GTP) to guanine diphosphate (GDP), activated G proteins are able to interact with effector systems (E), leading to clinically recognized responses. (From Schwinn DA. Adrenoceptors as models for G protein–coupled receptors: structure, function, and regulation. *Br J Anaesth* 1993;71:77–85; with permission.)

larized (become less negative), these ion channels undergo conformational changes so that the ion channel pore opens and ions pass through. The voltage-gated ion channels are protein complexes formed by the association of several individual subunits.

Ligand-Gated Ion Channels

These channels include acetylcholine receptors (nAChRs), serotonin receptors ($5HT_3$), gamma-aminobutyric acid receptors ($GABA_A$), and glycine receptors. A second family of ligand-gated ion channels is activated by glutamate, the principal excitatory neurotransmitter in the CNS. Ligand-gated ion channels are important targets for drugs administered during anesthesia (neuromuscular blocking drugs acting on nAChRs), barbiturates and benzodiazepines on $GABA_A$ receptors, and ketamine on N-methyl-D-aspartate (NMDA) receptors. Inhibitory neurotransmitters (GABA, glycine) open chloride ion channels and hyperpolarize cell membranes, thus preventing depolarization.

Transmembrane Receptors

Transmembrane receptors interact selectively with extracellular compounds (drugs, hormones, neurotransmitters) to initiate a cascade of biochemical changes that leads to the ultimate pharmacologic or physiologic response. Because transmembrane receptors are located in the lipid cell membrane, they are able to bind hydrophilic ligands located in the extracellular space. Thus, many water-soluble drugs do not have to cross lipid bilayers to interact with cells (see Fig. 1-6).

Receptor Families

Gamma-Aminobutyric Acid Receptors

The activation of the $GABA_A$-chloride channel (receptor) results in cell hyperpolarization or an increase in ion conductance that prevents depolarization, thereby inhibiting neuronal activity. Such activation by benzodiazepines, barbiturates, and propofol enhances the endogenous $GABA_A$-mediated inhibition in the CNS, providing a neurobiologic basis for the hypnotic and sedative effects of these drugs (Fig. 1-7). Approximately one-third of all synapses in the CNS are responsive to GABA. GABA is not pharmacologically active when administered systemically, because it cannot cross the blood-brain barrier.

Glycine Receptors

Glycine receptors are inhibitory receptors that are selectively permeable to anions and mediate rapid inhibitory synaptic transmission, primarily in the spinal cord.

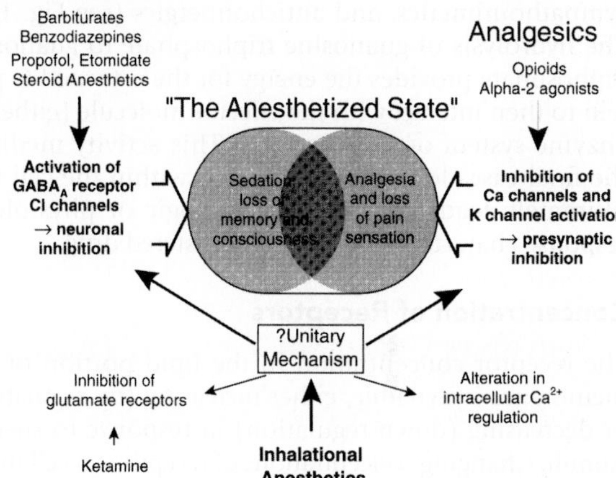

Figure 1-7. The major pathways for sedative-hypnotics and analgesics in generating the anesthetized state considered to be characteristic of volatile anesthetics. (From Lynch C, Pancrazio JJ. Snails, spiders, and stereospecificity—is there a role for calcium channels in anesthetic mechanisms? *Anesthesiology* 1994;81: 1–5; with permission.)

$5HT_3$ Receptors

$5HT_3$ receptors are excitatory, selectively permeable to cations, and exert a variety of effects in the CNS including anxiolysis, analgesia, and emesis.

Glutamate Receptors

The glutamate receptors (AMPA, NMDA, and kainate receptors) are widely expressed. The α-amino-3-hydroxy-5-methyl-4-isoxazole propionate (AMPA) receptors mediate fast excitatory transmission at most synapses in the CNS.

Guanine Nucleotide Proteins

G proteins are those essential intermediaries in cell communication that reflect the molecular mechanisms of actions of multiple classes of drugs including opioids, sympathomimetics, and anticholinergics (see Fig. 1-7). The hydrolysis of guanosine triphosphate to guanosine diphosphate provides the energy for the activated G protein to then interact with the effector molecule (either an enzyme system or ion channel). This activity mediates the final cascade of biological steps within the cell that ultimately leads to the pharmacologic or physiologic response characteristic of the administered drug.

Concentration of Receptors

The receptor concentration in the lipid portion of cell membranes is dynamic, either increasing (up-regulation) or decreasing (down-regulation) in response to specific stimuli. Changing concentrations of receptors in cell membranes emphasize that receptors determine that the pharmacologic responses to drugs are not static but rather dynamic.

Characteristics of Drug–Receptor Interaction

A drug or endogenous substance (ligand) is an *agonist* if the drug–receptor interaction elicits a pharmacologic effect by an alteration in the functional properties of receptors. A drug is an *antagonist* when it interacts with receptors but does not alter their functional properties and, at the same time, prevents their response to an agonist.

Receptor Occupancy Theory

Traditionally, it is assumed that the intensity of effect produced by the binding of drugs to receptors is proportional to the fraction of receptors occupied by the drug.

State of Receptor Activation

A modification of the receptor occupancy theory, consistent with differences in the intrinsic activity of drugs, is the concept of activated and nonactivated states for receptors.

In this theory, when an agonist binds to receptors, it converts the receptors from a nonactivated to an activated state.

Drug–Receptor Bond

The action of drugs on receptors requires binding between drugs and receptors by a physicochemical force (covalent bonding, ionic).

Plasma Drug Concentrations

Plasma drug concentrations are a reliable monitor of therapy only when interpreted in parallel with the clinical course of the patient. Furthermore, serial measurements of plasma drug concentrations at selected intervals are more informative than isolated determinations. It is misleading to measure the plasma concentrations of drugs during the rapidly changing distribution phase. Pharmacologic effects usually reflect only the free fraction of drug in the plasma.

Relationship of Plasma and Receptor Drug Concentration

In patients, the plasma concentration of a drug is the most practical measurement for monitoring the receptor concentration. Typically, a direct relationship exists between the (a) dose of drug administered, (b) resulting plasma concentration, and (c) intensity of drug effect.

Initial and Maintenance Doses

An initial loading dose is necessary to establish a prompt therapeutic concentration of drug. This initial dose will be larger than the subsequent maintenance dose.

PHARMACOKINETICS OF INHALED ANESTHETICS

The pharmacokinetics of inhaled anesthetics describes their (a) absorption (uptake) from alveoli into pulmonary capillary blood, (b) distribution in the body, (c) metabolism, and (d) elimination, principally via the lungs. A series of partial pressure gradients beginning at the anesthetic machine serve to propel the inhaled anesthetic across various barriers (alveoli, capillaries, cell membranes) to its sites of action in the CNS. The principal objective of inhalation anesthesia is to achieve a constant and optimal brain partial pressure of the inhaled anesthetic. The brain and all other tissues equilibrate with the partial pressures of inhaled anesthetics delivered to them by arterial blood (Pa) (Fig. 1-8). The PA of inhaled anesthetics mirrors the brain partial pressure (Pbr). Thus, the PA is used as an index of (a) depth of anesthesia, (b) recovery from anesthesia, and (c) anesthetic equal potency (MAC). Understanding those factors that determine the PA and thus the Pbr permits control over the doses of inhaled anesthetics delivered to the brain to maintain a constant and optimal depth of anesthesia.

Determinants of Alveolar Partial Pressure

The PA and ultimately the Pbr of inhaled anesthetics are determined by input (delivery) into alveoli minus uptake (loss) of the drug from alveoli into arterial blood (Table 1-7).

Inhaled Partial Pressure (PI)

A high PI delivered from the anesthetic machine is required during the initial administration of an anesthetic. A high initial input offsets the impact of uptake, thus accelerating the induction of anesthesia, as reflected by the rate of rise in the PA and thus the Pbr. With time,

$$P_A \rightleftharpoons P_a \rightleftharpoons P_{br}$$

Figure 1-8. The alveolar partial pressure (PA) of an inhaled anesthetic is in equilibrium with the arterial blood (Pa) and brain (Pbr). As a result, the PA is an indirect measurement of anesthetic partial pressure at the brain.

TABLE 1-7.
FACTORS DETERMINING PARTIAL PRESSURE GRADIENTS NECESSARY FOR ESTABLISHMENT OF ANESTHESIA

Transfer of inhaled anesthetic from anesthetic machine to alveoli (anesthetic input)
Inspired partial pressure
Alveolar ventilation
Characteristics of anesthetic breathing system
Functional residual capacity
Transfer of inhaled anesthetic from alveoli to arterial blood (anesthetic loss)
Blood:gas partition coefficient
Cardiac output
Alveolar-to-venous partial pressure difference
Transfer of inhaled anesthetic from arterial blood to brain (anesthetic loss)
Brain:blood partition coefficient
Cerebral blood flow
Arterial-to-venous partial pressure difference

as uptake into the blood decreases, the PI should be decreased to match the decreased anesthetic uptake and therefore maintain a constant and optimal Pbr. If the PI is maintained constant with time, the PA and Pbr will increase progressively as uptake diminishes.

Concentration Effect

The concentration effect states that the higher the PI, the more rapidly the PA approaches the PI.

Second-Gas Effect

The second-gas effect reflects the ability of a high-volume uptake of one gas (first gas) to accelerate the rate of increase of the PA for a concurrently administered "companion" gas (second gas).

Alveolar Ventilation

Increased alveolar ventilation, like PI, promotes the input of anesthetics to offset uptake. The net effect is a more rapid rate of increase in the PA toward the PI and thus the induction of anesthesia. Decreased alveolar ventilation decreases input and thus slows the establishment of that PA and a Pbr necessary for the induction of anesthesia.

Spontaneous Versus Mechanical Ventilation

Inhaled anesthetics influence their own uptake by virtue of dose-dependent depressant effects on alveolar ventilation. This, in effect, is a negative-feedback protective mechanism that prevents the establishment of an excessive depth of anesthesia (delivery of anesthesia is decreased when ventilation is decreased) when a high PI is administered during spontaneous breathing. This protective mechanism against the development of an excessive depth of anesthesia (anesthetic overdose) is lost when mechanical ventilation of the lungs replaces spontaneous breathing.

Impact of Solubility

The impact of changes in alveolar ventilation on the rate of increase in the PA toward the PI depends on the solubility of the anesthetic in blood.

Anesthetic Breathing System

Those characteristics of the anesthetic breathing system that influence the rate of increase of the PA are the (a) volume of the external breathing system, (b) solubility of the inhaled anesthetics in the rubber or plastic components of the breathing system, and (c) gas inflow from the anesthetic machine. The volume of the anesthetic breathing system acts as a buffer to slow the achievement of the PA. High gas inflow rates (5 to 10 L/min) from the anesthetic machine negate this buffer effect.

Solubility

The solubility of the inhaled anesthetics in blood and tissues is denoted by the *partition coefficient* (Table 1-8). A partition coefficient is a distribution ratio describing how the inhaled anesthetic distributes itself between two phases at equilibrium (partial pressures equal in both phases). A blood:gas partition coefficient of 0.5 means that the concentration of inhaled anesthetic in the blood is half that present in the alveolar gases when the partial pressures on the anesthetic in these two phases is identical.

Blood:Gas Partition Coefficients

The rate of increase of the PA towards the PI (maintained constant by mechanical ventilation of the lungs) is inversely related to the solubility of the anesthetic in blood. Based on their blood:gas partition coefficients, inhaled anesthetics are categorized traditionally as soluble, intermediately soluble, and poorly soluble (see Table 1-8). The impact of high blood solubility on the rate of PA increase can be offset to some extent by increasing the PI above that required for the maintenance of anesthesia. This is termed the *overpressure technique* and may be used to speed the induction of anesthesia, all the while recognizing that the sustained delivery of a high PI will result in an anesthetic overdose. When blood solubility is low, minimal amounts of inhaled anesthetic must be dissolved before equilibration is achieved; therefore, the rate of increase of PA and Pa, and thus onset-of-drug effects, such as the induction of anesthesia, are rapid. For example, the inhalation of a constant PI of nitrous oxide, desflurane, or sevoflurane for about 10 minutes results in a PA that is 80% of the PI. Associated with the rapid increase in the PA of nitrous oxide is the absorption of several liters (up to 10 liters during the first 10 to 15 minutes) of this gas, reflecting its common administration at inhaled concentrations of 60% to 70%. This high-volume absorption of nitrous oxide is responsible for several unique effects when it is

TABLE 1-8.
COMPARATIVE SOLUBILITIES OF INHALED ANESTHETICS

	Blood: Gas Partition Coefficient	Brain: Blood Partition Coefficient	Muscle: Blood Partition Coefficient	Fat: Blood Partition Coefficient	Oil: Gas Partition Coefficient
Soluble					
Methoxyflurane	12	2	1.3	48.8	970
Intermediately soluble					
Halothane	2.5	41.9	3.4	51.1	224
Enflurane	1.90	1.5	1.7	36.2	98
Isoflurane	1.4	61.6	2.9	44.9	98
Poorly soluble					
Nitrous oxide	0.46	1.1	1.2	2.3	1.4
Desflurane	0.42	1.3	2.0	27.2	18.7
Sevoflurane	0.69	1.7	3.1	47.5	55
Xexon	0.115				

administered in the presence of volatile anesthetics or air-containing cavities increase in the solubility of volatile anesthetics in blood.

Tissue:Blood Partition Coefficients

The tissue:blood partition coefficients determine the uptake of anesthetic into tissues and the time necessary for equilibration of these tissues with the Pa. For volatile anesthetics, equilibration between the Pa and Pbr depends on the anesthetic's blood solubility and requires 5 to 15 minutes (three time constants).

Oil:Gas Partition Coefficients

Oil:gas partition coefficients parallel anesthetic requirements (an estimated MAC can be calculated as 150 divided by the oil:gas partition coefficient).

Nitrous Oxide Transfer to Closed Gas Spaces

The blood:gas partition coefficient of nitrous oxide (0.46) is about 34 times greater than that of nitrogen (0.014). This differential solubility means that nitrous oxide can leave the blood to enter an air-filled cavity 34 times more rapidly than nitrogen can leave the cavity to enter blood. As a result of this preferential transfer of nitrous oxide, the volume or pressure of an air-filled cavity increases. The passage of nitrous oxide into an air-filled cavity surrounded by a compliant wall (intestinal gas, pneumothorax, pulmonary blebs, air bubbles) causes the gas space to expand. Conversely, passage of nitrous oxide into an air-filled cavity surrounded by a noncompliant wall (middle ear, cerebral ventricles, supratentorial space) causes an increase in intracavitary pressure. The magnitude of volume or pressure increase is influenced by the (a) partial pressure of nitrous oxide, (b) blood flow to the air-filled cavity, and (c) duration of nitrous oxide administration. Intraocular gas bubbles, such as those used for internal retinal tamponade (retinal detachment, macular hole repair, complicated vitrectomy), may persist in the eye for up to 10 weeks following ocular surgery. The administration of nitrous oxide for periods as brief as 1 hour during this time may result in rapid increases in the volume of intraocular gas within the rigid closed eye; this may be sufficient to compress the retinal artery and result in visual loss.

Cardiopulmonary Bypass

Cardiopulmonary bypass produces changes in blood-gas solubility that depend on the constituents of the priming solution and temperature. Volatile anesthetics initiated during cardiopulmonary bypass take longer to equilibrate, whereas the same drugs already present when cardiopulmonary bypass is initiated are diluted, potentially changing the depth of anesthesia.

Cardiac Output

A patient's cardiac output (pulmonary blood flow) influences the uptake, and therefore PA by carrying away either more or less anesthetic from the alveoli. An increased cardiac output results in a more rapid uptake, so the rate of increase in the PA (and thus the induction of anesthesia) is slowed. A decreased cardiac output speeds the rate of increase of the PA, because less uptake is present to oppose input. As with alveolar ventilation, changes in cardiac output most influence the rate of PA increase for a soluble anesthetic. A low cardiac output, as with shock, could produce an unexpectedly high PA of a soluble anesthetic. Volatile anesthetics that depress cardiac output can exert a positive feedback response that contrasts with the negative (protective) feedback response on spontaneous breathing that is exerted by these drugs; decreases in cardiac output due to an excessive dose of volatile anesthetic results in an increase in the PA, which further increases anesthetic depth and thus cardiac depression.

Impact of a Shunt

When a right-to-left shunt is present, the diluting effect of the shunted blood on the partial pressure of anesthetic in blood coming from ventilated alveoli results in a decrease in the Pa and a slowing in the induction of anesthesia. Left-to-right tissue shunts (arteriovenous fistulas, volatile anesthetic–induced increases in cutaneous blood flow) result in delivery of blood to the lungs containing a higher partial pressure of anesthetic than that present in blood that has passed through tissues. As a result, left-to-right shunts offset the dilutional effects of a right-to-left shunt on the Pa.

Alveolar-to-Venous Partial Pressure Differences (A-vD)

The A-vD reflects the tissue uptake of the inhaled anesthetic. Highly perfused tissues (brain, heart, kidneys) in the adult account for $<10\%$ of body mass but receive 75% of the cardiac output (see Table 1-3). As a result of the small mass and high blood flow, these tissues, known as *vessel-rich group tissues,* equilibrate rapidly with the Pa. Indeed, after about three time constants, approximately 75% of the returning venous blood is at the same partial pressure as the PA. For this reason, uptake of a volatile anesthetic is decreased greatly after three time constants (5 to 15 minutes, depending on the blood solubility of the inhaled anesthetic), as reflected by a narrowing of the inspired-to-alveolar partial pressure difference. Continued uptake of anesthetic after the saturation of vessel-rich group tissues reflects principally the entrance of anesthetic into skeletal muscles and fat.

Recovery From Anesthesia

The recovery from anesthesia is depicted by the rate of decrease in the Pbr, as reflected by the PA with tissue concentrations of zero at the initiation of the induction of anesthesia. The failure of certain tissues to reach equilibrium with the PA of the inhaled anesthetic during maintenance of anesthesia means that the rate of decrease of the PA during recovery from anesthesia will be more rapid than the rate of increase of the PA during induction. The impact of administration duration on time to recovery is minimal with poorly soluble anesthetics (sevoflurane and desflurane).

Context-Sensitive Half-Time

The pharmacokinetics of the elimination of inhaled anesthetics depend on the length of administration and the blood-gas solubility of the inhaled anesthetic. The time needed for a 50% decrease in the anesthetic concentration of enflurane, isoflurane, desflurane, and sevoflurane is <5 minutes and does not increase significantly with increasing duration of anesthesia.

Diffusion Hypoxia

Diffusion hypoxia occurs when the inhalation of nitrous oxide is discontinued abruptly, thus leading to a reversal of partial pressure gradients so that nitrous oxide leaves the blood to enter alveoli. This initial high-volume outpouring of nitrous oxide from the blood into the alveoli can so dilute the PAO_2 that the PaO_2 decreases. Outpouring of nitrous oxide into alveoli is greatest during the first 1 to 5 minutes after its discontinuation at the conclusion of anesthesia. Thus, it is common practice to fill the lungs with oxygen at the end of anesthesia to ensure that arterial hypoxemia will not occur as a result of PAO_2 dilution by nitrous oxide.

PHARMACODYNAMICS OF INHALED ANESTHETICS

Minimal Alveolar Concentration (MAC)

The MAC of an inhaled anesthetic is defined as that concentration at 1 atm that prevents skeletal muscle movement in response to a supramaximal painful stimulus (surgical skin incision) in 50% of patients (ED_{50}). The immobility produced by inhaled anesthetics, as measured by MAC, is mediated principally by the effects of these drugs on the spinal cord, and only a minor component of immobility results from cerebral effects. MAC is among the most useful concepts in anesthetic pharmacology, because it establishes a common measure of potency (partial pressure at steady state) for inhaled anesthetics. A unique feature of MAC is its consistency, varying only 10% to 15% among individuals. The use of equally potent doses (comparable MAC concentrations) of inhaled anesthetics is mandatory for comparing the effects of these drugs, not only at the spinal cord but at all other organs (Table 1-9).

Factors That Alter MAC

MAC values for inhaled anesthetics are additive. For example, 0.5 MAC of nitrous oxide plus 0.5 MAC isoflurane has the same effect at the brain as does a 1-MAC concentration of either anesthetic alone. The fact that 1 MAC for nitrous oxide is >100% means that this anesthetic cannot

TABLE 1-9.
COMPARATIVE MINIMUM ALVEOLAR CONCENTRATION (MAC) OF INHALED ANESTHETICS

MAC (%, 30 to 55 Years Old at 37°C, PB 760 mm Hg)	
Nitrous oxide*	104
Halothane	0.75
Enflurane	1.63
Isoflurane	1.17
Desflurane	6.6
Sevoflurane	1.80
Xenon	63–71

*Determined in a hyperbaric chamber in males 21 to 55 years old.

be used alone at 1 atm and still provide an acceptable inhaled concentration of oxygen. Dose–response curves for inhaled anesthetics, although not parallel, are all steep (Table 1-10). This is emphasized by the fact that a 1-MAC dose prevents skeletal muscle movement in response to a painful stimulus in 50% of patients, whereas a modest increase to about 1.3 MAC prevents movement in at least 95% of patients.

Mechanism of Immobility

MAC is based on the characteristic ability of inhaled drugs to produce immobility by virtue of the actions of these drugs principally on the spinal cord, rather than on higher centers. The observation that immobility during noxious stimulation does not correlate with electroencephalographic activity reflects the fact that cortical electrical activity does not control motor responses to noxious stimulation. The effects of inhaled anesthetics on the spinal cord that lead to immobility are diverse and likely reflect a drug-induced depression of excitation as well as enhancement of inhibition.

Ionotropic and Metabotropic Receptors

Neurotransmitters signal through two families of receptors, designated as *ionotropic* and *metabotropic* receptors. Ionotropic receptors are also known as ligand-gated ion channels because the neurotransmitter GABA binds directly to ion channel proteins, and this interaction causes the opening (gating) of the ion channels, thus allowing the transmission of specific ions (chloride ions), with resulting changes in membrane potentials. The binding of neurotransmitters (acetylcholine) to metabotropic receptors causes an activation of those guanosine triphosphate binding progestins (G-proteins) associated with the receptors, and these G-proteins act as second messengers to activate other signaling molecules, such as protein kinases, or potassium or calcium channels. Inhaled anesthetics do not seem to stimulate the release of endogenous opioids and do not suppress autonomic or

TABLE 1-10. IMPACT OF PHYSIOLOGIC AND PHARMACOLOGIC FACTORS ON MINIMUM ALVEOLAR CONCENTRATION (MAC)

- Increases in MAC
  - Hyperthermia
  - Excess pheomelanin production (red hair)
  - Drug-induced increases in central nervous system catecholamine levels
  - Cyclosporine
  - Hypernatremia
- Decreases in MAC
  - Hypothermia
  - Increasing age
  - Preoperative medication
  - Drug-induced decreases in central nervous system catecholamine levels
  - α-2 Agonists
  - Acute alcohol ingestion
  - Pregnancy
  - Postpartum (returns to normal in 24 to 72 hours)
  - Lithium
  - Lidocaine
  - Neuraxial opioids (?)
  - Ketanserin
  - PaO_2 < 38 mm Hg
  - Blood pressure < 40 mm Hg
  - Cardiopulmonary bypass
  - Hyponatremia
- No change in MAC
  - Anesthetic metabolism
  - Chronic alcohol abuse
  - Gender
  - Duration of anesthesia (?)
  - $PaCO_2$ 15 to 95 mm Hg
  - PaO_2 > 38 mm Hg
  - Blood pressure > 40 mm Hg
  - Hyperkalemia or hypokalemia
  - Thyroid gland dysfunction

ventilatory responses to surgical stimulation at those concentrations that suppress movement. The fact that small doses of opioids decrease MAC levels reflects their ability to provide an effect (analgesia) that is not present with inhaled anesthetics alone. Evidence that α-$_2$ receptors participate in the immobility produced by inhaled anesthetics is provided by decreases in MAC produced by clonidine.

Inhibitory Ligand-Gated and Voltage Gated Channels (Glycine and $GABA_A$ Receptors)

Glycine receptors are major mediators of inhibitory neurotransmission in the spinal cord and mediate part of the immobility produced by inhaled anesthetics.

Glutamate (NMDA, AMPA, and Kainate Receptors)

Glutamate is the principal excitatory neurotransmitter in the mammalian CNS. Glutamate receptors include G-protein–coupled receptors and the ligand-gated receptors (NMDA, AMPA, and kainate). NMDA receptors likely are important mediators of the immobilizing effects of inhaled anesthetics. AMPA receptors mediate the initial (fast) component of excitatory postsynaptic transmission and are likely targets for volatile anesthetic-induced immobility.

Sodium Channels

Inhaled anesthetics can inhibit the presynaptic terminal release of neurotransmitters, particularly glutamate (the intravenous administration of lidocaine decreases MAC).

Mechanism of Anesthesia-Induced Unconsciousness

Loss of consciousness (hypnosis and amnesia) and the response to skin incision (immobility as reflected by MAC) are unlikely to be a single continuum of increasing anesthetic depth but rather two separate phenomena. It has been proposed that general anesthesia is a process requiring a state of unconsciousness of the brain (produced by volatile or injected anesthetics) plus immobility in response to a noxious stimulus. These effects are mediated by the action of volatile anesthetics on the spinal cord, administered at concentrations equivalent to MAC for that drug. Immobility may also be produced by the action of opioids at opioid receptors in the spinal cord or the action of local anesthetics on peripheral nerves. The mechanism by which inhaled anesthetics produce progressive, and occasionally selective, depression of the CNS is not known, although the relationship between the anesthetic activity of gases and their molecular structure indicates that inhaled anesthetics must act through specific interactions with target molecules (presumably proteins) in the CNS. A single theory to explain the mechanism of anesthesia is no longer viewed as tenable, because multiple potential targets of anesthetic action now are recognized.

Molecular and Cellular Mechanisms

At the molecular level, anesthetics almost certainly act by binding directly to proteins rather than by perturbing lipid bilayers. Inhaled anesthetics are a heterogeneous group of drugs and do not all interact with the same molecular target.

Voltage-Gated Ion Channels

The voltage-gated ion channels (sodium, potassium, calcium) seem unlikely to play a substantial role in the production of the anesthetic state.

Ligand-Gated Ion Channels

The ligand-gated ion channels (glutamate, glycine) may be important sites of anesthetic action. With the exception of ketamine, almost all injected and inhaled anesthetics enhance by >50% the current flow induced by low concentrations of GABA.

Stereoselectivity

The most definitive evidence that general anesthetics act by binding directly to proteins and not to a lipid bilayer comes from observations of stereoselectivity (possibility of a specific protein receptor interaction as the basis for anesthesia). The steep slope of the dose–response curve (MAC) for inhaled anesthetics is possible evidence of a protein receptor in the CNS as a site and mechanism of action of inhaled anesthetics (a crucial degree of receptor occupancy is characteristic of a steep dose–response curve).

Meyer-Overton Theory (Critical Volume Hypothesis)

Correlation between the lipid solubility of inhaled anesthetics (the oil:gas partition coefficient) and anesthetic potency has historically been presumed to be evidence that inhaled anesthetics act by disrupting the structure or dynamic properties of the lipid portions of nerve membranes. The most compelling evidence against the Meyer-Overton theory of anesthesia is the fact that the effects on lipid bilayers produced by inhaled anesthetics are implausibly small and can generally be mimicked by temperature changes of 1°C.

PHARMACOECONOMICS

Pharmacoeconomics is the application of economics to drug selection and usage, relative to the expenditure of financial resources that could be used for other purposes. The recognized obstacles to cost-effective care are society's inability to accept the reality of limited resources and patient's who have unrealistic expectations regarding the role of medical care in their lives. Anesthesia-related medications account for 8% to 12% of a hospital's total drug expenditures.

Inhaled Anesthetics

2

HISTORY

Halothane (Fig. 2-1) was synthesized in 1951 and introduced for clinical use in 1956 (Stoelting RK, Hillier SC. Inhaled anesthetics. In: *Pharmacology and Physiology in Anesthetic Practice,* 4th ed. Philadelphia. Lippincott Williams & Wilkins, 2006:42–86). However, the tendency for alkane derivatives such as halothane to enhance the dysrhythmogenic effects of epinephrine led to the search for new inhaled anesthetics derived from ethers. Isoflurane, the isomer of enflurane, was introduced in 1981. This drug was resistant to metabolism, thus making organ toxicity an unlikely occurrence after its administration.

Inhaled Anesthetics for the Present and Future

The exclusion of all halogens except fluorine results in nonflammable liquids that are poorly lipid soluble and extremely resistant to metabolism. Desflurane, a totally fluorinated methyl ethyl ether, was introduced in 1992, and it was followed in 1994 by the totally fluorinated methyl isopropyl ether, sevoflurane The low solubility in blood of these newest anesthetics was desirable, because it would facilitate the rapid induction of anesthesia, permit precise control of anesthetic concentrations during maintenance of anesthesia, and favor prompt recovery at the end of anesthesia independent of the duration of administration. New risks [airway irritation, sympathetic nervous system stimulation, carbon monoxide production, complex vaporizer technology, fluoromethyl-2,2-difluro-1-(trifluoromethyl) vinyl ether or compound A production] and increased

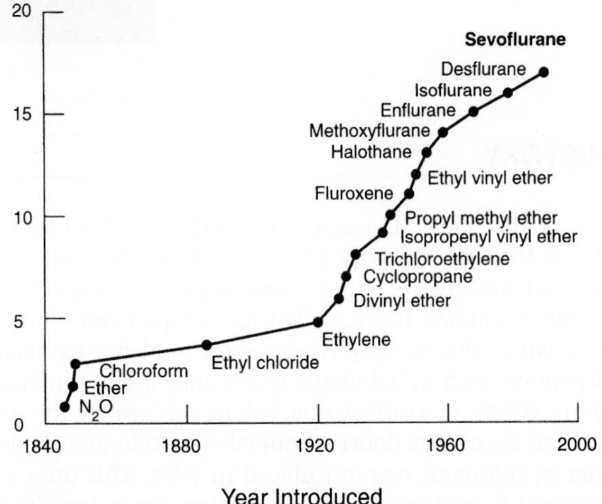

Figure 2-1. Inhaled anesthetics were introduced into clinical practice beginning with the successful use of nitrous oxide, in 1844, for dental anesthesia. This was followed by a recognition of the anesthetic properties of ether, in 1846, and of chloroform in 1847. Modern anesthetics, beginning with halothane, differ from prior anesthetics in being fluorinated and nonflammable. [Modified from Eger EI. *Desflurane (Suprane): A Compendium and Reference*. Nutley, NJ: Anaquest,1993:1–119; with permission.]

expense are associated with the administration of these new drugs.

Cost Considerations

Cost is an increasingly important consideration in the adoption of new drugs, including inhaled anesthetics, into clinical practice. The costs of new inhaled anesthetics can be decreased somewhat by using low flow rates. Less soluble anesthetics are more suitable for use with low gas flow rates, because their poor solubility permits better control of the delivered concentration. Furthermore, less depletion of these anesthetics from the inspired gases occurs, so that fewer molecules need to be added to the returning rebreathed gases.

CLINICALLY USEFUL INHALED ANESTHETICS (TABLE 2-1 AND FIG. 2-2)

Volatile liquids are administered as vapors, following their evaporation in devices known as *vaporizers*.

Nitrous Oxide

Nitrous oxide is a low-molecular-weight, odorless to sweet-smelling nonflammable gas of low potency and poor blood solubility (0.46). It is most commonly administered in combination with opioids or volatile anesthetics to produce general anesthesia. The analgesic effects of nitrous oxide are prominent, but it causes minimal skeletal muscle relaxation. The routine use of nitrous oxide must be balanced against its possible adverse effects related to its high-volume absorption, appreciation of potential toxic effects on organ function, and ability to inactivate vitamin B_{12}.

Halothane

Halothane is a halogenated alkane derivative that has a sweet, nonpungent odor. An intermediate solubility in blood, combined with a high potency, permits rapid onset and recovery from anesthesia using halothane alone or in combination with nitrous oxide or injected drugs, such as opioids.

Enflurane

Enflurane is a halogenated methyl ethyl ether that has a pungent, ethereal odor. Its intermediate solubility in blood, combined with a high potency, permits rapid

TABLE 2-1.
PHYSICAL AND CHEMICAL PROPERTIES OF INHALED ANESTHETICS

	Nitrous Oxide	Halothane	Enflurane	Isoflurane	Desflurane	Sevoflurane
Molecular weight	44	197	184	184	168	200
Boiling point (°C)		50.2	56.5	48.5	22.8	58.5
Vapor pressure (mmHg; 20°C)	Gas	244	172	240	669	170
Odor	Sweet	Organic	Ethereal	Ethereal	Ethereal	Ethereal
Preservative necessary	No	Yes	No	No	No	No
Stability in soda lime (40°C)	Yes	No	Yes	Yes	Yes	No
Blood:gas partition coefficient	0.46	2.54	1.90	1.46	0.42	0.69
MAC (37°C, 30 to 55 years old, PB 760 mmHg) (%)	104	0.75	1.63	1.17	6.6	1.80

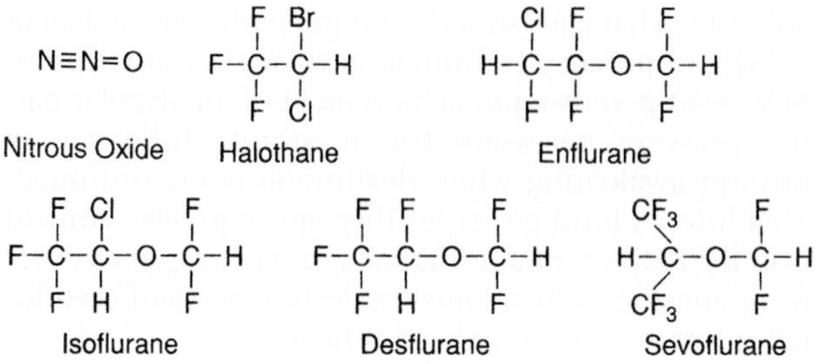

N≡N=O

Nitrous Oxide Halothane Enflurane

Isoflurane Desflurane Sevoflurane

Figure 2-2. Inhaled anesthetics.

onset and recovery from anesthesia using enflurane alone or in combination with nitrous oxide or injected drugs, such as opioids.

Isoflurane

Isoflurane is a halogenated methyl ethyl ether that has a pungent, ethereal odor. Its intermediate solubility in blood, combined with a high potency, permits rapid onset and recovery from anesthesia using isoflurane alone or in combination with nitrous oxide or injected drugs, such as opioids.

Desflurane

Desflurane is a fluorinated methyl ethyl ether that differs from isoflurane only by substitution of a fluorine atom for the chlorine atom found on the α-ethyl component of isoflurane. Fluorination rather than chlorination increases vapor pressure (decreases intermolecular attraction), enhances molecular stability, and decreases potency. Unlike halothane and sevoflurane, desflurane is pungent, making it unlikely that inhalation induction of anesthesia will be feasible or pleasant for the patient. Carbon monoxide results from the degradation of desflurane by the strong base present in carbon dioxide absorbents (most likely when desiccation is present).

Solubility characteristics (blood:gas partition coefficient 0.45) and potency (minimal alevolar concentration or MAC 6%) permit rapid achievement of an alveolar partial pressure necessary for anesthesia followed by prompt awakening when desflurane is discontinued. This lower blood-gas solubility, more precise control over the delivery of anesthesia, and more rapid recovery from anesthesia distinguishes desflurane (and sevoflurane) from earlier volatile anesthetics.

Sevoflurane

Sevoflurane is a fluorinated methyl isopropyl ether. The blood:gas partition coefficient of sevoflurane (0.69) resembles that of desflurane, thus ensuring prompt induction of anesthesia and recovery after discontinuation of the anesthetic. Sevoflurane is nonpungent, has minimal odor, produces bronchodilatation similar in degree to isoflurane, and causes the least degree of airway irritation among the currently available volatile anesthetics. Sevoflurane metabolism does not result in the formation of trifluoroacetylated liver proteins (as occurs with all other volatile anesthetics). Sevoflurane does not form significant amounts of carbon monoxide on exposure to carbon dioxide absorbents. In contrast to other volatile anesthetics, sevoflurane breaks down in the presence of the strong bases present in carbon dioxide absorbents to form compounds that are toxic in animals (compounds A).

Xenon

Xenon is an inert gas that is nonexplosive, nonpungent and odorless, and chemically inert, as reflected by an absence of metabolism and low toxicity. To date, its high cost has hindered its acceptance in anesthesia practice. Xenon is a potent hypnotic and analgesic, resulting in the suppression of hemodynamic and catecholamine responses to surgical stimulation.

COMPARATIVE PHARMACOLOGY

Measurements obtained from normothermic volunteers exposed to equal potent concentrations of inhaled anesthetics during controlled ventilation of the lungs to maintain normocapnia have provided the basis of comparison for the pharmacologic effects of these drugs on various organ systems. In this regard, it is important to recognize that surgically stimulated patients who have other confounding variables may respond in a way different from that of healthy volunteers (Table 2-2).

CENTRAL NERVOUS SYSTEM (CNS) EFFECTS

It is unlikely that the impairment of mental function in the personnel who work in the operating room can result from inhaling trace concentrations of anesthetics. Cerebral metabolic oxygen requirements are decreased in parallel with

TABLE 2-2.
VARIABLES INFLUENCING PHARMACOLOGIC EFFECTS OF INHALED ANESTHETICS

Anesthetic concentration
Rate of increase in anesthetic concentration
Spontaneous versus controlled ventilation
Variations from normocapnia
Surgical stimulation
Patient age
Coexisting disease
Concomitant drug therapy
Intravascular fluid volume
Preoperative medication
Injected drugs to induce and/or maintain anesthesia or skeletal muscle relaxation
Alterations in body temperature

drug-induced decreases in cerebral activity. Drug-induced increases in cerebral blood flow may increase intracranial pressure (ICP) in patients with space-occupying lesions.

Electroencephalogram (EEG)

Volatile anesthetics in concentrations of <0.4 MAC similarly increase the frequency and voltage on the EEG. At about 0.4 MAC, an abrupt shift of high-voltage activity occurs from posterior to anterior portions of the brain. Cerebral metabolic oxygen requirements also begin to decrease abruptly at about 0.4 MAC. It is likely that these changes reflect a transition from wakefulness to unconsciousness.

Seizure Activity

Enflurane can produce fast frequency and high voltage on the EEG. This often progresses to spike wave activity that is indistinguishable from the changes that accompany a seizure. This EEG activity may be accompanied by tonic-clonic twitching of skeletal muscles in the face and extremities. Isoflurane, desflurane, and sevoflurane do not evoke seizure activity on the EEG, even in the presence of deep levels of anesthesia, hypocapnia, or repetitive auditory stimulation.

Evoked Potentials

Volatile anesthetics cause dose-related decreases in the amplitude and increases in the latency of the cortical component of median nerve somatosensory evoked potentials, visual evoked potentials, and auditory evoked potentials.

Mental Function and Awareness

Inhaled anesthetics cause loss of response to verbal command at MAC-awake concentrations. Surgical stimulation may increase the anesthetic requirement to prevent awareness.

Cerebral Blood Flow

Volatile anesthetics produce dose-dependent increases in cerebral blood flow (CBF). The magnitude of this increase depends on the balance between the drug's intrinsic vasodilatory actions and vasoconstriction secondary to flow-metabolism uncoupling. Volatile anesthetics administered during normocapnia in concentrations of >0.6 MAC produce cerebral vasodilation, decreased cerebral vascular resistance, and resulting dose-dependent increases in CBF. Desflurane and isoflurane are similar in terms of increases in CBF and the preservation of reactivity to carbon dioxide.

Cerebral Metabolic Oxygen Requirements

When the EEG becomes isoelectric, an additional increase in the concentration of the volatile anesthetics does not produce further decreases in cerebral metabolic oxygen requirements. Desflurane and sevoflurane decrease cerebral metabolic oxygen requirements in a way similar to isoflurane.

Cerebral Protection

In animals experiencing temporary focal ischemia, no difference in neurologic outcome is noted when cerebral function is suppressed using isoflurane or thiopental if systemic blood pressure is maintained.

Intracranial Pressure

Inhaled anesthetics produce increases in the ICP that parallel increases in the CBF produced by these drugs. Patients with space-occupying intracranial lesions are most vulnerable to these drug-induced increases in ICP.

Cerebrospinal Fluid Production

Isoflurane does not alter the production of CSF and, at the same time, it decreases resistance to reabsorption of CSF.

CIRCULATORY EFFECTS

Inhaled anesthetics produce dose-dependent and drug-specific circulatory effects. The circulatory effects of inhaled anesthetics may differ in the presence of (a) controlled ventilation of the lungs, compared with spontaneous breathing; (b) preexisting cardiac disease; or (c) drugs that act directly or indirectly on the heart.

Mean Arterial Pressure

Halothane, isoflurane, desflurane, and sevoflurane produce similar and dose-dependent decreases in mean arterial pressure when administered to healthy human volunteers (Fig. 2-3). The magnitude of decrease in mean arterial pressure in volunteers is greater than that which occurs in the presence of surgical stimulation. In contrast with volatile anesthetics, nitrous oxide produces either

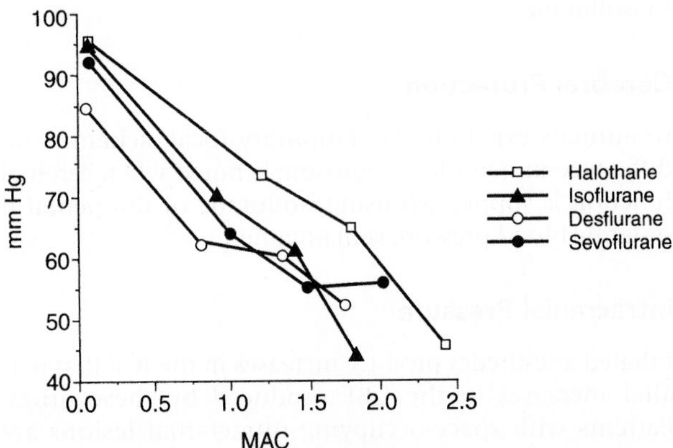

Figure 2-3. The effects of increasing concentrations (MAC) of halothane, isoflurane, desflurane, and sevoflurane on mean arterial pressure (mm Hg) when administered to healthy volunteers. [From Cahalan MK. Hemodynamic effects of inhaled anesthetics (review courses). Cleveland: International Anesthesia Research Society, 1996:14–18; with permission.]

no change or only modest increases in systemic blood pressure. The substitution of nitrous oxide for a portion of the volatile anesthetic decreases the magnitude of blood pressure decrease produced by the same MAC concentration of the volatile anesthetic alone. The decrease in blood pressure produced by halothane is, in part or in whole, a consequence of decreases in myocardial contractility and cardiac output, whereas with isoflurane, desflurane, and sevoflurane, the decrease in systemic blood pressure results principally from a decrease in systemic vascular resistance.

Heart Rate

Isoflurane, desflurane, and sevoflurane, but not halothane, increase heart rate when administered to healthy human volunteers (Fig. 2-4). Sevoflurane increases heart rate only at concentrations of >1.5 MAC, whereas isoflurane and

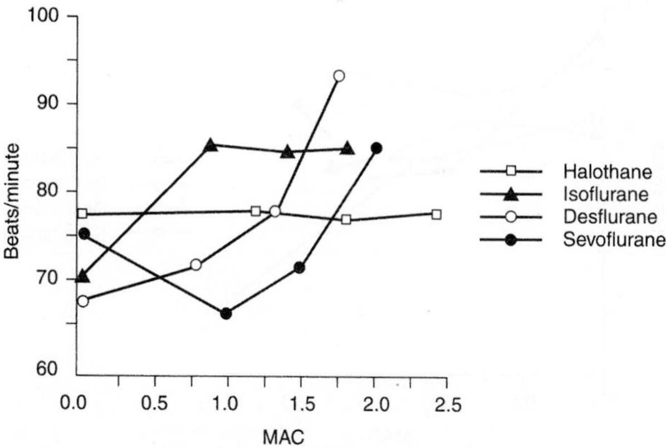

Figure 2-4. The effects of increasing concentrations (MAC) of halothane, isoflurane, desflurane, and sevoflurane on heart rate (beats/minute) when administered to healthy volunteers. [From Cahalan MK. Hemodynamic effects of inhaled anesthetics (review courses). Cleveland: International Anesthesia Research Society, 1996:14–18; with permission.]

desflurane tend to increase heart rate at lower concentrations. Heart rate effects seen in patients undergoing surgery may be quite different than those documented in volunteers, because so many confounding variables influence heart rate (opioids may prevent increases in heart rate).

Cardiac Output and Stroke Volume

Halothane, but not isoflurane, desflurane, and sevoflurane, produce dose-dependent decreases in cardiac output when administered to healthy human volunteers (Fig. 2-5). Cardiac output is modestly increased by nitrous oxide, possibly reflecting the mild sympathomimetic effects of this drug.

Right Atrial Pressure

Halothane, isoflurane, and desflurane, but not sevoflurane, increase right atrial pressure (central venous pressure)

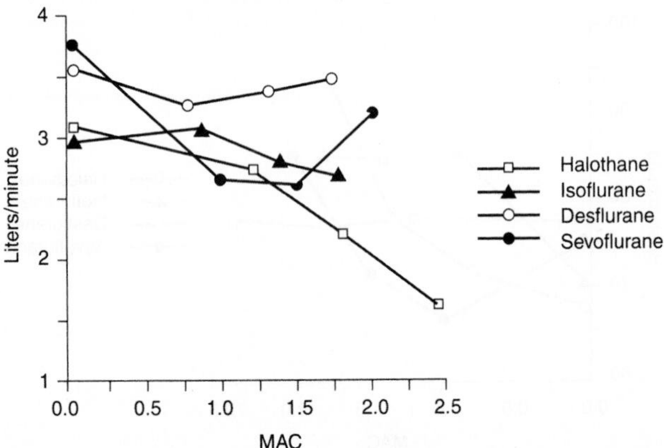

Figure 2-5. The effects of increasing concentrations (MAC) of halothane, isoflurane, desflurane, and sevoflurane on cardiac index (L/min) when administered to healthy volunteers. [From Cahalan MK. Hemodynamic effects of inhaled anesthetics (review courses). Cleveland: International Anesthesia Research Society, 1996:14–18; with permission.]

when administered to healthy human volunteers. The peripheral vasodilating effects of volatile anesthetics would tend to minimize the effects of the direct myocardial depression on right atrial pressure produced by these drugs. Increased right atrial pressure during the administration of nitrous oxide most likely reflects increased pulmonary vascular resistance due to the sympathomimetic effects of this drug.

Systemic Vascular Resistance

Isoflurane, desflurane, and sevoflurane, but not halothane, decrease systemic vascular resistance when administered to healthy human volunteers (Fig. 2-6). The absence of changes in systemic vascular resistance during the administration of halothane emphasizes that decreases in systemic blood pressure produced by this drug parallel decreases in myocardial contractility. The other volatile anesthetics decrease blood pressure principally by decreasing systemic vascular resistance. Nitrous oxide does not change systemic vascular resistance.

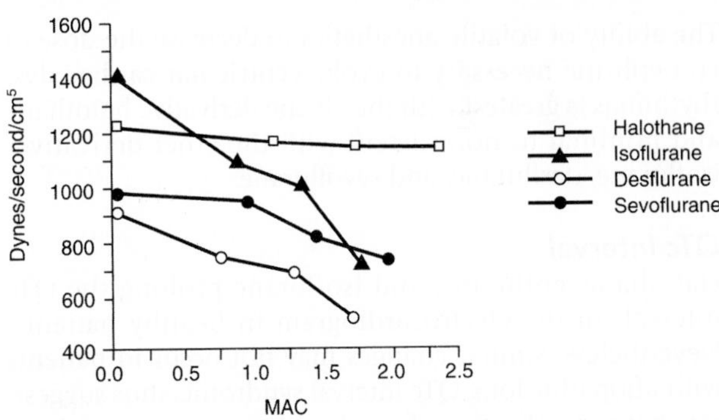

Figure 2-6. The effects of increasing concentrations (MAC) of halothane, isoflurane, desflurane, and sevoflurane on systemic vascular resistance (dynes/second/cm^5) when administered to healthy volunteers. [From Cahalan MK. Hemodynamic effects of inhaled anesthetics (review courses). Cleveland: International Anesthesia Research Society, 1996:14–18; with permission.]

Pulmonary Vascular Resistance

Volatile anesthetics appear to exert little or no predictable effect on pulmonary vascular smooth muscle. Conversely, nitrous oxide may produce increases in pulmonary vascular resistance that are exaggerated in patients with preexisting pulmonary hypertension.

Duration of Administration

Administration of a volatile anesthetic for 5 hours or longer is accompanied by recovery from the depressant effects of these drugs. For example, compared with measurements at 1 hour, the same MAC concentration after 5 hours is associated with a return of cardiac output toward predrug levels. After 5 hours, heart rate is also increased, but systemic blood pressure is unchanged, because the increase in cardiac output is offset by decreases in systemic vascular resistance. Increases in heart rate and peripheral vasodilation resembles a β-adrenergic agonist response.

Cardiac Dysrhythmias

The ability of volatile anesthetics to decrease the dose of epinephrine necessary to evoke ventricular cardiac dysrhythmias is greatest with the alkane derivative halothane and minimal to nonexistent with the ether derivatives isoflurane, desflurane, and sevoflurane.

QTc Interval

Halothane, enflurane, and isoflurane prolong the QTc interval on the electrocardiogram in healthy patients. Nevertheless, similar changes may not occur in patients with idiopathic long QTc interval syndrome, thus suggesting that generalizations from healthy patients to patients with long QTc interval syndrome may not be valid.

Accessory Pathway Conduction

Isoflurane, but not sevoflurane, increases the refractoriness of accessory pathways and the atrioventricular conduction system, thus interfering with interpretation of postablative studies.

Spontaneous Breathing

The circulatory effects produced by volatile anesthetics during spontaneous breathing are different from those observed during normocapnia and controlled ventilation of the lungs. This difference reflects the impact of sympathetic nervous system stimulation due to an accumulation of carbon dioxide (respiratory acidosis) and improved venous return during spontaneous breathing.

Coronary Blood Flow

Volatile anesthetics induce coronary vasodilation by preferentially acting on vessels with diameters from 20 μm to 200 μm, whereas adenosine has an additional pronounced impact on the small precapillary arterioles (coronary steal syndrome).

Neurocirculatory Responses

The solubility characteristics of desflurane make this volatile anesthetic a good choice to treat abrupt increases in systemic blood pressure and/or heart rate, such as may occur in response to sudden changes in the intensity of surgical stimulation. Nevertheless, abrupt increases in the alveolar concentrations of isoflurane and desflurane increase sympathetic nervous system and renin-angiotensin activity and cause transient increases in mean arterial pressure and heart rate. Fentanyl blunts the increase in heart rate and blood pressure, has minimal cardiovascular depressant effects, and imposes little postanesthetic sedation. In contrast to desflurane and isoflurane, neurocirculatory responses do not accompany abrupt increases in the delivered concentration of sevoflurane.

Pre-existing Diseases and Drug Therapy

Volatile anesthetics decrease the myocardial contractility of normal and failing cardiac muscle by similar amounts, but the significance is greater in diseased cardiac muscle because contractility is decreased even before the administration of depressant anesthetics. The peripheral vasodilation produced by isoflurane (presumably also by desflurane and sevoflurane) is undesirable in patients with aortic stenosis but may be beneficial in those with mitral or aortic regurgitation. Prior drug therapy that alters sympathetic nervous system activity (antihypertensives, β-adrenergic antagonists) may influence the magnitude of circulatory effects produced by volatile anesthetics.

Mechanisms of Circulatory Effects (Table 2-3)

Cardiac Protection (Anesthetic Preconditioning)

Brief episodes of myocardial ischemia occurring before a subsequent longer period of myocardial ischemia provide protection against myocardial dysfunction and necrosis. This is termed *ischemic preconditioning* (IPC). The opening of K_{ATP} channels is critical for the beneficial cardioprotective effects of IPC. Brief exposure to a volatile anesthetic

TABLE 2-3.
MECHANISMS OF CIRCULATORY EFFECTS PRODUCED BY INHALED ANESTHETICS

Direct myocardial depression
Inhibition of CNS sympathetic outflow
Peripheral autonomic ganglion blockade
Attenuate carotid sinus reflex activity
Decreased formation of cyclic adenosine monophosphate
Decreased release of catecholamines
Decreased influx of calcium ions through slow channels

(isoflurane, sevoflurane, desflurane) can activate K_{ATP} channels and result in cardioprotection. The manifestations of reversible reperfusion injury include cardiac dysrhythmias, contractile dysfunction ("stunning"), and microvascular injury. If anesthetic preconditioning is to be of clinical value, it is most likely because it affords additional time before the occurrence of dysfunction and/or infarction; this allows either spontaneous reperfusion or the application of therapies such as angioplasty to relieve a coronary occlusion. IPC is a fundamental endogenous protective mechanism against tissue injury (best characterized in the heart but also present in other tissues) ubiquitous to all species in which it has been studied. An early phase of IPC persists for 1 to 2 hours before disappearing and then reoccurring 24 hours later and persisting as long as an additional 72 hours. This second or late window of preconditioning may last for as long as 3 days.

VENTILATION EFFECTS

Pattern of Breathing

Inhaled anesthetics produce dose-dependent increases in the frequency of breathing. The effect of inhaled anesthetics on the frequency of breathing presumably reflects CNS stimulation. Tidal volume is decreased in association with anesthetic-induced increases in the frequency of breathing. The net effect of these changes is a rapid and shallow pattern of breathing during general anesthesia. The increase in frequency of breathing is insufficient to offset decreases in tidal volume, thus leading to decreases in minute ventilation and increases in $Paco_2$. The pattern of breathing during general anesthesia is also characterized as regular and rhythmic, in contrast to the awake pattern of intermittent deep breaths separated by varying intervals.

Ventilatory Response to Carbon Dioxide

Volatile anesthetics produce a dose-dependent depression of ventilation characterized by decreases in the

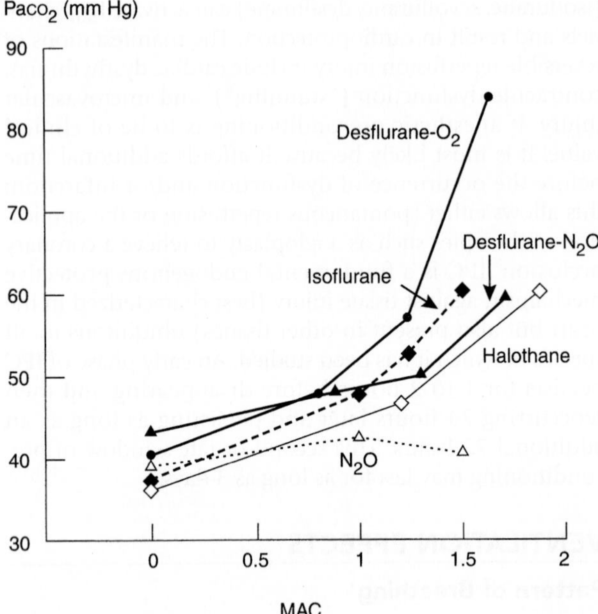

Figure 2-7. Inhaled anesthetics produce drug-specific and dose-dependent increases in Pa_{CO_2}. [From Eger EI. *Desflurane (Suprane): A Compendium and Reference.* Nutley, NJ: Anaquest, 1993:1–119; with permission.]

ventilatory response to carbon dioxide and increases in the Pa_{CO_2} (Fig. 2-7). Desflurane and sevoflurane depress ventilation and produce profound decreases in ventilation leading to apnea between 1.5 and 2.0 MAC. Nitrous oxide does not increase the Pa_{CO_2}, thus suggesting that the substitution of this anesthetic for a portion of the volatile anesthetic would result in less depression of ventilation (nitrous oxide combined with a volatile anesthetic produces less depression of ventilation and increase in Pa_{CO_2} than does the same MAC concentration of the volatile drug alone). The slope of the carbon dioxide response curve is decreased similarly and shifted

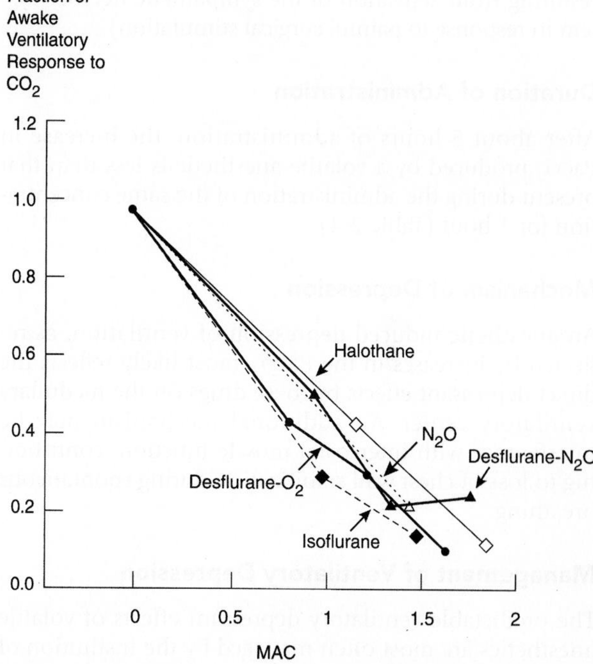

Figure 2-8. All inhaled anesthetics produce similar dose-dependent decreases in the ventilatory response to carbon dioxide. [From Eger EI. *Desflurane (Suprane): A Compendium and Reference*. Nutley, NJ: Anaquest, 1993:1–119; with permission.]

to the right by anesthetic concentrations of all inhaled anesthetics (Fig. 2-8).

Surgical Stimulation of Breathing

Surgical stimulation increases minute ventilation by about 40% because of increases in tidal volume and frequency of breathing. The $Paco_2$, however, decreases only about 10% (4 to 6 mm Hg), despite the larger increase in minute ventilation (reflects an increased production of carbon dioxide resulting from activation of the sympathetic nervous system in response to painful surgical stimulation).

Duration of Administration

After about 5 hours of administration, the increase in Pa_{CO_2} produced by a volatile anesthetic is less than that present during the administration of the same concentration for 1 hour (Table 2-4).

Mechanism of Depression

An anesthetic-induced depression of ventilation, as reflected by increases in the Pa_{CO_2}, most likely reflects the direct depressant effects by these drugs on the medullary ventilatory center. An additional mechanism may be interference with intercostal muscle function, contributing to loss of chest wall stabilization during spontaneous breathing.

Management of Ventilatory Depression

The predictable ventilatory depressant effects of volatile anesthetics are most often managed by the institution of mechanical (controlled) ventilation of the patient's lungs

TABLE 2-4.
EVIDENCE FOR RECOVERY FROM VENTILATORY DEPRESSANT EFFECTS OF VOLATILE ANESTHETICS

	Arterial P_{CO_2}	
Enflurane	**1 Hour of Administration (mm Hg)**	**5 Hours of Administration (mm Hg)**
1 MAC	61	46
2 MAC	Apnea	67

(the inherent ventilatory depressant effects of volatile anesthetics facilitate the initiation of controlled ventilation). Assisted ventilation of the lungs is a questionably effective method for offsetting the ventilatory depressant effects of volatile anesthetics.

Ventilatory Response to Hypoxemia

All inhaled anesthetics, including nitrous oxide, profoundly depress the ventilatory response to hypoxemia that is normally mediated by the carotid bodies (0.1 MAC produces 50% to 70% depression, and 1.1 MAC produces 100% depression of this response). This contrasts with the absence of significant depression of the ventilatory response to carbon dioxide during administration of 0.1 MAC of volatile anesthetics.

Airway Resistance and Irritability

Sevoflurane and isoflurane produce bronchodilation in patients with chronic obstructive pulmonary disease (Fig. 2-9).

Bronchoconstriction produced by desflurane is most likely to occur in patients who smoke. After tracheal intubation in patients without asthma, sevoflurane decreases airway resistance as much or more than isoflurane. The inhalation of sevoflurane degradation products produced by exposure of sevoflurane to desiccated carbon dioxide absorbent may cause airway irritation and impaired gas exchange Compound A is not an airway irritant.

HEPATIC EFFECTS

Hepatic Circulation

Hepatic blood flow during the administration of desflurane and sevoflurane is maintained similar to isoflurane. Maintenance of hepatic oxygen delivery relative to demand during exposure to anesthetics is uniquely important in view of the evidence that hepatocyte

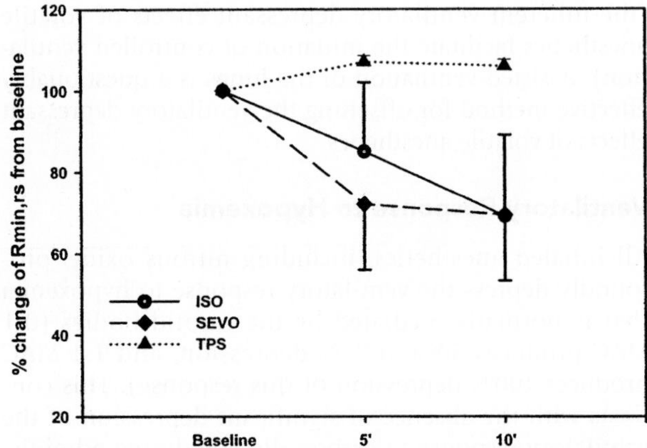

Figure 2-9. The percentage change (mean ± SD) in respiratory system resistance (Rmin, rs) after 5 and 10 minutes of maintenance of anesthesia using thiopental (TPS), 1.1 MAC isoflurane (ISO) or 1.1 MAC sevoflurane (SEVO) administered to patients with chronic obstructive pulmonary disease. (From Volta CA, Alvisi V, Petrini S, et al. The effect of volatile anesthetics on respiratory system resistance in patients with chronic obstructive pulmonary disease. *Anesth Analg* 2005;100:348–353; with permission.)

hypoxia is a significant mechanism in the multifactorial etiology of postoperative hepatic dysfunction.

Drug Clearance

Volatile anesthetics may interfere with the clearance of drugs from the plasma as a result of decreased hepatic blood flow or inhibition of drug-metabolizing enzymes.

Liver Function Tests

Transient increases in liver enzymes following surgery and anesthesia suggest that changes in hepatic blood flow evoked by painful stimulation can adversely alter hepatic function, independent of the volatile anesthetic.

Hepatotoxicity

Postoperative liver dysfunction has been associated with most volatile anesthetics, with halothane receiving the most attention. It is likely that inadequate hepatocyte oxygenation (oxygen supply relative to oxygen demand) is the principal mechanism responsible for hepatic dysfunction following anesthesia and surgery. Preexisting liver disease, such as hepatic cirrhosis, may be associated with marginal hepatocyte oxygenation, which would be further jeopardized by the depressant effects of anesthetics on hepatic blood flow and/or arterial oxygenation.

Halothane

Halothane produces two types of hepatotoxicity in susceptible patients. An estimated 20% of adult patients receiving halothane develop a mild, self-limited postoperative hepatotoxicity that is characterized by nausea, lethargy, fever, and minor increases in plasma concentrations of liver transaminase enzymes. The other and rarer type of hepatotoxicity (halothane hepatitis) is estimated to occur in 1 in 10,000 to 1 in 30,000 adult patients receiving halothane; it may lead to massive hepatic necrosis and death. It is likely that the more common self-limited form of hepatic dysfunction following halothane is a nonspecific drug effect due to those changes in hepatic blood flow that impair hepatic oxygenation. Conversely, the more rare, life-threatening form of hepatic dysfunction characterized, as *halothane hepatitis,* is most likely an immune-mediated hepatotoxicity.

Halothane Hepatitis

Clinical manifestations of halothane hepatitis suggest an immune-mediated response including eosinophilia, fever, rash, arthralgia, and prior exposure to halothane. The most compelling evidence for an immune-mediated mechanism is the presence of circulatory immunoglobulin G antibodies in at least 70% of those patients diagnosed with halothane hepatitis. These antibodies are directed against liver microsomal proteins on the surface of hepatocytes that have been covalently modified to form neoantigens by the reactive oxidative trifluoroacetyl halide metabolite of halothane.

Enflurane, Isoflurane, and Desflurane

The mild, self-limited postoperative hepatic dysfunction that is associated with all the volatile anesthetics most likely reflects anesthetic-induced alterations in hepatic oxygen delivery relative to demand; this results in inadequate hepatocyte oxygenation. The fact that enflurane, isoflurane, and desflurane are oxidatively metabolized by liver cytochrome P-450 to form acetylated liver protein adducts, by mechanisms similar to that of halothane, suggests that acetylated liver proteins capable of evoking an antibody response could occur after exposure to halothane, enflurane, isoflurane, or desflurane. This raises the possibility that enflurane, isoflurane, and desflurane could produce hepatotoxicity by a mechanism similar to that of halothane, but at a lower incidence, because the degree of anesthetic metabolism appears to be directly related to the potential for hepatic injury. Considering the magnitude of metabolism of these volatile anesthetics, it is predictable that the incidence of anesthetic-induced hepatitis would be greatest with halothane, intermediate with enflurane, and rare with isoflurane. Desflurane is metabolized even less than isoflurane, and from the standpoint of immune-mediated hepatotoxicity, desflurane should be very safe, because it would have the lowest level of adduct formation.

Sevoflurane

Sevoflurane metabolism does not result in the formation of trifluoroacetylated liver proteins and therefore cannot stimulate the formation of antitrifluoroacetylated protein antibodies. Therefore, unlike all the other fluorinated volatile anesthetics, sevoflurane would not be expected to produce immune-mediated hepatotoxicity or to cause cross-sensitivity in patients previously exposed to halothane.

RENAL EFFECTS

Volatile anesthetics produce similar dose-related decreases in renal blood flow, glomerular filtration rate, and urine output. These changes are not a result of the release of arginine vasopressin hormone, but rather most likely reflect the effects of volatile anesthetics on systemic blood pressure and cardiac output. Preoperative hydration attenuates or abolishes many of the changes in renal function associated with volatile anesthetics.

Fluoride-Induced Nephrotoxicity

Fluoride-induced nephrotoxicity is characterized by polyuria, hypernatremia, hyperosmolarity, increased plasma creatinine, and an inability to concentrate urine. A plasma fluoride concentration of 50 μm/L has been adopted as an indicator that renal toxicity may occur from other volatile anesthetics. The absence of renal toxicity despite peak plasma fluoride concentrations exceeding 50 μm/L after the administration of enflurane or sevoflurane suggests that this peak value alone cannot be accepted as an indicator for fluoride-induced nephrotoxicity after the administration of these volatile anesthetics.

Sevoflurane

Sevoflurane is metabolized to inorganic fluoride, yet sevoflurane anesthesia does not impair renal concentrating function. Despite reports failing to show renal impairment after the administration of sevoflurane, observations have been made of a transient impairment in renal concentrating ability and increased urinary excretion of β-N-acetylglucosaminidase (NAG) in patients exposed to sevoflurane and developing peak plasma inorganic fluoride concentrations >50 μm/L.

Concern that the administration of sevoflurane to patients with preexisting renal disease could accentuate renal dysfunction was not confirmed when this volatile anesthetic was administered to patients with chronic renal disease.

Vinyl Halide Nephrotoxicity

Carbon dioxide absorbents containing potassium and sodium hydroxide react with sevoflurane to form fluoromethyl-2,2-difluro-1-(trifluoromethyl) vinyl ether (compound A). Compound A is a dose-dependent nephrotoxin in rats. The rationale for utilizing at least a 2-L/min fresh gas flow rate when administering sevoflurane is intended to minimize the concentration of compound A that may accumulate in the anesthesia breathing circuit. The amount of compound A produced under clinical conditions has consistently been far below those concentrations associated with nephrotoxicity in animals. A proposed mechanism for nephrotoxicity is the metabolism of compound A to a reactive thiol via the β-lyase pathway. Because humans have less than one-tenth of the enzymatic activity for this pathway compared to rats, it is possible that humans should be less vulnerable to injury by this mechanism.

SKELETAL MUSCLE EFFECTS

Neuromuscular Junction

Volatile anesthetics produce a dose-dependent enhancement of the effects of neuromuscular-blocking drugs, with the effects of enflurane, isoflurane, desflurane, and sevoflurane being similar, and all being greater than halothane. Nitrous oxide does not significantly potentiate the in vivo effects of neuromuscular-blocking drugs.

Malignant Hyperthermia

Volatile anesthetics, including desflurane and sevoflurane, can trigger malignant hyperthermia in genetically susceptible patients even in the absence of the concomitant administration of succinylcholine. Among the volatile anesthetics, however, halothane is the most potent trigger. Nitrous oxide, when compared with volatile anesthetics, is a weak trigger for malignant hyperthermia.

OBSTETRIC EFFECTS

Volatile anesthetics produce similar and dose-dependent decreases in uterine smooth muscle contractility and blood flow. Anesthetic-induced uterine relaxation may be desirable to facilitate the removal of retained placenta. Conversely, uterine relaxation produced by volatile anesthetics may contribute to blood loss due to uterine atony. Inhaled anesthetics rapidly cross the placenta to enter the fetus, but these drugs are likewise rapidly exhaled by the newborn infant.

RESISTANCE TO INFECTION

Many of the immune changes seen in surgical patients are primarily the result of surgical trauma and endocrine responses (increased catecholamines and corticosteroids) rather than the result of the anesthetic exposure itself. Inhaled anesthetics, particularly nitrous oxide, produce a dose-dependent inhibition of polymorphonuclear leukocytes and their subsequent migration (chemotaxis) for phagocytosis, which is necessary for the inflammatory response to infection.

GENETIC EFFECTS

The *Ames test,* which identifies chemicals that act as mutagens and carcinogens, is negative for enflurane, isoflurane, desflurane, sevoflurane, and nitrous oxide, including their known metabolites. The increased incidence of spontaneous abortions in operating room personnel may reflect a teratogenic effect from chronic exposure to trace concentrations of inhaled anesthetics, especially nitrous oxide. Nitrous oxide irreversibly oxidizes the cobalt atom of vitamin B_{12} so that the activity of vitamin B_{12}–dependent enzymes (methionine synthetase and thymidylate synthetase) is decreased. The speculated but undocumented role of trace concentrations of nitrous oxide in the production of spontaneous abortions has led to the use of scavenging systems designed to remove waste anesthetic gases, including nitrous oxide, from the ambient air of the operating room. Nevertheless, animal studies using intermittent exposure to trace concentrations of nitrous oxide, halothane, enflurane, and isoflurane have not revealed harmful reproductive effects.

BONE MARROW FUNCTION

Interference with DNA synthesis is responsible for the megaloblastic changes and agranulocytosis that may follow the prolonged administration of nitrous oxide. Megaloblastic changes in bone marrow are consistently found in patients who have been exposed to anesthetic concentrations of nitrous oxide for 24 hours. Exposure to nitrous oxide lasting 4 days or longer results in agranulocytosis.

PERIPHERAL NEUROPATHY

Humans who chronically inhale nitrous oxide for nonmedical purposes may develop a neuropathy characterized by sensorimotor polyneuropathy; this is often combined with signs of a posterior lateral spinal cord degeneration resembling pernicious anemia.

TOTAL BODY OXYGEN REQUIREMENTS

Total body oxygen requirements are decreased by similar amounts by volatile anesthetics. The oxygen requirements of the heart decrease more than those of other organs, reflecting drug-induced decreases in cardiac work associated with decreases in systemic blood pressure and myocardial contractility.

METABOLISM

Intermediary metabolites, end-metabolites, or breakdown products from the exposure to desiccated carbon dioxide absorbents containing strong bases may be toxic to the kidneys, liver, or reproductive organs. A comparison of metabolite recovery and mass balance studies results in greatly different estimates of the magnitude of volatile anesthetic metabolism (Table 2-5).

Determinants of Metabolism

Chemical Structure

The ether bond and carbon-halogen bond are the sites in the anesthetic molecule most susceptible to oxidative

TABLE 2-5.
METABOLISM OF VOLATILE ANESTHETICS AS ASSESSED BY METABOLITE RECOVERY VERSUS MASS BALANCE STUDIES

	Magnitude of Metabolism	
Anesthetic	**Metabolite Recovery (%)**	**Mass Balance (%)**
Nitrous oxide	0.004	
Halothane	15–20	46.1
Enflurane	3	8.5
Isoflurane	0.2	0*
Desflurane	0.02	
Sevoflurane	5	

*Metabolism of isoflurane assumed to be 0 for this calculation.

metabolism. Two halogen atoms on a terminal carbon represent the optimal arrangement for dehalogenation, whereas a terminal carbon with fluorine atoms is very resistant to oxidative metabolism.

Hepatic Enzyme Activity

The activity of those hepatic cytochrome P-450 enzymes responsible for the metabolism of volatile anesthetics may be increased by a variety of drugs, including the anesthetics themselves.

Blood Concentration

The fraction of anesthetic that is metabolized on passing through the liver is influenced by the blood concentration of the anesthetic. Inhaled anesthetics that are not highly soluble in blood and tissues (nitrous oxide, enflurane, isoflurane, desflurane, sevoflurane) tend to be exhaled rapidly via the lungs at the conclusion of an anesthetic. As a result, less drug is available to pass continually through the liver at the low blood concentrations conducive to metabolism.

Genetics

Genetic factors appear to be the most important determinant of drug-metabolizing activity.

Metabolism of Inhaled Anesthetics

Nitrous Oxide

An estimated 0.004% of an absorbed dose of nitrous oxide undergoes reductive metabolism to nitrogen in the gastrointestinal tract.

Halothane

An estimated 15 to 20% of absorbed halothane undergoes metabolism (see Table 2-5).

Oxidative Metabolism

The oxidative metabolism of halothane produces trifluoroacetic acid, chloride, and bromide as the principal oxidative metabolites, resulting from metabolism by cytochrome P-450 enzymes. In genetically susceptible patients, a reactive trifluoroacetyl halide oxidative metabolite of halothane may interact with (acetylate) hepatic microsomal proteins on the surfaces of hepatocytes (neoantigens) to stimulate the formation of antibodies against this new foreign protein.

Reductive Metabolism

Reductive metabolism among the volatile anesthetics, which has been documented to occur only during the metabolism of halothane, is most likely to occur in the presence of hepatocyte hypoxia and enzyme induction. Data do not support a role for reductive metabolism in the initiation of halothane hepatitis.

Enflurane

An estimated 3% of absorbed enflurane undergoes oxidative metabolism by cytochrome P-450 enzymes to form inorganic fluoride and organic fluoride compounds (see Table 2-5). Like halothane, enflurane also undergoes P-450–mediated oxidative metabolism to adducts, which may cause the formation of neoantigens in susceptible patients.

Isoflurane

An estimated 0.2% of absorbed isoflurane undergoes oxidative metabolism by cytochrome P-450 enzymes (see Table 2-5). Trifluoroacetic acid is the principal organic fluoride metabolite of isoflurane. Like halothane, isoflurane also undergoes P-450–mediated oxidative metabolism to adducts, which may cause formation of neoantigens in susceptible patients.

Desflurane

An estimated 0.02% of absorbed desflurane undergoes oxidative metabolism by cytochrome P-450 enzymes (see Table 2-5). The metabolic pathways for desflurane likely parallel those for isoflurane, although the greater strength of the carbon–fluorine bond renders desflurane less vulnerable to metabolism than its chlorinated analog, isoflurane. The only evidence of desflurane metabolism is the presence of measurable concentrations of urinary trifluoroacetic acid equal to about one-fifth to one-tenth that produced by isoflurane metabolism. Neoantigens may be produced in susceptible patients.

Carbon Monoxide Toxicity

Carbon monoxide formation reflects the degradation of volatile anesthetics that contain a CHF2 moiety (desflurane, enflurane, and isoflurane) by the strong bases present in desiccated carbon dioxide absorbents (Table 2-6). Desflurane produces the highest carbon monoxide concentration (the package insert for desflurane describes this risk), followed by enflurane and isoflurane. Halothane and sevoflurane do not possess a vinyl group, thus carbon monoxide production on exposure to carbon dioxide absorbents has been considered unlikely. Nevertheless, carbon monoxide formation is a risk of sevoflurane administration in the presence of desiccated carbon dioxide absorbent, especially when an exothermic reaction between the volatile anesthetic and desiccated absorbent occurs. It is concluded that the potential for

TABLE 2-6.
FACTORS INFLUENCING CARBON MONOXIDE PRODUCTION FROM VOLATILE ANESTHETICS

Dryness of the carbon dioxide absorbent
High temperatures of the carbon dioxide absorbent (low fresh gas flows, increased metabolic production of carbon dioxide)
Prolonged high fresh gas flows through carbon dioxide absorbent
Type of carbon dioxide absorbent

carbon monoxide formation is a property of all modern volatile anesthetics contacting those dry carbon dioxide absorbents that contain potassium hydroxide and/or sodium hydroxide.

Diagnosing Carbon Monoxide Exposure

Intraoperative diagnosis of carbon monoxide exposure is difficult because pulse oximetry cannot differentiate between carboxyhemoglobin and oxyhemoglobin. Moderately decreased pulse oximetry readings despite adequate arterial partial pressures of oxygen (especially during the first case of the day, "Monday morning phenomena") should suggest the possibility of carbon monoxide exposure and the need to measure carboxyhemoglobin. Delayed neurophysiologic sequelae due to carbon monoxide (cognitive defects, personality changes, gait disturbances) may occur as late as 3 to 21 days after anesthesia.

Endogenous Carbon Monoxide Production

Endogenous carbon monoxide production reflects heme catabolism. Independent of volatile anesthetics and carbon dioxide absorbents, the exhaled carbon monoxide and carboxyhemoglobin concentrations are increased on the day following surgery; this suggests that oxidative stress associated with anesthesia and surgery may induce heme oxygenase-1, which catalyzes heme to produce carbon monoxide.

Sevoflurane

An estimated 5% of absorbed sevoflurane undergoes oxidative metabolism by cytochrome P-450 enzymes to form organic and inorganic fluoride metabolites (see Table 2-5). In addition, sevoflurane is degraded by carbon dioxide absorbents to potentially toxic compounds. Unlike all the other fluorinated volatile anesthetics, sevoflurane does not undergo metabolism to acetyl halide that could result in formation of trifluoroacetylated liver proteins. As a result, sevoflurane cannot stimulate the formation of antitrifluoroacetylated protein antibodies and lead to hepatotoxicity through this mechanism. Sevoflurane is absorbed and degraded by desiccated carbon dioxide absorbents, especially when the temperature of the absorbent is increased.

Carbon Dioxide Absorber Fires

Carbon dioxide absorber fires may occur with the use of sevoflurane. Sevoflurane reacts chemically with desiccated carbon dioxide absorbents to produce carbon monoxide

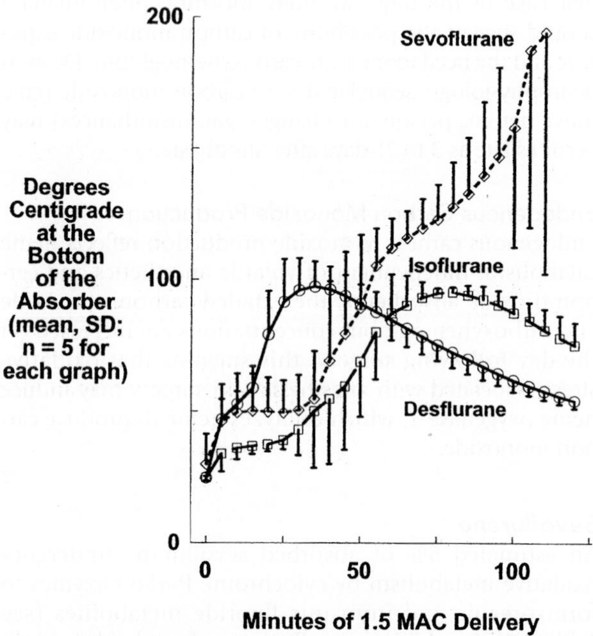

Figure 2-10. Temperatures recorded in the desiccated carbon dioxide absorbent exposed to 1.5 MAC sevoflurane increased progressively to >200C°. Temperature increases in the presence of 1.5 MAC isoflurane and desflurane were less and not sustained. (From Laster et al. Fires from the interaction of anesthetics with desiccated absorbent. *Anesth Analg* 2004;99:769–74; with permission.)

and flammable organic compounds, including methanol and formaldehyde. The reaction produces heat, and heat increases the reaction speed; thus, the rate of sevoflurane breakdown can accelerate rapidly (Fig. 2-10). Temperature increases in the carbon dioxide absorbent rise on exposure to isoflurane and desflurane, but the magnitude of the increase is less and is not sustained (see Fig. 2-10). At high temperatures, flammable metabolites can spontaneously combust (formaldehyde gas). Temperature increases are most likely to occur when sevoflurane is exposed to desiccated carbon dioxide absorbents. Spontaneous combustion and even explosions involving the carbon dioxide absorber and anesthesia breathing circuit have been described. These phenomena were associated with Baralyme® carbon dioxide absorbent (no longer clinically available), anesthesia machine use factors that contribute to desiccation of the absorbent (flow of dry gases through the absorber during a weekend, "Monday morning phenomena"), and the administration of sevoflurane. The critical observation regarding fires and the production of carbon monoxide is that desiccated absorbent allows these reactions to occur. Clinically, delayed increases or unexpected sudden decreases in inspired sevoflurane concentrations relative to the vaporizer setting may reflect excessive heating of the carbon dioxide absorber canister. Pulmonary injury has been observed following an exothermic reaction between sevoflurane and the carbon dioxide absorbent. Furthermore, formaldehyde alone, as a byproduct of sevoflurane breakdown, may cause pulmonary injury.

Opioid Agonists and Antagonists

3

The development of synthetic drugs with morphine-like properties has led to the use of the term *opioid* to refer to all exogenous substances, natural and synthetic, that bind specifically to any of several subpopulations of opioid receptors and produce at least some agonist (morphine-like) effects (Table 3-1) (Stoelting RK, Hillier SC. Opioid agonists and antagonists. In: *Pharmacology and Physiology in Anesthetic Practice*, 4th ed. Philadelphia. Lippincott Williams & Wilkins, 2006:87–126). Opioids are unique in producing analgesia without loss of touch, proprioception, or consciousness.

STRUCTURE–ACTIVITY RELATIONSHIPS

A close relationship exists between the stereochemical structure and potency of opioids, with levorotatory isomers being the most active.

Semisynthetic Opioids

Semisynthetic opioids result from a relatively simple modification of the morphine molecule (substitution of acetyl groups on carbons 3 and 6 results in diacetylmorphine, heroin).

Synthetic Opioids

Fentanyl, sufentanil, alfentanil, and remifentanil are semisynthetic opioids that are widely used to supplement

TABLE 3-1.
CLASSIFICATION OF OPIOID AGONISTS AND ANTAGONISTS

Opioids
Morphine
Morphine-6-glucuronide
Meperidine
Sufentanil
Fentanyl
Alfentanil
Remifentanil
Codeine
Hydromorphone
Oxymorphone
Oxycodone
Hydrocodone
Propoxyphene
Methadone
Tramadol
Heroin
Opioid agonists-antagonists
Pentazocine
Butorphanol
Nalbuphine
Buprenorphine
Nalorphine
Bremazocine
Dezocine
Meptazinol
Opioid antagonists
Naloxone
Naltrexone
Nalmefene

general anesthesia or as primary anesthetic drugs in very high doses during cardiac surgery. The major pharmacodynamic differences between these drugs are potency and rate of equilibration between the plasma and the site of drug effect (biophase).

MECHANISM OF ACTION

Opioids act as agonists on those stereospecific opioid receptors occurring at presynaptic and postsynaptic sites within the central nervous system (CNS) (principally the brainstem and spinal cord) and outside the CNS in peripheral tissues. Opioids mimic the actions of endogenous ligands by binding to opioid receptors, thus resulting in the activation of pain-modulating (antinoceptive) systems. The existence of the opioid in the ionized state appears to be necessary for strong binding at the anionic opioid receptor site. Only levorotatory forms of the opioid exhibit agonist activity. The principal effect of opioid receptor activation is a decrease in neurotransmission. The intracellular biochemical events initiated by occupation of opioid receptors with an opioid agonist are characterized by increased potassium conductance (leading to hyperpolarization), calcium channel inactivation, or both, which produce an immediate decrease in neurotransmitter release. It is assumed that increasing opioid receptor occupancy parallels opioid effects.

OPIOID RECEPTORS

Opioid receptors are classified as μ, δ, and κ receptors (Table 3-2). These opioid receptors belong to a superfamily of guanine (G) protein–coupled receptors. It is likely that distinct morphine-6-glucuronide receptors exist as a variants of the μ-receptor gene. μ or morphine-preferring receptors are principally responsible for supraspinal and spinal analgesia. Naloxone is a specific μ receptor antagonist, attaching to but not activating the receptor.

Endogenous Pain Suppression System

The obvious role of opioid receptors and endorphins is to function as an endogenous pain suppression system. Opioid receptors are located in those areas of the brain

TABLE 3-2.
CLASSIFICATION OF OPIOID RECEPTORS

	μ_1	μ_2	Kappa	Delta
Effect	Analgesia (supraspinal, spinal)	Analgesia (spinal)	Analgesia (supraspinal, spinal)	Analgesia (supraspinal, spinal)
	Euphoria		Dysphoria, sedation	
		Depression of ventilation		Depression of ventilation
	Low abuse potential	Physical dependence	Low abuse potential	Physical dependence
	Miosis		Miosis	
		Constipation (marked)		Constipation (minimal)
	Bradycardia			
	Hypothermia			
	Urinary retention		Diuresis	Urinary retention
Agonists	Endorphins*	Endorphins*	Dynorphins	Enkephalins
	Morphine	Morphine		
	Synthetic opioids	Synthetic opioids		
Antagonists	Naloxone	Naloxone	Naloxone	Naloxone
	Naltrexone	Naltrexone	Naltrexone	Naltrexone
	Nalmefene	Nalmefene	Nalmefene	Nalmefene

The existence of specific μ_1 and μ_2 receptors is not supported based on cloning studies of μ-receptors

* μ-Receptors seem to be a universal site of action for all endogenous opioid receptors.

(periaqueductal gray matter of the brain stem, amygdala, corpus striatum, and hypothalamus) and spinal cord (substantia gelatinosa) that are involved with pain perception, integration of pain impulses, and responses to pain. It is speculated that endorphins inhibit the release of excitatory neurotransmitters from the terminals of nerves carrying nociceptive impulses. As a result, neurons are hyperpolarized, which suppresses spontaneous discharges and evoked responses.

NEURAXIAL OPIOIDS

The placement of opioids in the epidural or subarachnoid space to manage acute or chronic pain is based on the knowledge that opioid receptors (principally μ receptors) are present in the substantia gelatinosa of the spinal cord. Analgesia produced by neuraxial opioids, in contrast to the intravenous administration of opioids or regional anesthesia with local anesthetics, is not associated with sympathetic nervous system denervation, skeletal muscle weakness, or loss of proprioception. Analgesia is dose related (epidural dose is 5 to 10 times the subarachnoid dose) and specific for visceral rather than somatic pain. Analgesia that follows the epidural placement of opioids reflects a diffusion of the drug across the dura to gain access to μ opioid receptors on the spinal cord, as well as a systemic absorption to produce effects similar to those that would follow intravenous administration of the opioid.

Pharmacokinetics

Opioids placed in the epidural space may undergo uptake into epidural fat, systemic absorption, or diffusion across the dura into the cerebrospinal fluid (CSF). Penetration of the dura is considerably influenced by lipid solubility. Fentanyl and sufentanil are, respectively, approximately 800 and 1,600 times as lipid soluble as morphine. After epidural administration, CSF concentrations of fentanyl peak in about 20 minutes and sufentanil in about 6 minutes. In contrast, CSF concentrations of morphine, after epidural administration, peak in 1 to 4 hours. Epidural administration of morphine, fentanyl, and sufentanil produces opioid blood concentrations that are similar to those produced by an intramuscular injection of an equivalent dose. The addition of epinephrine to the solution placed into the epidural space decreases systemic absorption of the opioid but does not influence the diffusion of morphine across the dura into the CSF. Cephalad movement of opioids in the CSF principally depends on lipid solubility (lipid-soluble opioids such as fentanyl and sufentanil are limited in their cephalad migration by uptake into the spinal cord, whereas less lipid-soluble morphine remains in the CSF for transfer to more cephalad locations). The underlying cause of morphine ascension is the bulk flow of CSF. CSF ascends in a cephalad direction from the lumbar region, reaching the cisterna magna in 1 to 2 hours and the fourth and lateral ventricles by 3 to 6 hours. Coughing or straining, but not body position, can affect the movement of CSF.

Side Effects

The four classic side effects of neuraxial opioids are pruritus, nausea and vomiting, urinary retention, and depression of ventilation (Table 3-3).

Pruritus

Pruritus is the most common side effect (often localized to face, neck, upper thorax) of neuraxial opioids. Pruritus usually occurs within a few hours of injection and may precede the onset of analgesia. Pruritus induced by neuraxial opioids is not due to histamine release but is likely due to the cephalad migration of the opioid in CSF and its subsequent interaction with opioid receptors in the trigeminal nucleus. An opioid antagonist, such as naloxone, is effective in relieving opioid-induced pruritus.

TABLE 3-3.
SIDE EFFECTS OF NEURAXIAL (EPIDURAL AND SPINAL) OPIOIDS

Pruritus
Nausea and vomiting
Urinary retention
Depression of ventilation
Sedation
Central nervous system excitation
Viral reactivation
Neonatal morbidity
Sexual dysfunction
Ocular dysfunction
Gastrointestinal dysfunction
Thermoregulatory dysfunction
Water retention

Paradoxically, antihistamines may be effective treatment for pruritus, likely secondary to their sedative effect.

Urinary Retention

Urinary retention occurring with neuraxial opioid administration is more common than after the intravenous or intramuscular administration of equivalent doses of the opioid and is most likely due to an interaction of the opioid with opioid receptors located in the sacral spinal cord. This interaction promotes the inhibition of sacral parasympathetic nervous system outflow, which causes detrusor muscle relaxation and an increase in maximum bladder capacity, thus leading to urinary retention.

Depression of Ventilation

The most serious side effect of neuraxial opioids is depression of ventilation, which may occur within minutes of administration or may be delayed for hours. The incidence of ventilatory depression requiring intervention after conventional doses of neuraxial opioids is about 1%, which is the same as that after conventional doses of intravenous or intramuscular opioids. Early depression of ventilation occurs within 2 hours of neuraxial injection of the opioid (most often fentanyl or sufentanil). This depression of ventilation most likely results from the systemic absorption of the lipid-soluble opioid, although cephalad migration of opioid in the CSF may also be responsible. Clinically significant early depression of ventilation after the intrathecal injection of morphine is unlikely. Delayed depression of ventilation occurs more than 2 hours after neuraxial opioid administration; this reflects cephalad migration of the opioid in the CSF and subsequent interaction with opioid receptors located in the ventral medulla (Table 3-4). Delayed depression of ventilation characteristically occurs 6 to 12 hours after the epidural or intrathecal administration of morphine. Factors that increase the risk of delayed depression of ventilation, especially concomitant use of any intravenous opioid or sedative, must be considered in determining the dose of neuraxial opioid (Table 3-4). Pulse oximetry reliably detects opioid-induced arterial hypoxemia, and supplemental oxygen (2 L/min) is an effective treatment. The most reliable clinical sign of ventilation depression appears to be a depressed level of consciousness, possibly caused by hypercarbia.

TABLE 3-4.
FACTORS THAT INCREASE THE RISK OF DEPRESSION OF VENTILATION

High opioid dose
Low lipid solubility of opioids
Concomitant administration of parenteral opioids or other sedatives
Lack of opioid tolerance
Advanced age
Patient position (?)
Increased intrathoracic pressure

Sedation

Sedation occurring after the administration of neuraxial opioids appears to be dose related. It occurs with all opioids but is most commonly associated with the use of sufentanil.

Central Nervous System Excitation

Tonic skeletal muscle rigidity resembling seizure activity is a well-known side effect of large intravenous doses of opioids, but this response is rarely observed after neuraxial administration.

Viral Reactivation

A link exists between the use of epidural morphine in obstetric patients and reactivation of herpes simplex labialis virus. The underlying mechanism causing herpes virus reactivation likely involves the cephalad migration of opioid in CSF and its subsequent interaction with the trigeminal nucleus.

Neonatal Morbidity

Systemic absorption after epidural administration of an opioid results in predictable blood levels of the drug in the neonate immediately after birth.

Miscellaneous Side Effects

Neuraxial opioids may delay gastric emptying, most likely reflecting an interaction of the opioid with spinal cord opioid receptors. Neuraxial opioids, by inhibiting shivering, may cause decreased body temperature.

OPIOID AGONISTS

The most notable feature of the clinical use of opioids is the extraordinary variation in dose requirements for pain management (see Table 3-1).

Morphine

Morphine is the prototype opioid agonist to which all other opioids are compared. In humans, morphine produces analgesia, euphoria, sedation, and a diminished ability to concentrate. Other sensations include nausea, a feeling of body warmth, heaviness of the extremities, dryness of the mouth, and pruritus, especially in the cutaneous areas around the nose. The cause of pain persists, but even low doses of morphine increase the threshold to pain and modify the perception of noxious stimulation so that it is no longer experienced as pain. In the absence of pain, however, morphine may produce dysphoria rather than euphoria.

Pharmacokinetics

Morphine is usually administered intravenously in the perioperative period, thus eliminating the unpredictable influence of drug absorption. The peak effect (equilibration time between the blood and brain) after the intravenous administration of morphine is delayed, compared with opioids such as fentanyl and alfentanil, and requires about 15 to 30 minutes (Table 3-5). Plasma morphine concentrations after rapid intravenous injections do not correlate closely with the opioid's pharmacologic activity. Presumably, this discrepancy reflects a delay in the penetration of morphine across the blood-brain barrier. Only a small amount of administered morphine gains access to the CNS. It is estimated that <0.1% of morphine that is administered intravenously has entered the CNS at the time of peak plasma concentrations.

Metabolism

The principal pathway of morphine metabolism is through conjugation with glucuronic acid in hepatic and extrahepatic sites, especially the kidneys. About 75% to 85% of a dose of morphine appears as morphine-3-glucuronide, and 5% to 10% as morphine-6-glucuronide

TABLE 3-5.
PHARMACOKINETICS OF OPIOID AGONISTS

	pK	Percent Nonionized (pH 7.4)	Protein Binding (%)	Clearance (ml/min)	Volume of Distribution (liters)	Partition Coefficient	Elimination Half-Time (hrs)	Context Sensitive Half-Time 4-hour Infusion (mins)	Effect-Site (Blood-Brain) Equilibration Time (mins)
Morphine	7.9	23	35	1,050	224	1	1.7–3.3		
Meperidine	8.5	7	70	1,020	305	32	3–5		
Fentanyl	8.4	8.5	84	1,530	335	955	3.1–6.6	260	6.8
Sufentanil	8.0	20	93	900	123	1,727	2.2–4.6	30	6.2
Alfentanil	6.5	89	92	238	27	129	1.4–1.5	60	1.4
Remifentanil	7.3	58	66–93	4,000	30		0.17–0.33	4	1.1

(a ratio of 9:1). Morphine-3-glucuronide is pharmacologically inactive, whereas morphine-6-glucuronide produces analgesia and depression of ventilation via its agonist actions at μ receptors. Renal metabolism makes a significant contribution to the total metabolism of morphine, which offers a possible explanation for the absence of any decrease in systemic clearance of morphine in patients with hepatic cirrhosis or during the anhepatic phase of orthotopic liver transplantation. The elimination of morphine glucuronides may be impaired in patients with renal failure, causing an accumulation of metabolites and unexpected ventilatory depressant effects even with small doses of opioids. The formation of glucuronide conjugates may be impaired by monoamine oxidase inhibitors, which is consistent with the exaggerated effects of morphine when administered to patients being treated with these drugs.

Elimination Half-Time (see Table 3-5)

Patients with renal failure exhibit higher plasma and CSF concentrations of morphine and morphine metabolites than do normal patients, reflecting a smaller volume of distribution (Vd).

Gender

Gender may affect opioid analgesia (morphine exhibits greater analgesic potency and slower speed of offset in women than men).

Side Effects

The side effects described for morphine also are characteristic of other opioid agonists, although the incidence and magnitude may vary.

Cardiovascular System

The administration of morphine, even in large doses (1 mg/kg IV), to supine and normovolemic patients is unlikely to cause direct myocardial depression or hypotension. Orthostatic hypotension, however, presumably reflecting a morphine-induced impairment of compensatory sympathetic nervous system responses, may occur in these patients. Morphine can also evoke decreases in systemic blood pressure due to drug-induced bradycardia or histamine release. The administration of opioids (morphine) in the preoperative medication or before the induction of anesthesia (fentanyl) tends to slow heart rate during exposure to volatile anesthetics, with or without surgical stimulation. The magnitude of morphine-induced histamine release and a subsequent decrease in systemic blood pressure can be minimized by (a) limiting the rate of morphine infusion to 5 mg/minute IV, (b) maintaining the patient in a supine to slightly head-down position, and (c) optimizing intravascular fluid volume.

Ventilation

All opioid agonists produce a dose-dependent and gender-specific depression of ventilation, primarily through an agonist effect at μ_2 receptors, which leads to a direct depressant effect on brainstem ventilation centers. An opioid-induced depression of ventilation is characterized by decreased responsiveness of these ventilation centers to carbon dioxide, as reflected by an increase in the resting $Paco_2$ and displacement of the carbon dioxide response curve to the right. Death from an opioid overdose is almost invariably attributable to depression of ventilation. Clinically, the ventilation depression produced by opioid agonists manifests as a decreased frequency of breathing that is often accompanied by a compensatory increase in tidal volume (although the compensatory increase in tidal volume is incomplete, as evidenced by increases in the $Paco_2$). Advanced age and the occurrence of natural sleep increases the ventilatory depressant effects of opioids, whereas pain from surgical stimulation counteracts the ventilation depression produced by opioids.

Cough Suppression

Opioids, such as codeine and dextromethorphan, depress cough through their effects on the medullary cough centers.

Nervous System

In the absence of hypoventilation, opioids decrease cerebral blood flow and possibly intracranial pressure (ICP). These drugs must be used with caution in patients with head injury because of their (a) associated effects on wakefulness, (b) production of miosis, and (c) depression of ventilation with associated increases in ICP if the $PaCO_2$ becomes increased. Skeletal muscle rigidity, especially of the thoracic and abdominal muscles, is common when large doses of opioid agonists are administered rapidly intravenously.

Sedation

The postoperative titration of morphine frequently induces a sedation that precedes the onset of analgesia. The usual recommendation for morphine titration includes a short interval between boluses (5 to 7 minutes) with no upper limit on the total dose administered.

Biliary Tract

Opioids can cause spasm of biliary smooth muscle, resulting in increases in intrabiliary pressure that may be associated with epigastric distress or biliary colic. This pain may be confused with angina pectoris. Naloxone will relieve the pain caused by biliary spasm but not myocardial ischemia. Conversely, nitroglycerin will relieve pain due to biliary spasm or myocardial ischemia. During surgery, opioid-induced spasm of the sphincter of Oddi may appear radiologically as a sharp constriction at the distal end of the common bile duct, and it may be misinterpreted as a common bile duct stone. Glucagon, 2 mg IV, also reverses opioid-induced biliary smooth muscle spasm and, unlike naloxone, does not antagonize the analgesic effects of the opioid.

Gastrointestinal Tract

Commonly used opioids such as morphine, meperidine, and fentanyl can produce spasm of the gastrointestinal smooth muscles, resulting in a variety of side effects including constipation, biliary colic, and delayed gastric emptying.

Nausea and Vomiting

Nausea and vomiting induced by opioids reflects their direct stimulation of the chemoreceptor trigger zone in the floor of the fourth ventricle. Nausea and vomiting are relatively uncommon in recumbent patients given morphine, suggesting that a vestibular component may contribute to opioid-induced nausea and vomiting.

Genitourinary System

Morphine can increase the tone and peristaltic activity of the ureter. The administration of morphine in the absence of painful surgical stimulation does not evoke the release of arginine vasopressin.

Cutaneous Changes

Morphine causes the cutaneous blood vessels of the face, neck, and upper chest to dilate.

Placenta

The placenta offers no real barrier to the transfer of opioids from mother to fetus. Therefore, depression of the neonate can occur as a consequence of opioid administration to the mother during labor.

Drug Interactions

The ventilatory depressant effects of some opioids may be exaggerated by amphetamines, phenothiazines, monoamine oxidase inhibitors, and tricyclic antidepressants.

Pharmacodynamic Tolerance and Physical Dependence

With repeated opioid administration, increasing pharmacodynamic tolerance and physical dependence are characteristic features of all opioid agonists and are among the major limitations of their clinical use.

TABLE 3-6.
TIME COURSE OF OPIOID WITHDRAWAL

	Onset	Peak Intensity	Duration
Morphine	6–18 hrs	36–72 hrs	7–10 days
Heroin	6–18 hrs	36–72 hrs	7–10 days
Meperidine	2–6 hrs	8–12 hrs	4–5 days
Fentanyl	2–6 hrs	8–12 hrs	4–5 day
Methadone	24–48 hrs	3–21 days	6–7 weeks

Tolerance develops to the analgesic, euphoric, sedative, ventilatory depression, and emetic effects of opioids but not to their effects on miosis and bowel motility (constipation). The potential for physical dependence (addiction) is an agonist effect of opioids. Physical dependence on morphine usually requires about 25 days to develop but may occur sooner in emotionally unstable persons (Table 3-6).

Hormonal Changes

The main effects of opioids on the hypothalamic-pituitary-gonadal axis involve modulation of hormone release.

Immune Modulation

Prolonged exposure to opioids appears more likely than short-term exposure to produce immunosuppression, especially in susceptible persons. Abrupt withdrawal also may induce immunosuppression.

Overdose

The principal manifestation of opioid overdose is ventilatory depression, manifesting as a slow breathing frequency, which may progress to apnea. Pupils are symmetric and miotic unless severe arterial hypoxemia is present, which results in mydriasis. Upper airway obstruction may occur, and pulmonary edema is common. Hypotension and seizures develop if arterial hypoxemia persists. The triad of myosis, hypoventilation and coma should suggest overdose with an opioid. Treatment of opioid overdose is mechanical ventilation of the patient's lungs with oxygen and administration of an opioid antagonist such as naloxone (may precipitate acute withdrawal).

Morphine-6-Glucuronide

Morphine and morphine-6-glucuronide bind to μ opioid receptors with comparable affinity, whereas the analgesic potency of morphine-6-glucuronide is 650-fold higher than morphine.

Meperidine

Meperidine is a synthetic opioid agonist at μ and κ opioid receptors (Fig. 3-1). The analogs of meperidine include fentanyl, sufentanil, alfentanil, and remifentanil. Meperidine shares several structural features that are present in local anesthetics, including a tertiary amine, an ester group, and a lipophilic phenyl group. Structurally, meperidine is similar to atropine, and it possesses a mild atropine-like antispasmodic effect.

Pharmacokinetics

Meperidine is about one-tenth as potent as morphine, with an 80 to 100 mg intramuscular dose being equivalent to about 10 mg of intramuscular morphine. In equal analgesic doses, meperidine produces as much sedation, euphoria, nausea, vomiting, and depression of ventilation as does morphine. Unlike morphine, meperidine is well absorbed from the gastrointestinal tract.

Metabolism

The hepatic metabolism of meperidine is extensive, with about 90% of the drug initially undergoing demethylation to normeperidine and hydrolysis to meperidinic acid. Normeperidine is about one-half as active as meperidine

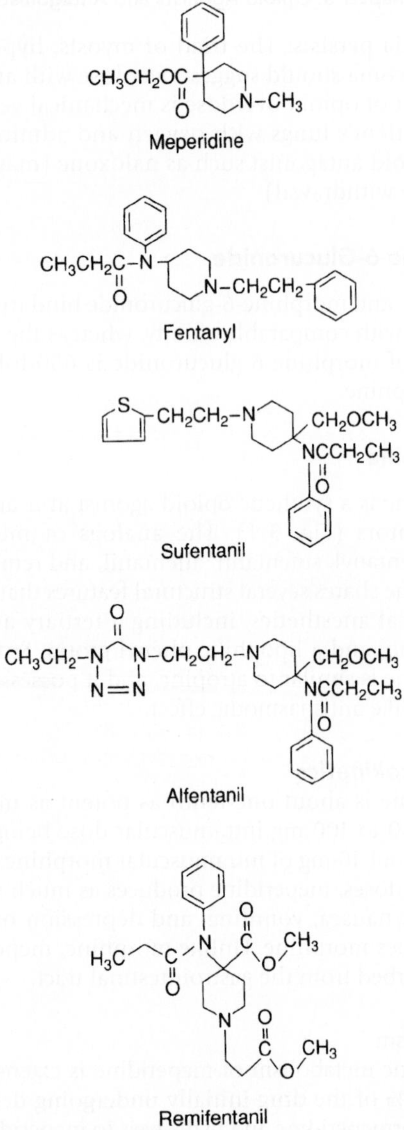

Meperidine

Fentanyl

Sufentanil

Alfentanil

Remifentanil

Figure 3-1. Synthetic opioid agonists.

as an analgesic but also produces CNS stimulation (myoclonus, seizures).

Elimination Half-Time (Table 3-5)

Clinical Uses

The principal use of meperidine is for analgesia during labor and delivery and after surgery. Meperidine may be effective in suppressing postoperative shivering that may result in detrimental increases in metabolic oxygen consumption. Unlike morphine, meperidine is not useful for the treatment of diarrhea and is not an effective antitussive. During bronchoscopy, the relative lack of meperidine's antitussive activity makes this opioid less useful.

Side Effects

The side effects of meperidine resemble those of morphine. Orthostatic hypotension suggests that meperidine, like morphine, interferes with compensatory sympathetic nervous system reflexes. Meperidine, in contrast to morphine, rarely causes bradycardia but instead may increase heart rate, thus reflecting its modest atropine-like qualities. Large doses of meperidine result in decreases in myocardial contractility, which, among opioids, is unique for this drug. Delirium and seizures, when they occur, presumably reflect an accumulation of normeperidine, which has stimulating effects on the CNS. Meperidine readily impairs ventilation and promptly crosses the placenta. Meperidine may produce less constipation and urinary retention than morphine. Meperidine does not cause miosis but rather tends to cause mydriasis, reflecting its modest atropine-like actions.

Fentanyl

Fentanyl is a phenyl piperidine-derivative synthetic opioid agonist that is structurally related to meperidine (see Fig. 3-1). As an analgesic, fentanyl is 75 to 125 times more potent than morphine.

Pharmacokinetics

A single dose of fentanyl administered intravenously has a more rapid onset and shorter duration of action than morphine. Despite the clinical impression that fentanyl produces a rapid onset, a distinct time lag occurs between the peak plasma fentanyl concentration and peak slowing on the EEG (the effect-site equilibration time between blood and the brain). When multiple intravenous doses of fentanyl are administered, or when there is continuous infusion of the drug, progressive saturation of inactive tissue sites occurs. As a result, the plasma concentration of fentanyl does not decrease rapidly, and the duration of analgesia, as well as depression of ventilation, may be prolonged.

Metabolism

Norfentanyl is structurally similar to normeperidine and is the principal metabolite of fentanyl in humans. Its pharmacologic activity is believed to be minimal.

Elimination Half-Time (Table 3-5)

Context-Sensitive Half-Time

As the duration of continuous infusion of fentanyl increases beyond about 2 hours, the context-sensitive half-time of this opioid becomes greater than that of sufentanil (Fig. 3-2). This reflects the saturation of inactive tissue sites with fentanyl during prolonged infusions and a return of the opioid from peripheral compartments to the plasma.

Cardiopulmonary Bypass

All opioids show a decrease in plasma concentration with the initiation of cardiopulmonary bypass.

Clinical Uses

Low doses of fentanyl, 1 to 2 μg/kg IV, are injected to provide analgesia. Fentanyl, 2 to 20 μg/kg IV, may be

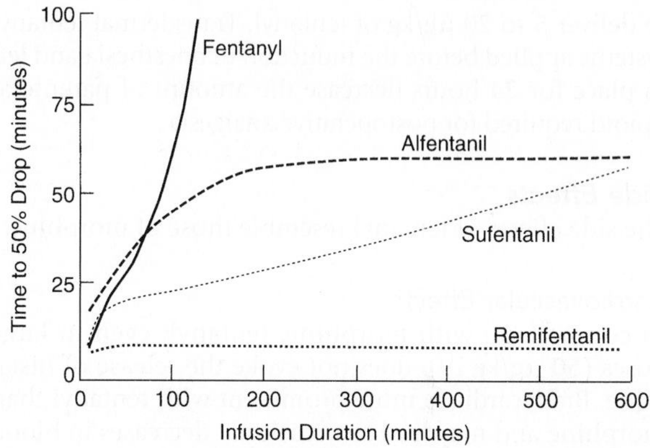

Figure 3-2. Computer simulation–derived context-sensitive half-times (time necessary for the plasma concentration to decrease 50% after discontinuation of the infusion) as a function of the duration of the intravenous infusion. [From Egan TD, Lemmens HJM, Fiset P, et al. The pharmacokinetics of the new short-acting opioid remifentanil (GI87084B) in healthy adult male volunteers. *Anesthesiology* 1993;79:881–892; with permission.]

administered as an adjuvant to inhaled anesthetics in an attempt to blunt circulatory responses to (a) direct laryngoscopy for intubation of the trachea, or (b) sudden changes in the level of surgical stimulation. Timing of the intravenous injection of fentanyl to prevent or treat such responses should consider the effect-site equilibration time, which for fentanyl is prolonged when compared with alfentanil and remifentanil. Large doses of fentanyl, 50 to 150 μg/kg IV, have been used alone to produce surgical anesthesia. These large doses of fentanyl as the sole anesthetic have the advantage of stable hemodynamics due principally to the (a) lack of direct myocardial depressant effects, (b) absence of histamine release, and (c) suppression of the stress responses to surgery. Fentanyl may be administered as a transmucosal preparation (oral transmucosal fentanyl) in a delivery device (lozenge mounted on a handle) designed to deliver 5 to 20 μg/kg of fentanyl. Transdermal fentanyl systems applied before the induction of anesthesia and left in place for 24 hours decrease the amount of parenteral opioid required for postoperative analgesia.

Side Effects

The side effects of fentanyl resemble those of morphine.

Cardiovascular Effects

In comparison with morphine, fentanyl, even in large doses (50 μg/kg IV), does not evoke the release of histamine. Bradycardia is more prominent with fentanyl than morphine and may lead to occasional decreases in blood pressure and cardiac output.

Seizure Activity

In the absence of EEG evidence of seizure activity, it is difficult to distinguish opioid-induced skeletal muscle rigidity or myoclonus from seizure activity.

Somatosensory Evoked Potentials and Electroencephalogram

Fentanyl, in doses exceeding 30 μg/kg IV, produces changes in somatosensory evoked potentials that, although detectable, do not interfere with the use and interpretation of this monitor during anesthesia.

Intracranial Pressure

The administration of fentanyl and sufentanil to head injury patients has been associated with modest increases (6 to 9 mm Hg) in ICP, despite the maintenance of an unchanged $PaCO_2$. These increases in ICP are typically accompanied by decreases in mean arterial pressure and cerebral perfusion pressure.

Drug Interactions

Analgesic concentrations of fentanyl greatly potentiate the effects of midazolam and decrease the dose requirements of propofol. The opioid-benzodiazepine combination displays marked synergism with respect to hypnosis and depression of ventilation.

Sufentanil

Sufentanil is a thienyl analog of fentanyl (see Fig. 3-1). The analgesic potency of sufentanil is five to ten times that of fentanyl, which parallels the greater affinity of sufentanil for opioid receptors, when compared with that of fentanyl.

Pharmacokinetics (see Table 3-5)

A high tissue affinity is consistent with the lipophilic nature of sufentanil, which permits a rapid penetration of the blood-brain barrier and onset of CNS effects. Its effect-site equilibration time of 6.2 minutes is similar to that of 6.8 minutes for fentanyl. A rapid redistribution to inactive tissue sites terminates the effect of small doses, but a cumulative drug effect can accompany large or repeated doses of sufentanil.

Metabolism

Sufentanil is rapidly metabolized by *N*-dealkylation to pharmacologically inactive products. Less than 1% of an administered dose of sufentanil appears unchanged in urine.

Context-Sensitive Half-Time

The context-sensitive half-time of sufentanil is less than that for alfentanil for continuous infusions of up to 8 hours in duration (see Fig. 3-2). This shorter context-sensitive half-time can be explained in part by the large Vd of sufentanil. After termination of a sufentanil infusion, the decrease in the plasma drug concentration is accelerated not only by metabolism but by a continued redistribution of sufentanil into peripheral tissue compartments.

Clinical Uses

A single dose of sufentanil, 0.1 to 0.4 μg/kg IV, produces a longer period of analgesia and less depression of ventilation than does a comparable dose of fentanyl (1 to 4 μg/kg IV). As observed with other opioids, sufentanil causes a decrease in cerebral metabolic oxygen requirements, and cerebral blood flow is also decreased or unchanged. Bradycardia produced by sufentanil may be sufficient to decrease cardiac output. As observed with fentanyl, delayed depression of ventilation has also been described after the administration of sufentanil. The use of large doses of opioids, including sufentanil or fentanyl, to produce the intravenous induction of anesthesia may result in rigidity of chest and abdominal musculature. This skeletal muscle rigidity makes ventilation of the patient's lungs with positive airway pressure difficult.

Alfentanil

Alfentanil is an analog of fentanyl that is less potent (one-fifth to one-tenth) and has one-third the duration of action of fentanyl (see Fig. 3-1). A unique advantage of alfentanil compared with fentanyl and sufentanil is the more rapid onset of action (rapid effect-site equilibration) after the intravenous administration of alfentanil. The effect-site equilibration time for alfentanil is 1.4 minutes, compared with 6.8 and 6.2 minutes for fentanyl and sufentanil, respectively.

Pharmacokinetics (see Table 3-5)

The rapid effect-site equilibration characteristic of alfentanil is a result of the low pK of this opioid, so that nearly 90% of the drug exists in the nonionized form at physiologic pH. The nonionized fraction readily crosses the blood-brain barrier. The rapid peak effect of alfentanil at the brain is useful when an opioid is required to blunt the response to a single, brief stimulus, such as tracheal intubation or the performance of a retrobulbar block.

Metabolism

Noralfentanil is the major metabolite recovered in urine, with <0.5% of an administered dose of alfentanil being excreted unchanged. The efficiency of hepatic metabolism is emphasized by a clearance of about 96% of alfentanil from the plasma within 60 minutes of its administration. Population variability in P-450 3A4 (CYP3A) activity is the most likely mechanistic explanation for the interindividual variability in alfentanil disposition.

Context-Sensitive Half-Time

The context-sensitive half-time of alfentanil is longer than that of sufentanil for infusions up to 8 hours in duration (see Fig. 3-2). The Vd of alfentanil equilibrates rapidly, and peripheral distribution of the drug away from the plasma is not a significant contributor to the decrease in its plasma concentration after discontinuation of the alfentanil infusion.

Clinical Uses

Alfentanil has a rapid onset and offset of intense analgesia, reflecting its very prompt effect-site equilibration. This characteristic of alfentanil is used to provide analgesia when the noxious stimulation is acute, but transient, as associated with laryngoscopy and tracheal intubation and the performance of a retrobulbar block. For example, the administration of alfentanil, 15 μg/kg IV, about 90 seconds before beginning direct laryngoscopy is effective in blunting the systemic blood pressure and heart rate response to tracheal intubation. Alfentanil, 150 to 300 μg/kg IV, administered rapidly, produces unconsciousness in about 45 seconds. After this induction, the maintenance of anesthesia can be provided with a continuous infusion of alfentanil, 25 to 150 μg/kg per hour, combined with an inhaled drug. Alfentanil increases biliary tract pressures similarly to fentanyl, but the duration of this increase is shorter than that produced by fentanyl.

Remifentanil

Remifentanil is a selective μ opioid agonist with an analgesic potency similar to that of fentanyl (15 to 20 times as potent as alfentanil) and a blood-brain equilibration (effect-site equilibration) time similar to that of alfentanil (see Table 3-5 and Fig. 3-1). Remifentanil is structurally unique because of its ester linkage, which renders it susceptible to hydrolysis to inactive metabolites by nonspecific plasma and tissue esterases (Fig. 3-3). This unique pathway of metabolism imparts to remifentanil (a) brevity of action, (b) precise and

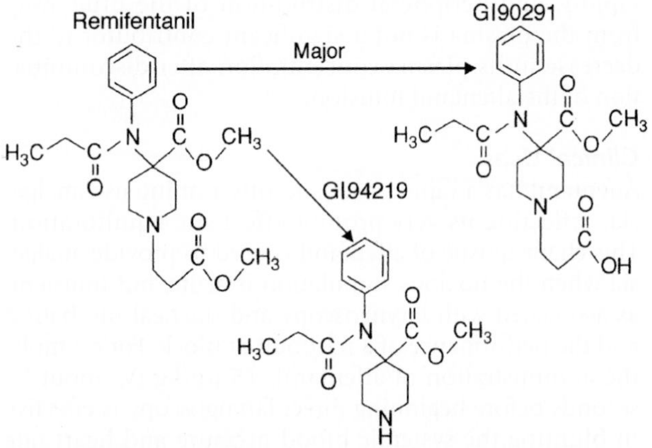

Remifentanil

Major

GI90291

GI94219

Figure 3-3. Remifentanil undergoes hydrolysis by nonspecific plasma and tissue esterases (major pathway) to a carboxylic acid metabolite (GI90291) that has no clinically significant agonist activity at opioid receptors. *N*-dealkylation of remifentanil to GI94219 is a minor pathway of metabolism. [From Egan TD, Lemmens HJM, Fiset P, et al. The pharmacokinetics of the new short-acting opioid remifentanil (GI87084B) in healthy adult male volunteers. *Anesthesiology* 1993;79:881–892; with permission.]

rapidly titratable effect due to its rapid onset (similar to that of alfentanil) and offset, (c) noncumulative effects, and (d) rapid recovery after discontinuation of its administration.

Ventilation

The combination of remifentanil and propofol is synergistic and may result in a severe depression of ventilation.

Pharmacokinetics (see Table 3-5)

The rapid metabolism of remifentanil and its small Vd mean that remifentanil will accumulate less than other opioids (predictable termination of drug effect). The combination of rapid clearance and small Vd produces a drug with a uniquely evanescent effect. The peak effect-site concentration of remifentanil will be present within 1.1 minutes, compared with 1.4 minutes for alfentanil. The effect, however, will be more transient after the administration of remifentanil than alfentanil.

Metabolism

Remifentanil is unique among the opioids in undergoing metabolism to inactive metabolites by nonspecific plasma and tissue esterases (see Fig. 3-3). Remifentanil does not appear to be a substrate for butyrylcholinesterases (pseudocholinesterase), and thus its clearance should not be affected by cholinesterase deficiency or anticholinergics. Esterase metabolism appears to be a very well-preserved metabolic system with little variability between individuals; this contributes to the predictability of drug effect associated with the infusion of remifentanil.

Elimination Half-Time

An estimated 99.8% of remifentanil is eliminated during the distribution (0.9 minute) and elimination (6.3 minutes) half-time.

Context-Sensitive Half-Time

The context-sensitive half-time for remifentanil is independent of the duration of infusion and is estimated to be about 4 minutes (see Fig. 3-2).

Clinical Uses

The clinical uses of remifentanil reflect the unique pharmacokinetic profile of this opioid, which allows rapid onset of drug effect, precise titration to the desired effect, the ability to maintain a sufficient plasma opioid concentration to suppress the stress response, and rapid recovery from the drug's effects. Anesthesia can be induced using remifentanil, 1 μg/kg IV administered over 60 to 90 seconds, or with a gradual initiation of the intravenous infusion at 0.5 to 1.0 μg/kg for about 10 minutes, before administration of a standard hypnotic before tracheal intubation. Before cessation of the remifentanil infusion, a longer-acting opioid may be administered to ensure analgesia when the patient awakens.

Side Effects

The advantage of remifentanil possessing a short recovery period may be considered a disadvantage if the infusion is stopped suddenly (it is important to administer a longer-acting opioid for postoperative analgesia). Histamine release does not accompany the administration of remifentanil. ICP and intraocular pressure are not changed by remifentanil. Placental passage of remifentanil is prompt, but neonatal effects do not occur.

Acute Opioid Tolerance

Postoperative analgesic requirements in patients receiving relatively large doses of remifentanil intraoperatively are often surprisingly high, thus suggesting that remifentanil may be associated with acute opioid tolerance (Fig. 3-4). Not all data support the development of acute opioid tolerance following remifentanil-based anesthesia.

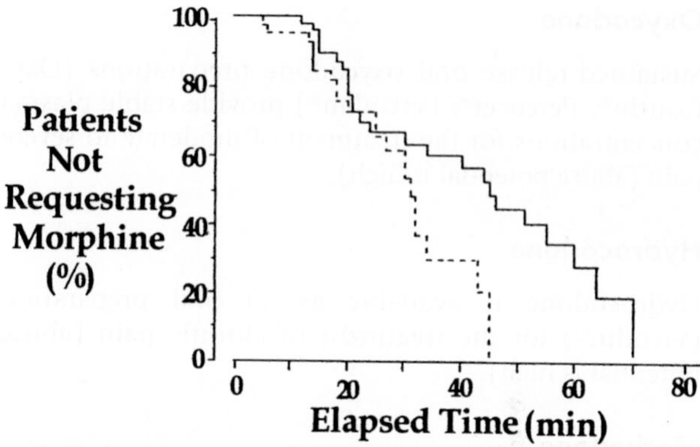

Figure 3-4. Cumulative curves for patients who did not request an additional morphine injection following discontinuation of remifentanil (dashed line) or desflurane (solid line). (From Guignard B, Bossard AE, Coste C, et al. Acute opioid tolerance. Intraoperative remifentanil increases postoperative pain and morphine requirement. *Anesthesiology* 2000;93:409–417; with permission.)

Codeine

Codeine is the result of the substitution of a methyl group for the hydroxyl group on carbon 3 of morphine. Codeine is an effective antitussive at oral doses of 15 mg. Maximal analgesia, equivalent to that produced by 650 mg of aspirin, occurs with 60 mg of codeine.

Hydromorphone

Hydromorphone is an effective alternative to morphine in the treatment of opioid-responsive moderate to severe pain.

Oxymorphone

Oxymorphone is about 10 times as potent as morphine and seems to cause more nausea and vomiting. Physical dependence liability is great.

Oxycodone

Sustained-release oral oxycodone preparations (OxyContin®; Percocet®; Percodan®) provide stable plasma concentrations for the treatment of moderate to severe pain (abuse potential is high).

Hydrocodone

Hydrocodone is available as an oral preparation (Vicodin®) for the treatment of chronic pain (abuse potential is high).

Methadone

Methadone is a synthetic opioid agonist that is highly effective by the oral route, thus making this an attractive drug for the suppression of withdrawal symptoms in physically dependent persons such as heroin addicts.

Opioid Withdrawal

Methadone can substitute for morphine in addicts at about one-fourth the dosage.

Treatment of Chronic Pain

Methadone has been proposed as an alternative to slow-release formulations for the treatment of chronic pain because of its low abuse potential. When methadone is administered more than once daily, as is common in the treatment of chronic pain syndromes, the drug may accumulate, resulting in high plasma concentrations and associated depression of ventilation.

Propoxyphene

Propoxyphene is structurally similar to methadone and binds to opioid receptors, as reflected by the antagonism of its pharmacologic effects by naloxone. The only clinical use of propoxyphene is in the treatment of mild to moderate pain that is not adequately relieved by aspirin.

Propoxyphene does not possess antipyretic or anti-inflammatory effects, and antitussive activity is not significant. Propoxyphene is about one-third as potent as codeine in depressing ventilation.

Tramadol

Tramadol is a centrally acting analgesic that has moderate affinity for μ receptors and weak κ and δ opioid receptor affinity but is 5 to 10 times less potent than morphine as an analgesic. The production of analgesia by tramadol with the absence of depression of ventilation and a low potential for the development of tolerance, dependence, and abuse may be a result of the complementary and synergistic antinociceptive interaction of its two enantiomers. Tramadol, 3 mg/kg administered orally, intramuscularly, or intravenously is effective for the treatment of moderate to severe pain.

Heroin

Heroin (diacetylmorphine) is a synthetic opioid produced by the acetylation of morphine. Heroin penetrates rapidly into the brain, where it is hydrolyzed to the active metabolites monoacetylmorphine and morphine. Compared with morphine, parenteral heroin has a (a) more rapid onset, (b) lack of a nauseating effect, and (c) greater potential for physical dependency.

OPIOID AGONIST-ANTAGONISTS

Opioid agonist-antagonists bind to μ receptors, where they produce limited responses (partial agonists) or no effect (competitive antagonists). The side effects are similar to those of opioid agonists, and, in addition, these drugs may cause dysphoric reactions. The advantages of opioid agonist-antagonists are the ability to produce analgesia with limited depression of ventilation and a low potential to produce physical dependence.

Pentazocine

Pentazocine possesses opioid agonist actions as well as weak antagonist actions. The agonist effects of pentazocine are antagonized by naloxone.

Pharmacokinetics

Pentazocine is well absorbed after oral or parenteral administration. The elimination half-time is 2 to 3 hours.

Clinical Uses

Pentazocine, 10 to 30 mg intravenous or 50 mg orally, is used most often for the relief of moderate pain. An oral dose of 50 mg is equivalent in analgesic potency to 60 mg of codeine.

Side Effects

The most common side effect of pentazocine is sedation. Dysphoria, including fear of impending death, is associated with high doses of pentazocine (limits physical dependence liability). Pentazocine crosses the placenta and may cause fetal depression. In contrast to morphine, miosis does not occur after the administration of pentazocine.

Butorphanol

Butorphanol is an agonist-antagonist opioid that resembles pentazocine.

Side Effects

The side effects of butorphanol include sedation, nausea, and diaphoresis. Dysphoria, reported frequently with other opioid agonist-antagonists, is infrequent after the administration of butorphanol. Depression of ventilation is similar to that produced by similar doses of morphine. The effects of opioid agonists are blunted by butorphanol (remember when considering the use of butorphanol or any other opioid-agonist for preoperative medication.)

Nalbuphine

Nalbuphine is an agonist-antagonist opioid that is equal in potency as an analgesic to morphine and is about one-fourth as potent as nalorphine as an antagonist. Sedation is the most common side effect, occurring in about one-third of patients treated with nalbuphine. The incidence of dysphoria is less than that with pentazocine or butorphanol.

Buprenorphine

Buprenorphine is an agonist-antagonist opioid, and its analgesic potency is great, with a 0.3-mg intramuscular dose being equivalent to 10 mg of morphine. Buprenorphine is effective in relieving moderate to severe pain, such as that present in the postoperative period and that associated with cancer, renal colic, and myocardial infarction.

Side Effects

The side effects of buprenorphine include drowsiness, nausea, vomiting, and depression of ventilation that are similar in magnitude to the side effects of morphine but may be prolonged and resistant to antagonism with naloxone. In contrast to other opioid agonist-antagonists, dysphoria is unlikely to occur in association with the administration of this drug. Because of its antagonist properties, buprenorphine can precipitate withdrawal in patients who are physically dependent on morphine.

Nalorphine

Nalorphine is equally as potent as morphine as an analgesic but is not clinically useful because of a high incidence of dysphoria.

Bremazocine

Bremazocine is twice as potent as morphine as an analgesic but, in animals, does not produce depression of ventilation or evidence of physical dependence.

Dezocine

Dezocine is an opioid agonist-antagonist comparable to morphine in analgesic potency, onset, and duration of action in the relief of postoperative pain. Like other opioid agonist-antagonists, dezocine exhibits a ceiling effect for depression of ventilation that parallels its analgesic activity.

Meptazinol

Meptazinol is a partial opioid agonist with relative selectivity at μ_1 receptors. As a result, depression of ventilation does not occur with analgesic doses of meptazinol. Physical dependence does not occur, miosis is slight, and constipation is absent. Nausea and vomiting are common side effects.

OPIOID ANTAGONISTS

Minor changes in the structure of an opioid agonist can convert the drug into an opioid antagonist at one or more of the opioid receptor sites (Fig. 3-5). The high affinity for the opioid receptors characteristic of pure opioid antagonists results in a displacement of the opioid agonist from μ receptors. After this displacement, the binding of the pure antagonist does not activate μ receptors and antagonism occurs.

Naloxone

Naloxone is a nonselective antagonist at all three opioid receptors. It is selective when used to (a) treat opioid-induced depression of ventilation, as may be present in the postoperative period, (b) treat opioid-induced depression of ventilation in the neonate due to maternal administration of an opioid, (c) facilitate treatment of deliberate opioid overdose, and (d) detect suspected physical dependence. Naloxone, 1 to 4 μg/kg IV, promptly reverses opioid-induced analgesia and depression of

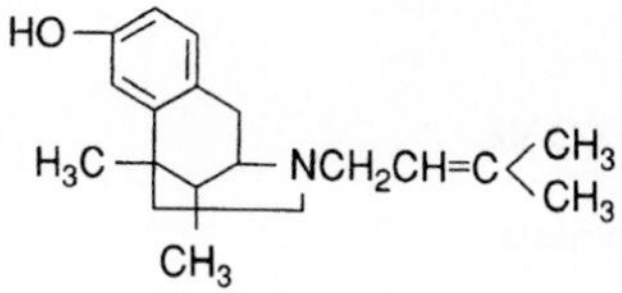

Pentazocine

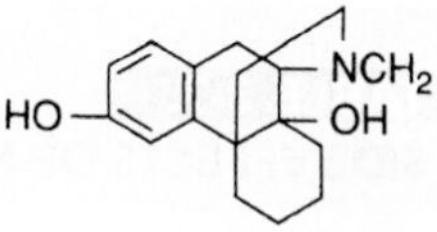

Butorphanol

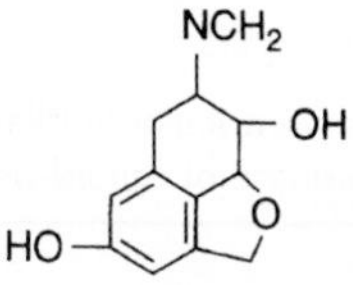

Nalbuphine

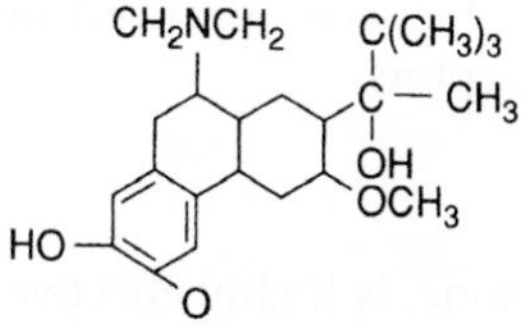

Buprenorphine

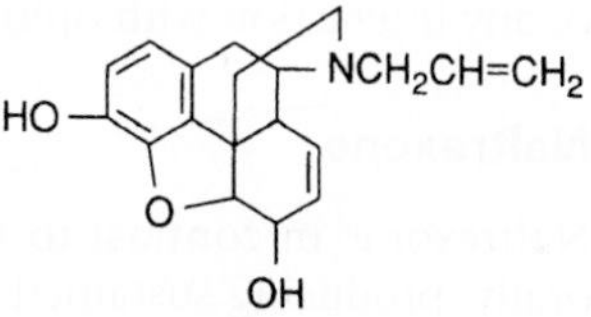

Nalorphine

Figure 3-5. Opioid antagonists.

ventilation. The short duration of action of naloxone (30 to 45 minutes) is presumed to be due to its rapid removal from the brain. This emphasizes that supplemental doses of naloxone will likely be necessary for sustained antagonism of opioid agonists. In this regard, a continuous infusion of naloxone, 5 μg/kg per hour, prevents depression of ventilation without altering the analgesia produced by neuraxial opioids.

Side Effects (Table 3-7)

Antagonism of General Anesthesia

The occasional observation that high doses of naloxone seem to antagonize the depressant effect of inhaled

TABLE 3-7.
SIDE EFFECTS OF NALOXONE

Reversal of opioid-induced analgesia
Nausea and vomiting
Cardiovascular stimulation
Tachycardia
Hypertension
Pulmonary edema
Cardiac dysrhythmias (ventricular fibrillation)
Opioid withdrawal in neonate of opioid-dependent parturients

anesthetics may represent a drug-induced activation of the cholinergic arousal system in the brain, independent of any interaction with opioid receptors.

Naltrexone

Naltrexone, in contrast to naloxone, is highly effective orally, producing sustained antagonism of the effects of opioid agonists for as long as 24 hours.

Nalmefene

Nalmefene is a pure opioid antagonist that is equipotent to naloxone. The primary advantage of nalmefene over naloxone is its longer duration of action, which might provide a greater degree of protection from delayed depression of ventilation due to residual effects of the opioid.

Methylnaltrexone

Methylnaltrexone is a quaternary opioid receptor antagonist. The highly ionized quaternary methyl group limits the transfer of methylnaltrexone across the blood-brain barrier. As a result, methylnaltrexone is active at peripheral rather than central opioid receptors. It attenuates morphine-induced changes in the rate of gastric emptying and also decreases the incidence of nausea whereas analgesia may remain intact.

ANESTHETIC REQUIREMENTS

The contribution of opioids to total anesthetic requirements can be quantitated by determining the decrease in MAC of a volatile anesthetic in the presence of opioids. Opioid agonist-antagonists are less effective than opioid agonists in decreasing MAC.

Barbiturates

4

The classification of barbiturates as long-, intermediate-, short-, and ultrashort-acting is not recommended, because it incorrectly suggests that the action of these drugs ends abruptly after specified time intervals (Stoelting RK, Hillier SC. Barbiturates. In: *Pharmacology and Physiology in Anesthetic Practice*, 4th ed. Philadelphia. Lippincott Williams & Wilkins, 2006:127–139).

COMMERCIAL PREPARATIONS

Barbiturates are prepared commercially as sodium salts that are readily soluble in water or saline from highly alkaline solutions (pH of a 2.5% solution of thiopental is 10.5). These highly alkaline solutions are incompatible for mixture with drugs such as opioids, catecholamines, and neuromuscular-blocking drugs, which are acidic in solution. Although the S(−) isomers of thiopental and thiamylal are twice as potent as the R(+) isomers, both drugs are commercially available only as racemic mixtures. Methohexital is also marketed as the racemic mixture of the S(−) and R(+) isomers, with the S(−) isomers being four to five times more potent than the R(+) isomers. Thiopental and thiamylal are usually prepared for clinical use in 2.5% solutions. Methohexital is used most often as a 1% solution.

STRUCTURE–ACTIVITY RELATIONSHIPS

Barbiturates are defined as any drug derived from barbituric acid. Barbituric acid, which lacks central nervous

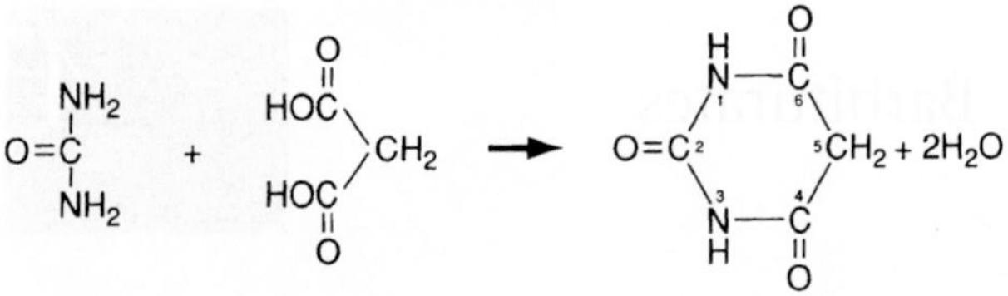

Figure 4-1. Barbituric acid is formed by the combination of urea and malonic acid.

system (CNS) activity, is a cyclic compound obtained by the combination of urea and malonic acid (Fig. 4-1). Barbiturates with sedative-hypnotic properties result from substitutions at the number 2 and 5 carbon atoms of barbituric acid (Fig. 4-2). Barbiturates that retain an oxygen atom on the number 2 carbon of the barbituric acid ring are designated as *oxybarbiturates*. Replacement of this oxygen atom with a sulfur atom results in *thiobarbiturates*, which are more lipid soluble than oxybarbiturates.

MECHANISM OF ACTION

Barbiturates most likely produce their sedative-hypnotic effects through an interaction with the inhibitory neurotransmitter γ-aminobutyric acid (GABA) in the CNS. When $GABA_A$ receptors are activated, transmembrane chloride conductance increases, resulting in hyperpolarization of the postsynaptic cell membranes and functional inhibition of postsynaptic neurons. The ability of barbiturates to uniquely depress the reticular activating system, which is presumed to be important in the maintenance of wakefulness, may reflect the ability of barbiturates to decrease the rate of dissociation of GABA from its receptors.

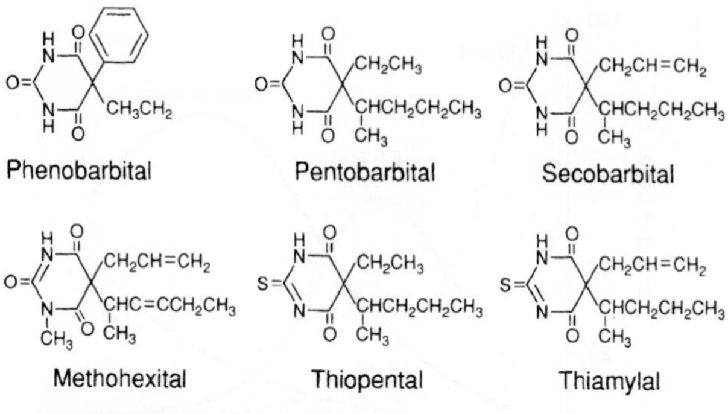

Phenobarbital

Pentobarbital

Secobarbital

Methohexital

Thiopental

Thiamylal

Figure 4-2. Barbiturates with sedative-hypnotic properties result from substitutions at the number 2 and 5 carbon atoms of barbituric acid (see Fig. 4-1).

PHARMACOKINETICS

Prompt awakening after a single intravenous dose of thiopental, thiamylal, or methohexital reflects the redistribution of these drugs from the brain to inactive tissues (Fig. 4-3). Ultimately, however, elimination from the body depends almost entirely on metabolism, because <1% of these drugs are recovered unchanged in urine. The time required for equilibration of the brain with the thiopental concentration in the blood (effect-site equilibration time) is rapid. Conversely, the time necessary for the plasma concentration of thiopental to decrease 50% after discontinuation of a prolonged infusion (context-sensitive half-time) is prolonged as the drug sequestered in fat and skeletal muscle reenters the circulation to maintain the plasma concentration (see Fig. 1-4).

Protein Binding

Protein binding of barbiturates parallels their lipid solubility (thiopental, as a highly lipid-soluble barbiturate, is avidly bound to plasma proteins). Decreased protein

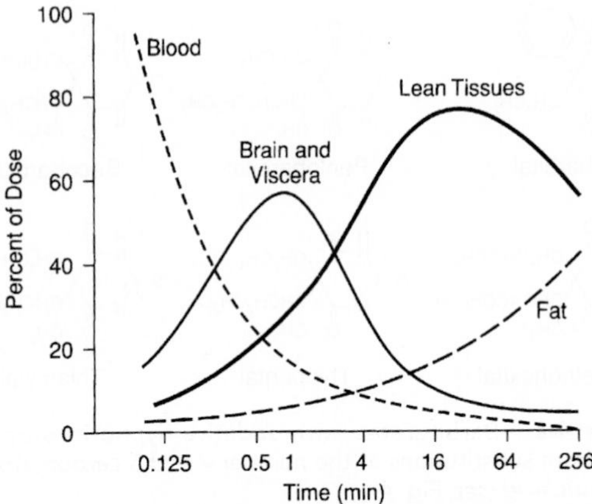

Figure 4-3. After a rapid intravenous injection, the percentage of thiopental remaining in the blood rapidly decreases as drug moves from the blood to tissues. Time to achievement of peak levels is a direct function of tissue capacity for barbiturate relative to blood flow. Initially, most thiopental is taken up by the vessel-rich group tissues because of their high blood flow. Subsequently, the drug is redistributed to skeletal muscles and, to a lesser extent, to fat. The rate of metabolism equals the early rate of removal by fat, and the sum of these two events is similar to the uptake of drug by skeletal muscles. (From Saidman LJ. Uptake, distribution, and elimination of barbiturates. In: Eger EI, ed. *Anesthetic Uptake and Action.* Baltimore: Williams & Wilkins, 1974; with permission.)

binding of thiopental may explain, in part, the increased drug sensitivity demonstrated by patients with uremia or cirrhosis of the liver. Decreased protein binding in patients with uremia may be partially due to competitive binding inhibitors, such as nitrogenous waste products. Hypoalbuminemia may account for decreased protein binding of barbiturates in patients with cirrhosis of the liver.

Distribution

Distribution of barbiturates in the body is determined by their lipid solubility (most important), protein binding, and degree of ionization.

Brain

Thiopental, thiamylal, and methohexital undergo maximal brain uptake within 30 seconds (rapid effect-site equilibration), thus accounting for the prompt onset of CNS depression (see Fig. 4-3). The brain receives about 10% of the total dose of thiopental in the first 30 to 40 seconds. This maximal brain concentration is followed by a decrease over the next 5 minutes to one-half the initial peak concentration, due to a redistribution of the drug from the brain to other tissues (redistribution is the principal mechanism accounting for early awakening after a single intravenous dose of these drugs).

Skeletal Muscles

Skeletal muscles are the most prominent sites for the initial redistribution of highly lipid-soluble barbiturates such as thiopental (see Fig. 4-3).

Fat

Fat is the only compartment in which thiopental content continues to increase 30 minutes after injection (see Fig. 4-3). Large or repeated doses of lipid-soluble barbiturates produce a cumulative effect because of the storage capacity of fat; thus, a dose of thiopental is best calculated according to lean body mass to avoid an overdose.

Cardiopulmonary Bypass

In the presence of an existing steady concentration of thiopental, the institution of cardiopulmonary bypass results in an abrupt 50% decrease in the plasma concentration, followed by a gradual increase to 70% of the prebypass concentration.

Ionization

Because the pK of thiopental (7.6) is near blood pH, acidosis will favor the nonionized fraction of drug, whereas alkalosis has the opposite effect. The nonionized form of drug has greater access to the CNS because of its higher lipid solubility. Acidosis will thus increase and alkalosis will decrease the intensity of the barbiturate effect.

Metabolism

Oxybarbiturates are metabolized only in hepatocytes, whereas thiobarbiturates also break down to a small extent in extrahepatic sites, such as the kidneys and possibly the CNS. Metabolites are usually inactive and are always more water soluble than the parent compound, which facilitates renal excretion.

Thiopental

Metabolism of thiopental occurs at a slow rate, with 10% to 24% being metabolized by the liver each hour. Ultimately, metabolism of thiopental is almost complete (99%).

Methohexital

Methohexital is metabolized more rapidly than thiopental, reflecting its lesser lipid solubility. Hepatic clearance of methohexital is three to four times that of thiopental. Despite this greater hepatic clearance, early awakening from a single intravenous dose of methohexital depends primarily on its redistribution to inactive tissue sites. Recovery from methohexital is predictably more rapid than that from thiopental when repeated doses of drug are administered, reflecting the greater role of metabolism in the clearance of methohexital from the plasma.

Renal Excretion

All barbiturates are filtered by the renal glomeruli, but the high degree of protein binding limits the magnitude of filtration, whereas high lipid solubility favors reabsorption of any filtered drug back into the circulation (<1% of administered thiopental, thiamylal, or methohexital is excreted unchanged in urine).

TABLE 4-1.
COMPARATIVE PHARMACOKINETICS

	Thiopental	Methohexital
Rapid distribution half-time (mins)	8.5	5.6
Slow distribution half-time (mins)	62.7	58.3
Elimination half-time (hrs)	11.6	3.9*
Clearance (ml/kg/min)	3.4	10.9
Volume of distribution (liters/kg)	2.5	2.2

*Significantly different from thiopental.

Elimination Half-Time (Table 4-1)

Elimination half-time of thiopental is prolonged in obese patients compared with nonobese patients, reflecting an increased volume of distribution (Vd) resulting from excess fat storage sites. Increasing age is associated with a slower passage of thiopental from the central compartment to peripheral compartments (approximately 30% slower in 80-year-old patients compared with young adults). Evidence that pharmacokinetics (intercompartmental clearance) are responsible for decreased thiopental dose requirements in elderly patients is the similar plasma concentration of thiopental in all adult-age patients required to suppress the electroencephalogram (EEG) to a similar degree.

CLINICAL USES

The principal clinical uses of barbiturates are for (a) induction of anesthesia and (b) treatment of increased intracranial pressure (ICP). The use of phenobarbital to treat hyperbilirubinemia and kernicterus reflects barbiturate-induced increases in hepatic glucuronyl transferase enzyme activity. Other clinical uses of barbiturates are declining in frequency because these drugs (a) lack specificity of effect in the CNS, (b) have a lower therapeutic index than do benzodiazepines, (c) result in tolerance more often than do benzodiazepines, (d) have a greater liability for abuse, and (e) have a high risk for drug interactions. Drowsiness may last for only a short time after a sedative-hypnotic dose of a barbiturate administered orally, but residual CNS effects, characterized as "hangover," may persist for several hours. Barbiturates have been replaced by benzodiazepines for preanesthetic medication. The rapid onset of action of barbiturates renders these drugs useful for the treatment of grand mal seizures, but, again, benzodiazepines are probably superior, providing a more specific site of action in the CNS.

Induction of Anesthesia

The supremacy of barbiturates for the intravenous induction of anesthesia remained virtually unchallenged from 1934, with the introduction of thiopental, until the approval of propofol for clinical use in 1989. Propofol, although more expensive than thiopental, has replaced barbiturates for induction of anesthesia in many patients, especially in those where rapid awakening is considered essential. The relative potency of barbiturates used for the intravenous induction of anesthesia, assuming that thiopental is 1, is thiamylal 1.1, and methohexital 2.5. The CNS is exquisitely sensitive to intravenous doses of these barbiturates, which produce minimal to no effects on skeletal, cardiac, or smooth muscles.

Treatment of Increased Intracranial Pressure

Barbiturates decrease ICP by decreasing cerebral blood volume through drug-induced cerebral vascular vasoconstriction and an associated decrease in cerebral blood flow. An isoelectric EEG confirms the presence of maximal barbiturate-induced depression of cerebral metabolic oxygen requirements by about 55%. Improved outcome after head trauma has not, however, been demonstrated in patients treated with barbiturates, despite the ability of these drugs to decrease and control ICP. A hazard of the high-dose barbiturate therapy used to lower ICP is hypotension, which can jeopardize the maintenance of an adequate cerebral perfusion pressure.

Cerebral Protection

The ability of barbiturate therapy to improve brain survival after global cerebral ischemia due to cardiac arrest is unlikely, because these drugs are effective only when the EEG remains active and metabolic suppression is possible. During cardiac arrest, the EEG becomes flat in 20 to 30 seconds, and barbiturates would not be expected to improve outcome. Patients at risk for incomplete cerebral ischemia who might benefit from prior production of an isoelectric EEG (metabolic suppression) with barbiturates include those undergoing cardiopulmonary bypass, those scheduled for carotid endarterectomy or thoracic aneurysm resection, and those managed with profound controlled hypotension.

SIDE EFFECTS

Cardiovascular System

The mild and transient decrease in systemic blood pressure that accompanies the induction of anesthesia with barbiturates is principally due to peripheral vasodilation, reflecting depression of the medullary vasomotor center and decreased sympathetic nervous system outflow from the CNS. The fact that blood pressure and cardiac output are minimally altered by the intravenous induction of anesthesia with barbiturates reflects the ability of carotid sinus–mediated baroreceptor reflex responses to offset the effects of peripheral vasodilation. Hypovolemic patients, who are less able to compensate for the peripheral vasodilating effects of barbiturates, are highly vulnerable to marked decreases in systemic blood pressure when these drugs are administered rapidly for the intravenous induction of anesthesia. Conceptually, the slow intravenous administration of thiopental should be more likely to permit compensatory reflex responses and thus minimize systemic blood pressure decreases, compared with rapid intravenous injection. This would be most important in the presence of hypovolemia. Nevertheless, rapid or slow intravenous administration of thiopental to normovolemic patients produces similar decreases in blood pressure and increases in heart rate.

Ventilation

Barbiturates administered intravenously for the induction of anesthesia produce dose-dependent depression of medullary and pontine ventilatory centers. The resumption of spontaneous ventilation after a single intravenous induction dose of barbiturate is characterized by slow frequency of breathing and decreased tidal volume. Laryngeal reflexes and the cough reflex are not depressed until large doses of barbiturates have been administered. Stimulation of the upper airway as by laryngoscopy, intubation of the trachea, or secretions in the presence of inadequate depression of laryngeal reflexes by barbiturate may result in laryngospasm or bronchospasm.

Electroencephalogram

A continuous infusion of thiopental, 4 mg/kg, produces an isoelectric EEG that is consistent with near-maximal decreases in cerebral metabolic oxygen requirements. Barbiturate-induced depression of cerebral metabolic oxygen requirements when the EEG is isoelectric is about 55%, reflecting a decrease in neuronal needs for oxygen. Hypothermia is the only reliable method for decreasing the basal cellular metabolic requirements for oxygen.

Somatosensory Evoked Responses

Doses of thiopental sufficient to produce an isoelectric EEG fail to render any component of these responses unobtainable (thiopental is an acceptable drug to administer when the ability to monitor somatosensory evoked potentials is desirable).

Liver

Thiopental, in the absence of other drugs, produces only modest decreases in hepatic blood flow. Induction doses of thiopental do not alter postoperative liver function tests.

Enzyme Induction

Barbiturates stimulate an increase in liver microsomal protein content (enzyme induction) after 2 to 7 days of sustained drug administration. Altered drug responses and drug interactions may reflect barbiturate-induced enzyme induction, resulting in accelerated metabolism of (a) other drugs, such as oral anticoagulants, phenytoin, and tricyclic antidepressants; or (b) endogenous substances, including corticosteroids, bile salts, and vitamin K. Barbiturates also stimulate the activity of a mitochondrial enzyme (in contrast to a microsomal enzyme) known as *D-aminolevulinic acid synthetase*. As a result, the production of heme is accelerated, and acute intermittent porphyria may be exacerbated in susceptible patients who receive barbiturates.

Kidneys

The renal effects of thiopental may include modest decreases in renal blood flow and glomerular filtration rate.

Placental Transfer

Barbiturates used for the intravenous induction of anesthesia readily cross the placenta, but fetal plasma concentrations of barbiturates are substantially less than those in maternal plasma. Clearance by the fetal liver and dilution by blood from the fetal viscera and extremities result in the fetal brain being exposed to lower barbiturate concentrations than those measured in the umbilical vein.

Tolerance and Physical Dependence

Acute tolerance to barbiturates occurs earlier than does barbiturate-induced induction of microsomal enzymes (required effective dose of barbiturate may be increased sixfold). As tolerance to barbiturate-induced sedation increases, the therapeutic index decreases. The severity of the barbiturate withdrawal syndrome relates to the degree of tolerance and the rate of elimination of the barbiturates. Slow elimination of the barbiturate allows time for the CNS to diminish its compensatory excitatory responses more nearly in phase with the diminution in barbiturate-induced depression of the CNS. Abrupt discontinuation of phenobarbital in patients being treated for epilepsy may result in status epilepticus.

Intraarterial Injection

The intraarterial injection of thiopental usually results in immediate, intense vasoconstriction and excruciating pain that radiates along the distribution of the artery. Vasoconstriction may obscure distal arterial pulses, and blanching of the extremity is followed by cyanosis. Gangrene and permanent nerve damage may occur.

Mechanism of Damage

The most likely mechanism of damage seems to be the precipitation of thiopental crystals in the arterial vessels, leading to an inflammatory response and arteritis, which, coupled with the microembolization that follows, eventually results in occlusion of the distal circulation.

Treatment

The treatment of an accidental intraarterial injection of a barbiturate includes immediate attempts to dilute the drug, prevention of arterial spasm, and general measures to sustain adequate blood flow. Dilution of the barbiturate is best accomplished by the injection of saline through the needle or catheter that still remains in the artery. At the same time, an injection of lidocaine, papaverine, or phenoxybenzamine may be administered to produce vasodilation. Sympathectomy of the upper extremity produced by a stellate ganglion block or brachial plexus block may relieve vasoconstriction.

Venous Thrombosis

Venous thrombosis occurring after the intravenous administration of a barbiturate for the induction of anesthesia presumably reflects deposition of barbiturate crystals in the vein.

Allergic Reactions

Allergic reactions associated with the intravenous administration of barbiturates for induction of anesthesia most likely represent anaphylaxis (antigen-antibody interaction).

Immunosuppression

The long-term administration of high doses of thiopental is associated with an increased incidence of nosocomial infections and associated mortality. Bone marrow suppression and leukopenia may accompany the long-term administration of thiopental to treat increased ICP. It is possible that thiopental could exert its permissive effect on nosocomial infections in part by inhibiting the function of immune cells.

Benzodiazepines

5

Benzodiazepines are drugs that exert, in slightly varying degrees, five principal pharmacologic effects: anxiolysis, sedation, anticonvulsant actions, spinal cord–mediated skeletal muscle relaxation, and anterograde (acquisition or encoding of new information) amnesia (Stoelting RK, Hillier SC. Benzodiazepines. In: *Pharmacology and Physiology in Anesthetic Practice,* 4th ed. Philadelphia. Lippincott Williams & Wilkins, 2006:140–154). The amnestic potency of benzodiazepines is greater than their sedative effects and results in a longer duration of amnesia than sedation. Stored information (retrograde amnesia) is not altered by benzodiazepines. Benzodiazepines do not produce adequate skeletal muscle relaxation for surgical procedures, nor does their use influence the dose requirements for neuromuscular-blocking drugs. Compared with barbiturates, benzodiazepines have less tendency to produce tolerance and addiction, less potential for abuse, a greater margin of safety after an overdose, and elicit fewer and less serious drug interactions. Unlike barbiturates, benzodiazepines do not induce hepatic microsomal enzymes. Benzodiazepines have replaced barbiturates for preoperative medication and the production of sedation during monitored anesthesia care (intravenous midazolam is likely to be used for continuous infusion). Unlike other drugs administered intravenously to produce central nervous system (CNS) effects, benzodiazepines, as a class of drugs, are unique in the availability of a specific pharmacologic antagonist, flumazenil.

STRUCTURE–ACTIVITY RELATIONSHIP

Structurally, benzodiazepines are similar and share many active metabolites. The term *benzodiazepine* refers to that portion of the chemical structure composed of a benzene ring fused to a seven-membered diazepine ring.

MECHANISM OF ACTION

Benzodiazepines appear to produce all their pharmacologic effects by facilitating the actions of γ-aminobutyric acid (GABA), the principal inhibitory neurotransmitter in the CNS (Fig. 5-1). Benzodiazepines do not activate $GABA_A$ receptors but rather enhance the affinity of the receptors for GABA. As a result of this drug-induced

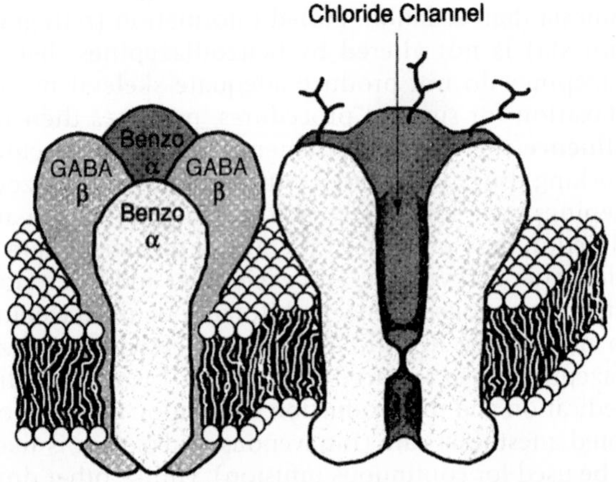

Figure 5-1. Model of the γ-aminobutyric acid (GABA) receptor forming a chloride channel. Benzodiazepines (Benzo) attach selectively to α-subunits and are presumed to facilitate the action of the inhibitory neurotransmitter GABA on α-subunits. (From Mohler H, Richards JG. The benzodiazepine receptor: a pharmacologic control element of brain function. *Eur J Anesthesiol Suppl* 1988;2:15–24; with permission.)

increased affinity of GABA receptors for the inhibitory neurotransmitter, an enhanced opening of chloride gating channels results in increased chloride conductance, thus producing hyperpolarization of the postsynaptic cell membrane and rendering postsynaptic neurons more resistant to excitation. The $GABA_A$ receptor is a large macromolecule that contains physically separate binding sites (principally α, β, and γ subunits) not only for GABA and the benzodiazepines but also for barbiturates, etomidate, propofol, neurosteroids, and alcohol. Acting on a single receptor through different mechanisms, benzodiazepines, barbiturates, and alcohol can produce synergistic effects to increase $GABA_A$ receptor–mediated inhibition in the CNS. This property explains the pharmacologic synergy of these substances and, likewise, the risks of combined overdose, which can produce life-threatening CNS depression. Benzodiazepines have a built-in ceiling effect that prevents them from exceeding the physiologic maximum of GABA inhibition. Differences in the onset and duration of action among commonly administered benzodiazepines reflect differences in potency (receptor binding affinity), lipid solubility (ability to cross the blood-brain barrier and redistribute to peripheral tissues), and pharmacokinetics (uptake, distribution, metabolism, and elimination).

Nucleoside Transporter Systems

Benzodiazepines decrease adenosine degradation by inhibiting the nucleoside transporter. Adenosine is an important regulator of cardiac function; it reduces cardiac oxygen demand by slowing heart rate, and it increases oxygen delivery by causing coronary vasodilation. Its physiologic effects convey cardioprotection during myocardial ischemia.

Electroencephalogram

The effects of benzodiazepines that appear on the electroencephalogram (EEG) resemble those of barbiturates in that α-activity is decreased and low-voltage, rapid β-activity is increased. Midazolam, in contrast to barbiturates and propofol, is unable to produce an isoelectric EEG.

SIDE EFFECTS (TABLE 5-1)

MIDAZOLAM

Midazolam is a water-soluble benzodiazepine with an imidazole ring in its structure that accounts for its stability in aqueous solutions and its rapid metabolism. Compared with diazepam, midazolam is two to three times as potent. As with other benzodiazepines, the amnestic effects of midazolam are more potent than its sedative effects. Thus,

TABLE 5-1.
SIDE EFFECTS OF BENZODIAZEPINES

- Fatigue
- Drowsiness
- Decreased motor coordination
- Impairment of cognitive function
- Anterograde amnesia (accentuated by concomitant ingestion of alcohol)
- Drug interactions
  - Synergistic effects with other CNS depressants
  - Decreased anesthetic requirements
  - Potentiation of ventilatory depressant effects of opioids
  - Reduced analgesic effects of opioids
  - Suppression of the hypothalamic-pituitary adrenal axis
  - Dependence (misleading to consider dependence as evidence of addiction in the absence of inappropriate drug-seeking behavior; withdrawal symptoms [irritability, insomnia, tremulousness] have a time of onset that reflects the elimination half-time of the drug being discontinued)
  - Inhibit platelet aggregation

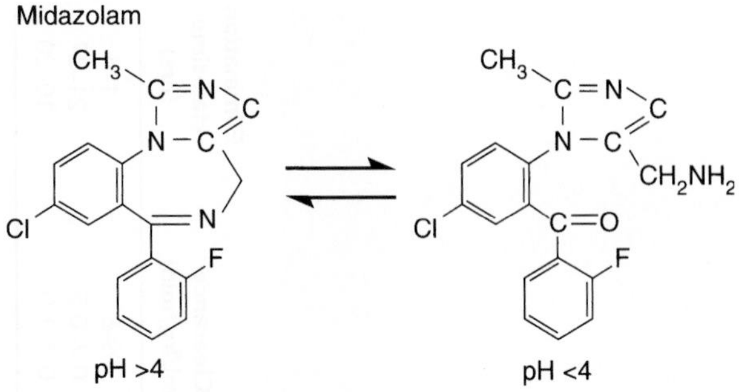

Midazolam

pH >4

pH <4

Figure 5-2. Reversible ring opening of midazolam above and below a pH of 4. The ring closes at a pH >4, converting midazolam from a water-soluble to a lipid-soluble drug.

patients may be awake following the administration of midazolam but remain amnestic for events and conversations (postoperative instructions) for several hours.

Commercial Preparation

Midazolam is characterized by a pH-dependent ring-opening phenomenon in which the ring remains open at pH values of <4, thus maintaining the water solubility of the drug (Fig. 5-2). The ring closes at pH values of >4, as when the drug is exposed to physiologic pH, thus converting midazolam to a highly lipid-soluble drug (see Fig. 5-2). The water solubility of midazolam obviates the need for a solubilizing preparation, such as propylene glycol, which can produce venoirritation. Midazolam is compatible with lactated Ringer's solution and can be mixed with the acidic salts of other drugs, including opioids and anticholinergics.

Pharmacokinetics (Table 5-2)

Midazolam undergoes rapid absorption from the gastrointestinal tract and achieves prompt passage across

TABLE 5-2.

COMPARATIVE PHARMACOLOGY OF BENZODIAZEPINES

	Equivalent Dose (mg)	Volume of Distribution (liters/kg)	Protein Binding (%)	Clearance (ml/kg/min)	Elimination Half-time (hrs)
Midazolam	0.15–0.3	1.0–1.5	96–98	6–8	1–4
Diazepam	0.3–0.5	1.0–1.5	96–98	0.2–0.5	21–37
Lorazepam	0.05	0.8–1.3	96–98	0.7–1.0	10–20

the blood-brain barrier. Despite this prompt passage into the brain, midazolam is considered to have a slow effect-site equilibration time (0.9 to 5.6 minutes) compared with other drugs such as propofol and thiopental. In this regard, intravenous doses of midazolam should be sufficiently spaced to permit the peak clinical effect to be appreciated before a repeat dose is considered.

Metabolism

Midazolam is rapidly metabolized by hepatic and small intestine cytochrome P-450 (CYP3A4) enzymes to active (1-hydroxymidazolam may accumulate in critically ill patients) and inactive metabolites (Fig. 5-3). The metabolism of midazolam is slowed in the presence of drugs that inhibit cytochrome P-450 enzymes (cimetidine, erythromycin, calcium channel blockers, antifungal drugs) and may result in unexpected CNS depression.

Renal Clearance

The elimination half-time, volume of distribution (Vd), and clearance of midazolam are not altered by renal failure.

Effects on Organ Systems

Central Nervous System

Midazolam, like other benzodiazepines, produces decreases in cerebral metabolic oxygen requirements ($CMRO_2$) and cerebral blood flow analogous to barbiturates and propofol. In contrast to these drugs, however, midazolam is unable to produce an isoelectric EEG, emphasizing that a ceiling effect exists with respect to the decrease in $CMRO_2$ produced by increasing doses of midazolam. Patients with decreased intracranial compliance show little or no change in intracranial pressure (ICP) when given midazolam as an alternative to barbiturates for the induction of anesthesia in patients with intracranial pathology. Similar to thiopental induction of anesthesia with midazolam does not prevent increases in ICP associated with direct laryngoscopy for tracheal

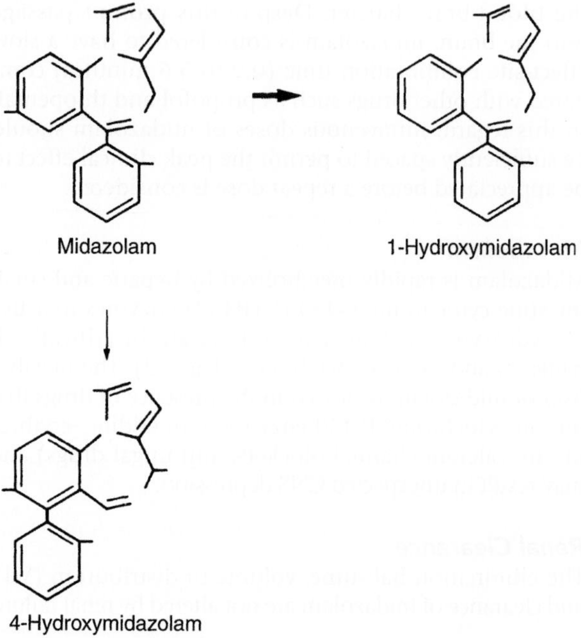

Midazolam

1-Hydroxymidazolam

4-Hydroxymidazolam

Figure 5-3. The principal metabolite of midazolam is 1-hydroxymidazolam. A lesser amount of midazolam is metabolized to 4-hydroxymidazolam. (From Reves JG, Fragen RJ, Vinik HR, et al. Midazolam: pharmacology and uses. *Anesthesiology* 1985;62: 310–324; with permission.)

intubation. Although midazolam may improve neurologic outcome after incomplete ischemia, benzodiazepines have not been shown to possess neuroprotective activity in humans. Midazolam is a potent anticonvulsant effective in the treatment of status epilepticus.

Ventilation

Patients with chronic obstructive pulmonary disease experience a greater midazolam-induced depression of ventilation. Transient apnea may occur after the rapid injection of large doses of midazolam, especially in the presence of preoperative medication that includes an opioid. Benzodiazepines also depress the swallowing reflex and decrease upper airway activity.

Cardiovascular System

In the presence of hypovolemia, the administration of midazolam results in enhanced blood pressure–lowering effects similar to those produced by other intravenous-induction drugs. Midazolam does not prevent the blood pressure and heart rate responses evoked by intubation of the trachea.

Clinical Uses

Preoperative Medication

Midazolam is the most commonly used oral preoperative medication for children; oral midazolam syrup (2 mg/mL) is effective for producing sedation and anxiolysis at a dose of 0.25 mg/kg with minimal effects on ventilation and oxygen saturation.

Intravenous Sedation

Midazolam in doses of 1.0 to 2.5 mg IV (onset within 30 to 60 seconds, time to peak effect 3 to 5 minutes, duration of sedation 15 to 80 minutes) is effective for sedation during regional anesthesia, as well as for brief therapeutic procedures. The effect-site equilibrium time for midazolam must be considered in recognizing the likely time of peak clinical effect and the need for supplemental doses of midazolam. Midazolam-induced depression of ventilation is exaggerated (synergistic effects) in the presence of opioids and other CNS depressant drugs. It is important to appreciate that increasing age greatly increases the pharmacodynamic sensitivity to the hypnotic effects of midazolam.

Induction of Anesthesia

Anesthesia can be induced by administration of midazolam, 0.1 to 0.2 mg/kg IV, over 30 to 60 seconds (thiopental usually produces induction of anesthesia 50% to 100% faster than midazolam). Onset of unconsciousness (synergistic interaction) is facilitated when a small dose of opioid (fentanyl, 50 to 100 μg IV or its equivalent) precedes the injection of midazolam by 1 to 3 minutes. In healthy patients receiving small doses of benzodiazepines, the cardiovascular depression associated with these drugs is minimal. When significant cardiovascular responses occur, it is most likely a reflection of benzodiazepine-induced peripheral vasodilation. As with depression of ventilation, cardiovascular changes produced by benzodiazepines may be exaggerated in the presence of other CNS depressant drugs, such as propofol and thiopental.

Maintenance of Anesthesia

Midazolam may be administered to supplement opioids, propofol, and/or inhaled anesthetics during maintenance of anesthesia. Anesthetic requirements for volatile anesthetics are decreased in a dose-dependent manner by midazolam.

Postoperative Sedation

The long-term intravenous administration of midazolam (loading dose 0.5 to 4 mg and maintenance dose 1 to 7 mg/hr) to produce sedation in intubated patients results in the relative saturation of peripheral tissues with midazolam, and clearance from the systemic circulation becomes less dependent on redistribution into peripheral tissues and more dependent on hepatic metabolism. Emergence time from midazolam is increased in elderly patients, obese patients, and in the presence of severe liver disease.

Paradoxical Vocal Cord Motion

Midazolam (0.5 to 1 mg IV) may be an effective treatment for the paradoxical vocal cord motion that may manifest postoperatively.

DIAZEPAM

Commercial Preparation

Diazepam is dissolved in organic solvents (propylene glycol, sodium benzoate) because it is insoluble in water. Dilution with water or saline causes cloudiness but does not alter the potency of the drug. Injection by either the intramuscular or intravenous route may be painful.

Pharmacokinetics

Diazepam has a rapid uptake into the brain, followed by redistribution to inactive tissue sites, especially fat, because this benzodiazepine is highly lipid soluble. The Vd of diazepam is large, reflecting extensive tissue uptake of this lipid-soluble drug (women with a greater body fat content are likely to have a larger Vd for diazepam than men). Diazepam rapidly crosses the placenta, achieving fetal concentrations equal to and sometimes greater than those present in the maternal circulation.

Protein Binding (see Table 5-2)

Protein binding of benzodiazepines parallels their lipid solubility. Cirrhosis of the liver or renal insufficiency with associated decreases in plasma concentrations of albumin may manifest as decreased protein binding of diazepam and an increased incidence of drug-related side effects. The high degree of protein binding limits the efficacy of hemodialysis in the treatment of diazepam overdose.

Metabolism

Diazepam is principally metabolized by hepatic microsomal enzymes using an oxidative pathway of *N*-demethylation. The two principal metabolites of diazepam are desmethyldiazepam and oxazepam, with a lesser amount metabolized to temazepam. Desmethyldiazepam is metabolized more slowly than oxazepam and is only slightly less potent than diazepam. Therefore, it is likely that this metabolite contributes to the return of drowsiness that manifests 6 to 8 hours after the administration of diazepam, as well as to the sustained effects usually attributed to the parent drug.

Cimetidine

Cimetidine inhibits P-450 hepatic microsomal enzymes and thus prolongs the elimination half-time of both diazepam and desmethyldiazepam.

Elimination Half-Time (see Table 5-2)

Cirrhosis of the liver is accompanied by up to fivefold increases in the elimination half-time of diazepam. Likewise, the elimination half-time of diazepam increases progressively with increasing age, which is consistent with the increased sensitivity of these patients to the drug's sedative effects. Desmethyldiazepam, the principal metabolite of diazepam, has an elimination half-time of 48 to 96 hours. As such, the elimination half-time of the metabolite may exceed that of the parent drug. This pharmacologically active metabolite can accumulate in plasma and tissues during the chronic use of diazepam. Prolonged somnolence associated with high doses of diazepam is likely to be caused by the sequestration of the parent drug and its active metabolite, desmethyldiazepam, in tissues, presumably fat, for subsequent release back into the circulation.

Effects on Organ Systems

Diazepam, like other benzodiazepines, produces minimal effects on ventilation and the systemic circulation. Diazepam does not increase the incidence of nausea and vomiting.

Ventilation

Diazepam produces minimal depressant effects on ventilation, with detectable increases in $PaCO_2$ not occurring until an intravenous dose of 0.2 mg/kg is administered. The combination of diazepam with other CNS depressants (opioids, alcohol) or the administration of this drug to patients with chronic obstructive airway disease may result in exaggerated or prolonged depression of ventilation. The ventilatory depressant effects of benzodiazepines are reversed by surgical stimulation but not by naloxone.

Cardiovascular System

Diazepam administered in doses of 0.5 to 1 mg/kg IV for the induction of anesthesia typically produces minimal decreases in systemic blood pressure, cardiac output, and systemic vascular resistance that are similar in magnitude to those observed during natural sleep (10% to 20% decreases). Diazepam appears to have no direct action on the sympathetic nervous system, and it does not cause orthostatic hypotension.

Skeletal Muscle

Skeletal muscle–relaxant effects of diazepam reflect its actions on spinal internuncial neurons and not actions at the neuromuscular junction (presumably diazepam diminishes the tonic facilitatory influence on spinal γ-neurons).

Overdose

Despite massive overdoses of diazepam, serious sequelae (coma) are unlikely to occur if cardiac and pulmonary function are supported and other drugs, such as alcohol, are not present.

Clinical Uses

Diazepam is the benzodiazepine most likely to be selected for the management of delirium tremens and the treatment of local anesthetic–induced seizures. Midazolam has largely replaced diazepam for intravenous sedation and the preoperative medication of children.

Anticonvulsant Activity

Diazepam, 0.1 mg/kg IV, is effective in abolishing seizure activity produced by lidocaine, delirium tremens, and status epilepticus. The efficacy of diazepam as an anticonvulsant may reflect its ability to facilitate the actions of the inhibitory neurotransmitter GABA. In contrast to barbiturates, which inhibit seizures through the nonselective depression of the CNS, diazepam selectively inhibits activity in the limbic system, particularly the hippocampus. If diazepam is administered to terminate seizures, a longer-acting antiepileptic drug, such as fosphenytoin, is also administered.

LORAZEPAM

Lorazepam is a more potent sedative and amnesic than midazolam and diazepam, whereas its effects on ventilation, the cardiovascular system, and skeletal muscles resemble those of other benzodiazepines.

Pharmacokinetics (see Table 5-2)

Lorazepam is conjugated with glucuronic acid in the liver to form pharmacologically inactive metabolites that are excreted by the kidneys. This contrasts with the formation of pharmacologically active metabolites after the administration of midazolam and diazepam. The metabolism of lorazepam is less likely than that of diazepam to be influenced by alterations in hepatic function, increasing age, or drugs that inhibit P-450 enzymes, such as cimetidine. Lorazepam has a slower onset of action than midazolam or diazepam because of its lower lipid solubility and slower entrance into the CNS.

Clinical Uses

The recommended oral dose of lorazepam for preoperative medication is 50 μg/kg, not to exceed 4 mg (produces maximal anterograde amnesia lasting up to 6 hours occurs). The prolonged duration of action of lorazepam limits its usefulness for preoperative medication when rapid awakening at the end of surgery is desirable. A slow onset limits the usefulness of lorazepam for (a) the intravenous induction of anesthesia, (b) intravenous sedation during regional anesthesia, or (c) use as an anticonvulsant.

OXAZEPAM

Oxazepam is a commercially available, pharmacologically active metabolite of diazepam. Its duration is slightly shorter than that of diazepam, because oxazepam is converted to pharmacologically inactive metabolites by conjugation with glucuronic acid. The oral absorption of oxazepam is relatively slow. As a result, this drug may not be useful for the treatment of insomnia characterized by difficulty falling asleep. Conversely, oxazepam may be used for treatment of insomnia characterized by nightly awakenings or shortened total sleep time.

ALPRAZOLAM

Alprazolam has significant anxiety-reducing effects in patients with primary anxiety and panic attacks.

CLONAZEPAM

Clonazepam is particularly effective in the control and prevention of seizures, especially myoclonic and infantile spasms.

FLURAZEPAM

Flurazepam is chemically and pharmacologically similar to other benzodiazepines but is used exclusively to treat insomnia. The principal metabolite of flurazepam is desalkylflurazepam. This metabolite is pharmacologically active and has a prolonged elimination half-time that may manifest as daytime sedation (hangover).

TEMAZEPAM

Temazepam is administered exclusively for the treatment of insomnia. Despite the relatively long elimination half-time, temazepam, as used to treat insomnia, is unlikely to be accompanied by residual drowsiness the following morning.

TRIAZOLAM

Triazolam is an orally absorbed benzodiazepine that is effective in the treatment of insomnia. The two principal metabolites of triazolam have little if any hypnotic activity, and their elimination half-time is <4 hours. For these reasons, residual daytime effects or cumulative sedation effects with repeated doses of triazolam seem less likely than with other benzodiazepines. Rebound insomnia may occur when this drug is discontinued. Marked anterograde amnesia has developed when this drug has been self-administered in attempts to facilitate sleep when traveling through several time zones. In otherwise healthy elderly patients, triazolam causes a greater degree of sedation or psychomotor impairment than in young persons.

FLUMAZENIL

Flumazenil is a specific and exclusive benzodiazepine antagonist with a high affinity for benzodiazepine receptors, where it exerts minimal agonist activity. As a competitive antagonist, flumazenil prevents or reverses, in a dose-dependent manner, all the agonist effects of benzodiazepines. The metabolism of flumazenil is through hepatic microsomal enzymes to inactive metabolites.

Dose and Administration

The recommended initial intravenous dose of flumazenil is 0.2 mg (8 to 15 μg/kg), which typically reverses the CNS effects of benzodiazepine agonists within about 2 minutes. If required, further doses of 0.1 mg (to a total of 1 mg IV) may be administered at 60-second intervals. The duration of action of flumazenil is 30 to 60 minutes, and supplemental doses of the antagonist may be needed to maintain the desired level of consciousness. An alternative to repeated doses of flumazenil to maintain wakefulness is a continuous low-dose infusion of flumazenil, 0.1 to 0.4 mg/hour. Administration of flumazenil to patients being treated with antiepileptic drugs for control of seizure activity is not recommended, because it could precipitate acute withdrawal seizures.

Side Effects

Flumazenil-induced antagonism of excess benzodiazepine agonist effects is not followed by acute anxiety, hypertension, tachycardia, or neuroendocrine evidence of a stress response in postoperative patients.

SHORT-ACTING HYPNOSEDATIVES

Short-acting hypnosedatives, such as zaleplon, zolpidem, and zopiclone, seem to have more selectivity for certain subunits of GABA receptors. This results in a clinical profile for the treatment of sleeping disorders that is more efficacious and has fewer side effects than occur with conventional benzodiazepines. *Zaleplon* (10 mg orally) has a rapid elimination and is utilized for patients who experience delayed onset of sleep. By comparison, *zolpidem* (10 mg orally) and *zopiclone* (7.5 mg orally) have a more delayed elimination, so there may be a prolonged drug effect (useful for the sustained treatment of insomnia with less waking during the night).

Nonbarbiturate Intravenous Anesthetic Drugs

6

PROPOFOL

Propofol is a substituted isopropyl phenol (2,6-diisopropylphenol) that is chemically distinct from all other drugs that act as intravenous sedative-hypnotics (Fig. 6-1) (Stoelting RK, Hillier, SC. Nonbarbiturate intravenous anesthetic drugs. In: *Pharmacology and Physiology in Anesthetic Practice,* 4th ed. Philadelphia. Lippincott Williams & Wilkins, 2006:155–178). The intravenous administration of propofol, 1.5 to 2.5 mg/kg (equivalent to thiopental, 4 to 5 mg/kg IV, or methohexital, 1.5 mg/kg IV) as a rapid injection (<15 s), produces unconsciousness within about 30 s. Awakening is more rapid and complete than that after induction of anesthesia with all other drugs used for the rapid intravenous induction of anesthesia—one of the most important advantages of propofol compared with alternative drugs administered for the same purpose.

Commercial Preparations

Propofol is an insoluble drug that requires a lipid vehicle for emulsification. The emulsifying agent is composed of long-chain triglycerides that support bacterial growth and cause increased plasma triglyceride concentrations, especially when prolonged intravenous infusions are utilized.

$$\text{2,6-}(CH(CH_3)_2)_2C_6H_3OH$$

Figure 6-1. Propofol.

Diprivan® utilizes the preservative disodium edetate (0.005%) and requires sodium hydroxide to adjust the pH level to 7 to 8.5. A generic formulation of propofol incorporates sodium metabisulfite (0.25 mg/ml) as the preservative and has a lower pH level (4.5 to 6.4). Propofol, unlike thiopental, etomidate, and ketamine, is not a chiral compound.

Mechanism of Action

Propofol is a relatively selective modulator of γ-aminobutyric acid ($GABA_A$) receptors and does not appear to modulate other ligand gated ion channels at clinically relevant concentrations. When $GABA_A$ receptors are activated, transmembrane chloride conductance increases, resulting in hyperpolarization of the postsynaptic cell membrane and functional inhibition of the postsynaptic neuron.

Pharmacokinetics

The clearance of propofol from the plasma exceeds hepatic blood flow, thus emphasizing that tissue uptake occurs (possibly into the lungs), as well as hepatic metabolism (Table 6-1; Fig 6-2). Although the glucuronide and sulfate conjugates of propofol appear to be pharmacologically inactive, 4-hydroxypropofol has about one-third the hypnotic activity of propofol. The context-sensitive half-time of propofol is minimally influenced by the duration of the infusion because of rapid metabolic clearance when the infusion is discontinued, so that drug that returns from tissue storage sites to the circulation is not available to retard the decrease in plasma concentrations

TABLE 6-1.

COMPARATIVE CHARACTERISTICS OF NONBARBITURATE INDUCTION DRUGS

	Elimination Half-time (hrs)	Volume of Distribution (liters/kg)	Clearance (ml/kg/min)	Systemic Blood	Heart Rate
Propofol	0.5–1.5	3.5–4.5	30–60	Decreased	Decreased
Etomidate	2–5	2.2–4.5	10–20	No change	No change to decreased
Ketamine	2–3	2.5–3.5	16–18	Increased	Increased

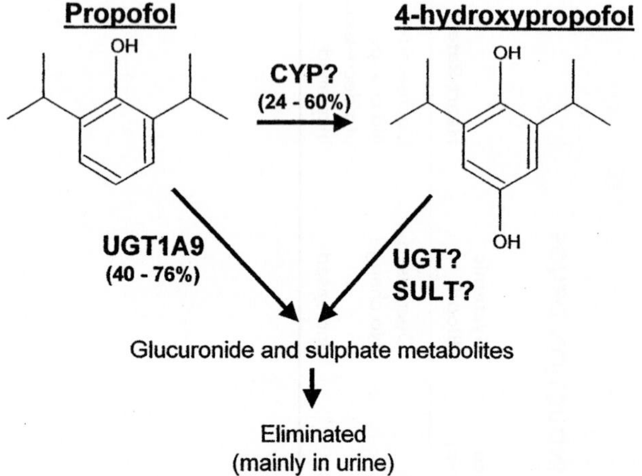

Figure 6-2. Major metabolic pathways for propofol. (From Court MH, Duan SX, Hesse LM, et al. Cytochrome P-450 2B6 is responsible for interindividual variability of propofol hydroxylation by human liver microsomes. *Anesthesiology* 2001;94:110–119; with permission.)

of the drug. Propofol, like thiopental and alfentanil, has a short effect-site equilibration time, so that effects on the brain occur promptly after intravenous administration. Despite the rapid clearance of propofol through metabolism, no evidence suggests impaired elimination in patients with cirrhosis of the liver. Renal dysfunction does not influence the clearance of propofol, despite the observation that nearly three-fourths of propofol metabolites are eliminated in urine in the first 24 hours. Propofol readily crosses the placenta but is rapidly cleared from the neonatal circulation.

Clinical Uses

Propofol has become the induction drug of choice for many forms of anesthesia, especially when rapid and complete awakening is considered essential. A continuous intravenous infusion of propofol, with or without other anesthetic drugs, has become a commonly used method for producing "conscious" sedation or as part of a balanced or total intravenous anesthetic. The administration of propofol as a continuous infusion may be used for sedation of patients in the intensive care unit (ICU).

Induction of Anesthesia

The induction dose of intravenous propofol in healthy adults is 1.5 to 2.5 mg/kg (children may require higher doses and elderly patients lower doses). The complete awakening without residual CNS effects that is characteristic of propofol is the principal reason this drug has replaced thiopental for the induction of anesthesia in many clinical situations.

Intravenous Sedation

The prompt recovery, without residual sedation and a low incidence of nausea and vomiting, make propofol particularly well suited to ambulatory conscious sedation techniques (25 to 100 μg/kg per minute IV produces minimal analgesic and amnestic effects). In selected patients, midazolam or an opioid may be added to propofol for continuous intravenous sedation. Propofol has been administered as a sedative during mechanical ventilation in the ICU. Increasing metabolic acidosis, lipemic plasma, bradycardia, and progressive myocardial failure has been described in a few children who were sedated with propofol during the management of acute respiratory failure in the ICU.

Maintenance of Anesthesia

Propofol (100 to 300 μg/kg per minute IV), often in combination with a short-acting opioid, has proved to be a valuable adjuvant during short ambulatory procedures. General anesthesia with propofol is generally associated with minimal postoperative nausea and vomiting, and awakening is prompt, with minimal residual sedative effects.

Nonhypnotic Therapeutic Applications

Antiemetic Effects

The incidence of postoperative nausea and vomiting is decreased when propofol is administered, regardless of the anesthetic technique or anesthetic drugs used. Subhypnotic doses of propofol (10 to 15 mg IV) may be used in the postanesthesia care unit to treat nausea and vomiting. Propofol in subhypnotic doses is effective against chemotherapy-induced nausea and vomiting. The mechanisms mediating the antiemetic effects of propofol remain unknown. Subhypnotic doses of propofol that are effective as an antiemetic do not inhibit gastric emptying, and propofol is not considered a prokinetic drug.

Antipruritic Effects

Propofol, 10 mg IV, is effective in the treatment of pruritus associated with neuraxial opioids or cholestasis.

Anticonvulsant Activity

Propofol possesses antiepileptic properties, presumably reflecting the GABA-mediated presynaptic and postsynaptic inhibition of chloride ion channels.

Attenuation of Bronchoconstriction

Compared with thiopental, propofol decreases the prevalence of wheezing after the induction of anesthesia and tracheal intubation in healthy and asthmatic patients. However, a generic formulation of propofol utilizes metabisulfite as a preservative. Metabisulfite may cause bronchoconstriction in asthmatic patients. Nevertheless, propofol-induced bronchoconstriction has been described in patients with allergy histories; the formulation of propofol administered to these patients was Diprivan® containing soybean oil, glycerin, yolk lecithin, and sodium edetate.

Effects on Organ Systems

Central Nervous System

Propofol decreases the cerebral metabolic rate for oxygen ($CMRo_2$), cerebral blood flow, and intracranial pressure (ICP). Cerebrovascular autoregulation (in response to changes in systemic blood pressure) and reactivity of the cerebral blood flow to changes in $Paco_2$ are not affected by propofol. Propofol produces cortical electroencephalographic (EEG) changes that are similar to those of thiopental, including the ability of high doses to produce burst suppression. Cortical somatosensory evoked potentials, as utilized for monitoring spinal cord function, are not significantly modified in the presence of propofol alone, but the addition of nitrous oxide or a volatile anesthetic results in decreased amplitude.

Cardiovascular System

Propofol produces decreases in systemic blood pressure (often accompanied by corresponding changes in cardiac output and systemic vascular resistance) that are greater than those evoked by comparable doses of thiopental. The stimulation produced by direct laryngoscopy and intubation of the trachea reverses the blood pressure effects of propofol. The blood pressure effects of propofol may be exaggerated in hypovolemic patients, elderly patients, and patients with compromised left ventricular function due to coronary artery disease. Adequate hydration before rapid intravenous administration of propofol is recommended to minimize the blood pressure effects of this drug. Despite decreases in systemic blood pressure, heart rate often remains unchanged, in contrast to the modest increases that typically accompany the rapid intravenous injection of thiopental. Propofol does not prolong the QTc interval on the electrocardiogram.

Bradycardia-related Death

Profound bradycardia and asystole after the administration of propofol have been described in healthy adult patients, despite prophylactic anticholinergics. Heart rate responses to intravenous administration of atropine are attenuated in patients receiving propofol compared with awake patients. This decreased responsiveness to atropine cannot be effectively overcome by large doses of atropine, thus suggesting that propofol may induce a suppression of sympathetic nervous system activity. The treatment of propofol-induced bradycardia may require the administration of a β-agonist, such as isoproterenol.

Lungs

Propofol produces a dose-dependent depression of ventilation, with apnea occurring in 25% to 35% of patients after the induction of anesthesia with propofol. Opioids administered with the preoperative medication may enhance this ventilatory depressant effect. Painful surgical stimulation is likely to counteract the ventilatory depressant effects of propofol. Propofol can produce bronchodilation and decrease the incidence of intraoperative wheezing in patients with asthma.

Hepatic and Renal Function

Propofol does not adversely affect hepatic or renal function, as reflected by measurements of liver transaminase enzymes or creatinine concentrations.

Intraocular Pressure

Propofol is associated with significant decreases in intraocular pressure that occur immediately after the induction of anesthesia and are sustained during tracheal intubation.

Coagulation

Propofol does not alter tests of coagulation or platelet function.

Side Effects

Allergic Reactions

Allergenic components of propofol include the phenyl nucleus and diisopropyl side chain. Patients who develop evidence of anaphylaxis on the first exposure to propofol may have been previously sensitized to the diisopropyl radical, which is present in many dermatologic preparations. Anaphylaxis to propofol during the first exposure to this drug has been observed, especially in patients with a history of other drug allergies, often to neuromuscular-blocking drugs. Propofol-induced bronchoconstriction has been described in patients with allergy histories.

Lactic Acidosis

Lactic acidosis or *propofol infusion syndrome* has been described in pediatric and adult patients receiving prolonged high-dose infusions of propofol (>75 μg/kg per minute) for longer than 24 hours. Unexpected tachycardia occurring during propofol anesthesia should prompt a laboratory evaluation for possible metabolic (lactic) acidosis. A measurement of arterial blood gases and serum lactate concentrations is recommended. Metabolic acidosis in its early stages is reversible with discontinuation of propofol administration. The mechanism for sporadic propofol-induced metabolic acidosis is unclear but may reflect a poisoning (cytopathic hypoxia) of the electron transport chain and impaired oxidation of long-chain fatty acids by propofol or a propofol metabolite in uniquely susceptible patients. The differential diagnosis when propofol-induced lactic acidosis is suspected includes hyperchloremic metabolic acidosis associated with large volume infusions of 0.9% saline and metabolic acidosis associated with the excessive generation of organic acids, such as lactate and ketones (diabetic acidosis, release of a tourniquet).

Proconvulsant Activity

The majority of reported propofol-induced seizures during the induction of anesthesia or emergence from anesthesia reflect spontaneous excitatory movements of subcortical origin. The incidence of excitatory movements and associated EEG changes are low after the administration of propofol. Propofol resembles thiopental in that it does not produce seizure activity on the EEG when administered to patients with epilepsy. There appears to be no reason to avoid propofol for sedation or the induction and maintenance of anesthesia in patients with known seizure disorders.

Abuse Potential

Intense dreaming activity, amorous behavior, and hallucinations have been reported during recovery from the effects of propofol.

Bacterial Growth

Propofol strongly supports the growth of *Escherichia coli* and *Pseudomonas aeruginosa*. For this reason, it is recommended that (a) an aseptic technique be used in handling propofol, as reflected by disinfecting the ampule neck surface or vial rubber stopper with 70% isopropyl alcohol; (b) the contents of the ampule containing propofol should be withdrawn into a sterile syringe immediately after opening and administered promptly; and (c) the contents of an opened ampule must be discarded if they are not used within 6 hours. In the ICU, the tubing and any unused portion of propofol must be discarded after 12 hours.

Antioxidant Properties

Propofol has potent antioxidant properties that resemble those of the endogenous antioxidant vitamin E. A neuroprotective effect of propofol may be at least partially related to the antioxidant potential of propofol's phenol ring structure.

Pain on Injection

Pain on injection is the most commonly reported adverse event associated with propofol administration to awake patients. Preceding the propofol with (using the same injection site as for propofol) 1% lidocaine or by prior administration of a potent short-acting opioid decreases the incidence of discomfort experienced by the patient.

Airway Protection

Inhaled and injected anesthetic drugs alter pharyngeal function and have the associated risk of impaired upper airway protection and pulmonary aspiration. Subhypnotic concentrations of propofol, isoflurane, and sevoflurane cause decreased pharyngeal contractions forces that are most marked in patients receiving propofol.

Miscellaneous Effects

Propofol does not trigger malignant hyperthermia or coproporphyria. The secretion of cortisol is not influenced by propofol, even when administered for prolonged periods in the ICU.

ETOMIDATE

Etomidate is a carboxylated imidazole–containing compound that is chemically unrelated to any other drug used for the intravenous induction of anesthesia (Fig. 6-3).

Commercial Preparation

Etomidate is prepared as a fat emulsion, and pain on injection and venous irritation is unlikely. Administration through the oral mucosa results in direct systemic absorption while bypassing hepatic metabolism. The result is an achievement of higher blood concentrations more rapidly, compared with drug that is administered orally for delivery to the gastrointestinal tract.

Mechanism of Action

Etomidate is unique among injected and inhaled anesthetics in being administered in a single isomer in clinical

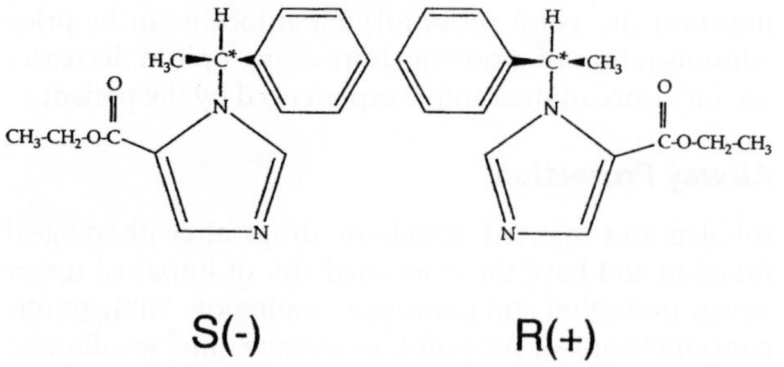

Figure 6-3. Structural isomers of etomidate. The asymmetric carbon atom is marked by an asterisk. R(+)-etomidate is the clinically useful isomer. (From Tomlin SL, Jenkins A, Lieb WR, et al. Stereoselective effects of etomidate optical isomers on gamma-aminobutyric acid type A receptors and animals. *Anesthesiology* 1998;88:708–717; with permission.)

practice (see Fig 6-3). The anesthetic effect of etomidate resides predominantly in the R(+) enantiomer, which is approximately five times as potent as the S(−) isomer. Etomidate is believed to exert its effects on $GABA_A$ receptors by binding directly to a specific site or sites on the protein and enhancing the affinity of the inhibitory neurotransmitter (GABA) for these receptors.

Pharmacokinetics

The volume of distribution (Vd) of etomidate is large, suggesting considerable tissue uptake (see Table 6-1). Etomidate penetrates the brain rapidly, reaching peak levels within 1 minute after intravenous injection. Prompt awakening after a single dose of etomidate principally reflects the redistribution of the drug from brain to inactive tissue sites. Rapid metabolism is also likely to contribute to prompt recovery.

Metabolism

Etomidate is rapidly metabolized through the hydrolysis of the ethyl ester side chain to its carboxylic acid ester, resulting in a water-soluble, pharmacologically inactive compound. The clearance of etomidate is about five times that for thiopental; this is reflected as a shorter elimination half-time of 2 to 5 hours. Likewise, the context-sensitive half-time of etomidate is less likely to be increased by continuous infusion, as compared with thiopental.

Cardiopulmonary Bypass

Institution of hypothermic cardiopulmonary bypass causes an initial decrease in the plasma etomidate concentration. Hepatic blood flow changes during cardiopulmonary bypass may be important, because etomidate is a high hepatic–extraction drug.

Clinical Uses

Etomidate (0.2 to 0.4 mg/kg IV) may be viewed as an alternative to propofol or barbiturates for the induction of anesthesia, especially in the presence of an unstable cardiovascular system. Involuntary myoclonic movements are common during the induction period as a result of alterations in the balance of inhibitory and excitatory influences on the thalamocortical tract. Awakening after a single intravenous dose of etomidate is more rapid than after barbiturates, and there is little or no evidence of a hangover or cumulative drug effect. Analgesia is not produced by etomidate. The principal limiting factor in the clinical use of etomidate for the induction of anesthesia is the ability of this drug to transiently depress adrenocortical function.

Side Effects

Central Nervous System

Etomidate is a potent direct cerebral vasoconstrictor that decreases cerebral blood flow and $CMRO_2$ (comparable to changes produced by thiopental). The frequency of excitatory spikes on the EEG is greater with etomidate than with thiopental and methohexital, suggesting caution in the administration of etomidate to patients with a history of seizures. Like methohexital, etomidate may activate seizure foci, manifesting as fast activity on the EEG. For this reason, etomidate should be used with caution in patients with focal epilepsy. Conversely, this characteristic has been observed to facilitate the localization of seizure foci in patients undergoing the cortical resection of epileptogenic tissue.

Cardiovascular System

Cardiovascular stability (minimal changes in heart rate, stroke volume, cardiac output) is characteristic of induction of anesthesia using 0.3 mg/kg IV of etomidate. A decrease in systemic blood pressure parallels changes in systemic vascular resistance; the administration of etomidate to acutely hypovolemic patients could result in sudden hypotension. Etomidate has been proposed for the induction of anesthesia in patients with little or no cardiac reserve. Etomidate may differ from most other intravenous anesthetics in that depressive effects on myocardial contractility are minimal at the concentrations needed for the production of anesthesia.

Ventilation

The depressant effects of etomidate on ventilation seem to be less than those of barbiturates, although apnea may occasionally accompany a rapid intravenous injection of the drug. The depression of ventilation may be exaggerated when etomidate is combined with inhaled anesthetics or opioids during continuous infusion techniques.

Pain on Injection

Pain on injection and venous irritation has been virtually eliminated with use of etomidate preparations utilizing a lipid emulsion vehicle rather than propylene glycol.

Myoclonus

Myoclonus (spontaneous movements) occurs in 50% to 80% of patients receiving etomidate in the absence of premedication. The prior administration of an opioid (fentanyl, 1 to 2 μg/kg IV) or a benzodiazepine may decrease the incidence of myoclonus associated with the administration of etomidate. The mechanism of etomidate-induced myoclonus appears to be disinhibition of subcortical structures that normally suppress extrapyramidal motor activity. The fact that etomidate-induced myoclonic activity may be associated with seizure activity (not all reports demonstrate this finding) on the EEG suggests caution in the use of this drug for the induction of anesthesia in patients with a history of seizure activity.

Adrenocortical Suppression

Etomidate causes adrenocortical suppression by producing a dose-dependent inhibition of the conversion of cholesterol to cortisol (Fig. 6-4). This enzyme inhibition lasts 4 to 8 hours after an intravenous induction dose of etomidate. Conceivably, patients experiencing sepsis or hemorrhage, and who might require an intact cortisol response, would be at a disadvantage should etomidate be administered. Conversely, the suppression of adrenocortical function could be considered desirable from the standpoint of "stress-free" anesthesia.

Allergic Reactions

Allergic reactions following the administration of etomidate are very rare.

KETAMINE

Ketamine is a phencyclidine derivative that produces "dissociative anesthesia," which resembles a cataleptic state in which the eyes remain open with a slow nystagmic gaze. The patient is noncommunicative, although wakefulness may appear to be present. Varying degrees of hypertonus and purposeful skeletal muscle movements often occur independently of surgical stimulation. The patient is amnesic, and analgesia is intense. Ketamine has advantages over propofol and etomidate in being water soluble

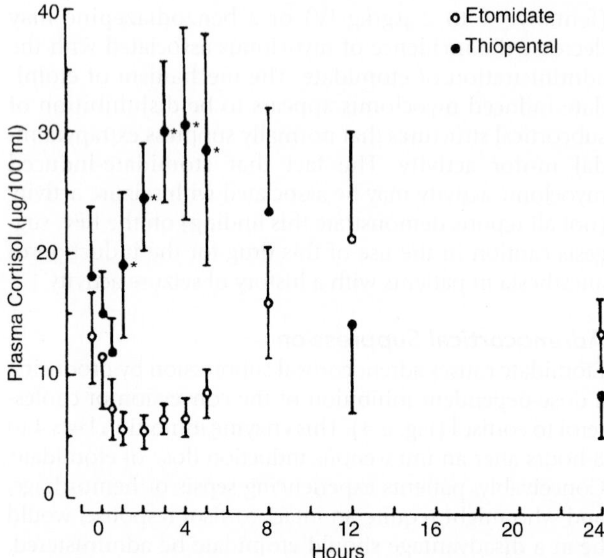

Figure 6-4. Etomidate, but not thiopental, is associated with decreases in the plasma concentrations of cortisol. (*P <.05 compared with thiopental; mean ± SD.) (From Fragen RJ, Shanks CA, Molteni A, et al. Effects of etomidate on hormonal responses to surgical stress. *Anesthesiology* 1984; 61:652–656; with permission.)

(it does not require a lipid emulsion vehicle) and in producing profound analgesia at subanesthetic doses. However, the possibility of emergence delirium limits the clinical usefulness of ketamine. Ketamine is considered a drug with abuse potential, thus emphasizing the need to take appropriate precautions against unauthorized nonmedical use.

Structure–Activity Relationships

The presence of an asymmetric carbon atom results in the existence of two optical isomers of ketamine (Fig 6-5). The racemic form of ketamine has been the most frequently used preparation although S(+)-ketamine is clinically

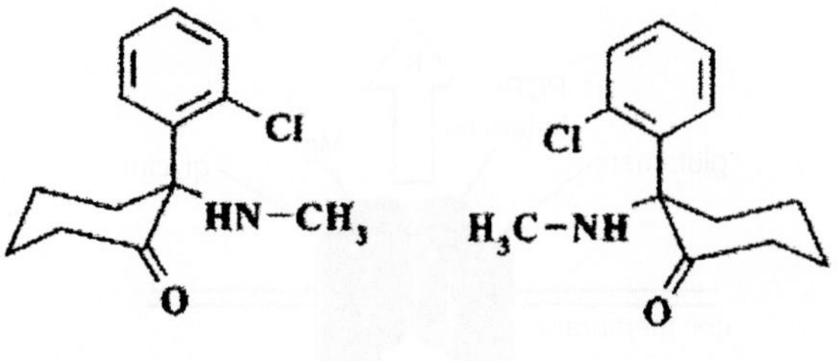

R (-) - ketamine

S (+) - ketamine

Figure 6-5. Structural formula of the two isomers of ketamine. (From Kohrs R, Durieux ME. Ketamine: Teaching an old drug new tricks. *Anesth Analg* 1998;87;1186–1193; with permission.)

available. S(+)-ketamine produces (a) more intense analgesia, (b) more rapid metabolism and thus recovery, (c) less salivation, and (d) a lower incidence of emergence reactions than the R(−)-ketamine. Both isomers of ketamine appear to inhibit the uptake of catecholamines back into postganglionic sympathetic nerve endings (cocaine-like effect). The fact that individual optical isomers of ketamine differ in their pharmacologic properties suggests that this drug interacts with specific receptors.

Mechanism of Action

Ketamine binds noncompetitively to the phencyclidine recognition site on *N*-methyl-D-aspartate (NMDA) receptors. Unlike propofol and etomidate, ketamine has only weak actions at $GABA_A$ receptors.

N-Methyl-D-Aspartate Receptor Antagonism

NMDA receptors (members of the glutamate receptors family) are ligand-gated ion channels that are unique in that channel activation requires the binding of the excitatory neurotransmitter glutamate with glycine as an obligatory coagonist (Fig. 6-6). This interaction with phencyclidine binding sites appears to be stereoselective, with the S(+) isomer of ketamine having the greatest affinity.

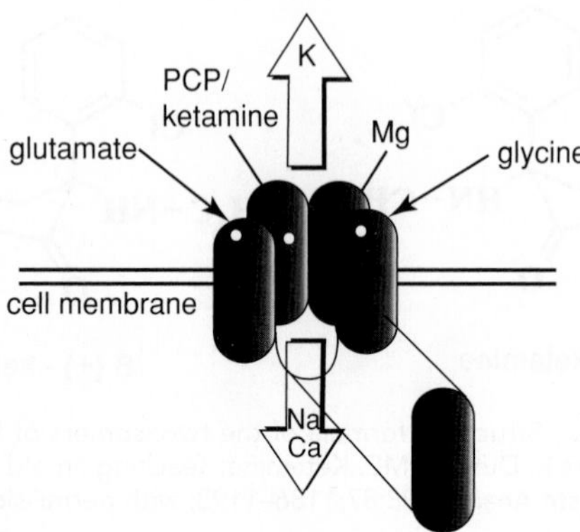

Figure 6-6. Schematic diagram of the *N*-methyl-D-aspartate (NMDA) glutamate receptor/channel complex. The receptor consists of five subunits surrounding a central ion channel that is permeable to calcium, potassium, and sodium. Binding sites for the agonist glutamate and the obligatory coagonist glycine are indicated. NMDA receptors are ligand-gated ion channels that are activated by the excitatory neurotransmitter, glutamate. Glutamate is the most abundant neurotransmitter in the central nervous system. One of the subunits has been removed to show the interior of the ion channel and binding sites for magnesium and ketamine, which produce noncompetitive NMDA receptor blockade. (From Kohrs R, Durieux ME. Ketamine: Teaching an old drug new tricks. *Anesth Analg* 1998;87;1186–1193; with permission.)

Opioid Receptors

Ketamine interacts with σ-receptors, although this receptor is no longer classified as an opioid receptor, and the interaction with ketamine is weak.

Muscarinic Receptors

The fact that ketamine produces anticholinergic symptoms (emergence delirium, bronchodilation, sympathomimetic action) suggests that an antagonist effect of ketamine at muscarinic receptors is more likely than an agonist effect.

Sodium Channels

Consistent with its mild local anesthetic-like properties, ketamine interacts with voltage-gated sodium channels sharing a binding site with local anesthetics.

Pharmacokinetics

The pharmacokinetics of ketamine resemble that of thiopental in rapid onset of action, relatively short duration of action, and high lipid solubility (see Table 6-1). The extreme lipid solubility of ketamine (five to ten times that of thiopental) ensures its rapid transfer across the blood-brain barrier. The high hepatic extraction ratio suggests that alterations in hepatic blood flow could influence ketamine's clearance rate.

Metabolism

Ketamine is metabolized through hepatic microsomal enzymes (demethylation of ketamine by cytochrome P-450 enzymes) to form norketamine (one-fifth to one-third as potent as ketamine) (Fig. 6-7). This active metabolite may contribute to the prolonged effects of ketamine (analgesia), especially with repeated doses or a continuous intravenous infusion. Norketamine is eventually hydroxylated and then conjugated to form more water-soluble and inactive glucuronide metabolites that are excreted by the kidneys. Tolerance may occur in burn patients receiving more than two short-interval exposures to ketamine.

Clinical Uses

Analgesia

Intense analgesia can be achieved with subanesthetic doses of ketamine, 0.2 to 0.5 mg/kg IV. Analgesia is thought to be greater for somatic than for visceral pain.

Neuraxial Analgesia

The neuraxial use of ketamine to produce analgesia is of limited value.

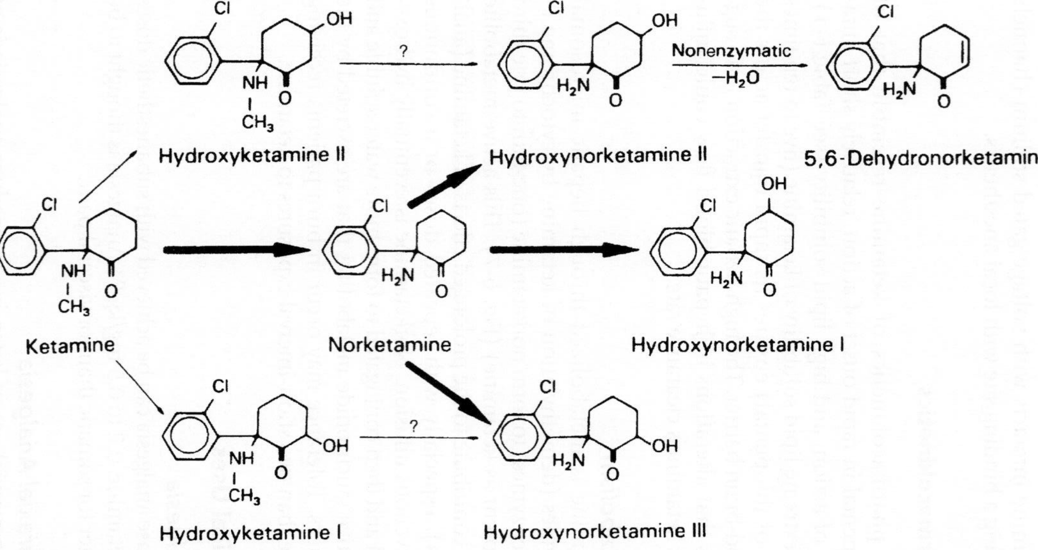

Figure 6-7. Metabolism of ketamine. (From White PF, Way WL, Trevor AJ. Ketamine: its pharmacology and therapeutic uses. *Anesthesiology* 1982;56:119–136; with permission.)

Induction of Anesthesia

The induction of anesthesia is produced by the administration of intravenous ketamine, 1 to 2 mg/kg or the intramuscular administration of 4 to 8 mg/kg. Intravenous injection of ketamine does not produce pain or venous irritation. Consciousness is lost in 30 to 60 seconds after an intravenous administration and in 2 to 4 minutes after an intramuscular injection. Unconsciousness is associated with the maintenance of normal or only slightly depressed pharyngeal and laryngeal reflexes. The return of consciousness usually occurs in 10 to 20 minutes after an injected induction dose of ketamine, but return to full orientation may require an additional 60 to 90 minutes. Amnesia persists for about 60 to 90 minutes after recovery of consciousness, but ketamine does not produce retrograde amnesia. Because of its rapid onset of action, ketamine has been used as an intramuscular induction drug in children and difficult-to-manage mentally retarded patients regardless of age.

Ketamine has been used extensively for burn dressing changes, débridements, and skin-grafting procedures. The excellent analgesia and ability to maintain spontaneous ventilation in an airway that might otherwise be altered by burn-scar contractures are important advantages of ketamine in these patients. Tolerance may develop, however, in burn patients receiving repeated, short-interval anesthesia with ketamine.

The induction of anesthesia in acutely hypovolemic patients is often accomplished using ketamine, taking advantage of the drug's cardiovascular-stimulating effects. The loss of cardioprotective effects (preconditioning) associated with racemic ketamine is a consideration when this drug is administered to patients with known coronary artery disease.

The beneficial effects of ketamine on airway resistance due to drug-induced bronchodilation make this a potentially useful drug for the rapid intravenous induction of anesthesia in patients with asthma.

Ketamine should be used cautiously or avoided in patients with systemic or pulmonary hypertension or increased ICP, although this recommendation may deserve reevaluation based on more recent data. Ketamine has been administered safely to patients with malignant hyperthermia and does not trigger the syndrome in susceptible swine.

Extensive experience with ketamine for pediatric cardiac catheterization has shown the drug to be useful, but its possible cardiac-stimulating effects must be considered in the interpretation of catheterization data.

Reversal of Opioid Tolerance

Subanesthetic doses of ketamine are effective in preventing and reversing morphine-induced tolerance.

Improvement of Mental Depression

As a NMDA antagonist, ketamine in small doses improved the postoperative depressive state in patients with mental depression.

Side Effects

Ketamine is unique among injected anesthetics in its ability to stimulate the cardiovascular system and produce emergence delirium.

Central Nervous System

Ketamine is traditionally considered to increase cerebral blood flow and $CMRO_2$, although evidence also suggests that this may not be a valid generalization.

Intracranial Pressure

Patients with intracranial pathology are commonly considered vulnerable to sustained increases in ICP after the administration of ketamine. Nevertheless, results in patients suggest that ketamine can be administered to anesthetized and mechanically ventilated patients with mildly increased ICP without adversely altering cerebral hemodynamics.

Neuroprotective Effects

The antagonist effect of ketamine on NMDA receptors suggests a possible neuroprotective role for this drug, although this remains an unproved hypothesis.

Electroencephalogram

Ketamine's effects on the EEG are characterized by the abolition of α-rhythm and dominance of θ-activity. Ketamine does not alter the seizure threshold in epileptic patients.

Somatosensory Evoked Potentials

Ketamine increases the cortical amplitude of somatosensory evoked potentials.

Cardiovascular System

Ketamine produces cardiovascular effects that resemble sympathetic nervous system stimulation.

Hemodynamic Effects

Systemic and pulmonary arterial blood pressure, heart rate, cardiac output, cardiac work, and myocardial oxygen requirements are increased after the intravenous administration of ketamine. The increase in systolic blood pressure in adults receiving clinical doses of ketamine is 20 to 40 mm Hg, with a slightly smaller increase in diastolic blood pressure. Typically, systemic blood pressure increases progressively during the first 3 to 5 minutes after an intravenous injection of ketamine and then decreases to predrug levels over the next 10 to 20 minutes. The cardiovascular-stimulating effects on the systemic and pulmonary circulations are blunted or prevented by the prior administration of benzodiazepines or the concomitant administration of inhaled anesthetics, including nitrous oxide. Critically ill patients occasionally respond to ketamine with unexpected decreases in systemic blood pressure and cardiac output, which may reflect a depletion of endogenous catecholamine stores and exhaustion of sympathetic nervous system compensatory mechanisms, thus leading to an unmasking of ketamine's direct myocardial depressant effects. In shocked animals, ketamine-induced vasoconstriction may maintain systemic blood pressure at the expense of tissue perfusion.

Cardiac Rhythm

The effect of ketamine on cardiac rhythm is inconclusive.

Mechanisms of Cardiovascular Effects

A direct stimulation of the CNS that leads to increased sympathetic nervous system outflow seems to be the most important mechanism for cardiovascular stimulation.

Ventilation and Airway

Ketamine does not produce significant depression of ventilation. The ventilatory response to carbon dioxide is maintained during ketamine anesthesia, and the $\text{Pa}CO_2$ is unlikely to increase to >3 mm Hg. Apnea, however, can occur if the drug is intravenously administered rapidly or an opioid is included in the preoperative medication. Upper airway skeletal muscle tone is well maintained, and upper airway reflexes remain relatively intact after the administration of ketamine. Despite the continued presence of upper airway reflexes, ketamine anesthesia does not negate the need for protection of the lungs against aspiration by placement of a cuffed tube in the patient's trachea. Salivary and tracheobronchial mucous gland secretions are increased following the intramuscular or intravenous administration of ketamine, leading to the frequent recommendation that an antisialagogue be included in the preoperative medication when use of this drug is anticipated.

Bronchomotor Tone

Ketamine has bronchodilatory effects and may be recommended as the intravenous induction drug of choice in patients with asthma. The mechanism by which ketamine produces airway relaxation is unclear.

Hepatic or Renal Function

Ketamine does not significantly alter laboratory tests that reflect hepatic or renal function.

Allergic Reactions

Ketamine does not evoke the release of histamine and rarely, if ever, causes allergic reactions.

Platelet Aggregation

Ketamine inhibits platelet aggregation.

Drug Interactions

The importance of an intact and normally functioning CNS in determining the cardiovascular effects of ketamine is emphasized by hemodynamic depression, rather than stimulation, that occurs when ketamine is administered in the presence of inhaled anesthetics. Diazepam, 0.3 to 0.5 mg/kg IV, or an equivalent dose of midazolam, is also effective in preventing the cardiac-stimulating effects of ketamine. Pancuronium may enhance the cardiac-stimulating effects of ketamine.

Emergence Delirium (Psychedelic Effects)

Emergence from ketamine anesthesia in the postoperative period may be associated with visual, auditory, proprioceptive, and confusional illusions, which may progress to delirium. Cortical blindness may be transiently present. Dreams and hallucinations can occur up to 24 hours after the administration of ketamine.

Mechanisms

Emergence delirium probably occurs secondary to ketamine-induced depression of the inferior colliculus and medial geniculate nucleus, thus leading to the misinterpretation of auditory and visual stimuli. Furthermore, the loss of skin and musculoskeletal sensations results in a decreased ability to perceive gravity, thereby

TABLE 6-2.
FACTORS ASSOCIATED WITH AN INCREASED INCIDENCE OF EMERGENCE DELIRIUM FOLLOWING ADMINISTRATION OF KETAMINE

Age greater than 15 years
Female gender
Dose greater than 2 mg/kg IV
History of frequent dreaming

producing a sensation of bodily detachment or floating in space.

Incidence

The observed incidence of emergence delirium after ketamine ranges from 5% to 30% (Table 6-2). Emergence delirium occurs less frequently when ketamine is used repeatedly. Inhaled anesthetics can also produce auditory, visual, proprioceptive, and confusional illusions, but the incidence of such phenomena, especially unpleasant experiences, is greater after anesthesia that includes the administration of ketamine.

Prevention (Table 6-3)

Preconditioning

The pharmacologic activation of adenosine triphosphate–regulated potassium (K_{ATP}) channels mimics ischemic preconditioning and decreases infarct size or improves the functional recovery of ischemic-reperfused viable (stunned) myocardium. Conversely, the pharmacologic blockade of K_{ATP} channels can antagonize the cardioprotective effects of ischemic preconditioning. In an animal model, ketamine blocked the cardioprotective effects of ischemic preconditioning, and this effect was due to the R(−) isomer. In patients at risk for myocardial infarction during the perioperative period, drugs known

TABLE 6-3.
PREVENTION OF KETAMINE-INDUCED EMERGENCE DELIRIUM

Midazolam (administer IV about 5 minutes before induction of anesthesia with ketamine)
Inclusion of thiopental or inhaled anesthetics
Prospective discussion with patient about side effects of ketamine
Awakening in quiet environment (no proof this is helpful)

to block preconditioning should be used with caution, whereas drugs know to elicit early and late preconditioning (opioids, volatile anesthetics) may be beneficial.

DEXTROMETHORPHAN

Dextromethorphan (a *d*-isomer of levorphanol) is a low affinity NMDA antagonist that is a common ingredient in over-the-counter cough suppressants. It is equal in potency to codeine as an antitussive but lacks analgesic or physical dependence properties.

Local Anesthetics

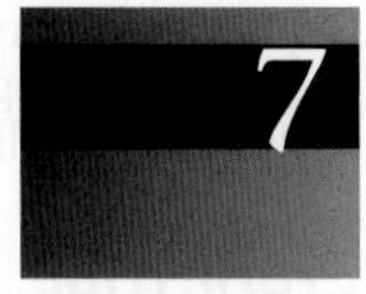

Local anesthetics are drugs that produce a reversible conduction blockade of impulses along central and peripheral nerve pathways after regional anesthesia (Stoelting RK, Hillier SC. Local Anesthetics. In: *Pharmacology and Physiology in Anesthetic Practice,* 4th ed. Philadelphia. Lippincott Williams & Wilkins, 2006:179–207). Removal of the local anesthetic is followed by spontaneous and complete return of nerve conduction, with no evidence of structural damage to nerve fibers as a result of the drug's effects.

COMMERCIAL PREPARATIONS

Local anesthetics are poorly soluble in water and therefore are marketed most often as water-soluble hydrochloride salts.

Liposomal Local Anesthetics

Drugs such as lidocaine, tetracaine, and bupivacaine have been incorporated into liposomes to prolong the duration of action and decrease toxicity. When infiltrated or applied topically, the extended-duration local anesthetics could have clinical use for prolonged postoperative analgesia and in the treatment of chronic pain.

Alkalinization

The alkalinization of local anesthetic solutions shortens the onset of neural blockade, enhances the depth of sensory and motor blockade, and increases the spread of epidural blockade. Alkalinization increases the percentage of local anesthetic existing in the lipid-soluble form that is available to diffuse across lipid cellular barriers.

STRUCTURE–ACTIVITY RELATIONSHIPS (FIG. 7-1)

Local anesthetics consist of a lipophilic (unsaturated aromatic ring such as para-aminobenzoic acid) and a hydrophilic (tertiary amine) portion separated by a connecting hydrocarbon chain. The lipophilic portion is essential for anesthetic activity. In almost all instances, an ester (–CO–) or an amide (–NHC–) bond links the hydrocarbon chain to the lipophilic aromatic ring. The nature of this bond is the basis for classifying drugs that produce a conduction blockade of nerve impulses as *ester* local anesthetics or *amide* local anesthetics (Fig. 7-2). The important differences between ester and amide local anesthetics relate to the site of metabolism and the potential to produce allergic reactions.

Modification of Chemical Structure

Modifying the chemical structure of a local anesthetic alters its pharmacologic effects (Table 7-1). Substituting a butyl group for the amine group on the benzene ring of procaine results in tetracaine. Compared with procaine, tetracaine is more lipid soluble, ten times more

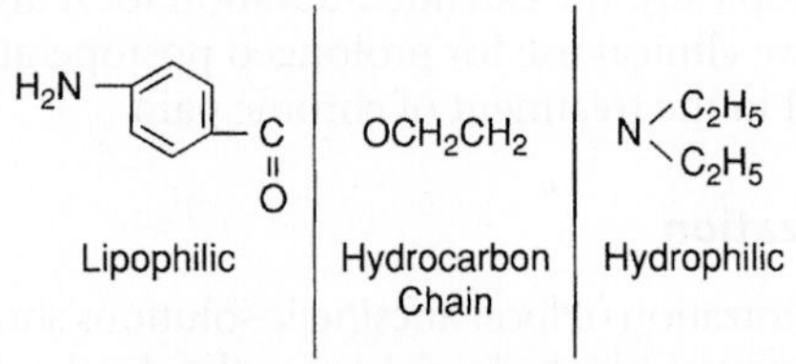

H_2N–C(=O) | OCH_2CH_2 | $N(C_2H_5)_2$

Lipophilic | Hydrocarbon Chain | Hydrophilic

Figure 7-1. Local anesthetics consist of a lipophilic and hydrophilic portion separated by a connecting hydrocarbon chain.

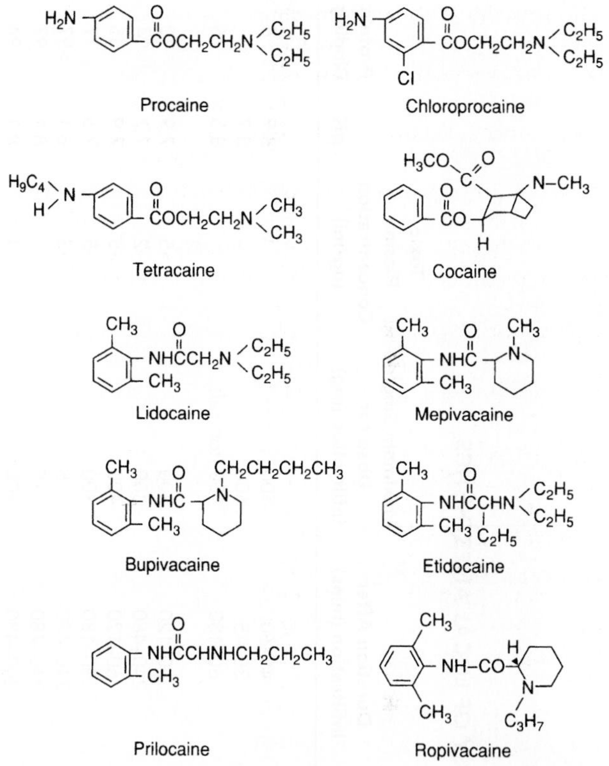

Procaine

Chloroprocaine

Tetracaine

Cocaine

Lidocaine

Mepivacaine

Bupivacaine

Etidocaine

Prilocaine

Ropivacaine

Figure 7-2. Ester and amide local anesthetics. Mepivacaine, bupivacaine, and ropivacaine are chiral drugs, because the molecules possess an asymmetric carbon atom.

potent, and has a longer duration of action, corresponding to a four- to fivefold decrease in the rate of metabolism. The halogenation of procaine to chloroprocaine results in a three- to fourfold increase in the hydrolysis rate of chloroprocaine by plasma cholinesterase. Mepivacaine, bupivacaine, and ropivacaine are characterized as *pipecoloxylidides* (see Fig. 7-2). The addition of a butyl group to the piperidine nitrogen of mepivacaine

TABLE 7-1.
COMPARATIVE PHARMACOLOGY OF LOCAL ANESTHETICS

Classification	Potency	Onset	Duration After Infiltration (mins)	Maximum Single Dose for Infiltration (mg)	Toxic Plasma Concentration (μg/ml)	pK	Protein Binding
Esters							
Procaine	1	Slow	45–60	500		8.9	6
Chloroprocaine	4	Rapid	30–45	600		8.7	
Tetracaine	16	Slow	60–180	100 (topical)		8.5	76
Amides							
Lidocaine	1	Rapid	60–120	300	>5	7.9	70
Etidocaine	4	Slow	240–480	300	~2	7.7	94
Prilocaine	1	Slow	60–120	400	>5	7.9	55
Mepivacaine	1	Slow	90–180	300	>5	7.6	77
Bupivacaine	4	Slow	240–480	175	>3	8.1	>97
Levobupivacaine	4	Slow	240–480	175		8.1	>97
Ropivacaine	4	Slow	240–480	200	>4	8.1	94

Classification	Fraction Nonionized (%)			Lipid Solubility	Volume of Distribution (liters)	Clearance (liters/min)	Elimination Half-Time (mins)
	pH 7.2	pH 7.4	pH 7.6				
Esters							
Procaine	2	3	5	0.6	65		9
Chloroprocaine	3	5	7		35		7
Tetracaine	5	7	11	80			
Amides							
Lidocaine	17	25	33	2.9	91	0.95	96
Etidocaine	24	33	44	141	133	1.22	156
Prilocaine	17	24	33	0.9	191		96
Mepivacaine	28	39	50	1	84	9.78	114
Bupivacaine	11	17	24	28	73	0.47	210
Levobupivacaine	11	17	24		55		156
Ropivacaine		17			59	0.44	108

results in bupivacaine, which is 35 times more lipid soluble and has a potency and duration of action three to four times that of mepivacaine. Ropivacaine structurally resembles bupivacaine and mepivacaine, with a propyl group on the piperidine nitrogen atom of the molecule.

Racemic Mixtures or Pure Isomers

The pipecoloxylidide local anesthetics (mepivacaine, bupivacaine, ropivacaine, levobupivacaine) are chiral drugs, because their molecules possess an asymmetric carbon atom (see Fig. 7-2). As such, these drugs may have a left- (S) or right- (R) handed configuration. Administering a racemic drug mixture is, in reality, the administration of two different drugs. The S enantiomers of bupivacaine and mepivacaine appear to be less toxic than the commercially available racemic mixtures of these local anesthetics.

Mepivacaine, bupivacaine, ropivacaine, and levobupivacaine have been developed as a pure S enantiomers. These S enantiomers are considered to produce less neurotoxicity and cardiotoxicity than racemic mixtures or the R enantiomers of local anesthetics, perhaps reflecting decreased potency at sodium ion channels.

MECHANISM OF ACTION

Local anesthetics prevent the transmission of nerve impulses (conduction blockade) by inhibiting the passage of sodium ions through ion-selective sodium channels in nerve membranes. The failure of sodium ion channel permeability to increase slows the rate of depolarization so that the threshold potential is not reached and thus an action potential is not propagated (Fig. 7-3). Local anesthetics do not alter the resting transmembrane potential or threshold potential.

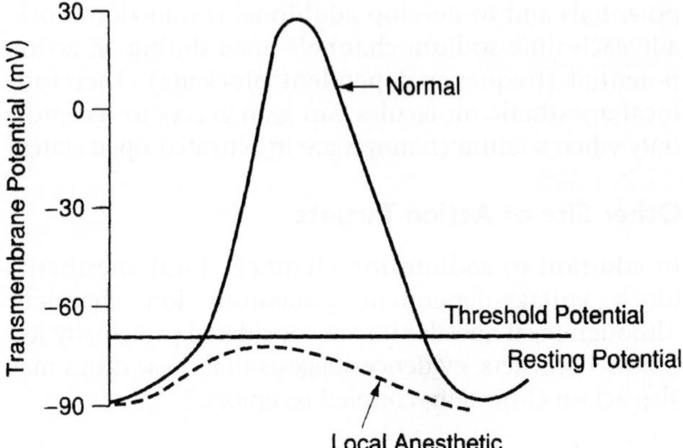

Figure 7-3. Local anesthetics slow the rate of depolarization of the nerve action potential so that the threshold potential is not reached. As a result, an action potential cannot be propagated in the presence of local anesthetic, and conduction blockade results.

Sodium Channels

The protein that forms sodium ion channels is a single polypeptide designated the α-subunit, and each channel consists of four subunits (DI–DIV). Sodium channels exist in activated-open, inactivated-closed, and rested-closed states during various phases of the action potential. By selectively binding to sodium channels in inactivated-closed states, local anesthetic molecules stabilize these channels in this configuration and prevent their change to the rested-closed and activated-open states in response to nerve impulses. Sodium channels in the inactivated-closed state are not permeable to sodium, and thus conduction of nerve impulses in the form of propagated action potentials cannot occur.

Frequency-Dependent Blockade

Sodium ion channels tend to recover from local anesthetic-induced conduction blockade between action potentials and to develop additional conduction blockade each time sodium channels open during an action potential (frequency-dependent blockade). Therefore, local anesthetic molecules can gain access to receptors only when sodium channels are in activated-open states.

Other Site of Action Targets

In addition to sodium ion channels, local anesthetics block voltage-dependent potassium ion channels. Although local anesthetics are considered principally ion channel blockers, evidence suggests that these drugs may also act on G-protein–coupled receptors.

MINIMUM CONCENTRATION

The minimum concentration of local anesthetic necessary to produce the conduction blockade of nerve impulses is termed the *Cm*. The Cm is analogous to the minimum alveolar concentration (MAC) for inhaled anesthetics. The Cm of motor fibers is approximately twice that of sensory fibers; thus, sensory anesthesia may not always be accompanied by skeletal muscle paralysis. A minimal length of myelinated nerve fiber must be exposed to an adequate concentration of local anesthetic for the conduction blockade of nerve impulses to occur in peripheral nerves. Both types of pain-conducting fibers (myelinated A-δ and nonmyelinated C fibers) are blocked by similar concentrations of local anesthetics, despite the differences in the diameters of these fibers. Preganglionic B fibers are more readily blocked by local anesthetics than any fiber, even though these fibers are myelinated.

Differential Conduction Blockade

A differential conduction blockade is illustrated by the selective blockade of preganglionic sympathetic nervous system B fibers in response to low concentrations of local anesthetics. Slightly higher concentrations of local anesthetics interrupt conduction in small C fibers and small- and medium-sized A fibers, with loss of sensation for pain and temperature. Nevertheless, touch, proprioception, and motor function are still present, so that the patient will sense pressure but not pain with surgical stimulation. In an anxious patient, however, any sensation may be misinterpreted as failure of the local anesthetic.

Changes during Pregnancy

Increased sensitivity (more rapid onset of conduction blockade) may be present during pregnancy.

PHARMACOKINETICS

Local anesthetics are weak bases that have pK values somewhat above physiologic pH levels (see Table 7-1). As a result, <50% of the local anesthetic exists in a lipid-soluble nonionized form at physiologic pH levels. Acidosis in the environment into which the local anesthetic is injected (as is present with tissue infection) further increases the ionized fraction of drug. This is consistent with the poor quality of local anesthesia that often results when a local anesthetic is injected into an acidic infected area. Local anesthetics with pK levels nearest to physiologic pH levels have the most rapid onset of action, reflecting the presence of an optimal ratio of ionized to nonionized drug fraction (see Table 7-1). Intrinsic vasodilator activity also will influence apparent potency and duration of action. The enhanced vasodilator action of lidocaine, compared with mepivacaine, results in the greater systemic absorption and shorter duration of action of lidocaine.

Absorption and Distribution

The absorption and distribution of a local anesthetic from its site of injection into the systemic circulation is influenced by the site of injection and dosage, use of epinephrine, and pharmacologic characteristics of the drug.

Lung Extraction

The lungs are capable of extracting local anesthetics such as lidocaine, bupivacaine, and prilocaine from the circulation.

Placental Transfer

Plasma protein binding influences the rate and degree of diffusion of local anesthetics across the placenta (see Table 7-1). Bupivacaine, which is highly protein bound (approximately 95%), has an umbilical vein–maternal arterial concentration ratio of about 0.32. Ester local anesthetics, because of their rapid hydrolysis, are not available to cross the placenta in significant amounts. Acidosis in the fetus, which may occur during prolonged labor, can result in accumulation of local anesthetic molecules in the fetus (ion trapping).

Clearance and Elimination Half-Times

Clearance values and elimination half-times for amide local anesthetics probably represent mainly hepatic metabolism, because renal excretion of unchanged drug is minimal (see Table 7-1). Pharmacokinetic studies of ester local anesthetics are limited because of a short elimination half-time due to their rapid hydrolysis in the plasma and liver.

Metabolism of Amide Local Anesthetics

Amide local anesthetics undergo varying rates of metabolism through microsomal enzymes located primarily in the liver. Prilocaine undergoes the most rapid metabolism; lidocaine and mepivacaine are intermediate; and etidocaine, bupivacaine, and ropivacaine undergo the slowest metabolism among the amide local anesthetics. Compared with that of ester local anesthetics, the metabolism of amide local anesthetics is more complex and slower. Slower metabolism means that sustained increases of the plasma concentrations of amide local anesthetics, and thus systemic toxicity, are more likely than with ester local anesthetics.

Lidocaine

The principal metabolic pathway of lidocaine is oxidative dealkylation in the liver to monoethylglycinexylidide, followed by hydrolysis of this metabolite to xylidide (Fig. 7-4). Monoethylglycinexylidide has approximately 80% of the activity of lidocaine for protecting against cardiac dysrhythmias in an animal model. This metabolite has a prolonged elimination half-time, accounting for its efficacy in controlling cardiac dysrhythmias after the infusion of lidocaine is discontinued. Hepatic disease or decreases in hepatic blood flow, which may occur during anesthesia, can decrease the metabolism rate of lidocaine. For example, the elimination half-time of lidocaine is increased more than fivefold in patients with liver dysfunction, compared with normal patients. The decreased hepatic metabolism of lidocaine should be anticipated when patients are anesthetized with volatile anesthetics.

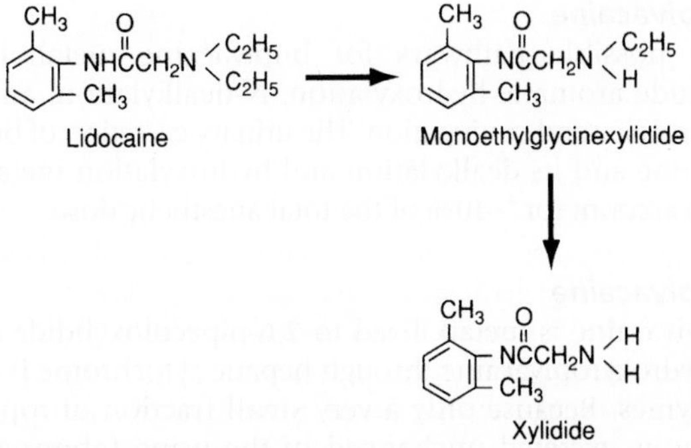

CH_3 O ‖ $NHCCH_2N\langle^{C_2H_5}_{C_2H_5}$ CH_3

Lidocaine

→

CH_3 O ‖ $NCCH_2N\langle^{C_2H_5}_{H}$ CH_3

Monoethylglycinexylidide

↓

CH_3 O ‖ $NCCH_2N\langle^{H}_{H}$ CH_3

Xylidide

Figure 7-4. Metabolism of lidocaine.

Etidocaine

A small amount (<1%) of etidocaine is excreted unchanged in the urine.

Prilocaine

Prilocaine is an amide local anesthetic that is metabolized to orthotoluidine. Orthotoluidine is an oxidizing compound capable of converting hemoglobin to its oxidized form, methemoglobin, thus resulting in a potentially life-threatening complication, methemoglobinemia. When the dose of prilocaine is >600 mg, sufficient methemoglobin may be present (3 to 5 g/dL) to cause the patient to appear cyanotic, and oxygen-carrying capacity is decreased. Methemoglobinemia is readily reversed by the administration of methylene blue, 1 to 2 mg/kg IV, over 5 minutes (total dose should not exceed 7 to 8 mg/kg).

Mepivacaine

Mepivacaine has pharmacologic properties similar to those of lidocaine, although the duration of action of mepivacaine is somewhat longer. In contrast to lidocaine, mepivacaine lacks vasodilator activity and is an alternate selection when the addition of epinephrine to the local anesthetic solution is not recommended.

Bupivacaine

The possible pathways for bupivacaine metabolism include aromatic hydroxylation, *N*-dealkylation, amide hydrolysis, and conjugation. The urinary excretion of bupivacaine and its dealkylation and hydroxylation metabolites account for >40% of the total anesthetic dose.

Ropivacaine

Ropivacaine is metabolized to 2,6-pipecoloxylidide and 3-hydroxyropivacaine through hepatic cytochrome P-450 enzymes. Because only a very small fraction of ropivacaine is excreted unchanged in the urine (about 1%) when the liver is functioning normally, dosage adjustments based on renal function do not seem necessary. Ropivacaine is highly bound to α_1-acid glycoprotein.

Dibucaine

Dibucaine is metabolized in the liver and is the most slowly eliminated of all the amide derivatives.

Metabolism of Ester Local Anesthetics

Ester local anesthetics undergo hydrolysis through the cholinesterase enzyme, principally in the plasma and to a lesser extent in the liver. The rate of hydrolysis varies, with chloroprocaine being most rapid, procaine being intermediate, and tetracaine being the slowest. The resulting metabolites are pharmacologically inactive, although para-aminobenzoic acid may be an antigen responsible for subsequent allergic reactions. The exception to the hydrolysis of ester local anesthetics in the plasma is cocaine, which undergoes significant metabolism in the liver. Systemic toxicity is inversely proportional to the rate of hydrolysis; thus, tetracaine is more likely than chloroprocaine to result in excessive plasma concentrations. Patients with atypical plasma cholinesterase may be at increased risk for developing excess systemic concentrations of an ester local anesthetic due to absent or limited plasma hydrolysis.

Procaine

Procaine is hydrolyzed to para-aminobenzoic acid, which is excreted unchanged in urine, and to dimethylaminoethanol, which is further metabolized, because only 30% is recovered in urine.

Chloroprocaine

The addition of a chlorine atom to the benzene ring of procaine to form chloroprocaine increases by 3.5 times the rate of hydrolysis of the local anesthetic by plasma cholinesterase as compared with procaine.

Tetracaine

Tetracaine undergoes hydrolysis by plasma cholinesterase, but the rate is slower than for procaine.

Benzocaine

Benzocaine is ideally suited for the topical anesthesia of mucous membranes prior to tracheal intubation, endoscopy, transesophageal echocardiography, and bronchoscopy. The onset of topical anesthesia is rapid and lasts 30 to 60 minutes. A brief spray of 20% benzocaine delivers the recommended dose of 200 to 300 mg. Cetacaine® is a combination of 14% benzocaine, 2% tetracaine, and 2% butamben. Methemoglobinemia is a rare but potentially life-threatening complication following the topical application of benzocaine, especially when the dose exceeds 200 to 300 mg.

Cocaine

Cocaine is metabolized by plasma and liver cholinesterases to water-soluble metabolites that are excreted in urine. Assays for the metabolites of cocaine in urine are useful markers of cocaine use or absorption.

Renal Elimination

The poor water solubility of local anesthetics usually limits the renal excretion of unchanged drug to <5% (exception is cocaine, of which 10% to 12% of unchanged drug can be recovered in urine). Water-soluble metabolites of local anesthetics, such as para-aminobenzoic acid resulting from metabolism of ester local anesthetics, are readily excreted in urine.

Use of Vasoconstrictors

The duration of action of a local anesthetic is proportional to the time the drug is in contact with nerve fibers. For this reason, epinephrine (1:200,000 or 5 μg/mL) may be added to local anesthetic solutions to produce vasoconstriction, which limits systemic absorption and

TABLE 7-2.
EFFECTS OF ADDITION OF EPINEPHRINE (1:200,000) TO LOCAL ANESTHETIC SOLUTIONS

	Increase Duration	Decrease Blood Levels (%)
Peripheral nerve block		
Lidocaine	++	20–30
Mepivacaine	++	20–30
Bupivacaine	++	10–20
Ropivacaine	—	0
Epidural		
Chloroprocaine	++	
Lidocaine	++	20–30
Mepivacaine	++	20–30
Bupivacaine	++	10–20
Levobupivacaine	—	0
Ropivacaine	—	0
Spinal*		
Lidocaine	++	
Tetracaine	++	
Bupivacaine	++	

* epinephrine dose, 0.2 mg

maintains the drug concentration in the vicinity of the nerve fibers to be anesthetized (Table 7-2). The impact of adding epinephrine to the local anesthetic solution is influenced by the specific local anesthetic selected and the level of sensory blockade required if a spinal or epidural anesthetic is chosen. The α-adrenergic effects of epinephrine may be associated with some degree of analgesia that could contribute to the effects of the conduction blockade. The addition of epinephrine to local anesthetic solutions has little, if any, effect on the onset rate of local anesthesia.

The decreased systemic absorption of local anesthetic due to the vasoconstriction produced by epinephrine increases the likelihood that the metabolism rate will match that of absorption, thus decreasing the possibility of systemic toxicity. Whenever local anesthetic solutions containing epinephrine are administered in the presence of inhaled anesthetics, the possibility of enhanced cardiac irritability should be considered. The systemic absorption of epinephrine may accentuate systemic hypertension in vulnerable patients.

Combinations of Local Anesthetics

Local anesthetics may be combined in an effort to produce a rapid onset (chloroprocaine) and prolonged duration (bupivacaine) of action. Tachyphylaxis to the local anesthetic mixture could also reflect local acidosis due to the low pH level of the bathing solution. The toxicity of combinations of local anesthetic drugs is additive rather than synergistic.

SIDE EFFECTS

The principal side effects related to the use of local anesthetics are allergic reactions and systemic toxicity due to excessive plasma and tissue concentrations of the local anesthetic.

Allergic Reactions

Allergic reactions to local anesthetics are rare despite the frequent use of these drugs (it is estimated that less than 1% of all adverse reactions to local anesthetics are due to an allergic mechanism). The overwhelming majority of adverse responses that are often attributed to an allergic reaction are instead manifestations of excess plasma concentrations of the local anesthetic. The ester local anesthetics that produce metabolites related to para-aminobenzoic acid are more likely to evoke an allergic reaction than are amide local anesthetics, which are not metabolized to para-aminobenzoic acid. An allergic reaction after the use of a local anesthetic may be due to the methylparaben or similar substances used as preservatives in commercial preparations of ester and amide local anesthetics. An allergic reaction may reflect prior stimulation of antibody production by the preservative and not a reaction to the local anesthetic.

Cross-Sensitivity

Cross-sensitivity between local anesthetics reflects the common metabolite para-aminobenzoic acid. A similar cross-sensitivity, however, does not exist between classes of local anesthetics. Therefore, a patient with a known allergy to an ester local anesthetic can receive an amide local anesthetic without an increased risk of an allergic reaction. It is important that the "safe" local anesthetic be preservative-free.

Documentation of Allergy

The documentation of allergy to a local anesthetic is based on the clinical history and perhaps the use of intradermal testing. The occurrence of rash, urticaria, and laryngeal edema, with or without hypotension and bronchospasm, is highly suggestive of a local anesthetic–induced allergic reaction. Conversely, hypotension associated with syncope or tachycardia when an epinephrine-containing local anesthetic solution is administered suggests an accidental intravascular injection of drug. The use of an intradermal test requires the injection of preservative-free preparations of local anesthetic solutions to eliminate the possibility that the allergic reaction was caused by a substance other than the local anesthetic.

Systemic Toxicity

Systemic toxicity from a local anesthetic is due to an excess plasma concentration of the drug. Plasma concentrations of local anesthetics are determined by the rate of drug entrance into the systemic circulation, relative to their redistribution to inactive tissue sites and clearance by metabolism. Accidental direct intravascular injection of local anesthetic solutions during the performance of peripheral nerve block anesthesia or epidural anesthesia is the most common mechanism for the production of excess plasma concentrations of local anesthetics. Less often, excess plasma concentrations of local anesthetics result from the absorption of the local anesthetic from the injection site.

Central Nervous System (Table 7-3)

Low plasma concentrations of local anesthetics are likely to produce numbness of the tongue and circumoral tissues, presumably reflecting the delivery of drug to these highly vascular tissues. As the plasma concentrations continue to increase, local anesthetics readily cross the blood-brain barrier and produce a predictable pattern of central nervous system (CNS) changes (skeletal muscle twitching signals the imminence of tonic-clonic seizures). Seizures are classically followed by CNS depression, which may be accompanied

TABLE 7-3.
DOSE-DEPENDENT EFFECTS OF LIDOCAINE

Plasma Lidocaine Concentration (μg/mL)	Effect
1–5	Analgesia
5–10	Circumoral numbness Tinnitus Skeletal muscle twitching Systemic hypotension Myocardial depression
10–15	Seizures Unconsciousness
15–25	Apnea Coma
>25	Cardiovascular depression

by hypotension and apnea. An inverse relationship exists between the $Paco_2$ level and seizure thresholds of local anesthetics, presumably reflecting variations in cerebral blood flow and the resultant delivery of drugs to the brain. Increases in the serum potassium concentration can facilitate depolarization and thus markedly increase local anesthetic toxicity. Conversely, hypokalemia, by creating hyperpolarization, can greatly decrease local anesthetic toxicity.

Treatment of Seizures

The treatment of local anesthetic–induced seizures includes ventilation of the patient's lungs with oxygen, because arterial hypoxemia and metabolic acidosis occur within seconds. The intravenous administration of a benzodiazepine, such as midazolam or diazepam, is effective in suppressing local anesthetic–induced seizures.

Neurotoxicity

Neurotoxicity from the placement of local anesthetic–containing solutions (especially lidocaine) into the epidural or subarachnoid space is an increasingly recognized phenomenon (transient neurologic symptoms). Symptoms of neurotoxicity may be erroneously attributed to myoskeletal discomfort secondary to positioning. Likewise, myofascial pain may be erroneously diagnosed as transient neurologic symptoms after the intrathecal placement of local anesthetics.

Transient Neurologic Symptoms

Transient neurologic symptoms manifest as moderate to severe pain in the lower back, buttocks, and posterior thighs that appears within 6 to 36 hours after complete recovery from uneventful single-shot spinal anesthesia. Sensory and motor neurologic examination is not abnormal and relief of pain with trigger point injections and nonsteroidal anti-inflammatory drugs suggests a musculoskeletal component. In some patients, the pain is sufficiently intense to require treatment with opioids. Full recovery from transient neurologic symptoms usually occurs within

1 to 7 days. The incidence of transient neurologic symptoms is not altered by decreasing spinal lidocaine concentrations from 2% to 1% or 0.5% and are similar to the incidence of symptoms described with 5% lidocaine. Spinal anesthesia produced with 0.5% bupivacaine or 0.5% tetracaine is associated with a lower incidence of transient neurologic symptoms compared with lidocaine.

Cauda Equina Syndrome

Cauda equina syndrome occurs when diffuse injury across the lumbosacral plexus produces varying degrees of (a) sensory anesthesia, (b) bowel and bladder sphincter dysfunction, and (c) paraplegia.

Anterior Spinal Artery Syndrome

Anterior spinal artery syndrome consists of lower-extremity paresis with a variable sensory deficit that is usually diagnosed as the neural blockade resolves. The etiology of this syndrome is uncertain, although thrombosis or spasm of the anterior spinal artery is possible, and the effects of hypotension or vasoconstrictor drugs effects also have been postulated. It may be difficult to distinguish symptoms due to anterior spinal artery syndrome from those caused by spinal cord compression produced by an epidural abscess or hematoma.

Cardiovascular System

The cardiovascular system is more resistant than the CNS to the toxic effects of high plasma concentrations of local anesthetics. Nevertheless, plasma lidocaine concentrations of 5 to 10 μg/mL and equivalent plasma concentrations of other local anesthetics may produce profound hypotension due to a relaxation of arteriolar vascular smooth muscle and direct myocardial depression (see Table 7-3).

Selective Cardiac Toxicity

The accidental intravenous injection of bupivacaine may result in precipitous hypotension, cardiac dysrhythmias,

TABLE 7-4.
ANIMALS MANIFESTING ADVERSE CARDIAC CHANGES AFTER ADMINISTRATION OF BUPIVACAINE OR LIDOCAINE

Cardiac Change	Bupivacaine (% of Animals)	Lidocaine (% of Animals)
Sinus tachycardia	0	100
Supraventricular tachycardia	60	9
Atrioventricular heart block	60	0
Ventricular tachycardia	80	0
Premature ventricular contractions	100	0
Wide QRS complexes	100	0
ST-T wave changes	60	40

and atrioventricular heart block (Table 7-4). Pregnancy may increase sensitivity to the cardiotoxic effects of bupivacaine, but not ropivacaine. All local anesthetics depress the maximal depolarization rate of the cardiac action potential (V_{max}) by virtue of their ability to inhibit sodium ion influx via sodium channels (bupivacaine depresses V_{max} considerably more than lidocaine, whereas ropivacaine is intermediate in its depressant effect on V_{max}). During diastole, highly lipid soluble bupivacaine dissociates from sodium ion channels at a slow rate when compared with lidocaine, thus accounting for the drug's persistent depressant effect on V_{max} and subsequent cardiac toxicity. At normal heart rates, diastolic time is sufficiently long for lidocaine dissociation, but bupivacaine block intensifies and depresses electrical conduction, causing reentrant-type ventricular dysrhythmias. Less lipid-soluble lidocaine dissociates rapidly from cardiac sodium channels, and cardiac toxicity is low. Ropivacaine is a pure S-enantiomer that is less lipid soluble and less cardiotoxic than bupivacaine but more cardiotoxic than lidocaine.

Methemoglobinemia

Methemoglobinemia is a rare but potentially life-threatening complication (decreased oxygen carrying capacity) that may follow the administration of certain drugs or chemicals that cause the oxidation of hemoglobin to methemoglobin more rapidly than methemoglobin is reduced to hemoglobin. Known oxidant substances include topical local anesthetics (prilocaine, benzocaine, Cetacaine®, lidocaine), nitroglycerin, phenytoin, and sulfonamides. The presence of methemoglobinemia is suggested by a difference between the calculated and measured arterial oxygen saturation. The diagnosis is confirmed by qualitative measurements of methemoglobin by co-oximetry. Methemoglobinemia is readily reversed through the administration of methylene blue, 1 to 2 mg/kg IV, over 5 minutes (total dose should not exceed 7 to 8 mg/kg).

Ventilatory Response to Hypoxia

Lidocaine at clinically useful plasma concentrations depresses the ventilatory responses to arterial hypoxemia.

Hepatotoxicity

Hepatic dysfunction following the administration of bupivacaine seems most likely to represent an allergic reaction.

Dysphoria

Vivid fear of imminent death and a delusional belief of having died have been described in patients experiencing toxic reactions to local anesthetics administered for regional anesthesia and pain relief.

USES OF LOCAL ANESTHETICS (TABLE 7-5)

Regional Anesthesia

Regional anesthesia is classified according to the following six sites of placement of the local anesthetic solution:

(a) topical or surface anesthesia, (b) local infiltration, (c) peripheral nerve block, (d) intervenous regional anesthesia (Bier block), (e) epidural anesthesia, and (f) spinal (subarachnoid) anesthesia.

Topical Anesthesia

Local anesthetics are used to produce topical anesthesia by placement on the mucous membranes of the nose, mouth, tracheobronchial tree, esophagus, or genitourinary tract. Nebulized lidocaine is used to produce surface anesthesia of the upper and lower respiratory tract before fiberoptic laryngoscopy and/or bronchoscopy. Local anesthetics are absorbed into the systemic circulation after topical application to mucous membranes. Systemic absorption of tetracaine, and to a lesser extent lidocaine, after placement on the tracheobronchial mucosa produces plasma concentrations similar to those present after an intravenous injection of the local anesthetic.

Eutectic Mixtures of Local Anesthetics

An eutectic mixture of local anesthetics (EMLA) is effective in relieving the pain of venipuncture, arterial cannulation, lumbar puncture, and myringotomy in children and adults. EMLA cream is not recommended for use on mucous membranes because lidocaine and prilocaine is absorbed faster through mucous membranes than through intact skin.

Other Topically Effective Local Anesthetics

Dyclonine (0.5% to 1.0%), *hexylcaine*, and *piperocaine* are effective for producing topical anesthesia of the mucous membranes (onset is 2 to 10 minutes and duration is 20 to 30 minutes), as required before direct laryngoscopy.

Local Infiltration Anesthesia

Local infiltration anesthesia involves the extravascular placement of local anesthetic in the area to be anesthetized (placement of an intravascular cannula). Lidocaine is the

TABLE 7-5. CLINICAL USES OF LOCAL ANESTHETICS

	Clinical Use	Concentration	Onset	Duration (min)	Recommended Maximum Single Dose (mg)
Lidocaine	Topical	4	Fast	30–60	300
	Infiltration	0.5–1	Fast	60–240	300 or 500 with epinephrine
	IVRA	0.25–0.5	Fast	30–60	300
	PNB	1–1.5	Fast	60–180	300 or 500 with epinephrine
	Epidural	1.5–2	Fast	60–120	300 or 500 with epinephrine
	Spinal	1.5–5	Fast	30–60	100
Mepivacaine	Infiltration	0.5–1	Fast	60–240	400 or 500 with epinephrine
	PNB	1–1.5	Fast	120–240	400 or 500 with epinephrine
	Epidural	1.5–2	Fast	60–180	400 or 500 with epinephrine
	Spinal	2–4	Fast	60–120	100
Etidocaine	Infiltration	0.5	Fast	120–480	300 or 400 with epinephrine
	PNB	0.5–1	Fast	180–720	300 or 400 with epinephrine
	Epidural	1–1.5	Fast	120–480	300 or 400 with epinephrine
Prilocaine	Infiltration	0.5–1	Fast	60–120	600
	IVRA	0.25–0.5	Fast	30–60	600
	PNB	1.5–2	Fast	90–180	600
	Epidural	2–3	Fast	60–180	600

Bupivacaine	Infiltration	0.25	Fast	120–480	175 or 225 with epinephrine
	PNB	0.25–0.5	Slow	240–960	175 or 225 with epinephrine
	Epidural	0.5–0.75	Moderate	120–300	175 or 225 with epinephrine
	Spinal	0.5–0.75	Fast	60–240	20
Levobupivacaine	Infiltration	0.25	Fast	120–480	150
	PNB	0.25–0.5	Slow	840–1020	150
	Epidural	0.5–0.75	Moderate	300–540	150
	Spinal	0.5–0.75	Fast	60–360	20
Ropivacaine	Infiltration	0.2–0.5	Fast	120–360	200
	PNB	0.5–1	Slow	300–480	250
	Epidural	0.5–1	Moderate	120–360	200
	Spinal?				
Chloroprocaine	Infiltration	1	Fast	30–60	800 or 1000 with epinephrine
	PNB	2	Fast	30–60	800 or 1000 with epinephrine
	Epidural	2–3	Fast	30–60	800 or 1000 with epinephrine
	Spinal	2–3	Fast	30–60	Preservative free*
Procaine	Spinal	10	Fast	30–60	1000
Tetracaine	Topical	2	Fast	30–60	20
	Spinal	0.5	Fast	120–360	20
Benzocaine	Topical	Up to 20%	Fast	30–60	200
Cocaine	Topical	4–10	Fast	30–60	150

*Off label use.

local anesthetic most often selected for infiltration anesthesia. Epinephrine-containing drugs should not be injected intracutaneously or into tissues supplied by end-arteries (fingers, ears, nose) because the resulting vasoconstriction can produce ischemia and even gangrene.

Peripheral Nerve Block Anesthesia

Peripheral nerve block anesthesia is achieved through the injection of local anesthetic solutions into tissues surrounding individual peripheral nerves or nerve plexuses, such as the brachial plexus. When local anesthetic solutions are deposited in the vicinity of a peripheral nerve, they diffuse from the outer surface (mantle) toward the center (core) of the nerve along a concentration gradient. Consequently, nerve fibers located in the mantle of the mixed nerve are anesthetized first. These mantle fibers usually are distributed to more proximal anatomical structures, in contrast to distal structures innervated by nerve fibers near the core of the nerve. This explains the initial development of anesthesia proximally, with subsequent distal spread as local anesthetic solution diffuses to reach more central core nerve fibers. Conversely, the recovery of sensation occurs in a reverse direction; nerve fibers in the mantle that are exposed to extraneural fluid are the first to lose local anesthetic, so that sensation returns initially to the proximal and last to the distal parts of the limb. The rapidity of onset of sensory anesthesia after the injection of a local anesthetic solution into tissues around a peripheral nerve depends on the pK level of the drug (amount of local anesthetic that exists in the active nonionized form at the pH level of the tissue) (see Table 7-1). The duration of action is prolonged by adding epinephrine to the local anesthetic solution.

Intravenous Regional Anesthesia (Bier Block)

The intravenous injection of a local anesthetic solution into an extremity isolated from the rest of the systemic circulation by a tourniquet produces a rapid onset of anesthesia and skeletal muscle relaxation. The duration of anesthesia is independent of the specific local anesthetic and is determined by how long the tourniquet is kept inflated. The mechanism by which local anesthetics produce intravenous regional anesthesia is unknown but probably reflects the action of the drug on nerve endings as well as nerve trunks. Normal sensation and skeletal muscle tone return promptly on release of the tourniquet, which allows blood flow to dilute the concentration of local anesthetic. Bupivacaine is not recommended for intravenous regional anesthesia, considering its greater likelihood than other local anesthetics for producing cardiotoxicity when the tourniquet is deflated at the conclusion of the anesthetic.

Epidural Anesthesia

Local anesthetic solutions placed in the epidural or sacral caudal space produce epidural anesthesia by diffusion across the dura to act on nerve roots and passage into the paravertebral area through the intervertebral foramina, thus producing multiple paravertebral nerve blocks. Despite a reasonable safety profile, bupivacaine is being replaced by levobupivacaine and ropivacaine for the production of epidural anesthesia, because these local anesthetics are associated with less risk for cardiac and CNS toxicity and are also less likely to result in unwanted postoperative motor blockade. In contrast to spinal anesthesia, during epidural anesthesia, often a zone of differential sympathetic nervous system blockade does not exist, and the zone of differential motor blockade may average up to four rather than two segments below the sensory level. Another difference from spinal anesthesia is the larger dose required to produce epidural anesthesia, leading to a substantial systemic absorption of the local anesthetic. The addition of 1:200,000 epinephrine solution decreases the systemic absorption of the local anesthetic by approximately one-third. Systemic absorption of epinephrine produces β-adrenergic stimulation, characterized by peripheral vasodilation and with resultant decreases in systemic blood pressure, even though cardiac output is increased by the inotropic and chronotropic effects of epinephrine. The addition of opioids to local anesthetic solutions placed in the epidural or intrathecal space results in synergistic analgesia. Combining local anesthetics and opioids for peripheral nerve blocks appears to be ineffective in altering the characteristics or results of the block.

Spinal Anesthesia

Spinal anesthesia is produced by the injection of local anesthetic solutions into the lumbar subarachnoid space. Local anesthetic solutions placed into lumbar cerebrospinal fluid act on superficial layers of the spinal cord, but the principal site of action is the preganglionic fibers as they leave the spinal cord in the anterior rami. Because preganglionic sympathetic nervous system fibers are blocked by concentrations of local anesthetics that are insufficient to affect sensory or motor fibers, the level of sympathetic nervous system denervation during spinal anesthesia extends approximately two spinal segments cephalad to the level of sensory anesthesia. For the same reasons, the level of motor anesthesia averages two segments below sensory anesthesia. Dosages of local anesthetics used for spinal anesthesia vary according to the (a) height of the patient, which determines the volume of the subarachnoid space, (b) segmental level of anesthesia desired, and (c) duration of anesthesia desired. The total dose of local anesthetic administered for spinal anesthesia is more important than the concentration of drug or the volume of the solution injected. Tetracaine, lidocaine, bupivacaine, ropivacaine, and levobupivacaine are the local anesthetics most likely to be administered for spinal anesthesia. The specific gravity of local anesthetic solutions injected into the lumbar cerebrospinal fluid is important in determining spread of the drugs. The addition of glucose to local anesthetic solutions increases the specific gravity of local anesthetic solutions above that of cerebrospinal fluid (hyperbaric). The addition of distilled water lowers the specific gravity of local anesthetic solutions below that of cerebrospinal fluid (hypobaric).

Physiologic Effects

The physiologic effects of spinal anesthesia reflect the accompanying level of sympathetic nervous system blockade, because plasma concentrations of local anesthetics after subarachnoid injection are too low to produce physiologic changes.

Cardiac Arrest

Cardiac arrest may accompany the hypotension and bradycardia associated with spinal anesthesia. Even when epinephrine is promptly administered, patients may be refractory to treatment because local anesthetic-induced sympathetic nervous system blockade, which decreases circulating blood volume, may also cause a defective neuroendocrine response to stress. The physiologic effect of spinal anesthesia on venous return emphasizes the risk of systemic hypotension if this technique is instituted in hypovolemic patients.

Apnea

Apnea that occurs with an excessive level of spinal anesthesia probably reflects the ischemic paralysis of the medullary ventilatory centers due to profound hypotension and associated decreases in cerebral blood flow. Concentrations of local anesthetics in ventricular cerebrospinal fluid are usually too low to produce pharmacologic effects on the ventilatory centers. Rarely is the cause of apnea due to phrenic nerve paralysis.

Analgesia

The administration of intravenous local anesthetics (lidocaine, procaine) for the production of analgesia is limited by the small margin of safety between intravenous analgesic doses and those that produce systemic toxicity.

Suppression of Ventricular Cardiac Dysrhythmias

In addition to suppressing ventricular cardiac dysrhythmias, the intravenous administration of lidocaine may increase the defibrillation threshold.

Suppression of Generalized Tonic-Clonic Seizures

Generalized tonic-clonic (grand mal) seizures have been suppressed by the intravenous administration of low doses of lidocaine or mepivacaine.

Anti-inflammatory Effects

Local anesthetics modulate inflammatory responses and may be useful in mitigating perioperative inflammatory injury. The beneficial effects attributed to epidural anesthesia (pain relief, decreased thrombosis from hypercoagulability) may reflect the anti-inflammatory effects of local anesthetics.

Local anesthetics may modulate inflammatory responses by inhibiting inflammatory mediator signaling. In addition, local anesthetics inhibit neutrophil accumulation at sites of inflammation and impair free radical and mediator release.

Bronchodilation

Inhaled lidocaine and ropivacaine attenuate histamine-induced bronchospasm and induce airway anesthesia (which reflects topical airway anesthesia).

Tumescent Liposuction

The tumescent technique for liposuction characterizes the subcutaneous infiltration of large volumes (5 or more liters) of solution containing highly diluted lidocaine (0.05% to 0.10%) with epinephrine (1:100,000). When highly diluted lidocaine solutions are administered for tumescent liposuction, the dose of lidocaine may range from 35 mg/kg to 55 mg/kg ("mega-dose lidocaine"). Despite the popularity and presumed safety of tumescent liposuction, reports exist of increased mortality associated with this technique, due to lidocaine toxicity or local anesthetic–induced depression of cardiac conduction and contractility.

COCAINE TOXICITY

Cocaine produces sympathetic nervous system stimulation by blocking the presynaptic uptake of norepinephrine

TABLE 7-6.
ADVERSE PHYSIOLOGIC EFFECTS OF COCAINE

Coronary vasospasm
Myocardial ischemia
Myocardial infarction
Ventricular cardiac dysrhythmias (ventricular fibrillation)
Hypertension and tachycardia (increased myocardial oxygen requirements)
Dose dependent decreases in uterine blood flow (fetal hypoxemia)

and dopamine, thus increasing their postsynaptic concentrations.

Pharmacokinetics

Peak venous plasma concentrations of cocaine are achieved at approximately 30 to 40 minutes after intranasal administration and approximately 5 minutes after intravenous and smoked cocaine administration. The maximum physiologic effects of intranasal cocaine occur within 15 to 40 minutes, and the maximum subjective effects occur within 10 to 20 minutes. The duration of effects is approximately 60 minutes or longer after peak effects.

Adverse Physiologic Effects (Table 7-6)

Treatment (Table 7-7)

TABLE 7-7.
TREATMENT OF COCAINE TOXICITY

Nitroglycerin
Esmolol (β-blockade may accentuate coronary artery vasospasm)
Nitroprusside
α-Adrenergic blocking drugs
Benzodiazepine (control seizures)

8

Neuromuscular-Blocking Drugs

The principal pharmacologic effect of neuromuscular-blocking drugs is to interrupt the transmission of nerve impulses at the neuromuscular junction (NMJ) (Stoelting RK, Hillier SC. Neuromuscular-blocking drugs. In: *Pharmacology and Physiology in Anesthetic Practice*, 4th ed. Philadelphia. Lippincott Williams & Wilkins, 2006: 208–250). On the basis of distinct electrophysiologic differences in their mechanisms of action and duration of action, these drugs can be classified as *depolarizing* neuromuscular-blocking drugs (mimic the actions of acetylcholine) and *nondepolarizing* neuromuscular-blocking drugs (interfere with the actions of acetylcholine). These are further subdivided into long-, intermediate, and short-acting drugs (Table 8-1 and Fig. 8-1). Neuromuscular-blocking drugs are either benzylisoquinolinium compounds or aminosteroid compounds (see Table 8-1). Neuromuscular-blocking drugs produce phase I depolarizing neuromuscular blockade, phase II depolarizing neuromuscular blockade, or nondepolarizing neuromuscular blockade.

PHARMACODYNAMICS

The pharmacodynamics of neuromuscular-blocking drugs are determined by measuring the speed of onset and duration of neuromuscular blockade (Fig. 8-2). Equal potency between neuromuscular-blocking drugs

TABLE 8-1.
CLASSIFICATION OF NEUROMUSCULAR-BLOCKING DRUGS

Clinical Classification	Chemical Classification
Depolarizers	
Succinylcholine	
Nondepolarizers	
Long-acting	
Pancuronium	Aminosteroid
Doxacurium	Aminosteroid
Pipecuronium	Aminosteroid
Intermediate-acting	
Atracurium	Benzylisoquinoline
Vecuronium	Aminosteroid
Rocuronium	Aminosteroid
Cisatracurium	Benzylisoquinoline
Short-acting	
Mivacurium	Benzylisoquinoline

is determined by measuring the dose needed to produce 95% suppression of the single twitch response (ED_{95}) (Table 8-2). The onset of neuromuscular blockade after the administration of a nondepolarizing neuromuscular blocking drug is more rapid but less intense at the laryngeal muscles (vocal cords) than the peripheral muscles (adductor pollicis). With intermediate- and short-acting nondepolarizing neuromuscular-blocking drugs, the period of laryngeal paralysis is brief and may be dissipating before a maximum effect is reached at the adductor pollicis. It is important to recognize that the dose of neuromuscular-blocking drug necessary to produce a given degree of neuromuscular blockade at the diaphragm is about twice the dose required to produce a similar blockade of the adductor pollicis muscle.

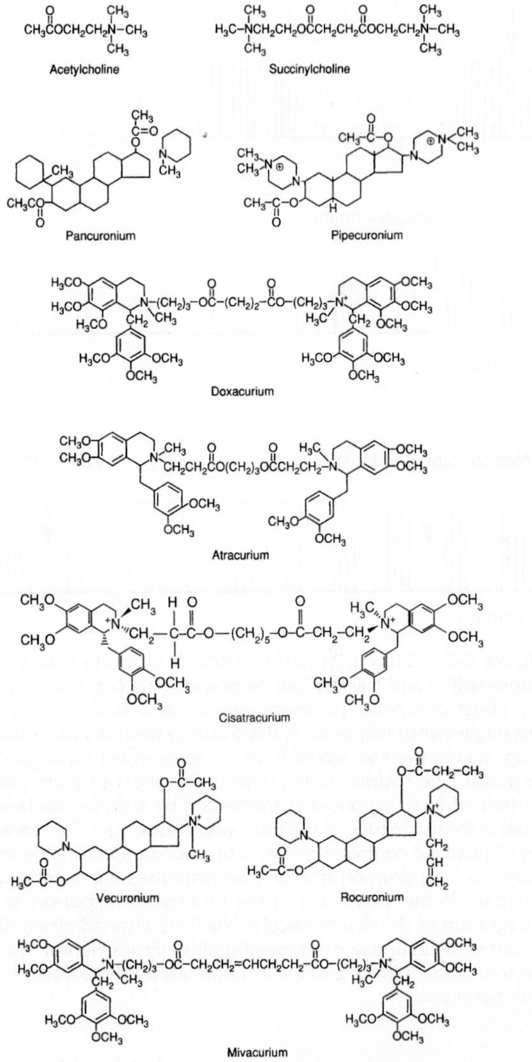

Acetylcholine

Succinylcholine

Pancuronium

Pipecuronium

Doxacurium

Atracurium

Cisatracurium

Vecuronium

Rocuronium

Mivacurium

Figure 8-1. Acetylcholine and neuromuscular-blocking drugs.

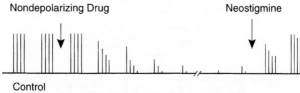

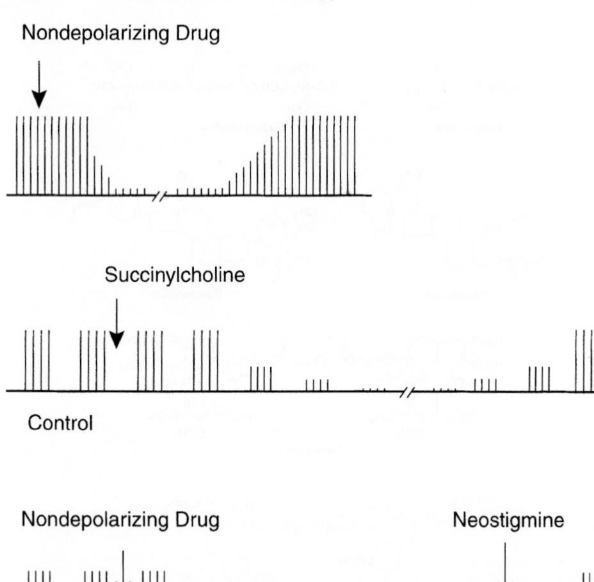

Figure 8-2. Effects of neuromuscular blocking-drugs on the single-twitch and train-of-four responses. The top tracing depicts the effect of a nondepolarizing neuromuscular-blocking drug on the single-twitch response. A depolarizing neuromuscular-blocking drug (succinylcholine) would have the same effect on single-twitch response. The middle tracing depicts the effect of succinylcholine on train-of-four responses characterized by a similar decrease (no fade) in the magnitude of the four-twitch responses. The lower tracing depicts the contrasting effects of a nondepolarizing neuromuscular-blocking drug on train-of-four responses characterized by a decrease in the magnitude of the four-twitch responses and the antagonism of the neuromuscular blockade after administration of an anticholinesterase drug neostigmine. (From Hunter JM. New neuromuscular blocking drugs. *N Engl J Med* 1996;332:1691–1699; with permission.)

TABLE 8-2.
DESCRIPTORS OF THE CLINICAL EFFECTS OF NEUROMUSCULAR BLOCKING DRUGS (SEE FIG. 8-2)

Potency	Effective dose (ED) necessary to depress single twitch depression 95% (ED95)
Onset	Time from injection to onset of maximal single twitch depression
Duration of Action	Time from injection to return of single twitch height to 25% or 95%
Recovery Index	Time from 25% return of single twitch heights to 75% return of single twitch height
Clinical Duration	Time from injection to recovery of the train-of-four ratio to ≥0.7 or ≥0.9

PHARMACOKINETICS (TABLE 8-3)

Neuromuscular-blocking drugs, because of their quaternary ammonium groups, are highly ionized, water-soluble compounds at physiologic pH and they possess limited lipid solubility. As a result of these two characteristics, the volume of distribution (Vd) of these drugs is limited, similar to the extracellular fluid volume. In addition, neuromuscular-blocking drugs cannot easily cross lipid membrane barriers such as the blood-brain barrier, renal tubular epithelium, gastrointestinal epithelium, or placenta. Therefore, neuromuscular-blocking drugs do not produce central nervous system (CNS) effects, renal tubular reabsorption is minimal, oral absorption is ineffective, and maternal administration does not affect the fetus.

HISTORY

The first use of d-tubocurarine (dTc) to produce surgical skeletal muscle relaxation during general anesthesia was

TABLE 8-3.

COMPARATIVE PHARMACOLOGY OF NONDEPOLARIZING NEUROMUSCULAR BLOCKING DRUG

	ED_{95} (mg/kg)	Intubating Dose (mg/kg)	Onset to Maximum Twitch Depression (min)	Duration to Return to ≥25% Control Twitch Height	Duration to Return to Train-of-Four >0.9 (min)	Continuous Infusion (μg/kg/min)
Pancuronium	0.06–0.07	0.1	3–5	60–90	130–220	
Doxacurium	0.03	0.05–0.08	4–6	60–90		
Pipecuronium	0.05–0.06	0.14	3–5	60–90		
Atracurium	0.25	0.4–0.5	3–5	20–35	55–80	4–12
Vecuronium	0.05–0.06	0.08–0.1	3–5	20–35	50–80	1
Rocuronium	0.3	0.6–1.2	1–2	20–35	55–80	3–12
Cisatracurium	0.05	0.1	3–5	20–35	60–90	0.4–4
Mivacurium	0.08	0.25	2–3	12–20	25–40	3–15

	Volume of Distribution (liters/kg)	Clearance (ml/kg/min)	Renal Excretion (% Unchanged)	Biliary Excretion (% Unchanged)	Hepatic Degradation (%)	Hydrolysis in Plasma
Pancuronium	0.26	1.8	80	5–10	10	No
Doxacurium	0.22	2.7	70	30	?	No
Pipecuronium	0.35	3.0	70	20	10	No
Atracurium	0.2	5.5	10	NS	?	Yes*
Vecuronium	0.27	5.2	15–25	40–75	20–30	No
Rocuronium	0.3	4.0	10–25	50–70	10–20	No
Cisatracurium	0.2	4.7–5.3	NS	NS	0	No*
Mivacurium			<10	NS	0	Yes

(continued)

TABLE 8-3.
(continued)

	Degradation Dependent on Body Temperature	Degradation Dependent on Blood pH	Elimination Dependent on Renal Function	Elimination Dependent on Hepatic Function	Elimination Half-Time (min)		
					Normal	Kidney Failure	Hepatic Failure
Pancuronium	Yes		Yes	Modest	132	240–1050	208–270
Doxacurium	Yes		Yes	No			
Pipecuronium	Yes		Yes	No			
Atracurium	Yes	Yes	No	No	21	18-25	20–25
Vecuronium	Yes	No	Yes	Yes	50–110	80–150	49–198
Rocuronium	Yes	No	Yes	Yes	87	97	97
Cisatracurium	Yes	Yes	No	No	22–30	25–34	21
Mivacurium	Yes	?	?	?	1–3		

NS, not significant.
*Also undergoes chemodegradation (Hofmann elimination).

reported in 1942. In 1906, the use of curarized animals in experiments to determine the parasympathomimetic effects of succinylcholine (SCh) masked the neuromuscular-blocking properties of this drug. It was not until 1949 that the neuromuscular-blocking effects of SCh were recognized.

CLINICAL USES

The principal uses of neuromuscular-blocking drugs are to provide skeletal muscle relaxation to facilitate tracheal intubation and to improve surgical working conditions during general anesthesia. A $2 \times ED_{95}$ dose of the nondepolarizing muscle relaxant is often recommended to facilitate tracheal intubation, whereas 90% suppression of single-twitch response is usually considered clinical evidence of adequate drug-induced skeletal muscle relaxation to optimize surgical working conditions. Neuromuscular-blocking drugs lack CNS depressant and analgesic effects. Therefore, these drugs cannot be substituted for anesthetic drugs. Furthermore, ventilation of the lungs must be provided mechanically whenever substantial neuromuscular blockade is produced by these drugs. Clinically, the degree of neuromuscular blockade is typically evaluated by monitoring the evoked skeletal muscle responses produced by an electrical stimulus delivered percutaneously to the ulnar or facial nerves by a peripheral nerve stimulator (see Table 8-2).

Drug Selection

The choice between depolarizing and nondepolarizing neuromuscular-blocking drugs is influenced by the speed of onset, duration of action, and possibility of drug-induced side effects due to the actions of these drugs at sites other than the NMJ. Rocuronium is the only nondepolarizing neuromuscular-blocking drug that mimics the rapid onset of SCh, but its duration of action is prolonged.

Sequence of Onset of Neuromuscular Blockade

Neuromuscular-blocking drugs affect small, rapidly moving muscles, such as those of the eyes and digits, before those of the trunk and abdomen. Ultimately, intercostal muscles and, finally, the diaphragm are paralyzed. The recovery of skeletal muscles usually occurs in the reverse order to that of paralysis, so that the diaphragm is the first to regain normal function. Relaxation of the small muscles of the middle ear improves acuity of hearing. Consciousness and sensorium remain undisturbed even in the presence of complete neuromuscular blockade.

STRUCTURE–ACTIVITY RELATIONSHIPS

Neuromuscular-blocking drugs are quaternary ammonium compounds that have at least one positively charged nitrogen atom that binds to the α-subunit of postsynaptic cholinergic receptors (see Fig. 8-1). In addition, these drugs have structural similarities to the endogenous neurotransmitter acetylcholine (succinylcholine is two molecules of acetylcholine linked through acetate methyl groups) (see Fig. 8-1). Pancuronium is the aminosteroid neuromuscular-blocking drug most closely related structurally to acetylcholine. The acetylcholine-like fragments of pancuronium give the steroidal molecule its high degree of neuromuscular-blocking activity and its plasma cholinesterase inhibiting action. Vecuronium and rocuronium are monoquaternary analogs of the bisquaternary nondepolarizing neuromuscular-blocking drug pancuronium. Aminosteroid neuromuscular-blocking drugs lack hormonal activity. Benzylisoquinolinium derivatives are more likely to evoke the release of histamine, compared with aminosteroid derivatives, presumably reflecting the presence of a tertiary amine.

NEUROMUSCULAR JUNCTION

The neuromuscular junction (NMJ) consists of a prejunctional motor nerve ending separated from a highly folded postjunctional membrane of the skeletal muscle fiber by a synaptic cleft that is 20 to 30 nm wide and filled with extracellular fluid (Fig. 8-3). The resting transmembrane potential of approximately −90 mv across nerve and skeletal muscle membranes is maintained by the unequal distribution of potassium and sodium ions across the

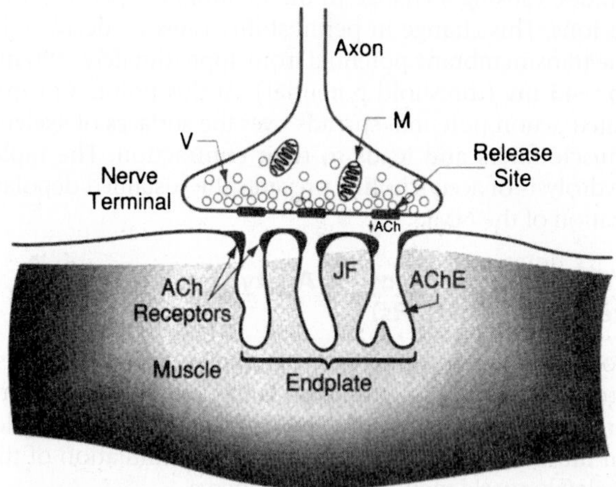

Figure 8-3. Schematic depiction of the neuromuscular junction. Acetylcholine (ACh) is present in vesicles (V) of the axon for release in response to nerve impulses. The neurotransmitter diffuses across the synaptic cleft to attach to receptors that are concentrated on the junctional folds (JF) of the skeletal muscle end-plate. Acetylcholinesterase (AChE) is present in the JF to facilitate rapid hydrolysis of ACh. (From Drachman DA. Myasthenia gravis. *N Engl J Med* 1978;298:136–142; with permission.)

membrane. The NMJ contains three types of nicotinic cholinergic receptors (nAChRs) designated as postsynaptic on the skeletal muscle surface (one junctional and the other extrajunctional) and presynaptic on the nerve ending. Extrajunctional receptors are not involved in normal neuromuscular transmission but may proliferate if the skeletal muscle is diseased, damaged, or denervated, thus altering the effect of neuromuscular-blocking drugs.

Acetylcholine

The neurotransmitter at the NMJ is the quaternary ammonium ester acetylcholine. The arrival of a nerve impulse causes the release of hundreds of quanta of acetylcholine that bind to α-subunits of nAChRs on postsynaptic membranes, causing a change in the membrane's permeability to ions. This change in permeability causes a decrease in the transmembrane potential from approximately −90 mv to −45 mv (threshold potential). At this point, a propagated action potential spreads over the surfaces of skeletal muscle fibers and leads to their contraction. The rapid hydrolysis of acetylcholine prevents the sustained depolarization of the NMJ.

Postjunctional Nicotinic Acetylcholine Receptors (nAChRs)

Postjunctional nicotinic acetylcholine receptors (nAChRs) are present in large numbers on postjunctional membranes. Extrajunctional nAChRs appear throughout skeletal muscles whenever there is deficient stimulation of the skeletal muscle membrane by the nerve.

Fetal Receptors

Fetal receptors oscillate between open (acetylcholine attached) and closed (acetylcholine dissociated) states.

Adult Receptors

Synapse maturation involves the gradual disappearance of fetal nAChRs from junctional and extrajunctional sites,

TABLE 8-4.
EVENTS ASSOCIATED WITH UP-REGULATION OR DOWN-REGULATION OF NICOTINIC ACETYLCHOLINE RECEPTORS

nAChR Up-Regulation	nAChR Down-Regulation
Spinal cord injury	Myasthenia gravis
Cerebral vascular accident	Anticholinesterase overdose
Thermal injury	Organophosphate poisoning
Prolonged immobility	
Prolonged exposure to neuromuscular-blocking drugs	
Multiple sclerosis	
Guillain-Barre syndrome	

nAChR; nicotinic acetylcholine receptor

and the formation of a motor nerve terminal with densely packed synaptic vesicles containing acetylcholine. Up-regulation and down-regulation of nAChRs occurs in response to physiologic, pathophysiologic, and pharmacologic stimulation (Table 8-4).

Structure and Function

The function of nAChR endplates depends on five subunit proteins that combine to form the pentameric unit. This pentameric unit consists of two α-subunits in association with single β-, δ-, and ε-subunits (Fig 8-4). These subunits form a transmembrane pore as well as the extracellular binding pockets for acetylcholine and other agonists (depolarizing neuromuscular-blocking drugs) or antagonists (nondepolarizing neuromuscular-blocking drugs). The two α-subunits, in addition to being the binding sites for acetylcholine, are the sites occupied by neuromuscular-blocking drugs. Nondepolarizing neuromuscular-blocking drugs bind to one or both α-subunits, but unlike acetylcholine, lack agonist activity (competitive blockade). Because SCh is not hydrolyzed

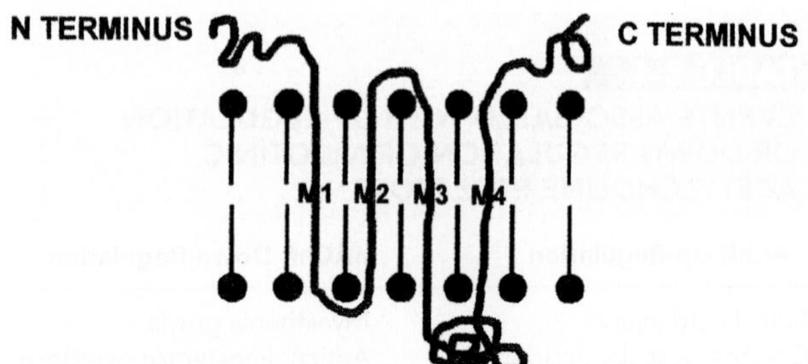

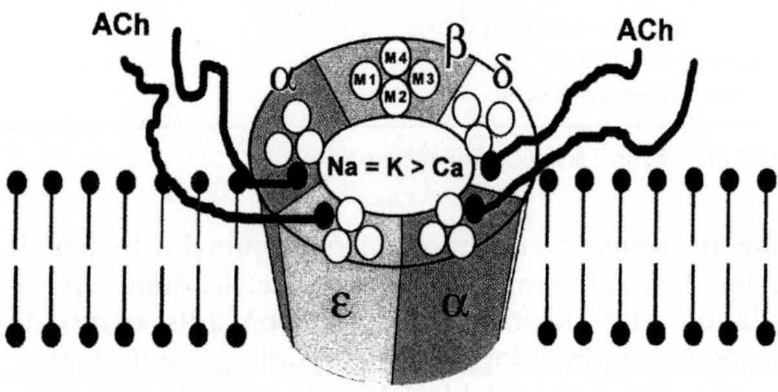

Figure 8-4. Subunit composition of the adult nicotinic acetylcholine receptor (nAChR) consisting of five (two α-, β-, δ-, ε-) protein subunits. Each subunit contains four helical domains (M1–M4), and the M2 domain forms the channel pore. A single α-subunit has its N and C termini on the extracellular surface of the membrane lipid bilayer (**Top**). Between the N and C termini, the α-subunit forms four helices (M1–M4) that span the membrane bilayer. The pentameric structure of the adult nAChR consists of the N termini of two α-subunits that form two distinct binding pockets for acetylcholine (**Bottom**). The ion channel has equal permeability for sodium and potassium ions, whereas calcium ion permeability contributes about 2.5% of the total permeability. (From Naguib M, Flood P, McArdle, et al. Advances in neurobiology of the neuromuscular junction: Implications for the anesthesiologist. *Anesthesiology* 2002;96:202–231; with permission).

by acetylcholinesterase, the channel remains open for a longer period than would be produced by acetylcholine and causes contractions known as *fasciculations*.

Extrajunctional nAChRs

Extrajunctional nAChRs normally are not present in large numbers, because their synthesis is suppressed by neural activity. Whenever motor nerves are less active, due to trauma or skeletal muscle denervation, these extrajunctional cholinergic receptors proliferate rapidly.

Prejunctional nAChRs

Prejunctional nAChRs on motor nerve endings influence the release of neurotransmitters.

DEPOLARIZING NEUROMUSCULAR-BLOCKING DRUGS

The only depolarizing neuromuscular-blocking drug in clinical use is SCh (see Fig. 8-1). SCh rapidly produces intense paralysis (30 to 60 s) and has a short duration of action (3 to 5 minutes). These characteristics make SCh a useful drug for providing skeletal muscle relaxation to facilitate the intubation of the trachea. SCh has several associated adverse effects that can limit or even contraindicate its use.

Dose

The traditional intravenous dose of SCh to facilitate tracheal intubation is 1 mg/kg. Conceptually, it is anticipated that administration of 1 mg/kg IV to a preoxygenated patient would be associated with the return of spontaneous breathing before arterial hypoxemia became significant. Considering the variability in response to SCh among patients, it is concluded that no single perfect intubating dose of SCh exists.

Mechanism of Action

SCh attaches to one or both of the α-subunits of nAChRs and mimics the action of acetylcholine (partial agonist), thus depolarizing the postjunctional membrane. Compared with acetylcholine, the hydrolysis of SCh is slow, resulting in sustained depolarization (opening) of the receptor ion channels. Neuromuscular blockade develops because a depolarized postjunctional membrane cannot respond to subsequent release of acetylcholine (depolarizing neuromuscular blockade). Depolarizing neuromuscular blockade is also referred to as *phase I blockade.* A single large intravenous dose of SCh (>2 mg/kg), repeated doses, or a prolonged continuous infusion of SCh may result in postjunctional membranes that do not respond normally to acetylcholine even when the postjunctional membranes have become repolarized (desensitization neuromuscular blockade). The mechanism for the development of desensitization neuromuscular blockade is unknown and, for this reason, designation as *phase II blockade,* which does not imply a mechanism, is the preferred terminology.

Characteristics of Phase I Blockade (Table 8-5)

Characteristics of Phase II Blockade

Electrically evoked mechanical responses, using a peripheral nerve stimulator, are characteristic of phase II blockade

TABLE 8-5.
CHARACTERISTICS OF PHASE I BLOCKADE

Decreased contraction in response to single twitch
Decreased amplitude but sustained response to continuous stimulation
Train-of-four ratio >0.7
Absence of posttetanic facilitation
Augmentation of neuromuscular blockade after administration of anticholinesterase drugs

and resemble those considered typical of the neuromuscular blockade produced by nondepolarizing neuromuscular-blocking drugs (see Fig. 8-2). When neuromuscular blockade is predominantly phase I, administering an anticholinesterase drug will enhance existing neuromuscular blockade. Conversely, an anticholinesterase drug will antagonize a predominant phase II blockade. If a small dose of edrophonium (0.1 to 0.2 mg/kg IV) improves neuromuscular transmission, it is likely that an additional dose of anticholinesterase drug will antagonize, rather than enhance, the neuromuscular blockade produced by SCh.

Duration of Action

The brief duration of action of SCh (3 to 5 minutes) is principally due to its hydrolysis by plasma cholinesterase (pseudocholinesterase) enzyme (Fig. 8-5). Plasma cholinesterase has an enormous capacity to hydrolyze SCh at a rapid rate so that only a small fraction of the original intravenous dose of drug actually reaches the NMJ. Because plasma cholinesterase is not present in significant amounts at the NMJ, the neuromuscular blockade produced by SCh is terminated by its diffusion away from the NMJ and into extracellular fluid. Therefore, plasma cholinesterase influences the duration of action of SCh by controlling the amount of neuromuscular-blocking drug that is hydrolyzed before reaching the NMJ.

Plasma Cholinesterase Activity

Decreases in the hepatic production of plasma cholines terase, drug-induced decreases in plasma cholinesterase activity, or the genetically determined presence of atypical plasma cholinesterase result in the slowed to absent hydrolysis of SCh and a corresponding prolongation of the neuromuscular blockade produced by the drug. Liver disease must be severe before decreases in plasma cholinesterase production sufficient to prolong SCh-induced neuromuscular blockade occur.

$$H_3C\overset{CH_3}{\underset{CH_3}{N}}CH_2CH_2O\overset{O}{\overset{\|}{C}}CH_2CH_2\overset{O}{\overset{\|}{C}}OCH_2CH_2\overset{CH_3}{\underset{CH_3}{N}}CH_3$$

Succinylcholine

↓ plasma cholinesterase

$$H_3C\overset{CH_3}{\underset{CH_3}{N}}CH_2CH_2O\overset{O}{\overset{\|}{C}}CH_2CH_2\overset{O}{\overset{\|}{C}}OH + HOCH_2CH_2\overset{CH_3}{\underset{CH_3}{N}}CH_3$$

Succinylmonocholine Choline

↓ plasma cholinesterase

$$HO\overset{O}{\overset{\|}{C}}CH_2CH_2\overset{O}{\overset{\|}{C}}OH + HOCH_2CH_2\overset{CH_3}{\underset{CH_3}{N}}CH_3$$

Succinic Acid Choline

Figure 8-5. The brief duration of action of succinylcholine is due principally to its rapid hydrolysis to inactive plasma metabolites by cholinesterase enzyme activity.

Atypical Plasma Cholinesterase

The presence of atypical plasma cholinesterase is often recognized only after an otherwise healthy patient experiences prolonged neuromuscular blockade (1 to 3 hours) after a conventional dose of SCh. A single cholinesterase gene is present, and nucleotide alterations in this gene are responsible for the numerous variants in the enzyme. Among the several genetically determined variants of plasma cholinesterase, the dibucaine-related variants seem to be the most important (Table 8-6). Dibucaine, a local anesthetic with an amide linkage, inhibits the activity of normal plasma cholinesterase enzyme by approximately 80% compared with only approximately 20% inhibition of the activity of atypical enzyme. A dibucaine number of 80, which reflects the 80% inhibition of enzyme activity,

TABLE 8-6.
HEREDITARY VARIANTS OF PLASMA CHOLINESTERASE

Genotype	Dibucaine Number	Fluoride Number	Response to Succinylcholine	Frequency
E^uE^u	80	60	Normal	96%
E^aE^a	20	20	Greatly prolonged	1 in 3,200
E^uE^a	60	45	Slightly prolonged	1 in 480
E^uE^f	75	50	Slightly prolonged	1 in 200
E^fE^a	45	35	Greatly prolonged	1 in 20,000

confirms the presence of normal plasma cholinesterase enzyme, whereas approximately 1 in every 3,200 patients is homozygous for an atypical plasma cholinesterase enzyme variant and has a dibucaine number of 20. In these patients, neuromuscular blockade after the administration of SCh, 1 mg/kg IV, may persist for 3 hours or longer. Approximately 1 in every 480 patients is heterozygous for the atypical plasma cholinesterase enzyme that results in a dibucaine number of 40 to 60. These heterozygous patients may manifest a modestly prolonged duration of neuromuscular blockade (up to 30 minutes) after the administration of SCh. It is important to recognize that the dibucaine number reflects the quality of cholinesterase enzyme (ability to hydrolyze SCh) and not the quantity of the enzyme that is circulating in the plasma. For example, decreases in the plasma cholinesterase activity due to liver disease or anticholinesterase drugs are associated with normal (near 80) dibucaine numbers.

Adverse Side Effects

Adverse side effects that may accompany the administration of SCh may limit or even contraindicate the administration of SCh (Table 8-7).

NONDEPOLARIZING NEUROMUSCULAR-BLOCKING DRUGS (TABLE 8-1)

Differences in onset, duration of action, rate of recovery, metabolism, and clearance influence the clinical decision to select one drug over another. Many of the variable patient responses evoked by nondepolarizing neuromuscular-blocking drugs can be explained by differences in pharmacokinetics.

Mechanism of Action

Nondepolarizing neuromuscular-blocking drugs are classically thought to act by combining with nicotinic

TABLE 8-7.
SIDE EFFECTS OF SUCCINYLCHOLINE

Cardiac dysrhythmias (sinus bradycardia reflects actions of SCh at muscarinic cholinergic receptors, where it mimics actions of acetylcholine)
Hyperkalemia (occurs in patients with clinically unrecognized skeletal muscle dystrophy, unhealed third-degree burns, denervation leading to skeletal muscle atrophy; occurs within 96 hours of denervation and persists for an indefinite period)
Myalgia (prominent in muscles of neck, back and abdomen, may mimic sore throat)
Myoglobinuria
Increased intragastric pressure
Increased intraocular pressure (transient)
Increased intracranial pressure (not a consistent observation)
Sustained skeletal muscle contractions (especially in children)

nAChRs without causing any activation of these ion receptor channels. Specifically, these drugs can act competitively with acetylcholine at the α-subunits of the postjunctional nAChRs without causing a change in the configuration of these receptors. Occupation of as many as 70% of the nicotinic cholinergic receptors by a neuromuscular-blocking drug does not produce evidence of neuromuscular blockade, as reflected by the twitch response to a single electrical stimulus. Neuromuscular transmission, however, fails when 80% to 90% of the receptors are blocked.

Characteristics of Nondepolarizing Neuromuscular Blockade (Table 8-8)

Cardiovascular Effects

Nondepolarizing neuromuscular-blocking drugs may exert cardiovascular effects through the drug-induced release of histamine, via effects at cardiac muscarinic

TABLE 8-8.
CHARACTERISTICS OF NONDEPOLARIZING NEUROMUSCULAR BLOCKADE

Decreased twitch response to a single stimulus
Unsustained response (fade) during continuous stimulation
Train-of-four ratio <0.7
Post-tetanic potentiation
Potentiation of other nondepolarizing neuromuscular-blocking drugs
Antagonism of neuromuscular blockade after administration of anticholinesterase drugs
Absence of fasciculations

receptors, or effects on nicotinic receptors at autonomic ganglia (Table 8-9). Despite the frequent reference to the cardiovascular effects of nondepolarizing neuromuscular-

TABLE 8-9.
MECHANISMS OF NEUROMUSCULAR-BLOCKING DRUG–INDUCED CARDIOVASCULAR EFFECTS

	Histamine Release	Cardiac Muscarinic Receptors	Nicotinic Receptors at Autonomic Ganglia
Succinylcholine	Slight	Modest stimulation	Modest stimulation
Pancuronium	None	Modest blockade	None
Doxacurium	None	None	None
Pipecuronium	None	None	None
Atracurium	Slight	None	None
Vecuronium	None	None	None
Rocuronium	None	None	None
Cisatracurium	None	None	None
Mivacurium	Slight	None	None

blocking drugs, it is rare that these changes achieve clinical significance.

Critical Illness Myopathy

A small fraction of patients with asthma or acutely injured patients with multiple-organ system failure and who require drug-induced skeletal muscle paralysis to facilitate mechanical ventilation of the lungs for prolonged periods (usually >6 days) manifest skeletal muscular weakness on recovery. When monitoring of neuromuscular blockade with a peripheral nerve stimulator is combined with clinical guidelines, including adequate sedation and analgesia, smaller doses of nondepolarizing neuromuscular-blocking drugs are used to facilitate mechanical ventilation of the lungs, and prolonged paralysis is less likely.

Causes of Altered Responses (Table 8-10)

Volatile Anesthetics

Volatile anesthetics produces dose-dependent enhancement of the magnitude and duration of neuromuscular blockade due to nondepolarizing neuromuscular-blocking drugs (greatest with enflurane, isoflurane, desflurane, and sevoflurane and least with nitrous oxide–opioid combinations). The advantage of lessened augmentation of intermediate-acting neuromuscular-blocking drugs by volatile anesthetics is a more predictable degree of neuromuscular blockade, without precise knowledge of the alveolar (brain) partial pressure of the anesthetic. Volatile anesthetics most likely enhance the effects of nondepolarizing neuromuscular-blocking drugs by virtue of anesthetic-induced depression of the CNS, which decreases the tone of skeletal muscles. The plasma concentrations of nondepolarizing neuromuscular-blocking drugs necessary to depress single-twitch responses are less in the presence of volatile anesthetics than in the presence of nitrous oxide–opioid combinations, confirming that the potentiation of neuromuscular blockade by volatile anesthetics

TABLE 8-10.
DRUGS AND EVENTS UNRELATED TO DRUG THERAPY THAT MAY ENHANCE THE EFFECTS OF NONDEPOLARIZING NEUROMUSCULAR BLOCKING DRUGS

Volatile anesthetics
Aminoglycoside antibiotics
Local anesthetics
Cardiac antidysrhythmic drugs
Anticonvulsants
Diuretics
Magnesium
Lithium
Cyclosporine
Hypothermia
Changes in serum potassium concentrations
Thermal (burn) injury
Paresis or hemiplegia
Allergic reactions
Prior administration of succinylcholine
Gender

represents a change in pharmacodynamics rather than a change in pharmacokinetics.

Antibiotics

The aminoglycoside antibiotics are prominent among those antibiotics that enhance the effects of nondepolarizing neuromuscular-blocking drugs. Antagonism of antibiotic-potentiated neuromuscular blockade by an anticholinesterase drug or calcium is unpredictable. The penicillins and cephalosporins are antibiotics devoid of neuromuscular-blocking effects.

Local Anesthetics

Small doses of local anesthetics can enhance the neuromuscular blockade produced by nondepolarizing neuromuscular-blocking drugs, whereas large doses of local anesthetics can block neuromuscular transmission.

Cardiac Antidysrhythmic Drugs

Intravenous lidocaine administered to treat cardiac dysrhythmias could augment preexisting neuromuscular blockade.

Diuretics

Furosemide, 1 mg/kg IV, enhances the neuromuscular blockade produced by nondepolarizing neuromuscular-blocking drugs. Mannitol does not influence the degree of neuromuscular blockade produced by nondepolarizing neuromuscular-blocking drugs, even in the presence of diuresis. This emphasizes that the renal clearance of neuromuscular-blocking drugs depends on glomerular filtration. Osmotic diuretics increase urine output, independent of glomerular filtration rate.

Magnesium

Magnesium enhances the neuromuscular blockade produced by nondepolarizing neuromuscular-blocking drugs and, to a lesser extent, enhances the neuromuscular blockade produced by SCh.

Lithium

Lithium, as used to treat psychiatric depression, may enhance the neuromuscular-blocking effects of depolarizing and nondepolarizing neuromuscular-blocking drugs.

Anticonvulsants

Patients treated chronically with anticonvulsants (phenytoin, carbamazepine) are relatively resistant to some (pancuronium, vecuronium, rocuronium, cisatracurium, pipecuronium, doxacurium) but not all (mivacurium, atracurium) nondepolarizing neuromuscular-blocking drugs.

Cyclosporine

Cyclosporine may prolong the duration of the neuromuscular blockade produced by nondepolarizing neuromuscular-blocking drugs.

Hypothermia

Hypothermia enhances the effects of nondepolarizing neuromuscular-blocking drugs at the NMJ.

Serum Potassium Concentration

An acute decrease in the extracellular concentration of potassium increases the transmembrane potential, causing hyperpolarization of cell membranes. This change manifests as resistance to the effects of depolarizing neuromuscular-blocking drugs and increased sensitivity to nondepolarizing neuromuscular-blocking drugs. Conversely, hyperkalemia decreases the resting transmembrane potential and thus partially depolarizes cell membranes. This change increases the effects of depolarizing neuromuscular-blocking drugs and opposes the action of nondepolarizing neuromuscular-blocking drugs.

Thermal (Burn) Injury

Thermal (burn) injury causes resistance to the effects of nondepolarizing neuromuscular-blocking drugs that manifests approximately 10 days after injury, peaks at approximately 40 days, and declines after approximately 60 days. Approximately 30% or more of the body must be burned to produce resistance. A pharmacodynamic explanation as the principal mechanism for this resistance is documented by the need to achieve higher plasma concentrations to produce a given degree of twitch suppression in thermal injury versus non–thermal injury patients.

Paresis or Hemiplegia

Monitoring neuromuscular blockade with a peripheral nerve stimulator attached to the paretic arm on the side affected by a cerebral vascular accident reveals resistance (decreased sensitivity) to the effects of the neuromuscular-blocking drug compared with the response observed on the unaffected side. The unaffected arm shows resistance to the effects of neuromuscular-blocking drugs compared with responses observed in normal patients. As a result, monitoring neuromuscular blockade with a peripheral nerve stimulator after a cerebral vascular accident may underestimate the degree of neuromuscular blockade present at the muscles of ventilation. Resistance to neuromuscular-blocking drugs after a cerebral vascular accident may reflect the proliferation of extrajunctional nAChRs that respond to acetylcholine.

Allergic Reactions

Cross-sensitivity may occur between all the neuromuscular-blocking drugs, reflecting the presence of a common antigenic component, the quaternary ammonium group. Anaphylactic reactions after the first exposure to a neuromuscular-blocking drug may reflect sensitization from prior contact with cosmetics or soaps that also contain antigenic quaternary ammonium groups (females have a greater incidence of allergic reactions to neuromuscular blocking drugs than do males).

Succinylcholine Followed by a Nondepolarizing Neuromuscular-Blocking Drug

The prior administration of SCh, 1 mg/kg IV, to facilitate tracheal intubation enhances the magnitude of twitch response suppression produced by the subsequently administered nondepolarizing neuromuscular-blocking drug, even when the evidence of neuromuscular blockade produced by SCh has waned.

Gender

Women seem to be more sensitive to the effects of nondepolarizing neuromuscular-blocking drugs than men.

LONG-ACTING NONDEPOLARIZING NEUROMUSCULAR-BLOCKING DRUGS

Pancuronium is the most commonly administered long-acting nondepolarizing neuromuscular-blocking drug. Doxacurium and pipecuronium resemble pancuronium but, unlike pancuronium, these drugs are devoid of cardiovascular side effects. The low cost of pancuronium has been cited as an advantage of this drug compared with newer and more expensive nondepolarizing neuromuscular-blocking drugs.

Pancuronium

Pancuronium is a bisquaternary aminosteroid nondepolarizing neuromuscular-blocking drug with an ED_{95} of 70 μg/kg that has an onset of action in 3 to 5 minutes and a duration of neuromuscular blockade lasting 60 to 90 minutes (see Fig. 8-1 and Table 8-3).

Clearance

An estimated 80% of a single dose of pancuronium is eliminated unchanged in the urine. An estimated 10% to 40% of a dose of pancuronium undergoes hepatic deacetylation of 3-desacetylpancuronium, 17-desacetylpancuronium, and 3,17-desacetylpancuronium. The 3-desacetylpancuronium metabolite is approximately 50% as potent as pancuronium at the NMJ, whereas the other metabolites have only minimal activity.

Cardiovascular Effects

Pancuronium typically produces a modest 10% to 15% increase in heart rate, mean arterial pressure, and cardiac output. These cardiovascular effects are attributed to selective cardiac vagal blockade (atropine-like effect limited to cardiac muscarinic receptors) and activation of the sympathetic nervous system. The magnitude of heart rate increase evoked by pancuronium seems more dependent on the preexisting heart rate (an inverse relationship) than the dose or rate of pancuronium administration. Marked increases in heart rate in response to pancuronium seem more likely to occur in patients with an altered atrioventricular conduction of cardiac impulses, as may occur in the presence of atrial fibrillation.

Doxacurium

Doxacurium is a benzylisoquinolinium nondepolarizing neuromuscular-blocking drug with an ED_{95} of 30 μg/kg that produces an onset in 4 to 6 minutes and a duration of neuromuscular blockade lasting 60 to 90 minutes (see Fig. 8-1 and Table 8-3). The pharmacokinetics of doxacurium resemble pancuronium with respect to dependence on renal clearance. Drug-induced histamine release does not occur, and, as a result, cardiovascular changes do not accompany the administration of doxacurium.

Pipecuronium

Pipecuronium is a bisquaternary aminosteroid nondepolarizing neuromuscular-blocking drug with an ED_{95} of 50 to 60 μg/kg that produces an onset in 3 to 5 minutes and a duration of neuromuscular blockade lasting 60 to 90 minutes (see Fig. 8-1 and Table 8-3). Drug-induced histamine does not occur, and, as a result, cardiovascular changes do not accompany the administration of pipecuronium.

INTERMEDIATE-ACTING NONDEPOLARIZING NEUROMUSCULAR-BLOCKING DRUGS

Atracurium, vecuronium, rocuronium, and cisatracurium are classified as intermediate-acting nondepolarizing neuromuscular-blocking drugs. In contrast to the long-acting nondepolarizing neuromuscular-blocking drugs, these drugs possess efficient clearance mechanisms that minimize the likelihood of significant cumulative effects with repeated injections or continuous infusions. As such, intermediate-acting nondepolarizing neuromuscular-blocking drugs are useful, although they are more expensive alternatives to SCh and pancuronium. The intermediate duration of action of these drugs is due to their rapid and efficient clearance from the circulation. The neuromuscular blockade produced by intermediate-acting nondepolarizing neuromuscular-blocking drugs is reliably antagonized by anticholinesterase drugs, often within 20 minutes of administering a paralyzing dose of these drugs. Pharmacologic antagonism of neuromuscular blockade is further enhanced by the concomitant spontaneous recovery due to rapid clearance of the drug.

Atracurium

Atracurium is a bisquaternary benzylisoquinolinium nondepolarizing neuromuscular-blocking drug (mixture of ten geometric isomers) with an ED_{95} of 0.2 mg/kg that produces an onset in 3 to 5 minutes and a duration of neuromuscular blockade lasting 20 to 35 minutes (see Fig. 8-1 and Table 8-3).

Clearance

Atracurium undergoes spontaneous nonenzymatic degradation at normal body temperature and pH by a base-catalyzed reaction termed *Hofmann elimination*. A second and simultaneously occurring route of metabolism is hydrolysis by nonspecific plasma esterases. Hofmann elimination represents a chemical mechanism of elimination, whereas ester hydrolysis is a biologic mechanism. These two routes of metabolism are independent of hepatic and renal function as well as plasma cholinesterase activity (duration of atracurium-induced neuromuscular blockade is similar in normal patients and those with absent or impaired renal or hepatic function or those with atypical plasma cholinesterase). The absence of prolonged neuromuscular blockade after the administration of atracurium to patients with atypical cholinesterase emphasizes the dependence of atracurium's ester hydrolysis on nonspecific plasma esterases that are unrelated to plasma cholinesterase. Hofmann elimination and ester hydrolysis also account for the lack of cumulative drug effects with repeated doses or continuous infusions of atracurium. Overall, ester hydrolysis accounts for an estimated two-thirds of degraded atracurium, whereas Hofmann elimination provides a "safety net," especially in patients with impaired hepatic and/or renal function.

Laudanosine

Laudanosine is the major metabolite of both pathways of metabolism of atracurium. Laudanosine depends on the liver for clearance, with approximately 70% excreted in the bile and the remainder in urine. Despite increases in plasma laudanosine concentrations during each stage of liver transplantation in patients receiving atracurium, these levels are considered to be far below clinically significant concentrations. Although inactive at the NMJ (in contrast to metabolites of many other nondepolarizing neuromuscular-blocking drugs), animal studies have shown laudanosine to be a CNS stimulant, to increase the MAC of volatile anesthetics, and to cause peripheral vasodilation. In patients receiving a full paralyzing dose of atracurium (0.5 mg/kg IV), the resulting peak plasma concentrations of laudanosine are approximately 0.3 μg/mL, which is approximately 20 times less than the plasma concentrations producing cardiovascular effects in animals. Laudanosine resulting from the metabolism of atracurium probably will not produce seizure activity in anesthetized patients, because skeletal muscle paralysis from atracurium would prevent movement.

Acid-Base Changes

Despite pH-dependent Hofmann elimination (accelerated by alkalosis and slowed by acidosis), it is unlikely that the range of pH changes encountered clinically is sufficiently great to alter the rate of Hofmann elimination and, thus, the duration of atracurium-induced neuromuscular blockade.

Cumulative Effects

Consistency of onset to recovery intervals after repeated supplemental doses of atracurium is characteristic of this drug and reflects the absence of significant cumulative drug effect.

Cardiovascular Effects

Systemic blood pressure and heart rate changes do not accompany the rapid intravenous administration of atracurium in doses up to $2 \times ED_{95}$ with background anesthetics including nitrous oxide, fentanyl, and isoflurane. Facial and truncal flushing in some patients suggests a release of histamine as the mechanism for the circulatory changes accompanying the rapid administration of high doses ($3 \times ED_{95}$) of atracurium. It is estimated that the plasma histamine concentration must double before cardiovascular changes manifest clinically.

Pediatric Patients

Effective doses of atracurium are similar in adults and children (2 to 16 years old), when differences in extracellular fluid volume are minimized by calculating the dose on a mg/m^2 rather than a mg/kg basis.

Elderly Patients

Increasing age has no effect on the continuous rate of atracurium infusion necessary to maintain a constant degree of neuromuscular blockade. This most likely reflects the independence of clearance mechanisms (Hofmann elimination and ester hydrolysis) from age-related effects on renal and hepatic function.

Vecuronium

Vecuronium is a monoquaternary aminosteroid nondepolarizing neuromuscular-blocking drug with an ED_{95} of

50 μg/kg that produces an onset of action in 3 to 5 minutes and a duration of neuromuscular blockade lasting 20 to 35 minutes (see Fig. 8-1 and Table 8-3). Structurally, vecuronium is pancuronium without the quaternary methyl group in the A-ring of the steroid nucleus. The absence of this quaternary methyl group decreases the acetylcholine-like character of vecuronium, as compared with pancuronium.

Clearance

Vecuronium undergoes both hepatic metabolism and renal excretion. The 3-desacetylvecuronium metabolite is approximately one-half as potent as the parent compound, but it is rapidly converted to the 3,17-desacetylvecuronium derivative. The 3,17-desacetylvecuronium and 17-desacetylvecuronium derivatives have less than one-tenth the neuromuscular blocking properties of vecuronium. Increased lipid solubility also facilitates the biliary excretion of vecuronium. Approximately 30% of an administered dose of vecuronium appears in urine as unchanged drug and metabolites in the first 24 hours. The extensive hepatic uptake of vecuronium may account for the rapid decrease in vecuronium plasma concentrations and the drug's short duration of action.

Renal Dysfunction

Despite the presumption that the liver is the main organ of elimination, the elimination half-time of vecuronium and 3-desacetylvecuronium is prolonged in patients with renal failure.

Hepatic Dysfunction

Vecuronium, 0.2 mg/kg IV, is associated with a prolonged elimination half-time and a corresponding prolonged duration of action in patients with hepatic cirrhosis.

Acid-Base Changes

Hypercarbia introduced after (but not before) the establishment of vecuronium-induced neuromuscular blockade significantly enhances the effects of vecuronium. For this reason, the onset of hypoventilation, which may occur in the early postoperative period, could enhance neuromuscular blockade.

Cumulative Effects

Vecuronium has a large Vd, reflecting its tissue uptake. After a single dose of vecuronium, the plasma concentration decreases rapidly because of redistribution from central to peripheral compartments. With subsequent doses, any vecuronium present in various peripheral tissue compartments will limit the distribution phase and thus also the rate of decrease in the plasma concentration of vecuronium. As a result, vecuronium can be demonstrated to have a cumulative effect that is less than for pancuronium and greater than for atracurium.

Cardiovascular Effects

Vecuronium is typically devoid of circulatory effects even with the rapid intravenous administration of doses that exceed $3 \times ED_{95}$ of the drug, emphasizing the lack of vagolytic effects or histamine release associated with the administration of vecuronium.

Pediatric Patients

The potency of vecuronium in infants (7 to 45 weeks old), children (1 to 8 years old), and adults (18 to 38 years old) is similar during nitrous oxide–halothane anesthesia.

Elderly Patients

Increasing age is associated with decreases in the continuous rate of infusion of vecuronium necessary to maintain a constant degree of neuromuscular blockade.

Obstetric Patients

Insufficient amounts of nondepolarizing neuromuscular-blocking drugs cross the placenta to produce clinically significant effects in the fetus.

Obesity

The duration of action of vecuronium, but not atracurium, is prolonged in obese (>130% of ideal body weight) compared with nonobese adults.

Intraocular Pressure

The administration of paralyzing doses of vecuronium or atracurium after the induction of anesthesia with thiopental does not change intraocular pressure.

Malignant Hyperthermia

Malignant hyperthermia does not follow the administration of vecuronium or atracurium to sensitive swine.

Rocuronium

Rocuronium is a monoquaternary aminosteroid nondepolarizing neuromuscular-blocking drug with an ED_{95} of 0.3 mg/kg that has an onset of action in 1 to 2 minutes and a duration of neuromuscular blockade lasting 20 to 35 minutes (see Fig. 8-1 and Table 8-3). The onset of maximum single-twitch depression after the administration of 3- to 4 $\times$ ED_{95} of rocuronium resembles the onset of action of SCh, 1 mg/kg IV. Rocuronium is the only nondepolarizing neuromuscular-blocking drug that may serve as an alternative to SCh when the rapid onset of neuromuscular blockade is needed to facilitate tracheal intubation and SCh is contraindicated. Complete suppression of the single-twitch response at the adductor pollicis muscle does not confirm that the laryngeal muscles and diaphragm are also paralyzed. The period of maximum laryngeal paralysis may be missed if the onset of complete suppression of single-twitch response at the adductor pollicis is used as the clinical sign of optimal conditions for tracheal intubation (see Fig. 8-3). Conversely, initiating direct laryngoscopy for tracheal intubation at the time of peak laryngeal muscle paralysis could result in abdominal muscle and diaphragmatic movement when the tracheal tube is placed, because these muscles are not yet fully paralyzed.

Clearance

Animal studies have suggested that rocuronium is largely excreted unchanged (up to 50% in 2 hours) in the bile. The renal excretion of rocuronium may be >30% in 24 hours, and the administration of this drug to patients in renal failure may produce a modestly prolonged duration of action.

Cardiovascular Effects

Cardiovascular effects or the release of histamine do not follow the rapid intravenous administration of even large doses of rocuronium.

Cisatracurium

Cisatracurium is a benzylisoquinolinium nondepolarizing neuromuscular-blocking drug with an ED_{95} of 50 μg/kg that has an onset of action of 3 to 5 minutes and a duration of neuromuscular blockade lasting 20 to 35 minutes (see Fig. 8-1 and Table 8-3). Structurally, cisatracurium is the purified form of one of the ten stereoisomers of atracurium. Cisatracurium has a similar neuromuscular-blocking profile to atracurium, except that the onset of cisatracurium is somewhat slower and its propensity to release histamine is dramatically less.

Clearance

Cisatracurium principally undergoes degradation by Hofmann elimination at physiologic pH and temperature to form laudanosine and a monoquaternary acrylate. The organ-independent clearance of cisatracurium means that this nondepolarizing neuromuscular-blocking drug, like atracurium, can be administered to patients with hepatic or renal dysfunction without a change in its neuromuscular-blocking profile. The metabolites resulting from the degradation of cisatracurium by Hofmann elimination are inactive at the NMJ. In contrast to atracurium, plasma concentrations of laudanosine after the administration of a $2 \times ED_{95}$ dose of cisatracurium are fivefold less than that present after a 1.5 × ED_{95} dose of atracurium.

Cardiovascular Effects

Cisatracurium, in contrast to atracurium, is devoid of histamine-releasing effects so that cardiovascular changes do not accompany the rapid intravenous administration of even large doses (8 × ED_{95}) of cisatracurium.

SHORT-ACTING NONDEPOLARIZING NEUROMUSCULAR-BLOCKING DRUGS (TABLE 8-1)

Mivacurium

Mivacurium is a benzylisoquinolinium nondepolarizing neuromuscular-blocking drug with an ED_{95} of 80 μg/kg that has an onset of neuromuscular blockade in 2 to 3 minutes lasting 12 to 20 minutes (see Fig. 8-1 and Table 8-3). Mivacurium consists of three stereoisomers: The two most active and equipotent are the trans-trans and cis-trans isomers, whereas the cis-cis isomer has only one-tenth the activity of the other isomers. Mivacurium does not trigger malignant hyperthermia in susceptible swine.

Clearance

The cis-trans and trans-trans isomers of mivacurium are hydrolyzed by plasma cholinesterase at a rate equivalent to 88% that of SCh.

Atypical Plasma Cholinesterase

The hydrolysis of mivacurium is decreased and its duration of action increased in patients with atypical plasma cholinesterase.

Inhibition of Plasma Cholinesterase Activity

Fluoride is a potent inhibitor of plasma cholinesterase, suggesting that fluoride production, as from the metabolism of fluorinated volatile anesthetics, especially sevoflurane, might impact on the rate of hydrolysis of mivacurium. Nevertheless, fluoride concentrations equivalent to 100 μmol/L do not alter the in vitro half-times of the cis-trans and trans-trans isomers of mivacurium. Pancuronium potentiates mivacurium more than other nondepolarizing neuromuscular-blocking drugs because it occupies postsynaptic acetylcholine receptors and also slows the hydrolysis of mivacurium by inhibiting the activity of plasma cholinesterase.

Renal Dysfunction

Renal excretion appears to be a minor pathway for the clearance of mivacurium, with an estimated 7% of an administered dose appearing unchanged in urine.

Hepatic Dysfunction

The speed of onset of mivacurium-induced neuromuscular blockade is similar in normal patients and those with cirrhosis of the liver, but the duration of action of mivacurium is prolonged in those patients in whom liver disease was associated with decreased plasma cholinesterase activity.

Pharmacologic Antagonism

Spontaneous recovery from the neuromuscular-blocking effects of mivacurium is rapid.

Cardiovascular Effects

The cardiovascular response to mivacurium is minimal at doses up to $2 \times ED_{95}$.

Bronchospasm

Although mivacurium is not a potent histamine releaser, the possibility of histamine release and bronchospasm is a consideration especially in patients with reactive airway disease.

Burn Injury

Plasma cholinesterase activity is decreased by burn injury, and it is possible that this effect could counter receptor-mediated resistance to the effects of nondepolarizing neuromuscular-blocking drugs, thus resulting in lack of resistance to mivacurium.

GW280430A

GW280430A is a representative of a new class on nondepolarizing neuromuscular-blocking drugs characterized by a rapid breakdown in plasma through chemical hydrolysis and inactivation through cysteine adduction. This results in a very short duration of action. The onset and duration of action resemble succinylcholine.

Anticholinesterase Drugs and Cholinergic Agonists

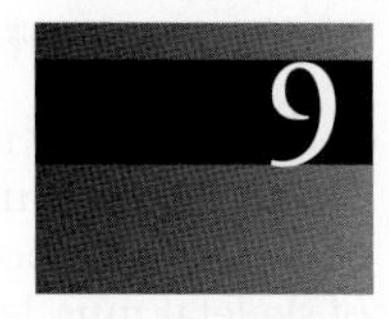

Anticholinesterase drugs (edrophonium, neostigmine, pyridostigmine) are most often administered to facilitate the speed of recovery from the skeletal muscle effects produced by nondepolarizing neuromuscular-blocking drugs (Stoelting RK, Hillier SC. Anticholinesterase drugs. In: Pharmacology and Physiology in Anesthetic Practice, 4th ed. Philadelphia. Lippincott Williams & Wilkins, 2006:251–265).

MECHANISM OF ACTION

Enzyme Inhibition

Edrophonium, neostigmine, and pyridostigmine inhibit the enzyme acetylcholinesterase (true cholinesterase), which is normally responsible for the rapid hydrolysis of the neurotransmitter acetylcholine to choline and acetic acid. The inhibition of acetylcholine hydrolysis secondary to the administration of an anticholinesterase drug results in greater availability at its sites of action, which include preganglionic sympathetic and parasympathetic nerve endings and the neuromuscular junction (NMJ). The increased availability acetylcholine at the NMJ is reflected by an increase in the size of the miniature end-plate potentials.

Presynaptic Effects

In the absence of nondepolarizing neuromuscular-blocking drugs, the administration of an anticholinesterase drug may produce spontaneous contractions (fasciculations) of skeletal muscles.

Direct Effects at the Neuromuscular Junction

It is possible that an excess of acetylcholine produced by acetylcholinesterase inhibition at the NMJ causes desensitization (end-plates no longer responsive to acetylcholine).

CLASSIFICATION

Anticholinesterase drugs are classified according to the mechanism by which they inhibit the activity of acetylcholinesterase.

Reversible Inhibition

Edrophonium is a quaternary ammonium anticholinesterase drug that produces inhibition of acetylcholinesterase through its electrostatic attachment to the anionic site on the enzyme. This binding is stabilized further by hydrogen bonding at the esteratic site on the enzyme. The duration of action of edrophonium is brief, reflecting its reversible binding with acetylcholinesterase. The predominant site of action of edrophonium appears to be presynaptic. The muscarinic effects of edrophonium are mild compared with longer-acting anticholinesterase drugs.

Formation of Carbamyl Esters

Drugs such as neostigmine, pyridostigmine, and physostigmine produce reversible inhibition of acetylcholinesterase by the formation of a carbamyl ester complex at the esteratic site of the enzyme. In contrast to edrophonium, these drugs act as competitive substrate substitutes for acetylcholine in the enzyme's normal interaction with acetylcholinesterase.

Irreversible Inactivation

Organophosphate anticholinesterase drugs (echothiophate) combine with acetylcholinesterase at the esteratic site to form a stable inactive complex that does not undergo hydrolysis. The spontaneous regeneration of acetylcholinesterase either requires several hours or does not occur, thus requiring synthesis of new enzyme.

STRUCTURE–ACTIVITY RELATIONSHIPS

Acetylcholinesterase consists of an anionic and esteratic site that are arranged complementary to the natural substrate acetylcholine. The anionic site of the enzyme binds the quaternary nitrogen of acetylcholine. This binding serves to orient the ester linkage of acetylcholine to the esteratic site of acetylcholinesterase. The esteratic site is responsible for the hydrolytic process. At the NMJ, acetylcholinesterase is responsible for a rapid hydrolysis of released acetylcholine, thereby controlling the duration of receptor activation. Approximately 50% of the released acetylcholine is hydrolyzed during the time of diffusion across the synaptic cleft to reach nicotinic cholinergic receptors (nAChRs).

PHARMACOKINETICS

In patients with normal renal function, no significant pharmacokinetic differences are present between anticholinesterase drugs (Table 9-1). The similarity in pharmacokinetics among the anticholinesterase drugs means that differences in potency and onset of action are most likely explained in terms of pharmacodynamics.

Lipid Solubility

Anticholinesterase drugs containing a quaternary ammonium group (edrophonium, neostigmine, pyridostigmine) are poorly lipid soluble and thus do not easily penetrate

TABLE 9-1.

COMPARATIVE CHARACTERISTICS OF ANTICHOLINESTERASE DRUGS ADMINISTERED TO ANTAGONIZE NONDEPOLARIZING NEUROMUSCULAR-BLOCKING DRUGS

	Elimination Half-Time (mins)		Volume of Distribution (L/kg)		Clearance (mL/kg/min)	
	Normal	Anephric	Normal	Anephric	Normal	Anephric
Edrophonium (0.5 kg/kg)	110	206	1.1	0.7	9.6	2.7
Neostigmine (0.043 mg/kg)	77	181	0.7	1.6	9.2	7.8
Pyridostigmine (0.35 mg/kg)	112	379	1.1	1.0	8.6	2.1

	Renal Contribution to Total Clearance (%)	Speed of Onset	Duration (mins)	Principal Site of Action	Anticholinergic Dose (μg/kg)	
					Atropine	Glycopyrrolate
Edrophonium (0.5 mg/kg)	66	Rapid	60	Presynaptic	7*	NR
Neostigmine (0.043 mg/kg)	54	Intermediate	54	Postsynaptic	20	10
Pyridostigmine (0.35 mg/kg)	76	Delayed	76	Postsynaptic	20	10

NR, not recommended.
*10–15 μg/kg if an opioid-based anesthetic.

lipid cell membranes (blood-brain barrier). Lipid-soluble drugs, such as tertiary amines (physostigmine) have predictable effects on the central nervous system (CNS).

Volume of Distribution

Presumably, the large volume of distribution (Vd) of acetylcholinesterase drugs reflects extensive tissue storage.

Onset of Action

During a steady-state infusion of a nondepolarizing muscle relaxant, the onset of action of edrophonium is 1 to 2 minutes, neostigmine 7 to 11 minutes, and pyridostigmine as long as 16 minutes.

Duration of Action

In clinical practice, acetylcholinesterase drugs are given when the effect of the nondepolarizing neuromuscular-blocking drug is waning, which makes determination of the actual duration of the reversal drug difficult to determine. During a steady-state infusion of a neuromuscular blocking drug, equivalent durations of action are provided by neostigmine 0.43 mg/kg IV, pyridostigmine 0.21 mg/kg IV, and edrophonium, 0.5 mg/kg IV.

Renal Clearance

Renal clearance accounts for approximately 50% of the elimination of neostigmine and approximately 75% of the elimination of edrophonium and pyridostigmine. As a result, the plasma clearance of anticholinesterase drugs is prolonged by renal failure (to a greater degree than that of most nondepolarizing-drugs, thus making the occurrence of recurarization unlikely).

Metabolism

In the absence of renal function, hepatic metabolism accounts for 50% of a dose of neostigmine, 30% of a dose of edrophonium, and 25% of a dose of pyridostigmine. The metabolites of anticholinesterase drugs are not pharmacologically active.

Influence of Patient Age

The duration of the maximum response produced by neostigmine and pyridostigmine is prolonged in elderly compared with younger patients, reflecting a smaller extracellular fluid volume and a slowed rate of plasma clearance in elderly patients.

PHARMACOLOGIC EFFECTS

The pharmacologic effects of anticholinesterase drugs are predictable and reflect the accumulation of acetylcholine at muscarinic receptors and nAChRs (bradycardia, salivation, miosis, hyperperistalsis). For this reason, using an anticholinesterase drug to reverse nondepolarizing neuromuscular-blocking drugs also includes administering an anticholinergic drug to prevent adverse muscarinic cholinergic effects. The anticholinergic drug selectively blocks the effects of acetylcholine at muscarinic cholinergic receptors and leaves intact the response to acetylcholine at nAChRs.

Cardiovascular Effects

The cardiovascular effects of anticholinesterase drugs reflect the effects of accumulated acetylcholine at the heart (bradycardia), blood vessels (decreased systemic vascular resistance), and postganglionic cholinergic nerve endings. The cardiac effects of anticholinesterase drugs can be attenuated by the administration of an anticholinergic drug that blocks muscarinic receptors but not nAChRs.

Gastrointestinal and Genitourinary Tract

Anticholinesterase drugs enhance gastric fluid secretion by parietal cells and increase the motility of the entire gastrointestinal tract, particularly the large intestine. Nausea and gastrointestinal disturbances associated with the use of anticholinesterase drugs to reverse nondepolarizing neuromuscular-blocking drugs are considerations when patients are to be discharged to home on the day of surgery.

Salivary Glands

Anticholinesterase drugs augment the secretion of glands that are innervated by postganglionic cholinergic fibers (bronchial, lacrimal, sweat, salivary). Cholinergic stimulation of the bronchi produces bronchoconstriction, and anticholinesterase drugs have the potential to increase airway resistance.

Eye

Anticholinesterase drugs applied topically to the cornea cause constriction of the sphincter of the iris (miosis) and ciliary muscle.

Myasthenia Gravis

Cholinergic crisis is the risk associated with the administration of anticholinesterase drugs to patients with myasthenia gravis who have also received nondepolarizing neuromuscular-blocking drugs.

β-Adrenergic Blockade

Bradycardia does not accompany the administration of mixtures of atropine and neostigmine to patients being treated with β-blockers.

CLINICAL USES

Antagonist-Assisted Reversal of Neuromuscular Blockade

Antagonist-assisted reversal of neuromuscular blockade using edrophonium, neostigmine, or pyridostigmine reflects the increased availability of acetylcholine at the NMJ due to inhibition of acetylcholinesterase, which is needed to hydrolyze acetylcholine. Increased amounts of the neurotransmitter acetylcholine in the region of the NMJ improves the chances that acetylcholine molecules will bind to the α-subunits of the nAChRs. Anticholinesterase drugs are typically administered during the time when spontaneous recovery from neuromuscular blockade is occurring, so that the effect of the pharmacologic antagonist adds to the rate of spontaneous recovery from the neuromuscular-blocking drug.

Onset and Duration of Action

Edrophonium has a more rapid onset of action than neostigmine and pyridostigmine, whereas the duration of action of these three anticholinesterase drugs is similar. Doses of anticholinesterase drugs that produce equivalent degrees of antagonism of neuromuscular blockade are edrophonium, 0.5 mg/kg IV (1 mg/kg IV if >90% twitch depression when reversal is initiated), neostigmine, 0.43 mg/kg IV, and pyridostigmine 0.21 mg/kg IV. Neostigmine appears preferable to either edrophonium or pyridostigmine when >90% twitch depression is to be antagonized.

Mixture with Anticholinergic Drugs

Reversal of nondepolarizing neuromuscular blockade requires only the nicotinic cholinergic effects of anticholinesterase drugs. Therefore, muscarinic cholinergic effects of the anticholinesterase drugs are attenuated or prevented by the concurrent administration of an anticholinergic drug, such as atropine or glycopyrrolate. It is desirable to administer an anticholinergic drug with a faster onset of action than the anticholinesterase drug to minimize the likelihood of drug-induced bradycardia (see Table 9-1). Thus, when edrophonium, 0.5 mg/kg IV, is administered, atropine, 7 μg/kg IV, is recommended. Neostigmine has a slower onset of action than edrophonium, and either atropine or glycopyrrolate may be administered as the anticholinesterase drug. The simultaneous administration of atropine and neostigmine leads to an initial tachycardia because of the more rapid onset of action of atropine. Conversely, the time course of action of glycopyrrolate more closely parallels the onset of action of neostigmine, so that the simultaneous administration of these two drugs may result in a more stable heart rate. Late bradycardia is more likely when short-acting atropine rather than long-acting glycopyrrolate is combined with neostigmine. The onset of action of pyridostigmine is slow, and an initial tachycardia may be expected with either atropine or glycopyrrolate.

Excessive Neuromuscular Blockade

Once acetylcholinesterase is maximally inhibited, administering additional anticholinesterase drug does not further antagonize nondepolarizing neuromuscular blockade. When twitch height is >10%, the administration of anticholinesterase drugs is more likely to produce predictable effects.

Events Influencing Reversal of Neuromuscular Blockade

The speed and extent to which neuromuscular blockade is reversed by anticholinesterase drugs are influenced by a number of factors, including the intensity of the neuromuscular blockade at the time pharmacologic reversal is initiated (train-of-four-twitches) and the nondepolarizing neuromuscular-blocking drug being reversed (Table 9-2). The continued administration of a volatile anesthetic may delay the drug-assisted antagonism of nondepolarizing muscle relaxants. Antagonism of neuromuscular blockade by anticholinesterase drugs may be inhibited or even prevented by certain antibiotics, hypothermia, respiratory acidosis associated with a $Pa{CO_2}$ >50 mmHg, hypokalemia and metabolic acidosis. Reversal of phase II block associated with the prolonged or repeated use of succinylcholine can be reversed using neostigmine or edrophonium.

TABLE 9-2.

RECOMMENDED DOSES OF NEOSTIGMINE OR EDROPHONIUM ACCORDING TO RESPONSES TO TRAIN-OF-FOUR (TOF) STIMULATION

TOF Visible Twitches	Fade	Anticholinesterase Drug	Dose (mg/kg)
None*	—	—	—
<2	++++	Neostigmine	0.07
3–4	+++	Neostigmine	0.04
4	++	Edrophonium	0.5
4	±	Edrophonium	0.25

*Postpone administration of anticholinesterase drug until some visible evoked response.

Treatment of Central Nervous System Effects of Certain Drugs

Central Anticholinergic Syndrome

Physostigmine (15 to 60 μg/kg IV), as a lipid soluble tertiary amine, is effective in antagonizing the restlessness and confusion caused by atropine or scopolamine. Presumably, physostigmine increases concentrations of acetylcholine in the brain, making more neurotransmitters available for nAChRs.

Opioids

Physostigmine abolishes the somnolent effects of opioids and may reverse the depression of the ventilatory response to carbon dioxide but not the analgesia produced by prior administration of morphine.

Treatment of Myasthenia Gravis

Neostigmine, pyridostigmine, and ambenonium are the standard anticholinesterase drugs used in the symptomatic treatment of myasthenia gravis. These drugs increase the response of skeletal muscles to repetitive impulses, presumably by increasing the availability of endogenous acetylcholine. In assessing the anticholinesterase drug therapy of myasthenia gravis, edrophonium 1 mg IV may be administered every 1 to 2 minutes until a change in symptoms is observed. Inadequate anticholinesterase drug therapy is diagnosed if a decrease in myasthenic symptoms occurs. Conversely, patients experiencing excessive anticholinesterase drug effect (cholinergic crisis) will manifest increased skeletal muscle weakness with the administration of edrophonium.

Treatment of Glaucoma

Anticholinesterase drugs decrease intraocular pressure in patients with narrow-angle and wide-angle glaucoma, reflecting a decrease in the resistance to outflow of aqueous humor.

Alzheimer's Disease

Cholinesterase inhibitors (tacrine, donepezil, rivastigmine, galantamine) are recommended for the treatment of patients with mild to moderate Alzheimer's disease. Compared with tacrine, the other centrally active anticholinesterase drugs are less toxic (lack hepatotoxicity) and their duration of action permits more convenient dosage regimens.

Diagnosis and Management of Cardiac Dysrhythmias

Edrophonium has been administered for the diagnosis and management of cardiac dysrhythmias, especially paroxysmal supraventricular tachycardias, including those due to Wolff-Parkinson-White syndrome.

Postoperative Analgesia

Intrathecal (50 to 100 μg) or epidural (1 to 4 μg/kg) injection of neostigmine produces analgesia in the postoperative period and in patients with chronic pain. Neostigmine probably produces analgesia by inhibiting the breakdown of spinally released acetylcholine, which is increased in the presence of pain. The disadvantages of intrathecal neostigmine to produce analgesia include a high incidence of nausea and vomiting, pruritus, and prolongation of the sensory and motor block produced by spinal anesthesia. Ventilatory depression characteristic of the analgesia produced by opioids does not accompany neostigmine-induced pain relief.

Postoperative Shivering

Administration of physostigmine, 40 μg/kg IV, at the conclusion of anesthesia decreases the incidence of postoperative shivering, similar to meperidine and clonidine. Physostigmine may enhance the secretion of neurotransmitters that are involved in the control of body temperature, especially at the hypothalamic thermoregulatory centers.

OVERDOSE OF ANTICHOLINESTERASE DRUGS

Overdoses of anticholinesterase drugs (organophosphates) manifest as muscarinic (bradycardia, bronchoconstriction, salivation, miosis, abdominal cramps, loss of bladder and bowel control) and nicotinic symptoms (skeletal muscle weakness) on peripheral and CNS (confusion, ataxia, coma, seizures, depression of ventilation) sites.

Treatment

The treatment of anticholinesterase drug overdose is with atropine, occasionally supplemented by an acetylcholinesterase reactivator, pralidoxime. Pralidoxime antagonizes the CNS effects of excessive amounts of acetylcholine. Atropine, 35 to 70 μg/kg IV, administered every 3 to 10 minutes until muscarinic symptoms disappear, is specific for antagonizing the muscarinic effects of acetylcholine at the NMJ. In addition to specific pharmacologic antagonism, treatment of anticholinesterase drug overdose includes supportive measures, such as intubation of the trachea and mechanical ventilation of the lungs.

SYNTHETIC CHOLINERGIC AGONISTS

Synthetic cholinergic agonist drugs (methacholine, carbachol, bethanechol) have as their primary action the activation of cholinergic (muscarinic) receptors that are innervated by postganglionic parasympathetic nerves. Asthma (bronchoconstriction), coronary artery disease (vasodilation and decreases in diastolic blood pressure), and peptic ulcer disease (enhanced secretion of acidic gastric fluid) are examples of diseases that could be exacerbated by cholinergic agonists. All the muscarinic effects of cholinergic agonists are blocked selectively by atropine.

Methacholine

Methacholine has a longer duration of action than acetylcholine because its rate of hydrolysis by acetylcholinesterase is slower. Furthermore, methacholine is almost totally resistant to hydrolysis by plasma cholinesterase.

Carbachol and Bethanechol

Carbachol and bethanechol are totally resistant to hydrolysis by acetylcholinesterase and both drugs act selectively on the smooth muscle of the gastrointestinal tract and urinary bladder (muscarinic actions). Oral administration of bethanechol may relieve adynamic ileus urinary retention. Carbachol is used as a topical drug to produce miosis.

Pilocarpine, Muscarine, and Arecoline

Pilocarpine, muscarine, and arecoline are examples of cholinomimetic alkaloids having dominant muscarinic actions (resemble vagal nerve stimulation). The clinical use of these drugs is limited to the topical administration of pilocarpine as a miotic.

Anticholinergic Drugs

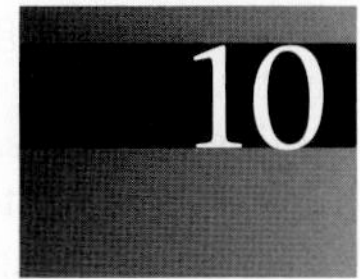

Anticholinergic drugs competitively antagonize the effects (parasympathetic) of the neurotransmitter acetylcholine at cholinergic postganglionic sites designated as muscarinic receptors (Stoelting RK, Hillier SC. Anticholinergic drugs. In: *Pharmacology and Physiology in Anesthetic Practice,* 4th ed. Philadelphia. Lippincott Williams & Wilkins, 2006:266–275). Muscarinic cholinergic receptors are present in the heart, salivary glands, and smooth muscles of the gastrointestinal and genitourinary tract. Acetylcholine is also the neurotransmitter at postganglionic nicotinic cholinergic receptors (nAChRs) located at the neuromuscular junction (NMJ) and autonomic ganglia. In contrast to the effects at muscarinic receptors, usual doses of anticholinergic drugs exert little or no effect at nAChRs. As such, anticholinergic drugs may be considered to be selectively antimuscarinic.

STRUCTURE–ACTIVITY RELATIONSHIPS

Naturally occurring anticholinergic drugs (atropine and scopolamine) are esters formed by the combination of tropic or mandelic acid and an organic base (tropine or scopine). Like acetylcholine, anticholinergic drugs contain a cationic portion that can fit into the muscarinic cholinergic receptor.

MECHANISM OF ACTION

Anticholinergic drugs combine reversibly with muscarinic cholinergic receptors and thus prevent access of the neurotransmitter acetylcholine to these sites. As competitive antagonists, the effect of anticholinergic drugs can be overcome by increasing the concentration of acetylcholine in the area of the muscarinic receptors. Five distinct muscarinic receptor subtypes, with recognized tissue distributions, are designated M1–M5 (Table 10-1). Muscarinic cholinergic receptors are examples of G protein–coupled receptors that also depend on second-messenger coupling. Muscarinic cholinergic receptors that control salivary and bronchial secretions (M3 receptors) are inhibited by lower doses of anticholinergic drugs than are necessary to inhibit receptors that regulate acetylcholine effects on the heart and eyes (M2 receptors). Even larger doses of anticholinergic drugs are needed to inhibit gastric secretion of hydrogen ions (M1 receptors). As a result, a dose of anticholinergic drug that inhibits the gastric secretion of hydrogen ions invariably affects salivary secretions, heart rate, ocular accommodation, and micturition. Examples of differences in anticholinergic potency between drugs are the greater antisialagogue and ocular effects of scopolamine compared with atropine (Table 10-2). Atropine, scopolamine, and glycopyrrolate do not discriminate among M1, M2, and M3 receptors; instead, they act as highly selective competitive antagonists of acetylcholine at all muscarinic receptors. The paradoxical slowing of heart rate that may follow the administration of anticholinergic drugs most likely reflects a blockade of presynaptic inhibitory M1 receptors on vagus nerve endings that usually provide negative feedback on further acetylcholine release.

PHARMACOKINETICS

Intravenous or intramuscular administration is used most often for the delivery of anticholinergic drugs. Atropine and scopolamine are lipid-soluble tertiary amines that easily penetrate the blood-brain barrier, whereas glycopyrrolate is a poorly lipid soluble quaternary ammonium compound with minimal ability to cross the blood-brain barrier and produce CNS effects.

TABLE 10-1.
MUSCARINIC RECEPTOR SUBTYPES

	M1	M2	M3	M4	M5
Location	CNS Stomach	Heart CNS Airway smooth muscles	CNS Salivary glands Airway smooth muscles Vascular endothelial cells	CNS Heart?	CNS
Clinical effects	Hydrogen ion secretion	Bradycardia	Salivation Bronchodilation Vasodilation	?	?
Clinically selective drugs available	Yes	No	No	No	No

TABLE 10-2.

COMPARATIVE EFFECTS OF ANTICHOLINERGIC DRUGS

	Sedation	Antisialagogue	Increase Heart Rate	Relax Smooth Muscle
Atropine	+	+	+++	++
Scopolamine	+++	+++	+	+
Glycopyrrolate	0	++	++	++

	Mydriasis, Cycloplegia	Prevent Motion-induced Nausea	Decrease Gastric Hydrogen Ion Secretion	Alter Fetal Heart Rate
Atropine	+	+	+	0
Scopolamine	+++	+++	+	?
Glycopyrrolate	0	0	+	0

0, none; +, mild; ++, moderate; +++, marked.

CLINICAL USES

The lack of selectivity of anticholinergic drugs makes it difficult to obtain desired therapeutic responses without concomitant side effects (see Table 10-1).

Preoperative Medication

When an anticholinergic drug is included in the preoperative medication, the most likely therapeutic goals are to produce sedation or an antisialagogue effect. Anticholinergic drugs in traditional doses used for preoperative medication in adults do not alter gastric fluid pH or volume.

Sedation

Scopolamine is selected when sedation is the reason for including an anticholinergic drug in the preoperative medication. Scopolamine also greatly enhances the sedative effects of concomitantly administered drugs, especially opioids and benzodiazepines. Glycopyrrolate, which does not easily cross the blood-brain barrier, is devoid of sedative effects. Occasionally, the CNS effects of anticholinergic drugs, especially scopolamine, cause symptoms ranging from restlessness to somnolence (delayed awakening from anesthesia especially in elderly patients).

Antisialagogue Effect

Scopolamine is approximately three times as potent as an antisialagogue than atropine. As an antisialagogue, glycopyrrolate is approximately twice as potent as atropine, and its duration for producing this effect is longer.

Treatment of Reflex-Mediated Bradycardia

Atropine, 15 to 70 μg/kg IV, is effective in treating intraoperative bradycardia resulting from increased parasympathetic nervous system activity. Equivalent doses of glycopyrrolate produce similar increases in heart rate, but the onset of effect is slower than after the administration of atropine. In young adults, in whom vagal tone is enhanced, the influence of atropine on heart rate is most evident, whereas in infants or elderly patients, even large doses may fail to increase heart rate.

Combination with Anticholinesterase Drugs

Pharmacologic-enhanced antagonism of nondepolarizing neuromuscular-blocking drugs with an anticholinesterase drug requires the concomitant administration of atropine or glycopyrrolate to prevent the parasympathomimetic effects that predictably accompany the intravenous administration of edrophonium, neostigmine, or pyridostigmine (see Chapter 9). Depending on the speed of onset of the anticholinesterase drug, atropine (rapid onset) or glycopyrrolate (slow onset) are selected for concomitant administration (see Chapter 9). The administration of anticholinergic drugs during pharmacologic antagonism of nondepolarizing neuromuscular blockade causes an impairment of parasympathetic nervous system control of heart rate that persists into the early postoperative period; the effects are shorter using glycopyrrolate than using atropine.

Bronchodilation

The effectiveness of anticholinergic drugs as bronchodilators reflects the antagonism of acetylcholine effects on airway smooth muscle via muscarinic receptors, present predominantly in large- and medium-sized airways, that respond to vagal nerve stimulation. The administration of anticholinergic drugs for preanesthetic medication could result in inspissation of secretions, possibly leading to airway obstruction rather than decreases in airway resistance.

Ipratropium

Ipratropium is the anticholinergic drug most often selected for aerosol administration (40 to 80 μg delivered by two to four actuations of the metered-dose inhaler) to produce bronchodilation in patients with chronic bronchitis or emphysema, thus emphasizing the role of cholinergic tone in these patients. Ipratropium provides only modest added bronchodilatory effect when administered with β-agonists being administered for the treatment of bronchial asthma.

The effects of aerosol ipratropium on heart rate and intraocular pressure, in contrast to atropine, do not occur, reflecting the minimal systemic absorption ($<1\%$ of the inhaled dose) of this quaternary ammonium drug.

Biliary and Ureteral Smooth Muscle Relaxation

Atropine may prevent spasm of the ureter produced by morphine.

Mydriasis and Cycloplegia

Anticholinergic drugs placed topically on the cornea block the action of acetylcholine at the circular muscles of the iris and the ciliary muscles, resulting in mydriasis and cycloplegia. Doses of atropine used for preoperative medication are probably inadequate to increase intraocular pressure even in susceptible patients, assuming medications being used to treat glaucoma are continued. The intravenous administration of atropine or glycopyrrolate to prevent or treat reflex- or drug-mediated bradycardia does not produce sufficient tissue levels of the drug in the eye to produce adverse effects in patients with glaucoma.

Antagonism of Gastric Hydrogen Ion Secretion

The efficacy of H_2 receptor antagonists has largely negated the use of anticholinergic drugs for the purpose of decreasing gastric hydrogen ion secretion. High doses of anticholinergic drugs prevent excess peristalsis of the gastrointestinal tract that would otherwise be associated with the administration of an anticholinesterase drug for the antagonism of nondepolarizing neuromuscular-blocking drugs.

Prevention of Motion-Induced Nausea

Transdermal absorption of scopolamine provides sustained therapeutic plasma concentrations that protect against motion-induced nausea (vestibular stimulation) without introducing prohibitive side effects such as sedation, cycloplegia, or drying of secretions. Morphine and synthetic opioids increase vestibular sensitivity, and transdermal scopolamine provides antiemetic effects in those treated with patient-controlled analgesia or epidural morphine for the management of postoperative pain. Anisocoria has been attributed to contamination of the eye after digital manipulation of the transdermal scopolamine patch.

Constituents of Nonprescription Cold Remedies

Anticholinergic drugs are common constituents of nonprescription cold remedies, reflecting their ability to inhibit the production of upper airway secretions.

Management of Parkinson's Disease

Benztropine and trihexyphenidyl are used in the management of Parkinson's disease for their effects on tremor, skeletal muscle rigidity, and dystonia.

CENTRAL ANTICHOLINERGIC SYNDROME

Scopolamine and, to a lesser extent, atropine can enter the CNS and produce symptoms characterized as the central anticholinergic syndrome (restlessness, hallucinations, somnolence, unconsciousness).

Presumably, these responses reflect a blockade of muscarinic cholinergic receptors and the competitive inhibition of the effects of acetylcholine in the CNS. Physostigmine, a lipid-soluble tertiary anticholinesterase drug, administered in doses of 15 to 60 μg/kg IV (may need to repeat every 1 to 2 hours) is a specific treatment of central anticholinergic syndrome. The central anticholinergic syndrome is often mistaken for delayed recovery from anesthesia.

OVERDOSE

Deliberate or accidental overdose with an anticholinergic drug produces a rapid onset of symptoms characteristic of muscarinic cholinergic receptor blockade (dry mouth, blurred vision, photophobia, tachycardia, increased body temperature due to inhibition of sweating). Small children are particularly vulnerable to drug-induced increases in body temperature. Physostigmine is the specific treatment.

DECREASED BARRIER PRESSURE

Administration of atropine, 0.6 mg IV or glycopyrrolate, 0.2 to 0.3 mg IV, decreases lower esophageal sphincter pressure and thus decreases barrier pressure (difference between gastric pressure and lower esophageal sphincter pressure) and the inherent resistance to reflux of acidic fluid into the esophagus (clinical significance undocumented).

11 Cyclooxygenase-2 Inhibitors and Nonspecific Nonsteroidal Antiinflammatory Drugs

Cyclooxygenase (COX) is an enzyme that catalyzes the synthesis of prostaglandins from arachidonic acid (Stoelting RK, Hillier SC. Cyclooxygenase-2 inhibitors and nonspecific nonsteroidal antiinflammatory drugs. In: *Pharmacology and Physiology in Anesthetic Practice*, 4th ed. Philadelphia. Lippincott Williams & Wilkins, 2006:276–291). Nonsteroidal antiinflammatory drugs (NSAIDs) block the action of COX enzyme, thus reducing the production of prostaglandin mediators, with resulting negative and positive effects (Tables 11-1 and 11-2).

CYCLOOXYGENASE ENZYMES

COX activity is associated with two isoenzymes designated COX-1 (gastric mucosa, renal parenchyma, platelets) and COX-2 (inducible and expressed mainly at sites of injury and inflammation).

CLASSIFICATION OF NONSTEROIDAL ANTIINFLAMMATORY DRUGS

NSAID is an all inclusive term denoting a varied group of drugs possessing analgesia, antiinflammatory, and

TABLE 11-1.
CHARACTERISTICS OF NONSTEROIDAL ANTIINFLAMMATORY DRUGS

Decrease activation and sensitization of peripheral nociceptors
Attenuate the inflammatory response
Absence of dependence or addiction potential
Synergistic effects with opioids
Preemptive analgesia (decreased neuronal sensitization)
Absence of depression of breathing
Less nausea and vomiting compared with opioids
Long duration of action
Less dose variability compared with opioids
No pupillary changes
Absence of cognitive effects

antipyretic effects. These drugs can be categorized into conventional nonspecific inhibitors of both isoforms of COX (ibuprofen, naproxen, aspirin, acetaminophen, ketorolac) and COX-2 selective inhibitors (celecoxib, rofecoxib, valdecoxib, parecoxib). Inhibition of COX-1 is responsible for many of the adverse effects associated with conventional NSAIDs. COX-2 inhibitors represent

TABLE 11-2.
POTENTIAL ADVERSE EFFECTS PRODUCED BY NONSTEROIDAL ANTIINFLAMMATORY DRUGS

Inhibition of platelet aggregation
Gastric ulceration
Renal dysfunction
Hepatocellular injury
Asthma exacerbation
Allergic reactions
Tinnitus
Urticaria

a significant therapeutic advance because of their improved side effect profile, when compared with conventional NSAIDs.

CYCLOOXYGENASE-2 SPECIFIC INHIBITORS

COX-2 specific inhibitors exhibit an analgesic efficacy comparable with that of conventional NSAIDs. These drugs lack effects on platelets and may be associated with decreased gastrointestinal side effects in patients with arthritis, compared with conventional NSAIDs.

Pharmacokinetics

As a class of drugs, the NSAIDs are well absorbed from the gastrointestinal tract and easily cross the blood-brain barrier (Table 11-3).

TABLE 11-3.
PHARMACOKINETICS OF CYCLOOXYGENASE-2 INHIBITORS

	Celecoxib	Rofecoxib*	Valdecoxib
Molecular weight	381.38	314.36	314.36
Elimination half-time (hrs)	12	17	8–11
Volume of distribution (L)	400	86–89	86
Protein binding (%)	98	87	98
Metabolism	Cytochrome P450	Cystsolic enzymes	Cytochrome P450
Metabolite	Inactive	Active	Active

*Not clinically available.

Because both parecoxib and valdecoxib are inhibitors of P-450, the potential exists for these COX-2 inhibitors to inhibit the metabolism of other drugs (propofol).

Clinical Uses

The perceived beneficial effects of COX-2 inhibitors have resulted in the wide-ranging use of these drugs for a variety of indications, especially for conditions associated with inflammation and pain (Table 11-4).

TABLE 11-4.
CLINICAL USES OF CYCLOOXYGENASE-2 INHIBITORS

Drug	Clinical Uses	Dosage
Celecoxib	Osteoarthritis	200 mg every day or 100 mg twice daily
	Rheumatoid arthritis	100–200 mg twice daily
	Familial adenomatous polyposis	400 mg twice daily
	Acute pain and primary dysmenorrhea	400 mg initially, followed by an additional 200 mg if needed, then 200 mg twice daily if needed
Rofecoxib*	Acute pain	50 mg every day
	Osteoarthritis	25 mg every day
	Rheumatoid arthritis	50 mg every day
	Primary dysmennorrhea	50 mg every day
Parecoxib	Acute pain	40 mg every day
Valdecoxib	Acute pain	40 mg every day
	Osteoarthritis	10 mg every day
	Rheumatoid arthritis	10 mg every day
	Primary dysmenorrhea	20 mg twice daily if needed

*Not clinically available.

TABLE 11-5.
FACTORS FAVORING NSAID-INDUCED NEPHROTOXICITY

Hypovolemia
Preexisting renal disease (patients who depend on prostaglandins for renal vasodilation)
Congestive heart failure
Sepsis
Combination with other potentially nephrotoxic drugs or radiographic contrast material
Diabetes mellitus
Cirrhosis
Elderly patients

Analgesic Efficacy

The COX-2 inhibitors are useful in the management of patients experiencing pain owing to osteoarthritis, rheumatoid arthritis, acute gout, and primary dysmenorrhea (see Table 11-2). The majority of adverse effects of NSAIDs appear in patients receiving these drugs chronically or in the treatment of arthritis (see Table 11-5). Acute postoperative pain, as associated with orthopedic surgery and arthroscopy, is responsive to COX-2 inhibitors, and the lack of platelet effects allows these drugs to be continued throughout the perioperative period.

Postoperative Pain Management

In contrast to the dose-dependent analgesic effects of opioids, NSAIDs appear to exhibit a ceiling effect when used for postoperative analgesia. NSAIDs are believed to reduce postoperative pain by suppressing COX-mediated production of prostaglandin E2, which is thought to be the primary inflammatory prostaglandin that directly activates and up-regulates the sensitivity of peripheral nociceptors to pain. Opioid requirements for postoperative pain are decreased 20% to 50% by the concomitant use of NSAIDs.

Postoperative Analgesia

Postoperative analgesia produced by COX-2 inhibitors is similar to conventional nonselective NSAIDs but without the effects on platelet function and bleeding.

Perioperative Inhibition of COX Enzyme

Perioperative inhibition of COX enzyme by NSAIDs may cause serious complications (renal injury, gastric ulceration, excessive bleeding). Brief perioperative NSAID use in otherwise healthy adults does not seem to cause significant renal dysfunction, but gastrointestinal ulceration or bleeding may occur after even brief use of NSAIDs.

Protection against Colorectal Cancer

COX-2 expression increases significantly in most human colorectal cancers, and the chronic use of aspirin and other conventional NSAIDs reduces the risk of colorectal cancer.

Protection against Dementia

The risk of developing Alzheimer's disease is decreased among those who use NSAIDs. This may reflect a decrease in inflammatory responses that result in neuronal destruction.

Side Effects

Gastrointestinal Toxicity

Because prostaglandins are involved in the maintenance of gastrointestinal integrity, and because only COX-1 is present in the gastrointestinal tract, it is presumed that the gastrointestinal toxicity produced by nonselective NSAIDs is due principally to inhibition of COX-1 activity. Prostaglandins normally protect gastrointestinal mucosa from damage by maintaining blood flow and increasing the secretion of mucus and bicarbonate. No evidence suggests that NSAIDs contribute to gastroesophageal reflux disease.

Coagulation Effects

Conventional nonspecific NSAIDs inhibit COX-1 (necessary for synthesis of thromboxane from A2 from prostaglandins in platelets) and impair the ability of platelets to aggregate. COX-2 inhibitors have no effect on platelet aggregation, bleeding time, or postoperative blood loss. Aspirin (75 to 325 mg/day) produces an irreversible inactivation of platelet COX-1 that lasts for the life of the platelet (7 to 10 days).

Cardiac Effects

The risk of experiencing a thrombotic episode, myocardial infarction, and congestive heart failure may be increased in patients treated with COX-2 inhibitors. COX-2 inhibitors may serve a protective role by mediating delayed preconditioning against myocardial infarction and stunning.

Hypertensive Effects

Prostaglandins modulate systemic blood pressure by virtue of effects on vascular tone in arteriolar smooth muscle and control of extracellular fluid volume. It is predictable that NSAIDs may interfere with the pharmacologic control of systemic hypertension, although the effect is usually small (about 5 mmHg).

Renal Effects

NSAIDs have no adverse effects on renal function in healthy individuals. When renal toxicity does manifest, it is likely due to NSAID-induced inhibition of prostaglandin synthesis, leading to renal medullary ischemia. Acetaminophen is a phenacetin metabolite that has been associated with an increased risk of end-stage renal disease. Hyperchloremic metabolic acidosis, often in association with hyperkalemia, is an effect of NSAID use, particularly in patients with pre-existing renal disease. There is general agreement that no NSAID other than aspirin can be prescribed with absolute safety with respect to adverse renal effects.

Hepatic Effects

Increases in plasma concentrations of liver transaminases may accompany treatment with NSAIDs.

Allergy

COX-2 inhibitors should not be administered to patients who have experienced asthma, urticaria, or allergic-type reactions to aspirin.

Asthma

NSAIDs may trigger bronchoconstriction in susceptible asthmatic patients by blocking COX-mediated conversion of arachidonic acid to prostaglandins, especially prostaglandin E_2, which is a potent antiinflammatory substance. A history of asthma exacerbation on exposure to aspirin is a reason to avoid NSAIDs that inhibit COX-1 and COX-2 (sodium salicylate and salicylamide may be safely administered to aspirin-sensitive patients).

Aseptic Meningitis

Drug-induced meningitis has been observed following administration of NSAIDs, especially ibuprofen.

Bone Healing

NSAIDs may impair bone healing; thus, these drugs are not recommended for patients undergoing spinal fusion surgery.

Drug Interactions (Table 11-6)

NONSPECIFIC CYCLOOXYGENASE INHIBITORS (TABLE 11-7)

Comparative trials have rarely revealed clinically important differences between these drugs, especially as utilized to treat patients with osteoarthritis or rheumatoid arthritis.

Aspirin

Aspirin is a salicylate that produces analgesia through its ability to irreversibly acetylate COX enzyme, leading to

TABLE 11-6.
DRUG INTERACTIONS IN PATIENTS BEING TREATED WITH NSAIDS

Oral anticoagulants (increased plasma warfarin concentrations)
Aspirin (increased risk of gastric ulceration)
Potassium-sparing diuretics (hyperkalemia)
Digoxin (decreased clearance)
β-Adrenergic antagonists (interfere with antihypertensive effects)
Angiotensin-converting enzyme inhibitors (interfere with antihypertensive effects)
Lithium (decreased clearance)

a decrease in the synthesis and release of prostaglandins.

Pharmacokinetics

Aspirin is rapidly absorbed from the small intestine and, to a lesser extent, from the stomach (acidic gastric pH slows absorption).

Clearance

Aspirin is rapidly hydrolyzed in the liver to salicylic acid, and the plasma concentration of this metabolite is increased in the presence of renal dysfunction.

TABLE 11-7.
CHEMICAL CLASSIFICATION OF NONSPECIFIC NONSTEROIDAL ANTIINFLAMMATORY DRUGS

Carboxylic acids
  Acetylated: aspirin
  Nonacetylated: sodium salicylate, salicylamide, diflunisal
Acetic acids: indomethacin, sulindac, tolmetin
Propionic acids: ibuprofen, naproxen, fenoprofen, ketoprofen
Enolic acids: phenylbutazone, piroxicam
Pyrrolopyrrole: ketorolac

TABLE 11-8.
CLINICAL USES OF ASPIRIN

Analgesia (headache, musculoskeletal pain)
Antipyretic (prevents pyrogen-induced release of prostaglandins in the CNS)
Antiplatelet effect (administered as soon as diagnosis of myocardial infarction is confirmed)

Clinical Uses (Table 11-8)

Side Effects (Table 11-9)

In contrast to other NSAIDs (especially acetaminophen), the chronic use of aspirin has not been shown to increase the incidence of end-stage renal disease.

TABLE 11-9.
SIDE EFFECTS OF ASPIRIN

Gastric irritation and ulceration (reflects inhibition of prostaglandin synthesis that normally inhibits gastric acid secretion)
Prolongation of bleeding time (reflects prevention of the formation of thromboxane, which is a potent stimulant for platelet aggregation; platelet inhibition lasts for the life of the platelet but effect on bleeding time largely disappears by 48 hours)
Central nervous system stimulation (hyperventilation and seizures, metabolic acidosis in children, hyperthermia and dehydration; sodium bicarbonate administration to produce metabolic alkalosis facilitates renal excretion)
Hepatic dysfunction (increased plasma transaminase concentrations)
Metabolic alterations (hyperglycemia)
Allergic reactions (laryngeal edema, bronchoconstriction, cross-tolerance with all NSAIDs)
Asthma

Acetaminophen

Acetaminophen is a useful alternative to aspirin as an analgesic and antipyretic, but it is not considered a true NSAID because it lacks significant antiinflammatory effects. Acetaminophen, unlike salicylates, does not produce gastric irritation or alter the aggregation characteristics of platelets.

Pharmacokinetics

Acetaminophen is converted by conjugation and hydroxylation in the liver to inactive metabolites.

Side Effects (Table 11-10)

Diflunisal

Diflunisal is a salicylic acid derivative that possesses prominent antiarthritic effects, and its effects on platelet aggregation are reversible.

Indomethacin

Indomethacin is a potent COX enzyme inhibitor, and its antiinflammatory effects are useful in the management of patients with arthritis. Cardiac failure in neonates caused by patent ductus arteriosus may be controlled with a single dose of indomethacin, emphasizing the ability of this drug to selectively inhibit the synthesis of prostaglandins.

TABLE 11-10.
SIDE EFFECTS OF ACETAMINOPHEN

Hepatic necrosis (formation of N-acetyl-p-benzoquinone normally scavenged by glutathione, which may be depleted by high doses of the drug; treatment is with acetylcysteine, which acts as a substitute for glutathione)
Methemoglobinemia (genetic deficiency of glucose-6-phosphate)
Hemolytic anemia (genetic deficiency of glucose-6-phosphate)

Side Effects

Side effects including gastrointestinal disturbances, inhibition of platelet aggregation, hepatotoxicity, and allergic reactions, limit the usefulness of this drug.

Sulindac

Sulindac is a substituted analog of indomethacin with similar analgesic, antipyretic, and antiinflammatory effects.

Tolmetin

Tolmetin is an analgesic, antipyretic, and antiinflammatory drug, that, like salicylates, causes gastric irritation and prolongs bleeding time.

Propionic Acid Derivatives

Propionic acid derivatives, such as ibuprofen, naproxen, and diclofenac, possess prominent analgesic, antipyretic, and antiinflammatory effects, reflecting the inhibition of prostaglandin synthesis.

Side Effects

Gastrointestinal irritation and ulceration are usually less severe than the irritation and ulceration that may accompany salicylate use. Platelet function is altered, but the duration varies with the specific drug, and the inhibition of prostaglandin synthesis may exacerbate renal dysfunction in patients with preexisting renal disease.

Drug Interactions

Drug interactions often reflect the extensive protein binding to albumin of propionic acid derivatives (warfarin displaced from protein binding sites).

Phenylbutazone

Phenylbutazone is an effective antiinflammatory drug that is useful in the therapy of acute gout and treatment of rheumatoid arthritis.

TABLE 11-11.
SIDE EFFECTS OF PHENYLBUTAZONE

Anemia and granulocytosis (limit usefulness of this drug)
Nausea, vomiting, and epigastric discomfort
Rashes
Sodium retention and decreased urine output
Increased plasma volume (weight gain, dilutional anemia, pulmonary edema in susceptible patients)
Displacement of warfarin from plasma protein binding sites
Inhibition of synthesis of organic iodide compounds

Pharmacokinetics

Phenylbutazone undergoes hepatic metabolism to oxyphenbutazone, which has an antiinflammatory activity similar to the parent drug. Phenylbutazone and oxyphenbutazone are excreted slowly in the urine, because extensive plasma protein binding limits glomerular filtration.

Side Effects (Table 11-11)

Piroxicam

Piroxicam inhibits prostaglandin synthesis and produces pharmacologic effects similar to other NSAIDs. Extensive protein binding may displace other drugs, such as aspirin and oral anticoagulants, from albumin-binding sites.

Ketorolac

Ketorolac is an NSAID that exhibits potent analgesic effects but only moderate antiinflammatory effects when administered intramuscularly or intravenously. This drug is useful for providing postoperative analgesia both as the sole drug (less painful ambulatory procedures) and to supplement opioids. In contrast to the dose-dependent analgesic effects of opioids, ketorolac and other NSAIDs appear to exhibit a ceiling effect with respect to postoperative analgesia. An important benefit of ketorolac analgesia is the absence of ventilatory or cardiac depression.

TABLE 11-12.
SIDE EFFECTS OF KETOROLAC

Inhibition of platelet aggregation (prolonged bleeding time)
Allergic reactions (bronchospasm in patients with aspirin sensitivity)
Renal toxicity (low risk)
Hepatic toxicity (modest increases in plasma transaminase concentrations)
Gastrointestinal irritation and perforation
Peripheral edema

Pharmacokinetics

After IM injection, maximum plasma concentrations of ketorolac are achieved within 45 to 60 minutes and the elimination half-time is about 5 hours.

Side Effects (Table 11-12)

MISCELLANEOUS ANTIARTHRITIC DRUGS

Colchicine

Colchicine decreases inflammation and thus decreases pain in acute gouty arthritis.

Mechanism of Action

Colchicine does not influence the renal excretion of uric acid but instead alters the fibrillar microtubules in granu-

TABLE 11-13.
SIDE EFFECTS OF COLCHICINE

Nausea, vomiting, diarrhea, and abdominal pain (discontinue drug when gastrointestinal symptoms appear)
Hemorrhagic gastroenteritis
Enhanced effects produced by CNS depressants and sympathomimetics
Depression of medullary ventilatory center
Bone marrow depression (leukopenia, thrombocytopenia)

TABLE 11-14.
SIDE EFFECTS OF ALLOPURINOL

Maculopapular rash (pruritus is an indication to discontinue therapy)
Fever and myalgia
Nephritis and vasculitis
Hepatic dysfunction
Inhibits enzymatic inactivation of 6-mercaptopurine and azathioprine
Inhibits hepatic drug metabolizing enzymes

locytes, thus inhibiting the migration of these cells into inflamed areas.

Side Effects (Table 11-13)

Allopurinol

Allopurinol is the preferred drug for the therapy of primary hyperuricemia of gout and hyperuricemia that occurs during therapy with chemotherapeutic drugs.

Mechanism of Action

Allopurinol interferes with the terminal steps of uric acid synthesis by inhibiting xanthine oxidase.

Side Effects (Table 11-14)

Uricosuric Drugs

Uricosuric drugs, such as probenecid and sulfinpyrazone, act directly on renal tubules to increase the rate of excretion of uric acid and other organic acids, including penicillin. These drugs are also useful in controlling hyperuricemia resulting from the use of chemotherapeutic drugs or from diseases associated with the accelerated destruction of erythrocytes. The biliary excretion of rifampin is decreased by probenecid, making it possible to achieve higher plasma concentrations of this antituberculosis drug.

Sympathomimetics

12

Sympathomimetics include naturally occurring (endogenous) catecholamines, synthetic catecholamines, and synthetic catecholamines (Table 12-1) (Stoelting RK, Hillier SC. Sympathomimetics. In: *Pharmacology and Physiology in Anesthetic Practice*, 4th ed. Philadelphia. Lippincott Williams & Wilkins, 2006:292–310). These drugs evoke physiologic responses similar to those produced by the endogenous activity of the sympathetic nervous system (see Table 12-2). The net effect of sympathomimetics on cardiac function is influenced by baroreceptor-mediated reflex responses.

CLINICAL USES (TABLE 12-3)

STRUCTURE–ACTIVITY RELATIONSHIPS

All sympathomimetics are derived from β-phenylethylamine (Fig. 12-1). The presence of hydroxyl groups on the 3 and 4 carbon positions of the benzene ring of β-phenylethylamine designates it as a catechol, and drugs with this composition are designated *catecholamines*. Synthetic noncatecholamines include the β-phenylethylamine structure but lack the hydroxyl groups on the 3 and 4 carbons of the benzene ring.

Receptor Selectivity

The receptor selectivity of sympathomimetics for various adrenergic receptors depends on the chemical structure of the drug. Maximal α- and β-adrenergic receptor activity

TABLE 12-1.
CLASSIFICATION OF SYMPATHOMIMETICS

Natural catecholamines
- Epinephrine
- Norepinephrine
- Dopamine

Synthetic catecholamines
- Isoproterenol
- Dobutamine

Synthetic noncatecholamines
- Indirect-acting
  - Ephedrine
  - Mephentermine
  - Amphetamines
  - Metaraminol
- Direct-acting
  - Phenylephrine
  - Methoxamine

TABLE 12-2.
PHARMACOLOGIC EFFECTS OF SYMPATHOMIMETICS

Vasoconstriction (especially in cutaneous and renal circulations)
Vasodilation (skeletal muscles)
Bronchodilation
Cardiac stimulation (increased heart rate, myocardial contractility and vulnerability to cardiac dysrhythmias)
Liberation of free fatty acids
Hepatic glycogenolysis
Modulation of insulin, renin, and pituitary hormone secretion
Central nervous system stimulation

TABLE 12-3.
CLINICAL USES OF SYMPATHOMIMETICS

Positive inotropic agents (ability to measure atrial filling pressures and cardiac output and calculate systemic vascular resistance is useful when used for this purpose)
Vasopressors (following sympathetic nervous system blockade produced by regional anesthesia, during time needed to eliminate excess volatile anesthetic or restore intravascular fluid volume, use as vasopressors only when pressure-dependent decreases in blood flow could result in tissue ischemia)
Bronchospasm
Allergic reactions
Retard systemic absorption of local anesthetics

depends on the presence of hydroxyl groups on the 3 and 4 carbon atoms of the benzene ring of β-phenylethylamine.

Central Nervous System Stimulation

Central nervous system (CNS) stimulation is prominent with synthetic noncatecholamines that lack substituents on the benzene ring (methamphetamine, ephedrine). Catecholamines have limited lipid solubility and thus are not likely to cross the blood-brain barrier in sufficient amounts to cause CNS stimulation.

MECHANISM OF ACTION

Sympathomimetics exert their pharmacologic effects by activating, either directly or indirectly, α-adrenergic, β-adrenergic, or dopaminergic receptors that belong to the family of G protein–coupled receptors. Once activated by binding with a ligand, G proteins diffuse into cell membranes to encounter an effector protein (an

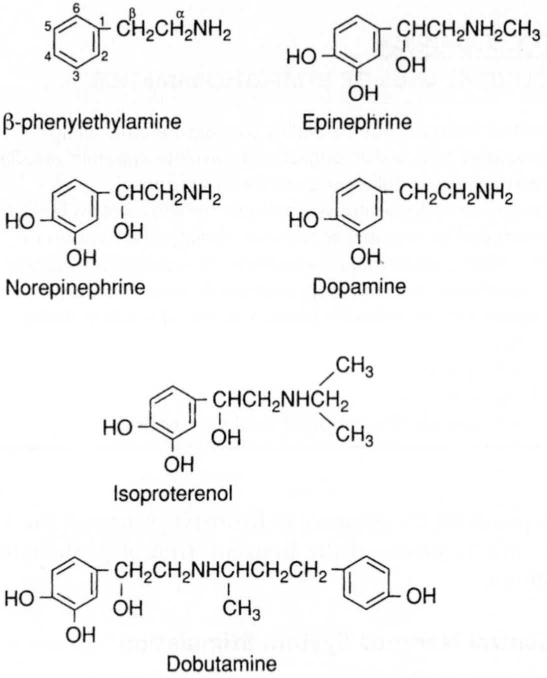

β-phenylethylamine

Epinephrine

Norepinephrine

Dopamine

Isoproterenol

Dobutamine

Figure 12-1. Sympathomimetics are derived from β-phenylethylamine, with a catecholamine being any compound that has hydroxyl groups on the 3 and 4 carbon positions of the benzene ring.

intracellular enzyme, such as adenylate cyclase) or an ion channel.

The production of cyclic adenosine monophosphate (cAMP, second messenger) by stimulating the enzyme adenylate cyclase is the speculated mechanism by which sympathomimetics produce pharmacologic effects. This is considered to reflect β-adrenergic receptor stimulation. An important factor in the pharmacologic response elicited by sympathomimetics is the distribution and density of α- and β-adrenergic receptors (Table 12-4).

Indirect-acting Sympathomimetics

Indirect-acting sympathomimetics are synthetic noncatecholamines that activate adrenergic receptors by evoking the release of the endogenous neurotransmitter norepinephrine from postganglionic sympathetic nerve endings.

Indirect-acting sympathomimetics are characterized mostly by α- and β-1-adrenergic agonist effects because norepinephrine is a weak β-2-agonist.

Direct-acting Sympathomimetics

Direct-acting sympathomimetics activate adrenergic receptors directly, although their potency is less than that of catecholamines. Most direct-acting sympathomimetics activate both α- and β-adrenergic receptors, but the magnitude of α- and β-activity varies greatly among drugs from almost pure α-agonist activity for phenylephrine to almost pure β-agonist activity for isoproterenol.

METABOLISM

Catecholamines

All drugs containing the 3,4-dihydroxybenzene structure are rapidly inactivated by the enzymes monoamine oxidase (MAO) or catechol-O-methyltransferase (COMT). The resulting inactive methylated metabolites are conjugated with glucuronic acid and appear in the urine as 3-methoxy-4-hydroxymandelic acid, metanephrine (derived from epinephrine), and normetanephrine (derived from norepinephrine). The lungs are efficient biochemical filters, as reflected by clearance of endogenous catecholamine from the central venous blood during pulmonary transit.

Synthetic Noncatecholamines

Synthetic noncatecholamines are not affected by COMT and thus depend on MAO for their metabolism

TABLE 12-4.

CLASSIFICATION AND COMPARATIVE PHARMACOLOGY OF SYMPATHOMIMETICS

	Receptors Stimulated			Mechanism of Action	Cardiac Effects		
	α	β1	β2		Cardiac Output	Heart Rate	Dysrhythmias
Natural catecholamines							
Epinephrine	+	++	++	Direct	++	++	+++
Norepinephrine	+++	++	0	Direct	–	–	+
Dopamine	++	++	+	Direct	+++	+	+
Synthetic catecholamines							
Isoproterenol	0	+++	+++		+++	+++	+++
Dobutamine	0	+++	0		+++	+	±
Synthetic noncatecholamines							
Indirect-acting							
Ephedrine	++	+	+	Indirect, some direct	++	++	++
Mephentermine	++	+	+	Indirect	++	++	++
Amphetamines	++	+	+	Indirect	+	+	+
Metaraminol	++	+	+	Indirect, direct	–	–	+
Direct-acting							
Phenylephrine	+++	0	0	Direct	–	–	NC
Methoxamine	+++	0	0	Direct	–	–	NC

0, none; +, minimal increase; ++, moderate increase; +++, marked increase; –, minimal decrease; – –, moderate decrease; – – – marked decrease; NC, no change.

(often slower than for catecholamines and inhibition of MAO) may even further prolong their duration of action.

ROUTE OF ADMINISTRATION

The oral administration of catecholamines is not effective, because of metabolism by enzymes in the gastrointestinal

Peripheral Vascular Resistance	Renal Blood Flow	Mean Arterial Pressure	Airway Resistance	Central Nervous System Stimulation	Single Intravenous Dose (70-kg Adult)	Continuous Infusion Dose (70-kg Adult)
±	−−	+	−−	Yes	2–8 μg	1–20 μg/min
+++	−−−	+++	NC	No	Not used	4–16 μg/min
+	+++	+	NC	No	Not used	2–20 μg/kg/min
−−	−	±	−−−	Yes	1–4 μg	1–5 μg/min
NC	++	+	NC		Not used	2–10 μg/kg/min
+	−−	++	−−	Yes	10–25 mg	Not used
+	−−	++	−	Yes	10–25 mg	Not used
++	−−	+	NC	Yes	Not used	Not used
+++	−−−	+++	NC	No	1.5–5.0 mg	40–500 μg/kg/min
+++	−−−	+++	NC	No	50–100 μg	20–50 μg/min
+++	−−−	+++	NC	No	5–10 mg	

mucosa and liver. For this reason, epinephrine is administered subcutaneously or intravenously. Dopamine, dobutamine, and norepinephrine are administered only intravenously.

NATURALLY OCCURRING CATECHOLAMINES (TABLE 12-1)

Epinephrine

Epinephrine is the prototype drug among the sympathomimetics. It is the most potent activator of α-adrenergic receptors (2 to 10 times more active than norepinephrine) and also activates β1 and β2 receptors.

Clinical Uses (Table 12-5)

Side Effects

Cardiovascular Effects

The cardiovascular effects of epinephrine result from epinephrine-induced stimulation of α- and β-adrenergic receptors (see Table 12-4). Small doses of epinephrine (1 to 2 μg/kg per minute IV) stimulate principally β2-receptors in peripheral vasculature. The stimulation of β1-receptors occurs at somewhat larger doses (4 μg/min IV), whereas larger doses of epinephrine (10 to 20 μg/kg per minute IV) stimulate both α- and β-adrenergic receptors with the effects of α-stimulation predominating in most vascular beds, including the cutaneous and renal circulations.

Airway Smooth Muscle

The smooth muscles of the bronchi are relaxed by virtue of epinephrine-induced activation of β2-receptors.

Metabolic Effects

Epinephrine has the most significant effects of all the catecholamines on metabolism (liver glycogenolysis, inhibition of insulin release).

TABLE 12-5.
CLINICAL USES OF EPINEPHRINE

Addition to local anesthetic solutions (decrease systemic absorption and prolong duration of action)
Treat life-threatening allergic reactions
Cardiopulmonary resuscitation (supraphysiologic doses not necessary)
Increase myocardial contractility (continuous infusion)

Electrolytes

Selective β2-adrenergic agonist effects following the low-dose infusion of epinephrine are speculated to reflect activation of the sodium-potassium pump in skeletal muscles, leading to the transfer of potassium ions into cells.

Ocular Effects

Epinephrine causes contraction of the radial muscles of the iris, producing mydriasis.

Gastrointestinal and Genitourinary Effects

Epinephrine, norepinephrine, and isoproterenol produce relaxation of gastrointestinal smooth muscle. Activation of β-adrenergic receptors relaxes the detrusor muscle of the bladder, whereas activation of α-adrenergic receptors contracts the trigone and sphincter muscles.

Coagulation

Blood coagulation is accelerated by epinephrine, and the hypercoagulable state present during the intraoperative and postoperative period may reflect a stress-associated release of epinephrine.

Treatment of Overdose

(See the section on phenylephrine, Treatment of Overdose.)

Norepinephrine

Norepinephrine is the endogenous neurotransmitter released from postganglionic sympathetic nerve endings. It is approximately equal in potency to epinephrine in the stimulation of β1-receptors, but unlike epinephrine, norepinephrine has little agonist effect at β2-receptors (see Table 12-4). Norepinephrine is a potent α-agonist that produces intense arterial and venous vasoconstriction.

Cardiovascular Effects

A continuous infusion of norepinephrine, 4 to 16 μg/kg per minute IV, may be used to treat the refractory hypotension that may occur in the early period after ligation of the vascular supply to a pheochromocytoma. Norepinephrine-induced peripheral vasoconstriction results in increased systemic vascular resistance and decreased venous return to the heart (when combined with baroreceptor-mediated reflex decreases in heart rate, this tends to decrease cardiac output).

Dopamine

Dopamine is an endogenous catecholamine that is the immediate precursor of norepinephrine. Dopamine regulates cardiac, vascular, and endocrine function and is an important neurotransmitter in the CNS and peripheral nervous system.

Depending on the dose, dopamine stimulates principally dopamine-1 receptors (0.5 to 3 μg/kg per minute IV) in the renal vasculature to produce renal vasodilation, β1 receptors (3 to 10 μg/kg per minute IV) in the heart to produce tachycardia and increased cardiac output and α-receptors (>10 μg/kg per minute IV) in the peripheral vasculature to produce vasoconstriction. Despite identical intravenous infusion rates, a 10- to 75-fold variability may occur in the plasma dopamine concentrations that are produced.

Clinical Uses

Dopamine is used clinically to increase cardiac output in patients with low systemic blood pressure, increased atrial filling pressures, and low urine output. It is unique among the catecholamines in being able to simultaneously increase myocardial contractility, renal blood flow, glomerular filtration rate, excretion of sodium, and urine output.

Renal Dose Dopamine

Renal-dose dopamine refers to a continuous infusion of small doses (1 to 3 μg/kg per minute IV) of dopamine to patients at risk for the development of acute renal failure. Data confirming the efficacy of dopamine in preventing acute renal failure (also true for mannitol and furosemide) are not available.

Side Effects

Cardiovascular Effects

Dopamine increases cardiac output by stimulation of β1-receptors. This increase in cardiac output is usually accompanied by only modest increases in heart rate, systemic blood pressure, and systemic vascular resistance. The divergent pharmacologic effects of dopamine and dobutamine make their use in combination potentially useful; the resulting increase in cardiac output and decrease in afterload mimics the effect achieved by the intraaortic balloon pump.

Ventilation Effects

The infusion of dopamine interferes with the ventilatory response to arterial hypoxemia, thus reflecting the role of dopamine as an inhibitory neurotransmitter at the carotid bodies (unexpected depression of ventilation).

SYNTHETIC CATECHOLAMINES (SEE TABLE 12-4)

Isoproterenol

Isoproterenol is the most potent activator of all the sympathomimetics at β1- and β2-receptors, being two to three times more potent than epinephrine and at least 100 times more active than norepinephrine. In clinical doses, isoproterenol is devoid of α-agonist effects. The metabolism of isoproterenol by the liver through the action of COMT is rapid, thus necessitating a continuous infusion.

Clinical Uses

The continuous infusion of isoproterenol at 1 to 5 μg/kg per minute is effective in increasing the heart rate in the presence of heart block. Isoproterenol is used to provide sustained increases in heart rate before the insertion of a temporary or permanent cardiac pacemaker in the treatment of bradydysrhythmias.

Cardiovascular Effects

The cardiovascular effects of isoproterenol reflect activation of β1-receptors in the heart and β2-receptors in the vasculature of skeletal muscles. The net effect of these changes is an increase in cardiac output that is sufficient to increase systolic blood pressure in the presence of decreases in systemic vascular resistance and associated decreases in diastolic blood pressure. Isoproterenol may decrease coronary blood flow at a time when myocardial oxygen requirements are increased by tachycardia and increased myocardial contractility.

Dobutamine

Dobutamine is a synthetic catecholamine that acts as a selective β1-agonist that undergoes rapid metabolism, thus necessitating its administration as a continuous intravenous infusion. Dobutamine administration results in increased myocardial contractility. Modest β2-agonist stimulation causes a modest degree of peripheral vasodilation.

Clinical Uses

Dobutamine is used to improve cardiac output in patients with congestive heart failure, particularly if heart rate and systemic vascular resistance are increased.

Cardiovascular Effects

Dobutamine produces dose-dependent increases in cardiac output and decreases in atrial filling pressures with associated significant increases in systemic blood pressure and heart rate. The small increase in heart rate, when compared with isoproterenol, reflects a lesser effect of dobutamine on the sinoatrial node. Vasoconstrictor activity and calculated systemic vascular resistance is usually not greatly altered; thus, dobutamine may be ineffective in patients who require increased systemic vascular resistance rather than augmentation of cardiac output to increase systemic blood pressure.

Dopexamine

Dopexamine is a synthetic catecholamine that activates dopaminergic and β2-receptors (unlike dopamine, dopexamine is devoid of α-effects).

SYNTHETIC NONCATECHOLAMINES (SEE TABLE 12-4)

Ephedrine

Ephedrine is an indirect-acting (through the stimulation of the endogenous release of norepinephrine) synthetic noncatecholamine that stimulates α- and β-adrenergic receptors. This drug also evokes pharmacologic effects by direct stimulant effects on adrenergic receptors. Ephedrine is resistant to metabolism by MAO in the gastrointestinal tract (thus it is effective orally). The slow inactivation and excretion of ephedrine are responsible for the prolonged duration of action of this sympathomimetic. Mydriasis accompanies the administration of ephedrine, and CNS stimulation does occur (but less than with amphetamine).

Clinical Uses (Table 12-6)

Cardiovascular Effects

The cardiovascular effects of ephedrine resemble those of epinephrine, but its systemic blood pressure-elevating response is less intense and lasts approximately 10 times longer. The intravenous administration of ephedrine results in increases in systolic and diastolic blood pressure, heart rate, and cardiac output, thus reflecting α-receptor mediated peripheral arterial and venous vasoconstriction and increased myocardial contractility due to activation of β1-receptors. A second dose of ephedrine produces a less

TABLE 12-6.
CLINICAL USES OF EPHEDRINE

Treat decreased blood pressure (10 to 25 mg IV) due to sympathetic nervous system blockade produced by regional anesthesia or inhaled or injected anesthetics
Treat decreased blood pressure in parturients due to spinal or epidural anesthesia (phenylephrine also acceptable)
Bronchial asthma (oral administration)
Decongestant nasal spray

intense systemic blood pressure response than the first dose (tachyphylaxis).

Mephentermine

Mephentermine is an indirect-acting synthetic noncatecholamine that stimulates α- and β-adrenergic receptors. Administered intravenously, mephentermine produces cardiovascular effects that resemble ephedrine.

Amphetamine and Related Sympathomimetics

Amphetamine and related sympathomimetics, such as *dextroamphetamine* and *methamphetamine*, resemble ephedrine in evoking α- and β-adrenergic receptors stimulation but differ from ephedrine in producing significant CNS stimulation and appetite suppression that reflects the release of endogenous norepinephrine.

Modafinil

Modafinil is a wakefulness-promoting drug that is useful for the treatment of narcolepsy and may be effective in countering the sedation and fatigue following recovery from general anesthesia.

Metaraminol

Metaraminol is a synthetic noncatecholamine that stimulates α- and β-adrenergic receptors by indirect and direct effects. Uptake into postganglionic sympathetic nerve endings occurs, because this drug substitutes for norepinephrine and acts as a weak neurotransmitter.

Cardiovascular Effects

Metaraminol produces more intense peripheral vasoconstriction and less increase in myocardial contractility than ephedrine. Sustained increases in systolic and diastolic blood pressure are due almost entirely to peripheral vasoconstriction.

Reflex bradycardia often accompanies these drug-induced increases in systemic blood pressure, resulting in a decrease in cardiac output.

Phenylephrine

Phenylephrine is a synthetic noncatecholamine that stimulates principally α1-adrenergic receptors by a direct effect, with only a small part of the pharmacologic response being due to its ability to evoke the release of norepinephrine (an indirect-action). Venoconstriction is greater than arterial constriction. Clinically, phenylephrine mimics the effects of norepinephrine but is less potent and longer lasting. CNS stimulation is minimal.

Clinical Uses (Table 12-7)

Obstetric Anesthesia

Phenylephrine is an alternative to ephedrine for the treatment of maternal hypotension. The intravenous administration of phenylephrine, but not ephedrine, to prevent maternal hypotension during combined spinal-epidural anesthesia for cesarean section decreases the rostral spread of spinal anesthesia; this may reflect the differential effects of these two drugs on epidural vein constriction.

Side Effects

Cardiovascular Effects

The rapid intravenous injection of phenylephrine to patients with coronary artery disease produces dose-

TABLE 12-7.
CLINICAL USES OF PHENYLEPHRINE

Treat decreased blood pressure (50 to 200 μg IV) due to sympathetic nervous system blockade produced by regional anesthesia or inhaled or injected anesthetics
Treat decreased blood pressure in parturients due to spinal or epidural anesthesia (phenylephrine is associated with a higher umbilical artery pH and less fetal acidosis at delivery compared with parturients receiving ephedrine)
Maintain perfusion pressure (continuous IV infusion during carotid endarterectomy)
Decongestant nasal spray
Prolong duration of spinal anesthesia when added to the local anesthetic solution (similar to epinephrine)

dependent peripheral vasoconstriction and increases in systemic blood pressure that are accompanied by decreases in cardiac output (reflects increased afterload and baroreceptor-mediated reflex bradycardia in response to drug-induced increases in diastolic blood pressure).

Metabolic Effects

Metabolic side effects include the stimulation of α-receptors by a continuous infusion of phenylephrine, which interferes with the movement of potassium ions across cell membranes into cells.

Treatment of Overdose

Systemic manifestations of sympathetic nervous system activation (systemic hypertension, tachycardia, baroreceptor-mediated bradycardia) may accompany the vascular absorption of α-agonists such as phenylephrine and epinephrine when they are utilized as topical or injected vasoconstrictors in the surgical field. Treatment of these systemic effects with β-adrenergic–blocking drugs (prevents compensatory increases in myocardial contractility and heart rate in response to abrupt increases in afterload) may be followed by pulmonary edema and irreversible cardiovascular collapse. Systemic hypertension induced by topically applied or injected α-agonists may not require treatment, because the duration of action of phenylephrine and epinephrine is brief. When pharmacologic intervention is deemed necessary, the administration of vasodilating drugs, such as nitroprusside or nitroglycerin, is recommended.

Methoxamine

Methoxamine is a synthetic noncatecholamine that acts directly and selectively on α-adrenergic receptors. It resembles phenylephrine but has a longer duration of action. Methoxamine, 5 to 10 mg IV, when administered to adults causes intense arterial vasoconstriction that manifests as increased systolic and diastolic blood pressure and baroreceptor-mediated reflex bradycardia that contributes to a decrease in cardiac output.

Milodrine

Milodrine is an α1-adrenergic agonist that activates receptors in arterioles and veins to increase systemic vascular resistance. It is used for the treatment of neurogenic orthostatic hypotension that may accompany diabetes mellitus.

SELECTIVE β2-ADRENERGIC AGONISTS

Selective β2-adrenergic agonists specifically relax bronchiole and uterine smooth muscle, but in contrast to isoproterenol, they generally lack stimulating (β1-adrenergic) effects on the heart. However, high concentrations of these drugs are likely to cause β1 stimulation.

Clinical Uses

β2-Adrenergic agonists are the preferred treatment for acute episodes of asthma and the prevention of exercise-

TABLE 12-8.

COMPARATIVE PHARMACOLOGY OF SELECTIVE β2-ADRENERGIC AGONIST BRONCHODILATORS

	β_2 Selectivity	Peak Effect (mins)	Duration of Action (hrs)	Concentration (μg per puff)	Method of Administration
Intermediate-acting (3–6 hrs)					
Albuterol	++++	30–60	4	90	MDI, oral
Metaproterenol	+++	30–60	3–4	200	Oral, subcutaneous
Terbutaline	++++	60	4	200	MDI, oral, subcutaneous
Isoetharine	++	15–60	2–3	340	MDI, solution
Bitolterol	++++	30–60	5	370	MDI
Long-acting (>12 hrs)					
Salmeterol	++++		>12	21	MDI

++, minimal stimulation; +++, moderate stimulation; ++++, marked stimulation; MDI, metered-dose inhaler; solution, solution of nebulization.

induced asthma (Table 12-8). In addition to the treatment of bronchospasm, β2-adrenergic agonists may also be administered as continuous infusions to stop premature uterine contractions (tocolytics).

Route of Administration (Table 12-8)

The inhaled route (through a nebulizer or metered-dose inhaler) is the preferred route of administration for β2-adrenergic agonists because the side effects from systemic absorption are fewer for any given degree of bronchodilation.

Side Effects (Table 12-9)

Albuterol

Albuterol is the preferred selective β2-adrenergic agonist for the treatment of acute bronchospasm due to asthma. Administration is most often by metered-dose inhaler, producing about 100 μg per puff (usual dose is two puffs during deep inhalations 1 to 5 minutes apart). This dose may be repeated every 4 to 6 hours. Alternatively, 2.5 to 5 mg of albuterol (0.5 to 1 mL of 0.5% solution in 5 mL of normal saline) may be administered by nebulization

TABLE 12-9.
SIDE EFFECTS OF β2 AGONISTS

Tremor (β2-receptors in skeletal muscles)
Tachycardia (reflects reflex tachycardia and direct stimulation of β2-receptors in the heart)
Transient decrease in arterial oxygenation (relaxation of compensatory pulmonary vascular vasoconstriction in areas of decreased ventilation)
Acute metabolic responses (hyperglycemia, hypokalemia, hypomagnesemia, not present with chronic treatment)
Lactic acidosis

TABLE 12-10.
SIDE EFFECTS OF RITODRINE

Tachycardia (stimulation of β2-receptors and reflex responses to decreased diastolic blood pressure)
Increased renin secretion (decreased excretion of sodium)
Pulmonary edema (restrict fluid intake)
Hypotension (exaggerated in presence of volatile anesthetics)
Hypokalemia (reflects translocation of potassium into cells)
Hyperglycemia (ketoacidosis may occur in diabetics)

every 15 minutes for three to four doses. The duration of action of an inhaled dose is about 4 hours.

Tachycardia and hypokalemia may accompany large doses of albuterol.

Bitolterol

Bitolterol is a selective β2-adrenergic agonist that resembles albuterol but is more potent and lasts longer.

Ritodrine

Ritodrine is the β2-adrenergic agonist most often use to stop the uterine contractions of premature labor.

Side Effects (Table 12-10)

Digitalis and Related Drugs

13

Digoxin, digitoxin, and ouabain are examples of clinically useful cardiac glycosides ("digitalis") (Stoelting RK, Hillier SC. Digitalis and related drugs. In: *Pharmacology and Physiology in Anesthetic Practice,* 4th ed. Philadelphia. Lippincott Williams & Wilkins, 2006:311–320). Nonglycoside and noncatecholamine drugs that may be administered for similar clinical purposes as cardiac glycosides include specific phosphodiesterase (PDE) III inhibitors, calcium, and glucagon.

CLINICAL USES

Cardiac glycosides are used most often during the perioperative period for the management of supraventricular tachydysrhythmias (paroxysmal atrial tachycardia, atrial fibrillation, atrial flutter) based on the ability of these drugs to slow the conduction of cardiac impulses through the atrioventricular node. The use of cardiac glycosides to treat acute decreases in left ventricular contractility is uncommon because of the availability of more potent and less toxic drugs. Nevertheless, cardiac glycosides continue to have an important therapeutic role in the treatment of chronic congestive heart failure. The intravenous administration of propranolol or esmolol combined with digoxin may provide more rapid control of supraventricular tachydysrhythmias and minimize the likelihood of toxicity by permitting decreases in the dose of both classes of drugs. Digitalis glycosides may be hazardous in the presence of direct-current cardioversion (cardiac dysrhythmias) and hypertrophic aortic stenosis (increased myocardial contractility intensifies resistance to ventricular ejection).

STRUCTURE–ACTIVITY RELATIONSHIPS

The basic structure of cardiac glycosides is that of a steroid cyclopentenophenanthrene nucleus that consists of a glycone portion (pharmacologically inactive but necessary for the fixation of cardiac glycosides to cardiac muscle) and an aglycone portion (produces pharmacologic effects).

MECHANISM OF ACTION

Direct Effects on the Heart

Cardiac glycosides selectively and reversibly inhibit the sodium-potassium adenosine triphosphate (ATP) ion transport system (sodium pump) located in the sarcolemma of cardiac cell membranes. The resulting increase in sodium ion concentration in cardiac cells leads to decreased extrusion of calcium ions by the sodium pump mechanism. It is presumed that this increased intracellular concentration of calcium ions is responsible for the positive inotropic effects of cardiac glycosides. Excessive digitalis-induced increases in intracellular calcium ion concentrations decrease the spread of excitatory current from one myocardial cell to another, manifesting as impaired conduction of cardiac impulses.

Alterations in Autonomic Nervous System Activity

The autonomic nervous system effects of cardiac glycosides include increased parasympathetic nervous system activity due to sensitization of arterial baroreceptors (carotid sinus) and activation of vagal nuclei and the nodose ganglion in the central nervous system (CNS), manifesting as a slowed heart rate, especially in the presence of atrial fibrillation.

PHARMACOKINETICS

At equilibrium, the concentration of cardiac glycosides in the heart is 15 to 30 times greater than those in the plasma.

Digoxin

The absorption of digoxin after oral administration is approximately 75% in the first hour, with peak plasma concentrations occurring in 1 to 2 hours (Table 13-1).

TABLE 13-1.
COMPARISON OF DIGOXIN AND DIGITOXIN

	Digoxin	Digitoxin
Average digitalizing dose		
Oral	0.75–1.50 mg	0.8–1.2 mg
Intravenous	0.5–1.0 mg	0.8–1.2 mg
Average daily maintenance dose		
Oral	0.125–0.500 mg	0.05–0.20 mg
Intravenous	0.25 mg	0.1 mg
Onset of effect		
Oral	1.5–6.0 hrs	3–6 hrs
Intravenous	5–30 mins	30–120 mins
Absorption from the gastrointestinal tract	75%	90–100%
Plasma protein binding	25%	95%
Route of elimination	Renal	Hepatic
Enterohepatic circulation	Minimal	Marked
Elimination half-time	31–33 hrs	5–7 days
Therapeutic plasma concentration	0.5–2.0 ng/ml	10–35 ng/ml

The clearance of digoxin from the plasma is primarily by the kidneys, with approximately 35% of the drug excreted daily. A guideline is to decrease the dose of digoxin by 50% when the serum creatinine concentration is 3 to 5 mg/dL. The principal inactive tissue reservoir site for digoxin is the skeletal muscles, therefore elderly patients with decreased skeletal muscle mass may develop increased plasma and myocardial digoxin levels of digoxin.

Digitoxin

The absorption of digitoxin after oral administration is 90% to 100%, reflecting the greater lipid solubility of this cardiac glycoside compared with digoxin (see Table 13-1).

Ouabain

Ouabain is administered in doses of 1.5 to 3.0 μg/kg IV to provide rapid increases in myocardial contractility or to decrease the heart rate in rapid ventricular response atrial fibrillation.

CARDIOVASCULAR EFFECTS

The principal cardiovascular effect of digitalis glycosides administered to patients with cardiac failure is a dose-dependent increase in myocardial contractility (increased stroke volume, decreased heart size, decreased left ventricular end-diastolic pressure). Improved renal perfusion due to an overall increase in cardiac output favors the mobilization and excretion of edema fluid, accounting for the diuresis that often accompanies the administration of cardiac glycosides to patients in cardiac failure. In addition to positive inotropic effects, cardiac glycosides enhance parasympathetic nervous system activity (negative dromotropic and chronotropic effect) leading to decreases in heart rate.

TABLE 13-2.
ELECTROCARDIOGRAPHIC EFFECTS OF CARDIAC GLYCOSIDES

Prolonged P-R interval (rarely >0.25 second)
Shortened QTc interval
ST segment depression (scaphoid or scooped out and may mimic myocardial ischemia)
Diminished amplitude or inversion of T waves

ELECTROCARDIOGRAPHIC EFFECTS (TABLE 13-2)

When digitalis is discontinued, the changes in the electrocardiogram (ECG) disappear in approximately 20 days.

DIGITALIS TOXICITY

Cardiac glycosides have a narrow therapeutic range; the therapeutic effects of cardiac glycosides develop at 35% of the fatal dose and cardiac dysrhythmias typically manifest at approximately 60% of the fatal dose. It is presumed that the increased intracellular calcium ion concentrations (inhibition of the sodium-potassium ATPase ion transport system) that accompany digitalis toxicity are responsible for associated ectopic cardiac dysrhythmias.

Causes (Table 13-3)

Diagnosis (Table 13-4)

Digitalis is often administered in situations in which the toxic effects of the drug are difficult to distinguish from the effects of the cardiac disease.

TABLE 13-3.
CAUSES OF DIGITALIS TOXICITY

Hypokalemia (diuretics, hyperventilation)
Hypercalcemia
Hypomagnesemia
Increased sympathetic nervous system activity (arterial hypoxemia)
Decreased skeletal muscle mass (elderly patients)
Renal dysfunction

TABLE 13-4.
DIAGNOSIS OF DIGITALIS TOXICITY

Plasma digoxin concentrations >3 ng/mL (higher in infants and children; lower in the presence of electrolyte disturbances and recent myocardial infarction)
Anorexia, nausea, and vomiting
Transitory amblyopia
Atrial or ventricular cardiac dysrhythmias (atrial tachycardia with block; ventricular fibrillation is most frequent cause of death from digitalis toxicity)

TABLE 13-5.
TREATMENT OF DIGITALIS TOXICITY

Correction of predisposing causes (hypokalemia, hypomagnesemia, arterial hypoxemia)
Treatment of cardiac dysrhythmias
Phenytoin 0.5 to 1.5 mg/kg IV over 5 minutes
Lidocaine 1 to 2 mg/kg IV
Atropine 35 to 70 μg/kg IV
Temporary artificial transvenous cardiac pacemaker (heart block)
Supplemental potassium (decreases binding of digitalis to cardiac muscle)
Propranolol (suppresses increased automaticity; not recommended when conduction blockade is present)
Fab antibodies (life-threatening digitalis toxicity)

Treatment (Table 13-5)

PREOPERATIVE PROPHYLACTIC DIGITALIS

The preoperative administration of prophylactic digitalis is controversial (narrow therapeutic range in the absence of an indication) but patients with limited cardiac reserve may benefit from it; for example, in elderly patients undergoing thoracic or abdominal surgery, it decreases the occurrence of postoperative supraventricular cardiac dysrhythmias. It is particularly important to continue digitalis therapy throughout the perioperative period in patients who are receiving the drug for heart rate control.

DRUG INTERACTIONS (TABLE 13-6)

SELECTIVE PHOSPHODIESTERASE INHIBITORS (NONCATECHOLAMINE, NONGLYCOSIDE CARDIAC INOTROPIC AGENTS)

These drugs exert a competitive inhibitory action on an isoenzyme fraction of PDE III, which decreases the

TABLE 13-6.
DRUG INTERACTIONS IN PATIENTS BEING TREATED WITH DIGITALIS

Quinidine (increases plasma concentrations of digoxin presumably by displacing from binding sites)
Succinylcholine (theoretical concern that is not supported by clinical experience)
β-Adrenergic agonists (cardiac dysrhythmias)
Calcium (cardiac dysrhythmias)

hydrolysis of cyclic adenosine monophosphate (cAMP) and cyclic guanosine monophosphate (cGMP). The overall effect of selective PDE III inhibitors is to combine positive inotropic effects with vascular smooth muscle relaxation. These drugs can be used in conjunction with digitalis without provoking digitalis toxicity. The PDE III inhibitors have their greatest clinical usefulness in the management of acute cardiac failure (as after a myocardial infarction) in patients who would benefit from combined inotropic and vasodilator therapy.

Amrinone

Amrinone is a bipyridine derivative that acts as a selective PDE III inhibitor and produces dose-dependent inotropic and vasodilator effects manifesting as increased cardiac output and decreased left ventricular end-diastolic pressure.

Route of Administration

Amrinone is effective when administered orally or intravenously (0.5 to 1.5 mg/kg increases cardiac output within 5 minutes, with detectable effects persisting for approximately 2 hours; a continuous infusion of 2 to 10 μg/kg/minute produces positive inotropic effects that persist for several hours after discontinuation of the infusion).

Side Effects

Side effects of amrinone include hypotension due to vasodilation and thrombocytopenia with chronic therapy. The therapeutic index of amrinone is approximately 100:1 compared with 1.2:1 for cardiac glycosides.

Milrinone

Milrinone is a bipyridine derivative that, like amrinone, produces positive inotropic and vasodilating effects (50 μg/kg followed by continuous infusion of 0.5 μg/kg/minute). Chronic oral therapy using milrinone may increase morbidity and mortality in patients with severe chronic heart failure.

Enoximone and Piroximone

Enoximone and Piroximone are imidazole derivatives that act as highly selective PDE III inhibitors to increase myocardial contractility.

NONSELECTIVE PHOSPHODIESTERASE INHIBITORS

Theophylline

Theophylline is a PDE inhibitor that, in contrast to selective PDE III inhibitors, is capable of inhibiting all fraction of PDE isoenzymes (I–V). Aminophylline is theophylline in complex with ethylenediamine to increase its solubility. Because methylxanthines also act as competitive antagonists of adenosine receptors, this could explain some of the effects of theophylline on the CNS and cardiac conduction system and may underlie the efficacy of theophylline in antagonizing bronchoconstriction.

Pharmacokinetics

Theophylline is metabolized by the liver and excreted by the kidneys (monitoring of plasma concentrations is indicated because of individual variation of liver metabolism).

Side Effects

Theophylline, unlike selective PDE III inhibitors has a very narrow therapeutic margin (therapeutic plasma concentrations are between 10 and 20 μg/mL, and cardiac dysrhythmias become more prevalent at plasma concentrations >20 μg/mL). Aminophylline readily crosses the placenta and may produce toxicity in infants of mothers receiving this drug during labor.

Clinical Uses

Administration of aminophylline (loading dose 5 mg/kg IV followed by 0.5 to 1.0 mg/kg per hour IV) has been recommended in the past for treatment of bronchospasm (selective β2-adrenergic agonists are equally effective).

Pentoxifylline

Pentoxifylline is a methylxanthine derivative that decreases the viscosity of blood, thus possibly improving intermittent claudication.

CALCIUM

When injected intravenously, calcium produces an intense positive inotropic effect lasting 10 to 20 minutes and manifesting as increases in stroke volume and decreases in left-ventricular end-diastolic pressure. Heart rate and systemic vascular resistance decrease. Calcium chloride, at 5 to 10 mg/kg IV to adults, may be administered to improve myocardial contractility and stroke volume at the conclusion of cardiopulmonary bypass.

GLUCAGON

Glucagon is a polypeptide hormone produced by the α-cells of the pancreas. Like catecholamines, glucagon enhances the formation of cGMP, but unlike catecholamines, it does not act via β-adrenergic receptors. The principal cardiac indication for glucagon is to increase myocardial contractility and heart rate in the presence of β-adrenergic blockade.

Cardiovascular Effects

Glucagon, as a rapid injection (1 to 5 mg IV to adults) or as a continuous infusion (20 mg/hour) reliably increases stroke volume and heart rate, independent of adrenergic receptor stimulation. Tachycardia may offset increases in cardiac output. Glucagon enhances automaticity in the sinoatrial and atrioventricular nodes without increasing automaticity in the ventricles.

TABLE 13-7.
SIDE EFFECTS OF GLUCAGON

Nausea and vomiting
Hyperglycemia
Paradoxical hypoglycemia (insufficient hepatic glycogen stores to offset the increased insulin release caused by glucagon)
Hypokalemia (increased secretion of insulin and intracellular transfer of potassium)
Systemic hypertension (evokes release of catecholamines and may be used as a provocative test in the differential diagnosis of pheochromocytoma)

Side Effects (Table 13-7)

MYOFILAMENT CALCIUM SENSITIZERS

Myofilament calcium sensitizers (pimobendan, sulmazole, and levosimendan) are positive inotropic drugs that improve myocardial contractility, independent of increases in intracellular cAMP or calcium concentrations. These drugs enhance the response of myofilament contractile elements to calcium without altering the availability of this ion.

The α- and β-Adrenergic Receptor Antagonists

14

The α- and β-adrenergic receptor antagonists prevent the interaction of the endogenous neurotransmitter norepinephrine or of sympathomimetics with the corresponding adrenergic receptors (Stoelting RK, Hillier SC. Alpha- and beta-adrenergic receptor antagonists. In: Pharmacology and Physiology in Anesthetic Practice. 4th ed. Philadelphia. Lipincott Williams & Wilkins, 2006:321–337). Interference with normal adrenergic receptor function attenuates sympathetic nervous system homeostatic mechanisms and evokes predictable pharmacologic responses.

α-ADRENERGIC RECEPTOR ANTAGONISTS

α-Adrenergic receptor antagonists bind selectively to α-adrenergic receptors and interfere with the ability of catecholamines to provoke α-responses on the heart and peripheral vasculature. Orthostatic hypotension, baroreceptor-mediated reflex tachycardia, and impotence are the invariable side effects of α-adrenergic blockade and this prevents the use of nonselective α-adrenergic antagonists in the management of ambulatory essential hypertension.

Mechanism of Action

Phentolamine, prazosin, and yohimbine are competitive (reversible binding with receptors) α-adrenergic antagonists; phenoxybenzamine binds covalently to α-adrenergic receptors to produce an irreversible α-receptor blockade.

Phentolamine

Phentolamine produces transient nonselective α-adrenergic blockade. Administered intravenously, phentolamine produces peripheral vasodilation (α1-receptor blockade and direct effect on vascular smooth muscle) and a decrease in systemic blood pressure that manifests within 2 minutes and lasts 10 to 15 minutes. Decreases in blood pressure elicit baroreceptor-mediated increases in sympathetic nervous system activity, manifesting as cardiac stimulation.

Clinical Uses (Table 14-1)

Phenoxybenzamine

Phenoxybenzamine acts as a nonselective α-adrenergic antagonist by combining covalently with α-adrenergic receptors (blockade at α1-receptors is more intense than at α2-receptors).

Pharmacokinetics

Absorption from the gastrointestinal tract is incomplete, and the onset of α-adrenergic blockade is slow, taking up

TABLE 14-1.
CLINICAL USES OF PHENTOLAMINE

Acute hypertensive emergencies (30 to 70 μg/kg IV)
Intraoperative manipulation of a pheochromocytoma
Autonomic nervous system hyperreflexia
Local infiltration (accidental extravascular injection of a sympathomimetic)

to 60 minutes to reach peak effect even after intravenous administration. This reflects the need to convert the drug molecule to a pharmacologically effective form. The elimination half-time is 24 hours, emphasizing the likelihood of cumulative effects with repeated doses.

Cardiovascular Effects

Orthostatic hypotension is prominent, especially in the presence of preexisting hypertension or hypovolemia.

Noncardiac Effects

Noncardiac effects include miosis, sedation (chronic therapy) and nasal stuffiness (unopposed vasodilation in mucous membranes).

Clinical Uses

Phenoxybenzamine, 0.5 to 1.0 mg/kg orally (or prazosin) is administered preoperatively to control blood pressure in patients with pheochromocytoma. Chronic α-adrenergic blockade, by relieving intense peripheral vasoconstriction, permits the expansion of intravascular fluid volume, as reflected by a decrease in the hematocrit.

Yohimbine

Yohimbine is a selective antagonist at presynaptic α2-receptors, leading to the enhanced release of norepinephrine from nerve endings. It is useful in the treatment of patients with idiopathic orthostatic hypotension.

Prazosin

Prazosin is a selective postsynaptic α1-receptor antagonist that leaves intact the inhibiting effect of α2-receptor activity on norepinephrine release from nerve endings. It is less likely than nonselective α-adrenergic antagonists to evoke reflex tachycardia.

Terazosin and Tamulosin

Terazosin and tamsulosin are orally effective α1-adrenergic antagonists that relax prostatic smooth muscle; they are useful in the treatment of benign prostatic hyperplasia.

Tolazoline

Tolazoline is a competitive nonselective α-adrenergic antagonist that has been used to treat persistent pulmonary hypertension of the newborn. It has been largely replaced by nitric oxide.

β-ADRENERGIC RECEPTOR ANTAGONISTS

β-Adrenergic receptor antagonists bind selectively to β-adrenergic receptors and interfere with the ability of catecholamines or other sympathomimetics to provoke β-responses. β-adrenergic antagonist therapy should be continued throughout the perioperative period to maintain desirable drug effects and to avoid the risk of sympathetic nervous system hyperactivity associated with abrupt discontinuation of these drugs. Propranolol is the standard β-antagonist drug to which all other β-adrenergic antagonists are compared.

Mechanism of Action

β-Adrenergic receptor antagonists exhibit selective affinity for β-adrenergic receptors, where they act by competitive inhibition. This inhibition is reversible if sufficiently large amounts of agonist become available. β-adrenergic receptors are G protein–coupled receptors, and their occupancy by agonists (norepinephrine, epinephrine) stimulates G proteins, which in turn activates adenylate cyclase to produce cyclic adenosine monophosphate (cAMP).

The net effect of β-adrenergic stimulation in the heart is to produce positive chronotropic, inotropic, and dromotropic effects; these responses are blunted by β-adrenergic receptor antagonists. It is estimated that 75% of β-receptors in the myocardium are β1-receptors.

Structure–Activity Relationships

β-Adrenergic receptor antagonists are derivatives of the β-agonist drug, isoproterenol, and substituents on the benzene ring determine whether the drug acts on β-adrenergic receptors as an antagonist or agonist.

Classification

β-Adrenergic receptor antagonists are classified as *nonselective* for β1 and β2 receptors (propranolol, nadolol, timolol, pindolol) and *cardioselective* (metoprolol, atenolol, acebutolol, betaxolol, esmolol, bisoprolol) for β1-receptors (Tables 14-2 and 14-3). It is important to recognize that β-receptor selectivity is dose dependent and is lost when large doses of antagonist are administered. Cardioselective drugs are better suited for administration to patients with asthma and reactive airway disease. β1-Receptor blockade is associated with a slowing of the sinus rate (increased diastolic perfusion time may enhance myocardial perfusion), slowing of conduction of cardiac impulses through the atrioventricular node, and a decrease in inotropy (effects are greater during activity than during rest).

Pharmacokinetics

The principal difference in pharmacokinetics among all the β-adrenergic receptor antagonists is the elimination half-time, ranging from brief for esmolol (about 10 minutes) to hours for other drugs (see Table 14-2). β-Receptor antagonists are eliminated by several different pathways, and this must be considered in the presence of renal and/or hepatic dysfunction (see Table 14-2). Interpatient variability in the response to β-adrenergic blockers is prominent (Table 14-4).

TABLE 14-2.

COMPARATIVE CHARACTERISTICS OF β-ADRENERGIC RECEPTOR ANTAGONISTS

	Propranolol	Nadolol	Pindolol	Timolol	Metoprolol	Aternolol	Acebutolol	Betaxolol	Esmolol
Cardiac selectivity	No	No	No	No	Yes	Yes	Yes	Yes	Yes
Partial agonist activity	No	No	Yes	No	No	No	Yes	No	No
Protein binding (%)	90–95	30	40–60	10	10	5	25		55
Clearance	Hepatic	Renal	Hepatic renal	Hepatic	Hepatic	Renal	Hepatic renal	Hepatic renal	Plasma hydrolysis
Active metabolites	Yes	No	No	No	No	No	Yes		No
Elimination half-time (hrs)	2–3	20–24	3–4	3–4	3–4	6–7	3–4	11–22	0.15

First-pass hepatic metabolism (estimate) (%)	75	Minimal	10–15	50	60	10	60		
Blood level variability	++++	+	++	+++	++++	+	++		
Adult oral dose (mg)	40–360	40–320	5–20	10–30	50–400	50–200	200–800	Topical	
Adult intravenous dose (mg)	1–10		0.4–2	0.4–1	1–15	5–10	12.5–50		10–80 50–300 μg/kg/min

+, minimal; ++, modest; +++, moderate; ++++, marked

TABLE 14-3.
COMPARATIVE CHARACTERISTICS OF β-ADRENERGIC RECEPTOR ANTAGONISTS EFFECTIVE IN THE TREATMENT OF CONGESTIVE HEART FAILURE

	Metoprolol (Extended Release)	Carvedilol	Bisoprolol
Cardiac selectivity	Yes	No	Yes
Partial agonist activity	No	No	No
Initial oral dose*	6.25 mg twice daily	3.125 mg twice daily	1.25 mg daily
Desired dosage range*	50–150 mg daily	25–50 mg twice daily	5 mg daily

*Recommended doses for treatment of patients with mild to moderate congestive heart failure.

TABLE 14-4.
EXPLANATIONS FOR INTERPATIENT VARIABILITY IN RESPONSES TO β-ADRENERGIC ANTAGONISTS

Differences in basal sympathetic nervous system activity
Flat dose response curves (changes in plasma concentrations of drug evoke minimal changes in pharmacologic effects)
Variations in magnitude of hepatic first-pass metabolism (20 fold differences in plasma concentrations after oral administration)
Active metabolites
Genetic differences in β-adrenergic receptors

Propranolol

Propranolol is a nonselective β-adrenergic antagonist that lacks intrinsic sympathomimetic activity and thus is a pure antagonist (effects similar to β1- and β2-receptors) (see Table 14-2). Typically, propranolol is administered in stepwise increments until physiologic plasma concentrations have been attained, as indicated by a resting heart rate of 55 to 60 beats/minute.

Cardiac Effects (Table 14-5)

Pharmacokinetics (Table 14-6)

Nadolol

Nadolol is a nonselective β-adrenergic receptor antagonist that is unique in that its long duration of action permits once-daily administration.

Pharmacokinetics

Nadolol does not undergo hepatic metabolism, with about 75% of the drug excreted unchanged in the urine.

TABLE 14-5.
CARDIAC EFFECTS OF PROPRANOLOL

Decreased heart rate (β1-effect, lasts longer than negative inotropic effect)
Decreased myocardial contractility (β1-effect)
Decreased cardiac output
Increased peripheral (and coronary) vascular resistance (β2-effect)
Decreased myocardial oxygen requirements (may relieve myocardial ischemia)
Sodium retention (intrarenal hemodynamic changes that accompany drug-induced decreases in cardiac output)

TABLE 14-6.
PHARMACOKINETICS OF PROPRANOLOL

Rapid oral absorption (systemic availability limited by hepatic first-pass metabolism; thus oral dose is greater than IV dose)
Extensive protein binding
Hepatic metabolism (4-hydroxypropranolol is an active metabolite)
Decreased clearance of amide local anesthetics (reflects decreases in hepatic blood flow and inhibition of hepatic metabolism)
Decreased pulmonary first-pass uptake of opioids

Timolol

Timolol is a nonselective β-adrenergic receptor antagonist that is effective in the treatment of glaucoma (as topical eye drops) because of its ability to decrease intraocular pressure, presumably by decreasing the production of aqueous humor.

Systemic absorption from topical administration may be sufficient to cause bradycardia and increased airway resistance.

Metoprolol

Metoprolol is a selective β1-adrenergic receptor antagonist that prevents inotropic and chronotropic responses to β-adrenergic stimulation. Conversely, the bronchodilator, vasodilator, and metabolic effects of β2-receptors remain intact, so that metoprolol is less likely to cause adverse effects in patients with chronic obstructive airway disease or peripheral vascular disease, and in patients vulnerable to hypoglycemia; however, large doses of metoprolol become nonselective, exerting antagonist effects at β2- as well as β1-receptors.

Pharmacokinetics

Metoprolol is readily absorbed from the gastrointestinal tract, but this is offset by substantial hepatic first-pass metabolism. Hepatic metabolites are not pharmacologically active, and <10% of the drug appears unchanged in the urine.

Atenolol

Atenolol is the most selective β1-adrenergic antagonist, and it may have specific value in patients in whom the continued presence of β2-receptor activity is desirable. The perioperative administration of atenolol to patients at high risk for coronary artery disease significantly decreases the incidence of postoperative myocardial infarction.

Pharmacokinetics

About 50% of an orally administered dose of atenolol is absorbed from the gastrointestinal tract. Atenolol undergoes little or no hepatic metabolism and is eliminated principally by renal excretion.

Betaxolol

Betaxolol is a cardioselective β1-adrenergic antagonist with no intrinsic sympathomimetic activity and weak membrane-stabilizing activity. A topical preparation is an alternative to timolol for the treatment of chronic open-angle glaucoma.

Bisoprolol

Bisoprolol is a β1 selective antagonist drug without intrinsic agonist activity that has been shown to improve survival in patients with mild to moderate congestive heart failure (see Table 14-3).

Esmolol

Esmolol is a rapid-onset and short-acting selective β1-adrenergic receptor antagonist that is administered only intravenously (0.5 mg/kg over about 60 seconds produces a therapeutic effect within 5 minutes that ceases within 10 to 30 minutes). Heart rate typically returns to predrug levels within 15 minutes. These characteristics make esmolol a useful drug for preventing or treating adverse systemic blood pressure and heart rate responses that occur intraoperatively in response to noxious stimulation (tracheal intubation). The treatment of excessive drug-induced sympathetic nervous system activity (cocaine, topical or subcutaneous epinephrine) with β-adrenergic receptor antagonists has been associated with fulminant pulmonary edema and irreversible cardiovascular collapse; these conditions are more safely treated with a peripheral vasodilator, such as sodium nitroprusside or nitroglycerin. It is possible that acute drug-induced β-receptor antagonism removes the ability of the heart to compensate for catecholamine-induced increases in left ventricular afterload.

Pharmacokinetics

The elimination half-time of esmolol is about 9 minutes, reflecting its rapid hydrolysis in the blood by plasma esterases; elimination is independent of renal and hepatic function and the activity of plasma cholinesterases. The duration of action of succinylcholine is not prolonged in patients treated with esmolol.

Side Effects of β-Adrenergic Antagonists

The side effects of β-adrenergic antagonists are similar for all available drugs, although the magnitude may differ depending on their selectivity and the presence or absence of intrinsic sympathomimetic activity (Table 14-7). β-Adrenergic antagonists exert their most prominent pharmacologic effects, as well as side effects, on the cardiovascular system. The principal contraindication to the administration of β-adrenergic receptor antagonists is preexisting atrioventricular heart block.

TABLE 14-7.
SIDE EFFECTS OF β-ADRENERGIC RECEPTOR ANTAGONISTS

Cardiovascular System (effects greatest when preexisting sympathetic nervous system activity is increased as during exercise or in patients in cardiac failure)
- Negative inotropic effects
- Negative chronotropic effects (may precipitate cardiac failure in a previously compensated patient)
- Slowed conduction of cardiac impulses through the atrioventricular node
- Decreased rate of spontaneous phase 4 depolarization
- Peripheral vasoconstriction (unopposed α-adrenergic receptor effects)
- Prevent dysrhythmogenic effects of catecholamines

Airway Resistance
- Bronchoconstriction (blockade of β2-receptors, accentuated in patients with preexisting obstructive airway disease)

Metabolism
- Interference with glycogenolysis (blockade of β2-receptors)
- Unrecognized hypoglycemia (tachycardia as a warning sign is blunted)

Distribution of Extracellular Potassium
- Plasma potassium concentrations increased (β-blockade inhibits uptake of potassium into cells)

Interaction with Anesthetics
- Additive myocardial depression is not excessive (treatment with β-adrenergic antagonists may be safely continued throughout the perioperative period)
- Bradycardia (may be exaggerated in presence of timolol)

Nervous System
- Fatigue and lethargy (β-adrenergic antagonists may cross the blood-brain barrier)

Fetus
- Bradycardia, hypotension, and hypoglycemia

Withdrawal Hypersensitivity
- Acute discontinuation may result in excess sympathetic nervous system activity within 24 to 48 hours (presumably reflects up-regulation of β-adrenergic receptors during chronic therapy)

Treatment of Excess Myocardial Depression (Table 14-8)

Clinical Uses (Table 14-9)

It is accepted that patients being treated with β-adrenergic receptor antagonists should have their medication continued uninterrupted throughout the perioperative period. It is also recommended that patients at high risk

TABLE 14-8.
TREATMENT OF EXCESS MYOCARDIAL DEPRESSION PRODUCED BY β-ADRENERGIC ANTAGONISTS

Clinical Manifestations
- Bradycardia
- Low cardiac output
- Hypotension
- Cardiogenic shock
- Bronchospasm
- Hypoglycemia

Treatment
- Atropine (incremental doses of 7 μg/kg IV)
- Isoproterenol (2 to 25 μg/minute IV if atropine is ineffective in increasing heart rate)
- Dobutamine (recommended if a pure β-adrenergic antagonist is responsible; isoproterenol could produce vasodilation before its inotropic effect develops; dopamine is not recommended because α-adrenergic-induced vasoconstriction is likely to occur with the high doses required to overcome β-blockade)
- Glucagon (1 to 10 mg IV, followed by 5 mg/hour IV, normal doses are effective to produce effects independent of β-adrenergic receptors)
- Calcium chloride (250 to 1000 mg IV, acts independently of β-adrenergic receptors)
- Transvenous artificial cardiac pacemaker (bradycardia that is unresponsive to pharmacologic therapy)

TABLE 14-9.
CLINICAL USES OF β-ADRENERGIC BLOCKERS

Treatment of essential hypertension
Management of angina pectoris
Treatment of acute coronary syndrome
Perioperative β-adrenergic receptor blockade
Treatment of intraoperative myocardial ischemia
Suppression of cardiac dysrhythmias
Management of congestive heart failure
Prevention of excessive sympathetic nervous system activity
Preoperative preparation of hyperthyroid patients
Treatment of migraine headache

for myocardial ischemia presenting for major surgery should be treated with β-adrenergic receptor antagonists beginning preoperatively and continuing into the postoperative period.

Treatment of Essential Hypertension

The antihypertensive effects of β-adrenergic blockade is largely dependent on decreases in cardiac output due to decreased heart rate.

Management of Angina Pectoris

A decreased likelihood of myocardial ischemia, manifesting as angina pectoris, reflects drug-induced decreases in myocardial oxygen consumption secondary to decreased heart rate (resting heart rate <60 beats/minute) and myocardial contractility.

Treatment of Acute Coronary Syndrome

It is recommended that all patients with acute myocardial infarction without complications (severe bradycardia, unstable left ventricular failure, atrioventricular heart block) receive intravenous β-adrenergic antagonists as early as possible, regardless of whether they receive reperfusion therapy.

β-Adrenergic antagonist prophylaxis after acute myocardial infarction is considered to be one of the most scientifically substantiated, cost-effective preventive medical measures.

Perioperative β-Adrenergic Receptor Blockade (Table 14-10)

The goal of preoperative therapy is a resting heart rate between 65 and 80 beats/min. Perioperative myocardial ischemia is the single most important potentially reversible risk factor for mortality and cardiovascular complications after noncardiac surgery. All β-adrenergic receptor antagonists, except those with intrinsic sympathetic nervous system activity, decrease mortality at 24 months (Table 14-11). The mechanism for the beneficial effects of perioperative β-adrenergic receptor blockade is not known but is most likely multifactorial (Table 14-12).

Treatment of Intraoperative Myocardial Ischemia

The goal in treatment of intraoperative myocardial ischemia is to decrease the heart rate to about 60 beats/min IV (esmolol, 1 to 1.5 mg/kg IV, followed by a continuous infusion of 50 to 300 μg/kg/minute).

Suppression of Cardiac Dysrhythmias

Esmolol and propranolol are effective in the treatment of cardiac dysrhythmias, owing to enhanced sympathetic

TABLE 14-10.
EXAMPLES OF PATIENTS AT RISK FOR MYOCARDIAL ISCHEMIA IN THE PERIOPERATIVE PERIOD

Coronary artery disease
Positive preoperative stress tests
Diabetes mellitus treated with insulin
Left ventricular hypertrophy
High risk surgery (vascular, thoracic intraperitoneal, anticipated large blood loss)

TABLE 14-11.
EXAMPLES OF β-ADRENERGIC BLOCKER DRUG REGIMENS IN THE PERIOPERATIVE PERIOD

Preoperative Oral Therapy
- Atenolol 50 mg daily (seven days before and after surgery)
- Bisoprolol 5 to 10 mg daily
- Metoprolol 25 to 50 mg twice daily

Day of Surgery
- Atenolol 5 to 10 mg IV (before induction of anesthesia and every 12 hours for 7 days)
- Metoprolol 5 to 10 mg IV

Intraoperatively and Postoperatively
- Esmolol IV
- Atenolol or metoprolol IV until oral intake possible

nervous system stimulation (ventricular response rate to atrial fibrillation).

Management of Congestive Heart Failure

Metoprolol, carvedilol, and bisoprolol improve ejection fraction and increase survival in patients in chronic heart

TABLE 14-12.
POSSIBLE EXPLANATIONS FOR CARDIOPROTECTIVE EFFECTS PRODUCED BY PERIOPERATIVE β-ADRENERGIC RECEPTOR BLOCKADE

Decreased myocardial oxygen consumption and demand
Less stress on potentially ischemic myocardium owing to decreased heart rate and myocardial contractility
Attenuation of effects of endogenous catecholamines
Redistribution of coronary blood flow to ischemic areas
Increased coronary blood flow owing to increased diastolic time
Plaque stabilization owing to decrease in shear forces
Cardiac antidysrhythmic effects
Antiinflammatory effects (?)

failure (see Table 14-3). When β-blocking drugs are used to treat congestive heart failure, the initial doses should be minimal and gradually increased.

Prevention of Excessive Sympathetic Nervous System Activity

β-Adrenergic blockade is associated with attenuated heart rate and blood pressure responses to direct laryngoscopy and tracheal intubation. The likelihood of cyanotic episodes in patients with tetralogy of Fallot is minimized by β-blockade.

Preoperative Preparation of Hyperthyroid Patients

Thyrotoxic patients can be prepared for surgery in an emergency by the intravenous administration of propranolol or esmolol.

COMBINED α- AND β-ADRENERGIC RECEPTOR ANTAGONISTS

Labetalol

Labetalol is a unique parenteral and oral antihypertensive drug that exhibits selective α1- and nonselective β1- and β2-adrenergic antagonist effects. Presynaptic α2-receptors are spared by labetalol, so that released norepinephrine can continue to inhibit the further release of catecholamines via the negative feedback mechanism resulting from stimulation of α2-receptors.

TABLE 14-13.
CLINICAL USES OF LABETALOL

Hypertensive emergencies (2 mg/kg IV)
Treatment of rebound hypertension after withdrawal of clonidine
Angina pectoris
Attenuate increases in heart rate and blood pressure related to abrupt increases in the level of surgical stimulation

Pharmacokinetics

Metabolism of labetalol is by conjugation of glucuronic acid, with 5% of the drug recovered unchanged in the urine.

Cardiovascular Effects

Administration of labetalol (0.1 to 0.5 mg/kg IV) lowers systemic blood pressure by decreasing systemic vascular resistance (α1-blockade), whereas reflex tachycardia triggered by vasodilation is attenuated by simultaneous β-blockade. Cardiac output remains unchanged.

Clinical Uses (Table 14-13)

Side Effects

Orthostatic hypotension is the most common side effect of labetalol therapy. Because fluid retention commonly occurs in patients treated chronically with labetalol, this drug is combined with a diuretic during prolonged therapy.

Carvedilol

Carvedilol is a nonselective β-adrenergic receptor antagonist with α1-blocking activity. Carvedilol is indicated for the treatment of mild to moderate congestive heart failure owing to ischemia or cardiomyopathy (see Table 14-3).

Antihypertensive Drugs

Drugs used to treat systemic hypertension include sympatholytics, angiotensin-converting enzyme (ACE) inhibitors, angiotensin receptor blockers, calcium channel blockers, vasodilators, and diuretics (Table 15-1) (Stoelting RK, Hillier SC. Antihypertensive drugs. In: Pharmacology and Physiology in Anesthetic Practice. 4th ed. Philadelphia. Lippincott Williams & Wilkins, 2006:338–351). The potential interaction between antihypertensive drugs and anesthetics has been exaggerated. When interactions are likely, they are usually predictable and can thus be avoided or their significance minimized (Table 15-2). The maintenance of antihypertensive drug therapy during the perioperative period is associated with fewer fluctuations in blood pressure and heart rate during anesthesia. It is an inescapable conclusion that previously effective antihypertensive drug therapy should be continued without interruption during the perioperative period. In this regard, the usual dose and unique pharmacology of each antihypertensive drug, as well as the physiologic reflexes that occur in response to drug-induced blood pressure changes, must be considered when planning the management of anesthesia.

SYMPATHOLYTICS

β-Adrenergic Blockers

β-Adrenergic blockers used as single-drug therapy for systemic hypertension seem to be most effective in young

TABLE 15-1.
DRUGS USED TO TREAT SYSTEMIC HYPERTENSION

Sympatholytics
- β-adrenergic blockers (acebutolol, atenolol, betaxolol, bisoprolol, carteolol, metoprolol, nadolol, penbutolol, pindolol, propranolol, timolol)
- Combined α-adrenergic blockers (labetalol)
- α-adrenergic blockers (prazosin, terazosin, doxazosin)
- Centrally acting blockers (clonidine, dexmedetomidine)

Angiotensin-converting enzyme inhibitors (captopril, enalapril, benazepril, fosinopril, lisinopril, quinapril, ramipril, spirapril, moexipril, perindopril, trandolapril)

Angiotensin II receptor inhibitors (losartan, valsartan, candesartan, eprosartan, irbesartan, telmisartan)

Calcium channel blockers (verapamil, diltiazem, nifedipine, nicardipine, isradipine, amlodipine, felodipine)

Vasodilating drugs (hydralazine, minoxidil)

Diuretics
- Thiazides (chlorothiazide, hydrochlorothiazide, bendroflumethiazide, hydroflumethiazide, methyclothiazide, polythiazide, trimethiazide, indapamide)
- Loop diuretics (bumetanide, ethacrynic acid, furosemide, torsemide)
- Potassium-sparing diuretics (amiloride, spironolactone, triamterene)

---

and middle-aged patients, as well as those with coronary artery disease.

Mechanism of Action

β-Blockers can be classified according to whether they exhibit selective (acting on β1-cardiac receptors) or nonselective (acting on β1- and β2-receptors associated with vascular and bronchial smooth muscle and metabolic receptors) properties and whether they possess intrinsic sympathomimetic activity. In contrast to nonselective β-blockers, selective β1-blockers (acebutolol, atenolol, metoprolol), administered in low doses are unlikely to

TABLE 15-2.
INTERACTIONS BETWEEN ANTIHYPERTENSIVE DRUGS AND ANESTHESIA

Attenuation of sympathetic nervous system activity
- Orthostatic hypotension
- Exaggerated systemic blood pressure responses to acute blood loss, body position change, decreased venous return as due to positive pressure ventilation of the lungs
- Decreased sensitivity to indirect-acting sympathomimetics (depletion of norepinephrine)
- Exaggerated responses to catecholamines and direct-acting sympathomimetics

Modification of response to sympathomimetic drugs

Sedation

produce bronchospasm, decrease peripheral blood flow, or mask hypoglycemia. For these reasons, β1-blockers are preferred drugs for patients with pulmonary disease, insulin-dependent diabetes mellitus, or symptomatic peripheral vascular disease.

Side Effects (Table 15-3)

Labetalol

Labetalol combines α1-adrenergic and β-adrenergic blocking properties and appears to also produce a direct vasodilating effect. The presence of α-adrenergic blocking properties results in less bradycardia and negative inotropic effects compared with β-blockers. These α properties may result in orthostatic hypotension. The incidence of bronchospasm is similar to that seen with timolol or metoprolol.

Prazosin

Prazosin is a selective postsynaptic α1-adrenergic receptor antagonist that results in vasodilating effects on both

TABLE 15-3.
SIDE EFFECTS OF β-BLOCKERS USED TO TREAT SYSTEMIC HYPERTENSION

Bradycardia (preexisting heart block a reason to avoid these drugs)
Congestive heart failure
Bronchospasm (especially in patients with asthma)
Claudication
Masking of hypoglycemia
Sedation
Impotence
Precipitation of angina pectoris with abrupt discontinuation

arterial and venous vasculature. In addition to treating essential hypertension, prazosin may be of value for decreasing afterload in patients with congestive heart failure.

Pharmacokinetics

Prazosin is nearly completely metabolized, and <60% bioavailability after oral administration suggests the occurrence of substantial first-pass hepatic metabolism.

Cardiovascular Effects

Prazosin decreases systemic vascular resistance without causing reflex-induced tachycardia or increases in renin activity. Failure to alter plasma renin activity reflects the continued activity of α2-receptors.

Side Effects (Table 15-4)

Terazosin and Doxazosin

Terazosin and Doxazosin resemble prazosin, acting as α1-receptor antagonists. Their advantage lies in their efficacy when taken once daily.

Clonidine

Clonidine is a centrally acting selective partial α2-adrenergic agonist (220:1 α2 to α1) that acts as an antihypertensive

TABLE 15-4.
SIDE EFFECTS OF PRAZOSIN

Vertigo
Fluid retention (administer with a diuretic)
Orthostatic hypotension
Sudden syncope (acute peripheral vasodilation)
Interference with antihypertensive effects by nonsteroidal antiinflammatory drugs
Dryness of the mouth
Exaggerated hypotension during epidural anesthesia (α1-blockade that prevents compensatory vasoconstriction in the unblocked portions of the body)

drug by virtue of its ability to decrease sympathetic nervous system output from the central nervous system (CNS). This drug has proved to be particularly effective in the treatment of patients with severe hypertension or renin-dependent disease. The usual daily adult dose is 0.2 to 0.3 mg orally. The availability of a transdermal clonidine patch designed for weekly administration is useful for patients who are unable to take oral medications.

Other Clinical Uses (Table 15-5)

Mechanism of Action

The α2-adrenergic agonists produce clinical effects by binding to α2-receptors Table 15-6. The quality of sedation produced by α2-agonists differs from the sedation produced by drugs (midazolam, propofol) that act on γ-aminobutyric acid (GABA) receptors. Sedation reflects decreased sympathetic nervous system activity, resulting in a calm patient who can be easily aroused to full consciousness.

Pharmacokinetics

Clonidine is rapidly absorbed after oral administration. The transdermal route requires about 48 hours to produce therapeutic concentrations.

TABLE 15-5.
OTHER CLINICAL USES OF CLONIDINE

Analgesia (epidural or subarachnoid 150 to 450 μg administered into epidural or subarachnoid space)
Preanesthetic medication (5 μg/kg orally blunts cardiovascular responses to sympathetic nervous system stimulation and decreases anesthetic requirements, prolonging the effects of regional anesthesia)
Protection against perioperative myocardial ischemia
Diagnosis of pheochromocytoma
Treatment of opioid and alcohol withdrawal syndrome
Treatment of shivering (75 μg IV)
Perioperative myocardial ischemia (decreases mortality following cardiovascular surgery)

Cardiovascular Effects

The decrease in systolic blood pressure produced by clonidine is more prominent than the decrease in diastolic blood pressure.

Respiratory Effects

The α2-agonists have minimal depressant effects on ventilation, and these agonists do not potentiate ventilatory depressant effects of opioids.

TABLE 15-6.
MECHANISM OF ACTION OF CLONIDINE

α2A-Receptors (sedation, analgesia, sympatholysis manifesting as peripheral vasodilation and decreases in systemic blood pressure, heart rate, and cardiac output)
α2B-Receptors (vasoconstriction, antishivering effects?)
α2C-Receptors (startle response?)

Side Effects (Table 15-7)

Rebound Hypertension

Rebound Hypertension may occur as soon as 8 hours after the abrupt discontinuation of clonidine (most likely in patients receiving >1.2 mg daily). The increase in systemic blood pressure may be associated with >100% increase in circulating concentrations of catecholamines and intense peripheral vasoconstriction (labetalol may be a useful treatment).

Transdermal clonidine provides a sustained therapeutic level of drug. Rebound hypertension presenting after the abrupt discontinuation of chronic treatment with antihypertensive drugs is not unique to clonidine. Antihypertensive drugs that act independently of central and peripheral sympathetic nervous system mechanisms (ACE inhibitors) do not seem to be associated with rebound hypertension after sudden discontinuation.

Dexmedetomidine

Dexmedetomidine is a highly selective, specific, and potent α2-adrenergic agonist (1,620:1 α2 to α1) that has a shorter duration of action than clonidine. Atipamezole is a specific and selective α2-receptor antagonist.

Pharmacokinetics

The elimination half-time of dexmedetomidine is 2 to 3 hours, compared with 6 to 10 hours for clonidine.

TABLE 15-7.
SIDE EFFECTS OF CLONIDINE

Sedation
Xerostomia
Decrease in anesthetic requirements
Bradycardia
Sodium and water retention
Skin rashes

Clinical Uses

As with clonidine, pretreatment with dexmedetomidine attenuates the hemodynamic responses to tracheal intubation, decreases plasma catecholamine concentrations during anesthesia, and decreases the perioperative requirements for inhaled anesthetics and opioids (plateau effect between 25% to 40%). Despite the marked dose-dependent analgesia and sedation produced by this drug, only mild depression of ventilation occurs.

Postoperative Sedation

Dexmedetomidine (200 to 700 μg/kg per hour IV) is useful for sedation of postoperative critical care patients in an intensive care unit environment, particularly when mechanical ventilation via a tracheal tube is necessary. Following tracheal extubation, dexmedetomidine-sedated patients breathe spontaneously and appear calm and relaxed.

ANGIOTENSIN-CONVERTING ENZYME INHIBITORS

ACE inhibitors represent a major advance in the treatment of all forms of hypertension because of their potency and minimal side effects (free of insomnia and rebound hypertension). These drugs have been established as first-line therapy in patients with systemic hypertension, congestive heart failure (remodeling the myocardium), and mitral regurgitation.

Mechanism of Action

ACE inhibitors block the conversion of angiotensin I to angiotensin II, a potent vasoconstrictor responsible for arterial smooth muscle constriction, increased aldosterone secretion, and sympathetic nervous system stimulation. The major difference among clinically used ACE inhibitors is in their duration of action (Table 15-8).

Side Effects (Table 15-9)

Preoperative Management

Adverse circulatory effects during anesthesia (prolonged hypotension especially in surgical procedures involving major body fluid shifts) are recognized in patients chronically treated with ACE inhibitors; some recommend these drugs be discontinued 12 to 24 hours before anesthesia and surgery. Hypotension attributed to continued ACE inhibitor therapy has been responsive to crystalloid fluid infusion and/or the administration of a sympathomimetic such as ephedrine or phenylephrine.

Captopril

Captopril is an orally effective antihypertensive drug that acts through the competitive inhibition of angiotensin I-converting enzyme.

Pharmacokinetics

Captopril is well absorbed after oral administration, and inhibition of converting enzyme occurs within 15 minutes.

Cardiovascular Effects

The antihypertensive effects of captopril are due to a decrease in systemic vascular resistance, as a result of decreased sodium and water retention. Typically, captopril decreases systemic blood pressure without concomitant alterations in cardiac output or heart rate.

Side Effects (Table 15-10)

Enalapril

Enalapril is an ACE inhibitor that resembles captopril with respect to pharmacologic effects. It is a prodrug that is metabolized in the liver to its active form, enalaprilat.

TABLE 15-8.

PHARMACOLOGIC EFFECTS OF SINGLE DOSES OF ANGIOTENSIN-CONVERTING ENZYME INHIBITORS

Drug	Dose (mg)	Prodrug	Time of Onset of Effect (min)	Time of Peak (hrs)	Duration of Effect (hrs)	Effect on Venous System	Effect on Arterial System
Captopril	100	No	15–30	1–2	6–10	++	+++
Enalapril	20	Yes	60–120	4–8	18–30	++	+++
Lisinopril	10	No	60	2–4	18–30	++	+++
Ramipril	20	Yes	30–60	3–8	24–60		

TABLE 15-9. SIDE EFFECTS OF ANGIOTENSIN-CONVERTING ENZYME INHIBITORS
Cough (reflects potentiation of effects of kinins)
Upper respiratory congestion
Rhinorrhea
Decreases in glomerular filtration (caution in patients with preexisting renal dysfunction)
Hyperkalemia (decreased production of aldosterone)

ANGIOTENSIN II RECEPTOR INHIBITORS

Angiotensin II receptor inhibitors produce antihypertensive effects by blocking the vasoconstrictive actions of angiotensin II without affecting ACE activity.

Losartan

Losartan is an orally effective antihypertensive drug that acts as an antagonist to angiotensin II (vasoactive hormone) at angiotensin II receptors found principally in vascular smooth muscles.

TABLE 15-10. SIDE EFFECTS OF CAPTOPRIL
Rash or pruritus
Alteration or loss of taste
Possible antagonism by nonsteroidal antiinflammatory drugs
Hyperkalemia (especially in patients with preexisting renal dysfunction)
Angioedema (drug-induced inhibition of metabolism of bradykinin)

Side Effects

Compared with ACE inhibitors, cough related to bradykinin accumulation is significantly less with losartan therapy. Hyperkalemia is a potential side effect, especially with the concomitant use of potassium-sparing diuretics. As with ACE inhibitors, hypotension following the induction of anesthesia has been observed in patients being treated with angiotensin II receptor blockers.

CALCIUM CHANNEL BLOCKERS

Calcium channel blockers, when used for the treatment of essential hypertension, are considered vasodilators.

VASODILATING DRUGS

Hydralazine

Hydralazine is a phthalazine derivative that activates guanylate cyclase to produce vascular relaxation. Decreases in systemic blood pressure reflect these direct relaxant effects on vascular smooth muscle, the dilatation effect on arterioles being greater than on veins. Concomitant administration of a β-blocker limits the reflex increase in sympathetic nervous system activity induced by hydralazine. The treatment of a hypertensive crisis can be accomplished with intravenous hydralazine, 2.5 to 10 mg. The antihypertensive effects begin within 10 to 20 minutes after intravenous administration and last 3 to 6 hours.

Pharmacokinetics

Extensive hepatic-first pass metabolism limits the availability of hydralazine after oral administration. Acetylation seems to be the major route of metabolism of hydralazine; rapid acetylators have lower bioavailability (about 30%)

than do slow acetylators (about 50%) after the oral administration of hydralazine.

Cardiovascular Effects

The preferential dilation of arterioles over veins minimizes the incidence of orthostatic hypotension and promotes an increase in cardiac output.

Side Effects (Table 15-11)

Minoxidil

Minoxidil is an orally active antihypertensive drug that decreases systemic blood pressure by the direct relaxation of arteriolar smooth muscle. It has little effect on venous capacitance vessels. ACE inhibitors and calcium-blocking drugs may be as effective, with fewer side effects.

Pharmacokinetics

Metabolism to inactive minoxidil glucuronide is extensive, and only 10% of the drug is recovered unchanged in the urine.

TABLE 15-11.
SIDE EFFECTS OF HYDRALAZINE

SIDE EFFECTS OF HYDRALAZINE
Sodium and water retention (administered with a diuretic)
Vertigo
Nausea
Tachycardia
Angina pectoris (myocardial stimulation)
Drug fever
Polyneuritis
Anemia
Systemic lupus erythematosus-like syndrome [10% to 20% of patients treated chronically (>6 months; >200 mg daily, slow acetylators)

Cardiovascular Effects

The hypotensive effects of minoxidil are accompanied by marked increases in heart rate and cardiac output, and orthostatic hypotension is prominent.

Side Effects (Table 15-12)

TABLE 15-12.
SIDE EFFECTS OF MINOXIDIL

Fluid retention (weight gain, edema)
Pulmonary hypertension (reflects fluid retention)
Pericardial effusion and cardiac tamponade
Abnormalities on the electrocardiogram (flattening or inversion of the T-wave, increased voltage of the QRS complex)
Hypertrichosis

Peripheral Vasodilators—Nitric Oxide and Nitrovasodilators

16

Peripheral vasodilators that act on the systemic circulation are most frequently used clinically to treat hypertensive crises, produce controlled hypotension, and facilitate left ventricular forward stroke volume, as in patients with regurgitant valvular heart lesions or acute cardiac failure (Stoelting RK, Hillier SC. Peripheral vasodilators-nitric oxide and nitrovasodilators. In: Pharmacology and Physiology in Anesthetic Practice. 4th ed. Philadelphia. Lippincott Williams & Wilkins, 2006:352–369). Preload-reducing vasodilators (nitroglycerin) alleviate pulmonary and systemic congestive symptoms, whereas arterial vasodilators (sodium nitroprusside, SNP) reverse the deleterious effects of peripheral vasoconstriction. Nitrovasodilators produce systemic and pulmonary vasodilation through the intercellular generation of nitric oxide (NO).

NITRIC OXIDE

NO is an endogenous gas that is recognized as a chemical messenger in a multitude of biological systems; it has effects as a vasorelaxant, in platelet regulation, and in neurotransmitter function in the central nervous system [CNS]). NO may be administered by inhalation to produce selective relaxation of the pulmonary vasculature.

Synthesis and Transport

NO is synthesized in endothelial cells and, as a gas, diffuses from these cells into target cells where it activates guanylate cyclase to increase cGMP concentrations. This in turn results in vasodilation. NO has a half-time of <5 seconds (inactivated by hemoglobin), which ensures a relatively localized action.

Physiologic Effects (Table 16-1)

Pathophysiology (Table 16-2)

Mechanism of Anesthesia

NO appears to be involved in excitatory neurotransmission in the CNS; the suppression of NO formation by anesthetics could decrease excitatory neurotransmission and increase inhibitory neurotransmission.

TABLE 16-1.
PHYSIOLOGIC EFFECTS OF NITRIC OXIDE

Cardiovascular system
Regulates systemic and pulmonary vascular resistance
Determines distribution of cardiac output
Autoregulation
Pulmonary system
Bronchodilation
Ventilation-to-perfusion matching
Platelets
Inhibits platelet activation
Nervous system
Neurotransmitter (brain, spinal cord, peripheral nervous system)
Immune function

TABLE 16-2.
EFFECTS OF INCREASED OR DECREASED NITRIC OXIDE RELEASE

Decreased nitric oxide release
- Essential hypertension
- Platelet aggregation associated with atherosclerosis
- Pulmonary hypertension
- Pyloric stenosis and achalasia
- Infection

Increased nitric oxide release
- Hypotension associated with septic shock
- Hyperdynamic state associated with cirrhosis
- Epilepsy
- Inflammation

Clinical Uses (Table 16-3)

The use of inhaled NO for the therapy of pulmonary disease is based on the finding that NO rapidly binds and is inactivated by hemoglobin (selective pulmonary vasodilator without systemic effects). The outcome benefit of

TABLE 16-3.
POTENTIAL BENEFICIAL EFFECTS OF INHALED NITRIC OXIDE

Bronchodilation
Improved ventilation/perfusion matching
Decreased right ventricular pressures
Decreased intracardiac shunt
Increased right ventricular ejection fraction
Decreased pulmonary artery pressures
Decreased pulmonary vascular resistance
Increased cardiac output
Increased arterial oxygenation

inhaled NO has been limited to the decreased need for extracorporeal membrane oxygenation in newborns with pulmonary hypertension.

Acute Lung Injury and Adult Respiratory Distress Syndrome

Clinical trials suggests that NO is not indicated in the routine therapy of patients with acute lung injury or adult respiratory distress syndrome (ARDS). In severe cases of ARDS, NO may have a role as "salvage" therapy to provide short-term physiologic improvements and allow time for the lungs to heal.

Cardiac Transplantation

NO may be a useful intervention following cardiac transplantation, because the donor heart has not been previously exposed to increased pulmonary vascular resistance—such as may be present in the recipient.

Toxicity

Inhaled NO increases methemoglobin levels as NO combines with hemoglobin. Rebound arterial hypoxemia and pulmonary hypertension may accompany discontinuation of inhaled NO therapy (slowly wean patients). NO is oxidized to nitrogen dioxide (NO_2) and is also a possible product of the interaction of NO with oxygen. Continuous monitoring of inspired NO and NO_2 concentrations is important to provide an early warning of possible pulmonary toxicity.

SODIUM NITROPRUSSIDE

SNP is a direct-acting, nonselective peripheral vasodilator that causes relaxation of arterial and venous vascular smooth muscle. Its onset of action is almost immediate, and its duration of action is transient, requiring continuous intravenous infusion to maintain a therapeutic effect.

Mechanism of Action

SNP interacts with oxyhemoglobin, dissociating immediately and forming methemoglobin while releasing cyanide and NO. NO is the active mediator responsible for the direct vasodilating effect of SNP.

Metabolism

Metabolism of SNP begins with the transfer of an electron from the iron of oxyhemoglobin to SNP, yielding methemoglobin and an unstable SNP radical. The unstable SNP radical breaks down, resulting in the nonenzymatic release of all five cyanide ions, one of which reacts with methemoglobin to form cyanomethemoglobin.

Toxicity

Cyanide Toxicity

Cyanide toxicity reflects the cyanide binding of tissue cytochrome oxidase, resulting in prevention of oxidative phosphorylation. Increased cyanide concentrations may precipitate tissue anoxia, anaerobic metabolism, and lactic acidosis. Cyanide toxicity should be suspected in any patient who is resistant to the hypotensive effects of the drug despite maximum infusion rates (>2 μg/kg/minute or 10 μg/kg/minute for longer than 10 minutes) or in a previously responsive patient. Mixed venous Po_2 is increased in the presence of cyanide toxicity, thus indicating paralysis of cytochrome oxidase. Plasma lactate concentrations are increased. No evidence suggests that preexisting hepatic or renal disease increases the likelihood of cyanide toxicity.

Treatment (Table 16-4)

Thiocyanate Toxicity

Thiocyanate toxicity is rare, because thiocyanate is 100-fold less toxic than cyanide. Clinical evidence of neurotoxicity produced by thiocyanate includes hyperreflexia, confusion, and psychosis.

TABLE 16-4.
TREATMENT OF CYANIDE TOXICITY

Immediate discontinuation of SNP when tachyphylaxis appears in a previously responsive patient in association with metabolic acidosis and increased mixed venous Po_2
Sodium bicarbonate
Sodium thiosulfate (provides sulfur donor to convert cyanide to thiocyanate)

Methemoglobinemia

Methemoglobinemia is unlikely, as it requires doses of SNP that exceed 10 mg/kg. Patients receiving high doses of SNP who present with evidence of impaired oxygenation despite an adequate cardiac output and arterial oxygenation should have methemoglobinemia considered in the differential diagnosis.

Phototoxicity

When protected from light, the in vitro breakdown of SNP to cyanide is not excessive in the first 24 hours after the solution of SNP is prepared.

Dose and Administration (Table 16-5)

Effects on Organ Systems

Cardiovascular System

SNP produces direct venous and arterial vasodilation, resulting in prompt decreases in systemic blood pressure. Systemic vascular resistance is decreased, as evidenced by arterial vasodilation, whereas venous return is decreased because of vasodilation of venous capacitance vessels. Although decreased venous return would tend to decrease cardiac output, the net effect is often an increase in cardiac output due to reflex-mediated increases in peripheral sympathetic nervous system

TABLE 16-5.
DOSE AND ADMINISTRATION OF SODIUM NITROPRUSSIDE

Initial dose 0.3 to 0.5 μg/kg/min IV titrated to the desired systemic blood pressure (should not exceed 2 μg/kg/min or a maximum rate of 10 μg/kg/min for no longer than 10 minutes)
Immediate onset and short duration of action
Continuous infusion required to produce sustained pharmacologic effect
Continuous monitoring of systemic blood pressure recommended (indwelling arterial catheter a consideration)
Infusion protected from light by aluminum foil
Decrease risk of cyanide toxicity by combining SNP with another drug (volatile anesthetic, beta-adrenergic blocker) to decrease dose of SNP needed

activity (tachycardia) combined with decreased impedance to left ventricular ejection. SNP-induced decreases in systemic blood pressure may result in decreases in renal function. SNP may increase the area of damage associated with a myocardial infarction (coronary steal).

Vasodilator Effects

SNP is a direct vasodilator, leading to increased cerebral blood flow and cerebral blood volume. In patients with decreased intracranial compliance this may cause undesirable increases in intracranial pressure.

Hypoxic Pulmonary Vasoconstriction

Decreases in PaO_2 may accompany the infusion of SNP and other peripheral vasodilators used to produce controlled hypotension (attenuation of hypoxic pulmonary vasoconstriction is the presumed mechanism).

Platelet Aggregation

Increased intracellular concentrations of cGMP, as produced by SNP and nitroglycerin, may inhibit platelet aggregation. Infusion rates of SNP >3 μg/kg/minute may result in increased bleeding times. Increased bleeding time could also be the result of vasodilation secondary to a direct effect of SNP on vascular tone.

Clinical Uses

Controlled Hypotension

The ability of SNP to rapidly and predictably decrease mean arterial pressure to desired levels makes this vasodilator a useful drug, especially during operations requiring nearly a bloodless field. Mean arterial pressures of 50 to 60 mmHg can be maintained in healthy patients without apparent complications (see Table 16-5).

Hypertensive Emergencies

SNP is more likely to be administered as a temporary initial treatment, with replacement by longer-lasting medications as soon as feasible.

Cardiac Disease

SNP infusion, by virtue of decreasing left ventricular afterload, may be of benefit in the management of patients with mitral or aortic regurgitation or congestive heart failure and after acute myocardial infarction complicated by left ventricular failure.

Aortic Surgery

The surgical repair of thoracic aortic aneurysms, dissections, and coarctations may include SNP to attenuate the proximal hypertension associated with cross-clamping the aorta.

Cardiac Surgery

Systemic hypertension during cardiac surgery is often treated with SNP, whereas SNP-induced vasodilation during the rewarming phase of cardiopulmonary bypass permits increased flow rates and improved heat delivery to peripheral tissues.

NITROGLYCERIN

Nitroglycerin is an organic nitrate that acts principally on venous capacitance vessels and large coronary arteries (in contrast to the arteriolar and venous dilating effects of SNP) to produce peripheral pooling of blood and decreased cardiac wall tension. Nitroglycerin can produce pulmonary vasodilation equivalent to the degree of systemic arterial vasodilation.

Route of Administration

Nitroglycerin is most frequently administered by the sublingual route, but is also available as an oral tablet, a buccal or transmucosal tablet, a lingual spray, and a transdermal ointment or patch. Sublingual administration of nitroglycerin results in peak plasma concentrations within 4 minutes.

Mechanism of Action

Nitroglycerin, like SNP, generates NO, which stimulates the production of cGMP to cause peripheral vasodilation. In contrast to SNP, which spontaneously produces NO, nitroglycerin requires the presence of thio-containing compounds.

Pharmacokinetics

Nitroglycerin has an elimination half-time of about 1.5 minutes, and the volume of distribution (Vd) is large (estimated that only 1% of the drug is in the plasma).

Methemoglobinemia

The nitrite metabolite of nitroglycerin is capable of oxidizing the ferrous ion in hemoglobin to the ferric state, thus producing methemoglobin. Treatment of the resulting methemoglobinemia is with methylene blue, 1 to 2 mg/kg IV, administered over 5 minutes, to facilitate the conversion of methemoglobin to hemoglobin.

Tolerance

A limitation to the use of all nitrates is the development of tolerance to their vasodilating effects. This usually manifests within 24 hours of sustained treatment. A drug-free interval of 12 to 24 hours is recommended to reverse tolerance to nitroglycerin and other nitrates.

Effects on Organ Systems (Table 16-6)

Cardiovascular Effects

Nitroglycerin in doses up to 2 μg/kg/minute IV produces dilatation of veins that predominates over that produced in arterioles. In normal individuals, nitroglycerin decreases cardiac output, reflecting decreased venous return. Nitroglycerin-induced decreases in systemic blood pressure depend more on blood volume than do blood pressure changes produced by SNP. Decreases in diastolic blood pressure may evoke baroreceptor-mediated reflex increases in sympathetic nervous system activity, manifesting as tachycardia and increased myocardial contractility.

Nitroglycerin primarily dilates the larger conductance vessels of the coronary circulation, often leading to an

TABLE 16-6.
EFFECTS OF NITROGLYCERIN ON ORGAN SYSTEMS

Venous dilatation
Relaxation of bronchial smooth muscle
Relaxation of gastrointestinal smooth muscle (sphincter of Oddi)
Relaxation of esophageal and ureteral smooth muscle tone
Cerebral vasodilation (may increase intracranial pressure)

increase in coronary blood flow to ischemic subendocardial areas (SNP may produce an opposite effect).

Nitroglycerin produces a dose-related prolongation of bleeding time that parallels the decrease in systemic blood pressure. Increased bleeding time could also be the result of vasodilation secondary to a direct effect of nitroglycerin on vascular tone.

Clinical Uses

Angina Pectoris

Sublingual nitroglycerin is the most useful of the organic nitrates for the acute and chronic treatment of angina pectoris due to atherosclerotic coronary artery disease or coronary artery vasospasm. Failure of three sublingual tablets within a 15-minute period to relieve angina pectoris may reflect myocardial infarction.

Mechanism of Action

The ability of nitroglycerin to decrease myocardial oxygen requirements (decreased preload and afterload) is the most likely mechanism by which this drug relieves angina pectoris. Nitroglycerin does not increase total coronary blood flow in patients with angina pectoris due to atherosclerosis. The ability of nitroglycerin to selectively dilate large conductive coronary arteries may be an important mechanism in the relief of angina pectoris due to vasospasm.

Side Effects (Table 16-7)

Acute Coronary Syndrome

The routine administration of intravenous nitroglycerin to patients receiving early thrombolytic therapy is probably not beneficial. Intravenous administration of nitroglycerin is most likely to be beneficial in patients with persistent or recurrent angina pectoris after reperfusion therapy and in patients in whom reperfusion therapy is not administered. Nitroglycerin should be

TABLE 16-7.
SIDE EFFECTS OF NITROGLYCERIN

Headache (dilation of meningeal vessels)
Facial flushing
Tolerance
Decreased sensitivity to heparin (interferes with binding of heparin to antithrombin III)

administered cautiously in patients with suspected right ventricular infarction, because these patients are highly dependent on preload and may become acutely hypotensive when vasodilation from nitroglycerin occurs.

Cardiac Failure

Nitroglycerin decreases preload and relieves pulmonary edema in cardiac failure.

Controlled Hypotension

Nitroglycerin can be used to produce controlled hypotension, but it is less potent than SNP. Because nitroglycerin acts predominantly on venous capacitance vessels, the production of controlled hypotension using this drug may be more dependent on intravascular fluid volume, compared with SNP.

Sphincter of Oddi Spasm

Nitroglycerin can relax vascular smooth muscles, including those in the gastrointestinal tract, and it may have a dilating effect on the sphincter of Oddi. Pain that mimics angina pectoris but which is due to opioid-induced biliary tract spasm may be relieved by nitroglycerin resulting in the erroneous diagnosis of myocardial ischemia.

ERECTILE DYSFUNCTION DRUGS

Erectile dysfunction drugs act as selective inhibitors of cGMP-specific phosphodiesterase type 5, which is the predominant enzyme metabolizing cGMP in the corpus cavernosum. These drugs may potentiate the hypotensive effects of nitrates, and concurrent administration of nitroglycerin and erectile dysfunction drugs within 24 hours is not recommended.

ISOSORBIDE DINITRATE

Isosorbide dinitrate is a commonly administered oral nitrate for the prophylaxis of angina pectoris. The predominant effect is the venous circulation, and it also improves the regional distribution of myocardial blood flow in patients with coronary artery disease.

HYDRALAZINE

Hydralazine is a direct systemic arterial vasodilator that activates guanylate cyclase to produce vasorelaxation. Arterial vasodilation may produce reflex sympathetic nervous system stimulation, with resulting increases in heart rate and myocardial contractility.

DIPYRIDAMOLE

Dipyridamole is most often administered orally in combination with warfarin to patients with prosthetic heart valves, as prophylaxis against thromboembolism. This clinical use reflects the ability of dipyridamole, like aspirin, to inhibit platelet aggregation. Dipyridamole may also be administered orally as prophylaxis against angina pectoris.

PAPAVERINE

Papaverine is a nonspecific smooth muscle relaxant present in opium but unrelated chemically or pharmacologically to the opioid alkaloids.

TRIMETHAPHAN

Trimethaphan is a peripheral vasodilator and ganglionic blocker that acts rapidly but so briefly that it must be administered as a continuous infusion. Its use has been abandoned in favor of drugs such as SNP and nitroglycerin. In contrast to SNP, trimethaphan-induced decreases in blood pressure are not associated with increases in plasma concentrations of catecholamines. As a quaternary ammonium drug, trimethaphan has a limited ability to cross the blood-brain barrier, and CNS effects are unlikely. Drug-induced mydriasis interferes with the neurologic evaluation of patients after intracranial surgery.

DIAZOXIDE

Diazoxide is chemically related to thiazide diuretics and is used to treat acute systemic blood pressure increases, as in patients with accelerated and severe hypertension associated with glomerulonephritis. The drug is administered intravenously (30 mg mini boluses up to 150 mg in a single injection) and produces a blood pressure response in 1 to 2 minutes that lasts 6 to 7 hours. Although excessive systemic blood pressure decreases are unlikely, a disadvantage of diazoxide, compared with SNP, is the inability to titrate the drug in accordance with the patient's response.

Cardiovascular Effects

Diazoxide-induced decreases in systemic blood pressure are associated with significant increases in cardiac output and often an increase in heart rate. It is not recommended

TABLE 16-8.
SIDE EFFECTS OF DIAZOXIDE

Sodium and water retention (risk of congestive heart failure in susceptible patients)
Uterine relaxant (can stop labor)
Hyperglycemia
Catecholamine release

for the treatment of hypertension associated with dissecting aortic aneurysm.

Side Effects (Table 16-8)

PURINES

Adenosine

Adenosine is an endogenous nucleoside present in all cells of the body. It is a potent dilator of coronary arteries and is capable of decreasing myocardial oxygen consumption through its antiadrenergic and negative chronotropic actions. As a locally acting metabolite, it protects the heart against hypoxia. The elimination half-time of endogenously released adenosine is very brief (0.6 to 1.5 seconds).

The principal electrophysiologic actions of adenosine on supraventricular tissues are mediated by the stimulation of potassium channels (identical to acetylcholine) that results in hyperpolarization of atrial myocytes and a decrease in the diastolic depolarization (phase 4) of the pacemaker cells in the sinoatrial node. Ventricular myocytes do not possess these adenosine-sensitive potassium channels.

Clinical Uses

Supraventricular Tachycardia

Adenosine is administered clinically as an alternative to verapamil to terminate paroxysmal supraventricular tachycardia and narrow complex regular tachycardia when the diagnosis is in doubt (atrial or junctional). For adult patients, the initial dose is 6 mg IV, followed by 12 mg IV if the first dose is ineffective. Because of its very short elimination half-time, intervals between doses can be as brief as 60 seconds. Continuous ECG monitoring and the availability of equipment for cardioversion are necessary in patients being treated with adenosine. Adenosine is not effective in the treatment of atrial flutter, atrial fibrillation, and ventricular tachycardia. In the absence of a functioning artificial cardiac pacemaker, adenosine should not be administered in the presence of second- or third-degree atrioventricular heart block or in the presence of sick sinus syndrome.

Controlled Hypotension

Adenosine-induced controlled hypotension is characterized by a rapid onset and stable level of hypotension (tachyphylaxis does not occur) that is promptly reversed when the infusion is discontinued. The rate of adenosine infusion required to produce controlled hypotension is unlikely to result in plasma concentrations that alter cardiac automaticity or the conduction of cardiac impulses.

Acadesine

Acadesine is a purine nucleoside analog that may decrease myocardial ischemic injury by selectively increasing the availability of adenosine in ischemic tissues.

Cardiac Antidysrhythmic Drugs

The use of antidysrhythmic drugs for the treatment and prevention of cardiac dysrhythmias is limited by the potential for these drugs to depress left ventricular contractility and the triggering of new dysrhythmias (Stoelting RK, Hillier SC. Cardiac antidysrhythmic drugs. In: *Pharmacology and Physiology in Anesthetic Practice*, 4th ed. Philadelphia: Lippincott Williams & Wilkins, 2006: 370–386). For these reasons, the pharmacologic treatment of cardiac dysrhythmias is principally used to treat atrial fibrillation and atrial flutter that is not responsive to catheter ablation treatment and for patients with implantable cardioverter-defibrillator devices who are receiving frequent but needed electrical shocks. The pharmacologic treatment of cardiac dysrhythmias and disturbances in the conduction of cardiac impulses using antidysrhythmic drugs is based on an understanding of the electrophysiologic basis of the abnormality and the mechanism of action of the therapeutic drug to be administered. The two major physiologic mechanisms that cause ectopic cardiac dysrhythmias are *reentry* and *enhanced automaticity* (Table 17-1). In many patients, the correction of identifiable precipitating events is not sufficient to suppress cardiac ectopic dysrhythmias, and therefore specific cardiac antidysrhythmic drugs may be administered. Drugs administered for the chronic suppression of cardiac dysrhythmias pose little threat to the uneventful course of anesthesia and should be continued

TABLE 17-1.
FACTORS UNDERLYING CARDIAC DYSRHYTHMIAS

Arterial hypoxemia
Electrolyte abnormalities (hypokalemia or hypomagnesemia as produced by diuretics predispose to ventricular dysrhythmias)
Acid-base abnormalities (alkalosis more likely than acidosis to trigger cardiac dysrhythmias)
Altered autonomic nervous system activity (increased activity predisposes to ventricular fibrillation)
Bradycardia (predisposes to ventricular dysrhythmias)
Drugs

up to the time of anesthesia induction. The majority of cardiac dysrhythmias that occur during anesthesia do not require therapy (Table 17-2).

MECHANISM OF ACTION

Cardiac antidysrhythmic drugs produce pharmacologic effects by blocking the passage of ions across the sodium, potassium, and calcium ion channels present in the heart.

CLASSIFICATION

Cardiac antidysrhythmic drugs are most commonly classified into four groups based primarily on the ability of

TABLE 17-2.
EXAMPLES OF CARDIAC DYSRHYTHMIAS THAT REQUIRE TREATMENT

Persists despite removing the precipitating cause
Hemodynamic function is compromised
Predisposes to more serious cardiac dysrhythmias

the drug to control dysrhythmias by blocking specific ion channels and current during the cardiac action potential (Tables 17-3 and 17-4). Antidysrhythmic drugs differ in their pharmacokinetics and efficacy in treating specific types of cardiac dysrhythmias (Tables 17-5 and 17-6).

TABLE 17-3.
CLASSIFICATION OF CARDIAC ANTIDYSRHYTHMIC DRUGS

Class I (inhibit fast sodium ion channels)
Class IA
- Quinidine
- Procainamide
- Disopyramide
- Moricizine

Class IB
- Lidocaine
- Tocainide
- Mexiletine

Class IC
- Flecainide
- Propafenone

Class II (decrease rate of depolarization)
- Esmolol
- Propranolol
- Acebutolol

Class III (inhibit potassium ion channels)
- Amiodarone
- Sotalol
- Ibutilide
- Dofetilide
- Bretylium

Class IV (inhibit slow calcium channels)
- Verapamil
- Diltiazem

TABLE 17-4.

ELECTROPHYSIOLOGIC AND ELECTROCARDIOGRAPHIC EFFECTS OF CARDIAC ANTIDYSRHYTHMIC DRUGS

	Class IA	Class IB	Class IC	Class II	Class III	Class IV
Depolarization rate (phase 0)	Decreased	No effect	Greatly decreased	No effect	No effect	No effect
Conduction velocity	Decreased	No effect	Greatly decreased	Decreased	Decreased	No effect
Effective refractory period	Greatly increased	Decreased	Increased	Decreased	Greatly increased	No effect
Action potential duration	Increased	Decreased	Increased	Increased	Greatly increase	Decreased
Automaticity	Decreased	Decreased	Decreased	Decreased	Decreased	No effect
P-R duration	No effect	No effect	Increased	No effect or Increased	Increased	No effect
QRS duration	Increased	No effect	Greatly increased	No effect	Increased	No effect
QTc duration	Greatly increased	No effect or decreased	Increased	Decreased	Greatly increased	No effect

TABLE 17-5.
PHARMACOKINETICS OF CARDIAC ANTIDYSRHYTHMIC DRUGS

	Principal Clearance Mechanism	Protein Binding (%)	Elimination Half-Time (hrs)	Therapeutic Plasma Concentration
Quinidine	Hepatic	80–90	5–12	1.2–4.0 μg/mL
Procainamide	Renal/hepatic	15	2.5–5.0	4–8 μg/mL
Disopyramide	Renal/hepatic	15	8–12	2–4 μg/mL
Lidocaine	Hepatic	55	1.4–8.0	1–5 μg/mL
Tocainide	Hepatic/renal	10–30	12–15	4–10 μg/mL
Mexiletine	Hepatic	60–75	6–12	0.75–2.00 μg/mL
Flecainide	Hepatic	30–45	13–30	0.3–1.5 μg/mL
Propafenone	Hepatic	>95	5–8	
Propranolol	Hepatic	90–95	2–4	10–30 ng/mL
Amiodarone	Hepatic	96	68–107 days	1.5–2.0 μg/mL
Sotalol	Renal			
Verapamil	Hepatic	90	4.5–12.0	100–300 ng/mL

TABLE 17-6.

EFFICACY OF CARDIAC ANTIDYSRHYTHMIC DRUGS

	Conversion of Atrial Fibrillation	Paroxysmal Supraventricular Tachycardia	Premature Ventricular Contractions	Ventricular Tachycardia
Quinidine	+	++	++	+
Procainamide	+	++	++	++
Disopyramide	+	++	++	++
Lidocaine	+	0	++	++
Tocainide	0	0	++	++
Mexiletine	0	0	++	++
Moricizine	0	0	++	++
Flecainide	0	+	++	++
Propafenone	0	+	++	++
Propranolol	+	++	+	+
Amiodarone	+	++	++	++
Sotalol	++	+	+	+
Verapamil	+	++	0	0
Diltiazem	+	++	0	0
Digitalis	++	++	0	0
Adenosine	0	++	0	0

0, no effect; +, effective; ++, highly effective.

PRODYSRHYTHMIC EFFECTS

The prodysrhythmic effects of these drugs describe those bradydysrhythmias or tachydysrhythmias that represent new cardiac dysrhythmias associated with chronic antidysrhythmic drug treatment.

Torsade de Pointes

Torsade de pointes—a polymorphic ventricular tachycardia and ventricular fibrillation—is associated with class IA drugs (quinidine, disopyramide) and class III drugs (amiodarone) that prolong the QTc interval by potassium channel blockade. Predisposing factors include hypokalemia, hypomagnesemia, poor left ventricular function, and the concomitant administration of other QTc-prolonging drugs.

Incessant Ventricular Tachycardia

Incessant ventricular tachycardia may be precipitated by cardiac antidysrhythmic drugs that slow the conduction of cardiac impulses (class IA and class IC drugs) sufficiently to create a continuous ventricular tachycardia reentry circuit.

Wide Complex Ventricular Tachycardia

Wide complex ventricular tachycardia is usually associated with class IC cardiac antidysrhythmic drugs in the setting of structural heart disease.

EFFICACY AND RESULTS OF TREATMENT USING CARDIAC ANTIDYSRHYTHMIC DRUGS

Suppression of ventricular ectopy using a cardiac antidysrhythmic drug does not prevent future life-threatening dysrhythmias and may increase mortality. In fact, patients treated with class IC cardiac antidysrhythmic drugs experienced a higher incidence of sudden cardiac arrest, reflecting the protodysrhythmic effects of these drugs. Survivors of cardiac arrest have a high risk of subsequent ventricular fibrillation, and the treatment of these patients with amiodarone results in fewer life-threatening cardiac events.

PROPHYLACTIC ANTIDYSRHYTHMIC THERAPY

Lidocaine is not recommended as a prophylactic treatment for patients in the early stages of acute myocardial infarction and without malignant ventricular ectopy. Calcium channel antagonists are not recommended as routine treatment of patients with acute myocardial infarction, because mortality is not decreased by these drugs. Treatment with magnesium is indicated in those patients who, following an acute myocardial infarction, develop torsade de pointes ventricular tachycardia.

DECISION TO TREAT CARDIAC DYSRHYTHMIAS

The benefit of antidysrhythmic drugs is clearest when it results in the immediate termination of a sustained tachycardia (as in ventricular tachycardia suppressed by lidocaine or supraventricular tachycardia suppressed by adenosine or verapamil). Conversely, it has been difficult to demonstrate that antidysrhythmic drugs alleviate those symptoms related to chronic cardiac dysrhythmias, a situation in which the risk of side effects is greater. The mechanism by which β-adrenergic antagonists decrease mortality after an acute myocardial infarction is not known.

QUINIDINE

Quinidine is a class IA drug that is effective in the treatment of acute and chronic supraventricular dysrhythmias. It slows the atrial rate in the presence of atrial fibrillation and suppresses tachydysrhythmias associated with Wolff-Parkinson-White syndrome.

Mechanism of Action

Quinidine decreases the slope of phase 4 depolarization, which explains its effectiveness in suppressing the cardiac dysrhythmias caused by enhanced automaticity.

Metabolism and Excretion

Quinidine is hydroxylated in the liver to inactive metabolites, which are excreted in the urine. The accumulation of quinidine or its metabolites may occur in the presence of hepatic and/or renal dysfunction.

Side Effects

Quinidine has a low therapeutic ratio, and its side effects are predictable if the plasma concentration becomes excessive (Table 17-7).

PROCAINAMIDE

Procainamide is as effective as quinidine for the treatment of ventricular tachydysrhythmias but is not as effective in abolishing atrial tachydysrhythmias. Although procainamide and quinidine have a broader spectrum of antidysrhythmic effects than lidocaine (useful in the treatment of supraventricular and ventricular cardiac dysrhythmias), they are rarely used during anesthesia because of their propensity to produce hypotension.

TABLE 17-7.
SIDE EFFECTS OF QUINIDINE

Prolongation of the P-R and QTc interval and widening of the QRS complex (heart block may occur)
Syncope (may reflect ventricular dysrhythmias)
Hypotension (vasodilation especially if administered IV)
Atropine-like action
Allergic reactions
Thrombocytopenia
Nausea and vomiting
Tinnitus and blurring of vision
Accentuate effects of neuromuscular blocking drugs (quinine like effects)

Mechanism of Action

Procainamide is an analog of the local anesthetic procaine and possesses an electrophysiologic action similar to that of quinidine; however, it produces less prolongation of the QTc interval.

Metabolism and Excretion

Procainamide is eliminated by renal (unchanged) and hepatic metabolism (acetylated to N-acetyl procainamide—activity of the necessary enzyme is genetically determined). The acetylated metabolite of procainamide is pharmacologically active.

Side Effects

The incidence of side effects is high when procainamide is used as an antidysrhythmic drug. These effects include hypotension due to direct myocardial depression.

DISOPYRAMIDE

Disopyramide is comparable to quinidine in effectively suppressing atrial and ventricular tachydysrhythmias. Prolongation of the QTc interval and paradoxical ventricular tachycardia (similar to quinidine) may occur. The potential for direct myocardial depression, especially in patients with preexisting left ventricular dysfunction, seems to be greater with this drug than with quinidine and procainamide.

MORICIZINE

Moricizine is a phenothiazine derivative with modest efficacy in the treatment of sustained ventricular dysrhythmias; it is best reserved for the treatment of life-threatening ventricular dysrhythmias, in view of its prodysrhythmic effects.

LIDOCAINE

Lidocaine is used principally for the suppression of ventricular dysrhythmias (premature ventricular contractions, ventricular tachycardia), having minimal effects on supraventricular tachydysrhythmias. The efficacy of prophylactic lidocaine therapy for preventing ventricular fibrillation after acute myocardial infarction has not been documented, and its use is no longer recommended. In adult patients with normal cardiac output, hepatic function, and hepatic blood flow, an initial intravenous administration of lidocaine, 2 mg/kg, followed by a continuous infusion of 1 to 4 mg/min should provide therapeutic plasma lidocaine concentrations of 1 to 5 μg/mL.

Mechanism of Action

Lidocaine delays the rate of spontaneous phase 4 depolarization by preventing or diminishing the gradual decrease in potassium ion permeability that normally occurs during this phase.

Metabolism and Excretion

Lidocaine is metabolized in the liver, and the resulting metabolites may possess cardiac antidysrhythmic activity.

Side Effects

Lidocaine is essentially devoid of effects on the ECG or cardiovascular system when the plasma concentration remains <5 μg/mL (Table 17-8).

TOCAINIDE

Tocainide, like mexiletine, is an orally effective amine analog of lidocaine that is used for the chronic suppression of ventricular cardiac tachydysrhythmias.

MEXILETINE

Mexiletine is an orally effective amine analog of lidocaine that is used for the chronic suppression of ventricular cardiac tachydysrhythmias.

TABLE 17-8. SIDE EFFECTS OF LIDOCAINE

Hypotension (peripheral vasodilation and myocardial depression when plasma concentrations 5 to 10 μg/mL)
Bradycardia (slowing of conduction of cardiac impulses, prolonged P-R interval, widened QRS complex)
Seizures (plasma concentrations 5 to 10 μg/mL)
CNS depression, apnea, cardiac arrest (plasma concentrations >10 μg/mL)

PHENYTOIN

Phenytoin is particularly effective in the suppression of ventricular dysrhythmias associated with digitalis toxicity. Phenytoin may be useful in the treatment of paradoxical ventricular tachycardia or torsade de pointes that is associated with a prolonged QTc.

Mechanism of Action

The effects of phenytoin on automaticity and velocity of conduction of cardiac impulses resemble those of lidocaine.

Metabolism and Excretion

Phenytoin is hydroxylated and then conjugated with glucuronic acid for excretion in the urine.

Side Effects (Table 17-9)

FLECAINIDE

Flecainide is a fluorinated local anesthetic analog of procainamide that is more effective in suppressing ventricular premature beats and ventricular tachycardia than quinidine and disopyramide. Flecainide is also effective in the treatment of atrial tachydysrhythmias.

TABLE 17-9.
SIDE EFFECTS OF PHENYTOIN

Cerebellar disturbances (ataxia, nystagmus, confusion)
Hyperglycemia (inhibition of insulin secretion)
Thrombocytopenia (bone marrow depression)
Skin rash

Side Effects

Prodysrhythmic side effects occur in a significant number of treated patients, especially in the presence of left ventricular dysfunction.

PROPAFENONE

Propafenone, like flecainide, is an effective antidysrhythmic drug for the suppression of ventricular and atrial tachydysrhythmias. Prodysrhythmic effects are more likely to occur in patients with preexisting ventricular dysrhythmias.

β-ADRENERGIC ANTAGONISTS

β-Adrenergic antagonists are effective for the treatment of cardiac dysrhythmias related to enhanced activity of the sympathetic nervous system (perioperative stress, thyrotoxicosis, pheochromocytoma). Propranolol and esmolol are effective for controlling the rate of ventricular response in patients with atrial fibrillation and atrial flutter. Multifocal atrial tachycardia may respond to esmolol or metoprolol but is best treated with amiodarone. Acebutolol is effective in the treatment of frequent premature ventricular contractions. β-Adrenergic antagonists, especially propranolol, may be effective in controlling torsade de pointes for patients with prolonged QTc intervals. Acebutolol, propranolol, and metoprolol are approved for the prevention of sudden death following myocardial infarction.

Mechanism of Action

The antidysrhythmic effects of β-adrenergic antagonists most likely reflect a blockade of the responses to β-receptors in the heart to sympathetic nervous system stimulation, as well as the effects of circulating catecholamines. As a result, the rate of spontaneous phase 4 depolarization is decreased and the rate of sinoatrial node discharge is decreased.

The usual oral dose of propranolol for the chronic suppression of ventricular dysrhythmias is 10 to 80 mg every 6 to 8 hours. Effective β-blockade is usually achieved in an otherwise normal person when the resting heart rate is 55 to 60 beats/minute.

Metabolism and Excretion

Orally administered propranolol is extensively metabolized in the liver, and a hepatic first-pass effect is responsible for the variation in plasma concentration; the therapeutic plasma concentration of propranolol may vary from 10 to 30 ng/mL. Propranolol readily crosses the blood-brain barrier. The principal metabolite of propranolol is 4-hydroxypropranolol, which possesses weak β-adrenergic antagonist activity.

Side Effects (Table 17-10)

TABLE 17-10.
SIDE EFFECTS OF BETA-ADRENERGIC ANTAGONISTS

Bradycardia
Hypotension
Myocardial depression
Bronchospasm
Congestive heart failure (especially in patients dependent on sympathetic nervous system activity as a compensatory mechanism)
Heart block (do not administer these drugs to patients with preexisting heart block)
Worsening of Raynaud's disease
Mental depression
Up-regulation of β-adrenergic receptors (manifests as supraventricular tachycardia when treatment is abruptly discontinued)

AMIODARONE

Amiodarone is a potent antidysrhythmic drug with a wide spectrum of activity against refractory supraventricular and ventricular tachydysrhythmias. In the presence of ventricular tachycardia or fibrillation that is resistant to electrical defibrillation, amiodarone (300 mg IV) is recommended. Lidocaine or procainamide are recommended during cardiopulmonary resuscitation only when amiodarone has been ineffective. Administered over 2 to 5 minutes, a dose of 5 mg/kg IV produces a prompt antidysrhythmic effect that lasts up to 4 hours. After discontinuation of chronic oral therapy, the pharmacologic effect of amiodarone lasts for a prolonged period (up to 60 days), reflecting the prolonged elimination half-time of this drug.

Mechanism of Action

Amiodarone, a benzofluorene derivative, is 37% iodine by weight and structurally resembles thyroxine. It prolongs the effective refractory period of all cardiac tissues, including the sinoatrial node, atrium, atrioventricular node, His-Purkinje system, and ventricle. Amiodarone has an antiadrenergic effect (noncompetitive blockade of α-and β-receptors) and a minor negative inotropic effect.

Metabolism and Excretion

Amiodarone has a prolonged elimination half-time (29 days) and large volume of distribution (Vd). This drug is minimally dependent on renal excretion. The principal metabolite, desethylamiodarone, is pharmacologically active and has a longer elimination half-time than the parent drug, resulting in an accumulation of this metabolite following chronic therapy.

Side Effects

Side effects in patients treated chronically with amiodarone are common, especially when the daily maintenance dose exceeds 400 mg (Table 17-11).

TABLE 17-11.
SIDE EFFECTS OF CHRONIC AMIODARONE THERAPY

Pulmonary toxicity
- Pulmonary alveolitis (occurs in 5% to 15% of treated patients)
- Slow insidious onset characterized by dyspnea, cough, and pulmonary infiltrates on x-ray
- Acute onset of dyspnea, cough, and arterial hypoxemia

Cardiotoxicity
- Prolongation of QTc interval
- Atrioventricular heart block (potential need for a temporary artificial pacemaker)

Ocular, Dermatologic, Neurologic, and Hepatic
- Corneal micro deposits
- Photosensitivity
- Peripheral neuropathy
- Increases in plasma transaminase concentrations

Pharmacokinetic
- Inhibition of P-450 enzymes (increased plasma concentrations of digoxin, warfarin)

Endocrine
- Hypothyroidism
- Hyperthyroidism (as late as 5 months after discontinuing therapy)

SOTALOL

Sotalol is administered for the treatment of sustained ventricular tachycardia or ventricular fibrillation. Sotalol is a nonselective β-adrenergic antagonist drug at low doses, and at higher doses, it prolongs the cardiac action potential in the atria, ventricles, and accessory bypass tracts. Because of its prodysrhythmic effects (torsade de pointes), this drug is usually restricted for patients with life-threatening ventricular dysrhythmias. Excretion is mainly through the kidneys.

IBUTILIDE

Ibutilide is effective for the conversion of recent onset atrial fibrillation or atrial flutter to normal sinus rhythm. Hepatic metabolism is extensive. Polymorphic ventricular tachycardia, with or without prolongation of the QTc interval, may occur.

DOFETILIDE

Dofetilide is effective for the conversion of recent-onset atrial fibrillation or atrial flutter to normal sinus rhythm. This drug is excreted unchanged in the urine. Torsade de pointes occurs, especially in patients with preexisting left ventricular dysfunction.

BRETYLIUM

Bretylium is no longer recommended for the treatment of ventricular fibrillation during cardiopulmonary resuscitation, because it is less effective than amiodarone and has more side effects.

VERAPAMIL AND DILTIAZEM

Among the calcium channel blockers, verapamil and diltiazem have the greatest efficacy for the treatment of cardiac dysrhythmias. Intravenous verapamil is highly effective in terminating paroxysmal supraventricular tachycardia (75 to 150 μg/kg over 1 to 3 minutes, followed by a continuous infusion of about 5 μg/kg per minute to maintain a sustained effect). This drug also effectively controls the ventricular rate in most patients who develop atrial fibrillation or flutter. Verapamil does not have a depressant effect on accessory tracts and thus will not slow the ventricular response rate in patients with Wolff-Parkinson-White syndrome.

Mechanism of Action

Verapamil and the other calcium channel blockers inhibit the flux of calcium ions across the slow channels of smooth muscle and cardiac cells. This effect manifests as a decreased rate of spontaneous phase 4 depolarization. Verapamil has a substantial depressant effect on the atrioventricular node and a negative chronotropic effect on the sinoatrial node.

Metabolism and Excretion

An estimated 70% of an injected dose of verapamil is eliminated by the kidneys.

Side Effects (Table 17-12)

OTHER CARDIAC ANTIDYSRHYTHMIC DRUGS

Digitalis Preparations

Digitalis preparations, such as digoxin, are effective cardiac antidysrhythmics for the stabilization of atrial electrical activity and the treatment and prevention of atrial tachydysrhythmias.

Adenosine

Adenosine is an endogenous nucleoside that slows the conduction of cardiac impulses through the atrioventricular node, making it an effective alternative to calcium channel blockers (verapamil) for the treatment of paroxysmal supraventricular tachycardia, including that due to conduction through accessory pathways in patients with Wolff-Parkinson-White syndrome. This drug is not effective in the treatment of atrial fibrillation, atrial flutter, or ventricular tachycardia. The usual dose of adenosine is 6 mg IV followed, if necessary, by a repeat injection of 6 to 12 mg IV about 3 minutes later.

TABLE 17-12.
SIDE EFFECTS OF CALCIUM CHANNEL BLOCKERS USED TO TREAT CARDIAC DYSRHYTHMIAS

Atrioventricular heart block
Direct myocardial depression
Hypotension (vasodilation)
Potentiation of anesthetic-induced myocardial depression
Exaggeration of effects of neuromuscular-blocking drugs

Mechanism of Action

Adenosine stimulates cardiac adenosine$_1$ receptors to increase potassium ion currents, shorten the action potential duration, and hyperpolarize cardiac cell membranes. Short-lived cardiac effects (elimination half-time 10 seconds) are due to carrier-mediated cellular uptake and metabolism to inosine by adenosine deaminase.

Side Effects (Table 17-13)

TABLE 17-13.
SIDE EFFECTS OF ADENOSINE

Flushing
Headache
Dyspnea
Chest discomfort
Nausea
Atrioventricular heart block
Bronchospasm

Calcium Channel Blockers

18

Calcium channel blockers (calcium entry blockers or calcium antagonists) are a diverse group of structurally unrelated compounds that selectively interfere with inward calcium ion movement across myocardial and vascular smooth muscle (Table 18-1) (Stoelting RK, Hillier SC. Calcium channel blockers. In: *Pharmacology and Physiology in Anesthetic Practice*, 4th ed. Philadelphia: Lippincott Williams & Wilkins, 2006:387–397). The various calcium channel blockers differ in terms of side effects, usual doses, metabolism, and duration of action (Tables 18-2 and 18-3).

MECHANISM OF ACTION

Calcium channel blockers bind to receptors on voltage-gated calcium channels (L-, N-, and T-subtypes) resulting in the maintenance of these channels in an inactive (closed) state. As a result, calcium influx is decreased, and a reduction in intracellular calcium occurs. All clinically utilized calcium channel blockers bind to unique sites on the $\alpha 1$ subunit of L-type calcium channels and thus diminish entry of calcium ions into cells. Calcium influx through L-type calcium channels is responsible for phase 2 of the cardiac action potential, which is important in excitation–contraction coupling in cardiac and vascular smooth muscle and depolarization in sinoatrial and atrioventricular nodal tissue. Thus blockade of slow calcium channels by calcium channel blockers predictably results in a slowing of the

TABLE 18-1.
CLASSIFICATION OF CALCIUM CHANNEL BLOCKERS

Phenylalkylamines (selective for atrioventricular node)
Verapamil
Dihydropyrimidines (selective for arterial beds)
Nifedipine
Nicardipine
Nimodipine
Isradipine
Felodipine
Amlodipine
Benzothiazepines (selective for atrioventricular node)
Diltiazem

heart rate, reduction in myocardial contractility, decreased speed of conduction of cardiac impulses through the atrioventricular node, and vascular smooth muscle relaxation (associated decrease in systemic blood pressure).

PHARMACOLOGIC EFFECTS (TABLE 18-2)

PHENYLALKYLAMINES

Verapamil

Verapamil is a synthetic derivative of papaverine that is supplied as a racemic mixture. The dextroisomer of verapamil is devoid of activity at slow calcium channels and instead acts on fast sodium channels, accounting for the local anesthetic effects of verapamil (1.6 times as potent as procaine). The levoisomer of verapamil is specific for slow calcium channels, and the predominance of this action accounts for the classification of verapamil as a calcium blocking drug.

TABLE 18-2.
COMPARATIVE PHARMACOLOGIC EFFECTS OF CALCIUM CHANNEL BLOCKERS

	Verapamil	Nifedipine	Nicardipine	Diltiazem
Systemic blood pressure	Decrease	Decrease	Decrease	Decrease
Heart rate	Decrease	Increase to no change	Increase to no change	Decrease
Myocardial depression	Moderate	Moderate	Slight	Moderate
Sinoatrial node depression	Moderate	None	None	Slight
Atrioventricular node conduction	Marked depression	None	None	Moderate
Coronary artery dilation	Moderate	Marked	Greatest	Moderate
Peripheral artery dilation	Moderate	Marked	Marked	Moderate

TABLE 18-3.
PHARMACOKINETICS OF CALCIUM CHANNEL BLOCKERS

	Verapamil	Nifedipine	Nicardipine	Nimodipine	Diltiazem
Dosage					
Oral	80–160 mg every 8 hrs	10–30 mg every 8 hrs	20 mg every 8 hrs	30–60 mg every 4–6 hrs	60-90 mg every 8 hrs
Intravenous	75–150 μg/kg	5–15 μg/kg		10 μg/kg	75–150 μg/kg
Absorption (%)					
Oral	> 90	> 90			> 90
Bioavailability (%)	10–20	65–70	30	5–10	40
Onset of effect (mins)					
Oral	< 30	< 20	20–60	30–90	30
Sublingual		3			
Intravenous	1–3	1–3		1–3	1–3
First-pass hepatic extraction after oral administration (%)	75–90	40–60	20–40	90	70–80
Protein binding (%)	83–93	92–98	95	99	98
Clearance					
Renal (%)	70	80	55	20	35
Hepatic (%)	15	<15	45	80	60
Active metabolites	Yes	No			Yes
Therapeutic plasma concentration (ng/ml)	50–250	10–100	5–100	10–30	100–250
Elimination half-time (hrs)	3–7	3–7	3–5	2	4–6

TABLE 18-4.
CLINICAL USES OF VERAPAMIL

Supraventricular tachydysrhythmias (action on atrioventricular node)
Vasospastic angina pectoris (mild vasodilating effects)
Essential hypertension (mild vasodilating effects)
Hypertrophic cardiomyopathy

Side Effects

Verapamil has a major depressant effect on the atrioventricular node, a negative chronotropic effect on the sinoatrial node, and a negative inotropic effect on cardiac muscle (exaggerated in patients with preexisting left ventricular dysfunction).

Clinical Uses (Table 18-4)

Calcium channel antagonists should not be routinely administered for acute myocardial infarction, because postinfarction mortality is not decreased.

Pharmacokinetics (See Table 18-3)

Pharmacologic effects following the intravenous administration of verapamil appear within 2 to 3 minutes and may last 6 hours. The demethylated metabolite of verapamil, norverapamil, possesses sufficient activity to contribute to the antidysrhythmic properties of the parent drug.

DIHYDROPYRIMIDINES

Dihydropyrimidines have a primary affinity for peripheral arterioles, whereas the vasodilating effects of these drugs on venous capacitance vessels are minimal.

Nifedipine

Nifedipine is a dihydropyridine derivative with greater coronary and peripheral arterial vasodilator properties than verapamil. Unlike verapamil, nifedipine has little or no direct depressant effect on sinoatrial or atrioventricular node activity.

The peripheral vasodilation and the resulting decrease in systemic blood pressure produced by nifedipine activate baroreceptors, leading to an increased peripheral sympathetic nervous system activity most often manifesting as an increased heart rate. This increased sympathetic nervous system activity counters the direct negative inotropic, chronotropic, and dromotropic effects of nifedipine.

Clinical Uses

Nifedipine is used to treat patients with angina pectoris, especially that due to coronary artery spasm.

Pharmacokinetics (See Table 18-3)

The absorption of an oral or sublingual dose of nifedipine is about 90%, with onset of an effect being detectable within 20 minutes after administration.

Side Effects (Table 18-5)

Nicardipine

Nicardipine lacks effects on the sinoatrial node and atrioventricular node and has minimal myocardial depressant effects. This drug has the greatest vasodilating effects of all the calcium channel blockers, with vasodilation being particularly prominent in the coronary arteries.

Nimodipine

Nimodipine is a highly lipid-soluble analog of nifedipine. Lipid solubility facilitates its entrance into the central nervous system, where it blocks the influx of the extracellular calcium ions necessary for contraction of large cerebral arteries.

TABLE 18-5.
SIDE EFFECTS OF NIFEDIPINE

Flushing
Vertigo
Headache
Peripheral edema (venodilation)
Hypotension
Paresthesias
Skeletal muscle weakness
Hepatic and renal dysfunction (rare)
Coronary artery vasospasm (abrupt discontinuation of treatment)

Clinical Uses

The lipid solubility of nimodipine and its ability to cross the blood-brain barrier is responsible for the potential value of this drug in treating patients with subarachnoid hemorrhage.

Cerebral Vasospasm

Cerebral vasospasm is also treatable using nimodipine. The vasodilating effect of nimodipine on cerebral arteries is uniquely valuable in preventing or attenuating the cerebral vasospasm that often accompanies subarachnoid hemorrhage.

Cerebral Protection

Nimodipine also has been evaluated for cerebral protection after global ischemia, as associated with cardiac arrest.

Amlodipine

Amlodipine is a dihydropyridine derivative that is available for only oral administration. It has minimal detrimental effects on myocardial contractility, and it provides anti-ischemic effects comparable to β-blockers in patients with acute coronary syndrome.

BENZOTHIAZEPINES

Diltiazem

Diltiazem, like verapamil, blocks predominantly the calcium channels of the atrioventricular node and is therefore a first-line medication for the treatment of supraventricular tachydysrhythmias.

Clinical Uses

The clinical uses and drug interactions for diltiazem are similar to those of verapamil.

Pharmacokinetics (Table 18-3)

DRUG INTERACTIONS

The known pharmacologic effects of calcium channel blockers on cardiac, skeletal, and vascular smooth muscle, as well as on the conduction velocity of cardiac impulses, make drug interactions possible (Table 18-6).

RISKS OF CHRONIC TREATMENT

Despite the popularity of calcium channel blockers in the treatment of cardiovascular diseases (essential hypertension, angina pectoris), increasing concern has surfaced about the long-term safety of these drugs, especially the short-acting dihydropyrimidine derivatives. For example, the risk of developing cardiovascular complications has been described as being greater in patients treated with nifedipine, compared with those receiving placebo or conventional therapy. The risk of developing cancer may be increased in those treated with calcium channel blockers, compared with β-adrenergic antagonists or angiotensin-converting enzyme (ACE) inhibitors.

TABLE 18-6.
CALCIUM CHANNEL BLOCKERS AND DRUG INTERACTIONS

Anesthetic drugs (common negative inotropic and chronotropic effects and peripheral vasodilating effects; no evidence of an increased risk when patients being treated chronically with calcium channel blockers receive anesthesia)
Neuromuscular blocking drugs (potentiated by calcium channel blockers)
Local anesthetics (possible increased risk of local anesthetic toxicity, as verapamil and diltiazem possess local anesthetic activity)
Potassium-containing solutions (hyperkalemia as calcium channel blockers slow inward movement of potassium ions as present in whole blood or with infusion of exogenous potassium chloride to treat hypokalemia)
Dantrolene (hyperkalemia)
Platelet function
Digoxin
H-2 antagonists (may increase plasma concentrations of calcium channel blockers)

CYTOPROTECTION

Drug-induced calcium channel blockade may provide protection against ischemic reperfusion injury.

19

Drugs Used for Psychopharmacologic Therapy

Antidepressants and anxiolytics are the drugs most likely to be prescribed for the treatment of depression in adults (Stoelting RK, Hillier SC. Drugs used for psychopharmacologic therapy. In: *Pharmacology and Physiology in Anesthetic Practice*, 4th ed. Philadelphia: Lippincott Williams & Wilkins, 2006:398–419). Lithium and antipsychotic drugs are used for the treatment of bipolar disorders and psychotic disorders including schizophrenia. It is now accepted that anesthesia can be safely administered to patients being treated with drugs used to treat mental illness (drug interactions between psychopharmacologic drugs and drugs administered in the perioperative period are less than previously perceived).

ANTIDEPRESSANTS

Considering the wide rage of disorders for which antidepressant drugs are effective, the term *antidepressant* has become a misnomer (Table 19-1). Antidepressants are logically classified on the basis of their chemical structures and their acute neuropharmacologic effects (Table 19-2). The precise mechanism by which antidepressants work is unknown, but they appear to act by altering noradrenergic neurotransmission and/or serotoninergic neurotransmission. Neurobiologically, reuptake blockade or monoamine oxidase (MAO) inhibition (necessary for

TABLE 19-1.
CLINICAL USES OF ANTIDEPRESSANT DRUGS

Unipolar and bipolar depression
Panic disorder
Social phobia
Post-traumatic stress syndrome
Neuropathic pain
Migraine prophylaxis
Obsessive-compulsive disorder
Bulimia
Childhood attention-deficit hyperactivity disorder

the breakdown of free norepinephrine and serotonin) occurs promptly after the initiation of antidepressant therapy, but clinical improvement typically does not occur for 2 to 4 weeks.

Selective Serotonin Reuptake Inhibitors

Selective serotonin reuptake inhibitors (SSRIs) are the most broadly prescribed class of antidepressants and are the drugs of choice for the treatment of mild to moderate depression. SSRIs are the first line of pharmacotherapy for panic disorder and obsessive-compulsive disorder. Compared with tricyclic antidepressants, SSRIs lack anticholinergic properties, do not cause postural hypotension or delayed conduction of cardiac impulses, and do not appear to have a major effect on the seizure threshold. Perhaps the most important advantage of SSRIs, when compared with tricyclic antidepressants, is the safety of SSRIs when taken in overdose. A small increased risk of suicidality may be present in children and adolescents treated with SSRIs.

Fluoxetine

Fluoxetine is commonly administered once daily in the morning to decrease the risk of associated insomnia.

TABLE 19-2.
COMPARATIVE PHARMACOLOGY OF ANTIDEPRESSANT DRUGS

	Sedative Potency	Anticholinergic Potency	Orthostatic Hypotension
Selective serotonin uptake inhibitors			
Fluoxetine	+	+	+
Sertraline	+	+	+
Paroxetine	+	+	+
Fluvoxamine	+	+	+
Citalopram	+	+	+
Escitalopram	+	+	+
Bupropion	+	+	+
Venlafaxine	+	+	May cause hypertension in some individuals
Trazodone	+++	+	+++; associated with cardiac dysrhythmias
Nefazodone	++	+	++
Tricyclic and related cyclic compounds*			
Amitriptyline	+++	++++	+++

(*continued*)

TABLE 19-2.
(continued)

	Sedative Potency	Anticholinergic Potency	Orthostatic Hypotension
Amoxapine	+	+	++
Clomipramine	+++	+++	+++
Desipramine	+	+	++
Doxepin	+++	++	++
Imipramine	++	++	+++
Nortriptyline	+	+	0
Protriptyline	+	+++	+
Trimipramine	+++	++	++
Mirtazapine			
Monoamine oxidase inhibitors			
Phenelzine	+	+	+++
Tranylcypromine	+	+	+++
Isocarboxazid	+	+	+++

0, none; +, mild; ++, moderate; +++, marked; ++++, greatest.
*All tricyclic and related cyclic compounds may produce cardiac dysrhythmias.

Because fluoxetine has a prolonged elimination half-time (1 to 3 days for acute administration and 4 to 6 days for chronic administration), the drug may be taken every other day.

Side Effects (Table 19-3)

Fluoxetine does not cause hypotension, and changes in the conduction of cardiac impulses seem infrequent. Because of its long elimination half-time, fluoxetine should be discontinued for about 5 weeks before initiating treatment with an MAO inhibitor. The long elimination half-time of fluoxetine appears to prevent the withdrawal symptoms induced by abrupt discontinuation of the drug. An overdose with fluoxetine alone is not associated with the risk of cardiovascular and central nervous system (CNS) toxicity.

Drug Interactions

Among the SSRIs, fluoxetine is the most potent inhibitor of certain hepatic cytochrome P-450 enzymes. As a result, this drug may increase the plasma concentrations of drugs that depend on hepatic metabolism for clearance (tricyclic antidepressants, some cardiac antidysrhythmic drugs, some β-adrenergic antagonist drugs). MAO inhibitors combined with fluoxetine may cause the development of a serotonin syndrome characterized by anxiety, restlessness, chills, ataxia, and insomnia.

TABLE 19-3.
SIDE EFFECTS OF FLUOXETINE

Nausea
Anorexia
Insomnia
Sexual dysfunction
Agitation
Neuromuscular restlessness
Appetite suppression
Analgesic for treatment of chronic pain

Sertraline

Sertraline has a spectrum of efficacy similar to fluoxetine. This drug has a shorter elimination half-time (25 hours) than fluoxetine and is a less potent inhibitor of hepatic microsomal enzymes.

Paroxetine

Paroxetine has an efficacy similar to that of fluoxetine. This drug has a relatively short elimination half-time (24 hours), and no active metabolites are produced.

Fluvoxamine

Fluvoxamine is effective in the management of obsessive-compulsive disorders.

Bupropion

Bupropion, which is structurally related to amphetamine, is effective in the treatment of major depression, producing improvement in 2 to 4 weeks. In addition, bupropion is effective for smoking cessation. Bupropion is associated with a greater incidence of seizures (about 0.4%) than other antidepressants.

Venlafaxine

Venlafaxine is perceived to have a profile of efficacy similar to that of the tricyclic antidepressants but has a more favorable side effect profile.

Trazodone

Trazodone inhibits serotonin uptake and may also act as a serotonin agonist via an active metabolite. Although effective in the management of depression, its greatest efficacy may be in the treatment of insomnia induced by SSRIs or bupropion.

Nefazodone

Nefazodone is chemically related to trazodone but with fewer $\alpha 1$-adrenergic–blocking properties. Like trazodone, this drug inhibits the reuptake of serotonin and norepinephrine. Nefazodone-induced inhibition of cytochrome

P-450 results in elevated plasma concentrations of benzodiazepines, antihistamines, and/or protease inhibitors used in the treatment of HIV infection.

Tricyclic and Related Antidepressants (See Table 19-2)

Although tricyclic antidepressants are highly effective, they have been supplanted as first-line drugs in many clinical situations because of their unfavorable side effect profile (largely resulting from anticholinergic, antiadrenergic, and antihistaminic properties). Tricyclic antidepressants also have a narrow therapeutic index and are lethal in overdose, resulting in part from the inhibition of sodium ion channels causing a slowing of conduction of cardiac impulses and potentially fatal cardiac dysrhythmias.

Chronic Pain Syndromes

The tricyclic antidepressants (especially amitriptyline and imipramine), in doses lower than those used to treat depression, may be useful in the treatment of chronic neuropathic pain.

Structure–Activity Relationships

The structure of tricyclic antidepressants resembles that of local anesthetics and phenothiazines.

Mechanism of Action

Tricyclic antidepressants act at several transporters and receptors, but their antidepressant effect is likely produced by blocking the reuptake (uptake) of serotonin and/or norepinephrine at presynaptic terminals, thereby increasing the availability of these neurotransmitters. It seems likely that the potentiation of monoaminergic neurotransmission in the brain is only an early event in a complex cascade of events that eventually results in an antidepressant effect.

Pharmacokinetics

Tricyclic antidepressants are efficiently absorbed from the gastrointestinal tract after oral administration, reflecting their high lipid solubility. Peak plasma concentrations occur within 2 to 8 hours after oral administration.

Metabolism

Tricyclic antidepressants are oxidized by microsomal enzymes in the liver, with subsequent conjugation with glucuronic acid.

Side Effects (See Table 19-2)

Anticholinergic Effects

Amitriptyline causes the highest incidence of anticholinergic effects (dry mouth, blurred vision, tachycardia, urinary retention, slowed gastric emptying, ileus), whereas desipramine produces the fewest such effects. Anticholinergic delirium may occur in elderly patients even at therapeutic doses of these drugs.

Cardiovascular Effects

Orthostatic hypotension and modest increases in heart rate are the most common side effects of tricyclic antidepressants, presumably reflecting a drug-induced inhibition of norepinephrine reuptake into presynaptic nerve terminals. Previous suggestions that tricyclic antidepressants increase the risk of cardiac dysrhythmias and sudden death have not been substantiated in the absence of drug overdose. Tricyclic antidepressants produce a depression of conduction of cardiac impulses through the atria and ventricles, manifesting on the electrocardiogram (ECG) as prolongation of the P-R interval, widening of the QRS complex, and flattening or inversion of the T wave. Nevertheless, these changes on the ECG are probably benign and gradually disappear with continued therapy. Direct cardiac depressant effects may reflect the quinidine-like actions of tricyclic antidepressants on the heart.

Central Nervous System Effects

Sedation associated with tricyclic antidepressant therapy may be desirable for the management of agitated patients. Amitriptyline and doxepin produce the greatest degree of sedation (see Table 19-2). Tricyclic antidepressants, especially maprotiline and clomipramine, lower the seizure threshold, thus raising the question of the advisability of administering these drugs to patients with seizure disorders (especially children) or to those receiving drugs that may produce seizures. The combination of a tricyclic antidepressant and an MAO inhibitor may result in CNS toxicity manifesting as hyperthermia, seizures, and coma.

Drug Interactions (Table 19-4)

Tolerance

Tolerance to anticholinergic effects (dry mouth, blurred vision, tachycardia) and orthostatic hypotension develops during chronic therapy with tricyclic antidepressants.

Overdose

Tricyclic antidepressant overdose is life-threatening, because the progression from an alert state to unresponsiveness may

TABLE 19-4.
DRUG INTERACTIONS IN PATIENTS BEING TREATED WITH TRICYCLIC ANTIDEPRESSANTS

Sympathomimetics
- Acute tricyclic antidepressant therapy (exaggerated pressor responses to indirect-acting sympathomimetics such as ephedrine; recommendation is titration of smaller than usual doses of a direct-acting sympathomimetic)
- Chronic (>6 weeks) tricyclic antidepressant therapy (decrease initial dose of direct- or indirect-acting sympathomimetic to about one-third the usual dose)

Anesthetics (induction may be associated with an increased incidence of cardiac dysrhythmias)

Anticholinergics (increased risk of central anticholinergic syndrome; glycopyrrolate may be less likely to evoke this response)

Antihypertensives (rebound hypertension after discontinuation of clonidine)

Opioids (enhanced analgesic and ventilatory depressant effects)

TABLE 19-5.
PHARMACOLOGIC TREATMENT OF TRICYCLIC ANTIDEPRESSANT OVERDOSE

Symptom	Treatment
Seizures	Diazepam Sodium bicarbonate Phenytoin
Ventricular cardiac dysrhythmias	Sodium bicarbonate Lidocaine Phenytoin
Heart block	Isoproterenol
Hypotension	Crystalloid or colloid solutions Sodium bicarbonate Sympathomimetics Inotropics

be rapid. Intractable myocardial depression or ventricular cardiac dysrhythmias are the most frequent terminal events. The comatose phase of tricyclic antidepressant overdose lasts 24 to 72 hours. Treatment of a life-threatening overdose of a tricyclic antidepressant is directed toward the management of CNS and cardiac toxicity (Table 19-5). Gastric lavage may be useful in the early treatment, but this is most safely performed with a cuffed tracheal tube already in place.

Monoamine Oxidase Inhibitors

Monoamine oxidase (MAO) inhibitors constitute a heterogeneous group of drugs that block the enzyme that metabolizes biogenic amines, thus increasing the availability of these neurotransmitters in the CNS and peripheral autonomic nervous system. MAO inhibitors are rarely used because their administration is complicated by side effects (hypotension), lethality in overdose, and lack of simplicity in dosing.

TABLE 19-6.
DIETARY RESTRICTIONS IN PATIENTS TREATED WITH MONOAMINE OXIDASE INHIBITORS

Prohibited foods
- Cheese
- Liver
- Fava beans
- Avocados
- Chianti wine

Prohibited drugs
- Cyclic antidepressants
- Fluoxetine
- Cold or allergy medications
- Nasal decongestants
- Sympathomimetic drugs
- Opioids (especially meperidine)

Patients treated with MAO inhibitors must follow a specific tyramine-free diet because of the potential for pharmacodynamic interactions with tyramine that can result in systemic hypertension (Table 19-6). Patients who do not respond to cyclic antidepressants may improve with MAO inhibitors. MAO inhibitors are also effective in the treatment of panic disorder.

Monoamine Oxidase Enzyme System

MAO is a flavin-containing enzyme found principally on outer mitochondrial membranes. The enzyme functions via oxidative deamination to inactivate several monoamines, including dopamine, serotonin (5-hydroxytryptamine), norepinephrine, and epinephrine. MAO is divided into MAO-A (preferentially deaminates serotonin, norepinephrine, epinephrine) and MAO-B (preferentially deaminates phenylethylamine) subtypes.

Mechanism of Action

MAO inhibitors act by forming a stable, irreversible complex with MAO enzyme; as a result, the amount of neurotransmitter (norepinephrine) available for release from CNS neurons increases. Concentrations of norepinephrine also increase in the sympathetic nervous system. Because MAO inhibitors cause irreversible enzyme inhibition, their effects are prolonged, as the synthesis of new enzyme is a slow process.

Side Effects (Table 19-7)

The effects of MAO inhibitors on the electroencephalogram (EEG) are minimal and not seizure-like, which contrasts with those of tricyclic antidepressants. Also in contrast with tricyclic antidepressants is the failure of MAO inhibitors to produce cardiac dysrhythmias.

Dietary Restrictions

MAO enzymes present in the liver, gastrointestinal tract, kidneys, and lungs seems to perform a protective function in activating circulating monoamines. This produces an initial defense against monoamines absorbed from foods, such as tyramine and β-phenylethanolamine, which would otherwise produce an indirect sympathomimetic response and precipitous hypertension (hyperadrenergic crisis), including hyperpyrexia and cerebral vascular accident. Treatment of hypertension is with a peripheral vasodilator such as nitroprusside.

TABLE 19-7.
SIDE EFFECTS OF MONOAMINE OXIDASE INHIBITORS

Orthostatic hypotension (accumulation of false neurotransmitter, octopamine)
Anticholinergic effects
Sedation
Impotency
Anorgasmy
Weight gain
Hepatitis (rare)

Drug Interactions

In addition to interacting with foods (see Table 19-6), MAO inhibitors can interact adversely with opioids, sympathomimetic drugs, tricyclic antidepressants, and SSRIs.

Opioids and Monoamine Oxidase Inhibitors

The administration of meperidine to a patient treated with MAO inhibitors may result in an excitatory (type I) response (agitation, headache, skeletal muscle rigidity, hyperpyrexia) or a depressive (type II) response characterized by hypotension, depression of ventilation, and coma. Enhanced serotonin activity in the brain is presumed to be responsible for the excitatory reactions evoked by meperidine.

A decelerated breakdown of meperidine due to N-demethylase inhibition by MAO inhibitors is the presumed explanation for hypotension and depression of ventilation. Derivatives of meperidine (fentanyl, sufentanil, alfentanil) have been associated with adverse reactions in patients treated with MAO inhibitors.

Morphine does not inhibit the uptake of serotonin, but its opioid effects may be potentiated in the presence of MAO inhibitors

Sympathomimetics and Monoamine Oxidase Inhibitors

The most consistent observations have been in occasional patients who experienced an exaggerated systemic blood pressure response after the administration of an indirect-acting vasopressor, such as ephedrine. The hypertensive response is presumed to reflect an exaggerated release of norepinephrine from neuronal nerve endings. If needed, the use of a direct-acting sympathomimetic (phenylephrine) is preferable to an indirect-acting drug, keeping in mind that receptor hypersensitivity may enhance the systemic blood pressure response to these drugs as well. Regardless of the drug selected, the recommendation is to decrease the dose to about one-third of normal, with additional titration of doses based on cardiovascular responses.

Overdose

Overdose with an MAO inhibitor is reflected by signs of excessive sympathetic nervous system activity (tachycardia, hyperthermia, mydriasis), seizures, and coma. Treatment is supportive, with gastric lavage.

Management of Anesthesia

There is growing appreciation that anesthesia can be safely administered in most patients being chronically treated with MAO inhibitors. The anesthetic technique should minimize the possibility of sympathetic nervous system stimulation or drug-induced hypotension. Regional anesthesia (may avoid epinephrine added to the local anesthetic solution), as used in parturients is acceptable, recognizing the disadvantage of these techniques should hypotension require the administration of a sympathomimetic. An advantage of regional anesthesia is postoperative analgesia such that the need for opioids is negated or minimized.

ANXIOLYTICS

Benzodiazepines

Benzodiazepines have less of a tendency to produce tolerance, less potential for abuse, and a large margin of safety if taken in an overdose.

Buspirone

Buspirone is a nonbenzodiazepine that is effective in the treatment of generalized anxiety disorders (onset of anxiolytic effect over several days) but not panic disorder. This drug is a partial agonist at serotonin receptors, resulting in decreased serotonin turnover and anxiolytic effects.

LITHIUM

Lithium is considered the drug of choice for the treatment of bipolar disorders. Full therapeutic effects of lithium take several weeks. The goal for treatment of acute mania is to maintain plasma lithium concentrations between 1.0

and 1.2 mEq/liter. Plasma lithium concentrations should be measured 10 to 12 hours after the last oral dose, and levels should not be drawn sooner than 4 to 5 days after the latest change in dose.

Pharmacokinetics

Lithium is distributed throughout the total body water and is excreted almost entirely by the kidneys. Lithium, like sodium, if filtered by the glomerulus and reabsorbed by the proximal, but not distal, renal tubules. Thus, its renal excretion is not enhanced by thiazide diuretics, which act selectively on the distal renal tubules. In fact, because proximal reabsorption of lithium and sodium is competitive, depletion of sodium as produced by dehydration, decreased sodium intake, and thiazide and loop diuretics may increase reabsorption of lithium by proximal renal tubules, resulting in as much as a 50% increase in the plasma concentration of lithium.

Side Effects (Table 19-8)

Drug Interactions (Table 19-9)

Toxicity

Many symptoms and signs of toxicity are closely correlated with the plasma lithium concentration (Table 19-10).

TABLE 19-8.
SIDE EFFECTS OF LITHIUM

Polydipsia and polyuria (reflects inhibitory effect of lithium on adenosine monophosphate formation in the renal tubules)
T-wave flattening on ECG (benign)
Hypothyroidism (5% of treated patients, more common in women than men)
Dermatological toxicities (acne, exacerbation of psoriasis)
Sedation (possible impact on anesthetic requirements)
Possible prolongation of effects of neuromuscular blocking drugs

TABLE 19-9.
DRUG INTERACTIONS WITH LITHIUM

Drug	Interaction
Thiazide diuretics	Increased plasma lithium concentration due to decreased renal clearance
Furosemide	Usually no change in the plasma lithium concentration
Nonsteroidal antiinflammatory drugs	Increased plasma lithium concentration due to decreased renal clearance (exceptions are aspirin and sulindac)
Aminophylline	Decreased plasma lithium concentration due to increased renal clearance
Angiotensin-converting enzyme inhibitors	May increase plasma lithium concentration
Neuroleptic drugs	Lithium may exacerbate extrapyramidal symptoms or increase the risk of the neuroleptic malignant syndrome
Anticonvulsant drugs (carbamazepine)	Concurrent use with lithium may result in additive neurotoxicity
β-Adrenergic antagonists	Decrease lithium-induced tremor
Neuromuscular blocking drugs	Lithium may prolong the duration of action

Treatment-Resistant Bipolar Disorder

An estimated 30% of patients with bipolar disorder cannot tolerate or do not respond to lithium. In these individuals, the anticonvulsants carbamazepine and valproic acid may be efficacious.

TABLE 19-10.
SIGNS AND SYMPTOMS OF LITHIUM TOXICITY

Toxic Effects	Plasma Lithium Concentration (mEq/liter)	Signs and Symptoms
Mild	1.0–1.5	Lethargy Irritability Skeletal muscle weakness Tremor Slurred speech Nausea
Moderate	1.6–2.5	Confusion Drowsiness Restlessness Unsteady gait Coarse tremor Dysarthria Skeletal muscle fasciculations Vomiting
Severe	>2.5	Impaired consciousness (coma) Delirium Ataxia Extrapyramidal symptoms Seizures Impaired renal function

ANTIPSYCHOTIC (NEUROLEPTIC) DRUGS

Antipsychotic (neuroleptic) drugs are a chemically diverse group of compounds (phenothiazines, thioxanthenes, butyrophenones) that are useful in the treatment of schizophrenia, mania, depression with psychotic features, and certain organic psychoses (Table 19-11).

TABLE 19-11.
COMPARATIVE PHARMACOLOGY OF ANTIPSYCHOTIC (NEUROLEPTIC) DRUGS

Category and Drug	Sedative Potency	Anticholinergic Potency	Orthostatic Hypotension Potency	Extrapyramidal Potency
Phenothiazines				
Chlorpromazine	+++	++	+++	+
Triflupromazine	+++	++	+++	++
Thioridazine	+++	+++	+++	+
Fluphenazine	++	+	+	+++
Perphenazine	+	+	+	+++
Trifluoperazine	++	+	+	+++
Thioxanthenes				
Chlorprothixene	+++	+++	+++	+
Thiothixene	+	+	+	+++
Dibenzodiazepines				
Clozapine	+++	+++	+++	0
Loxapine	++	++	++	+++
Butyrophenones				
Haloperidol	+	+	+	+++
Droperidol	+	+	+	+++
Diphenylbutylpiperidines				
Primozide	+	+	+	+++
Benzisoxazole				
Risperidone	+	+	++	+

0, none; +, mild; ++, moderate; +++, marked.

Structure–Activity Relationships

Phenothiazines have a three-ring structure in which two benzene rings are linked by a sulfur and a nitrogen atom. If the nitrogen atom at position 10 is replaced by a carbon atom with double bond to the side chain, the compound becomes a thioxanthene.

Mechanism of Action

The mechanism of action of antipsychotic drugs is thought to be due to the blockade of dopamine receptors (especially dopamine-2 receptors) in the basal ganglia and limbic portions of the forebrain. Blockade of dopamine receptors in the chemoreceptor trigger zone of the medulla is responsible for the antiemetic effect of these drugs.

Pharmacokinetics

Phenothiazines and thioxanthenes often display erratic and unpredictable patterns of absorption after oral administration. These drugs are highly lipid soluble and accumulate in well-perfused tissues such as the brain.

Metabolism

The metabolism of phenothiazines and thioxanthenes is principally by oxidation in the liver, followed by conjugation. Most oxidative metabolites are pharmacologically inactive, with a notable exception being 7-hydroxychlorpromazine.

Side Effects

With the exception of clozapine, the chronic use of phenothiazines and thioxanthenes may be complicated by serious side effects, most likely reflecting the drug-induced blockade of dopamine receptors, especially in the forebrain.

Extrapyramidal Effects

Tardive dyskinesia may occur in 20% of patients who receive antipsychotic drugs for >1 year. Manifestations of tardive dyskinesia include abnormal involuntary movements that may affect the tongue, facial and neck muscles, upper and lower extremities, truncal musculature, and occasionally, skeletal muscle groups involved in breathing and swallowing. Tardive dyskinesia only rarely remits, and no treatment exists. Acute dystonic reactions occur in approximately 2% of treated patients and are most likely to occur within the first 72 hours of therapy. Opisthotonos and oculogyric crises may occur. The sudden onset of respiratory distress in an patient on neuroleptics may reflect laryngeal dyskinesia (laryngospasm). Acute dystonia responds dramatically to diphenhydramine, 25 to 50 mg IV.

Cardiovascular Effects

The intravenous administration of chlorpromazine causes a decrease in systemic blood pressure (through peripheral α-adrenergic blockade, direct vasodilation, and direct cardiac depression).

Neuroleptic Malignant Syndrome

Neuroleptic malignant syndrome occurs in 0.5% to 1.0 of all patients treated with antipsychotic drugs and is more likely in the presence of dehydration and intercurrent illness (Table 19-12). Mortality is 20% to 30%, with common causes of death being ventilatory failure, cardiac failure and/or dysrhythmias, renal failure, and thromboembolism. The cause of neuroleptic malignant syndrome is not known and, as a result, treatment is empirical and includes supportive measures and the administration of the direct-acting muscle relaxant dantrolene and the dopamine agonists bromocriptine or amantadine. Malignant hyperthermia, as well as central anticholinergic syndrome, may mimic the neuroleptic malignant syndrome.

A distinguishing feature is the ability of nondepolarizing muscle relaxants to produce flaccid paralysis in

TABLE 19-12.
MANIFESTATIONS OF NEUROLEPTIC MALIGNANT SYNDROME

Hyperthermia
Hypertonicity of skeletal muscles (may require mechanical ventilation of the lungs, may result in myonecrosis and renal failure)
Autonomic nervous system instability
- Alterations in systemic blood pressure
- Tachycardia
- Cardiac dysrhythmias

Fluctuating levels of consciousness

---

patients experiencing the neuroleptic malignant syndrome but not in those experiencing malignant hyperthermia.

Endocrine Effects

Prolactin levels are increased as a result of the blockade of dopamine receptors and loss of the normal inhibition of prolactin secretion. Galactorrhea and gynecomastia may accompany excess prolactin secretion.

Sedation

The sedation produced by antipsychotic drugs appears to be due to α1-adrenergic, muscarinic, and histamine (H1) receptors.

Antiemetic Effects

The antiemetic effects of the antipsychotic drugs reflect their interaction with dopaminergic receptors in the chemoreceptor trigger zone of the medulla. These drugs seem most effective in preventing opioid-induced nausea and vomiting (perphenazine, 5 mg IV, is as effective as intravenous ondansetron, 4 mg IV, and droperidol, 1.25 mg IV). Unlike other antiemetics, perphenazine was not associated with sedation or hypotension.

Obstructive Jaundice

Obstructive jaundice, which is considered to be an allergic reaction, occurs rarely 2 to 4 weeks after the administration of phenothiazines or thioxanthenes.

Hypothermia

An effect of chlorpromazine on the hypothalamus is most likely responsible for the poikilothermic effect of this drug.

Seizure Threshold

Many antipsychotic drugs decrease the seizure threshold and produce a pattern on the EEG similar to that associated with seizure disorders.

Skeletal Muscle Relaxation

Skeletal muscle relaxation is presumed to reflect the actions of antipsychotic drugs on the CNS.

Drug Interactions

The ventilatory depressant, miotic, sedative, and analgesic effects of opioids are likely to be exaggerated by antipsychotic drugs.

Clozapine

Clozapine is the only antipsychotic that does not seem to cause tardive dyskinesia or extrapyramidal side effects. Orthostatic hypotension and sedation are prominent and paradoxical salivation (despite the fact that this is a strongly anticholinergic drug) may occur. Clozapine has been combined safely with lithium and antidepressant drugs, but a risk of excessive sedation may occur if this drug is combined with a benzodiazepine.

Butyrophenones

Butyrophenones, such as droperidol and haloperidol, structurally resemble and evoke pharmacologic effects similar to those of phenothiazines and thioxanthenes. The principal use of haloperidol is as a long-acting antipsychotic drug; it lacks significant α-adrenergic antagonist effects, so decreases in systemic blood pressure are unlikely.

Pharmacokinetics

The total body clearance of droperidol is similar to hepatic blood flow (perfusion dependent), emphasizing the importance of hepatic metabolism rather than hepatic enzyme activity (capacity dependent) in the elimination of this drug.

Side Effects

Central Nervous System

The outwardly calming effect of droperidol may mask an overwhelming fear of surgery (dysphoria). Akathisia (restlessness in the legs) may accompany the administration of droperidol. As a dopamine antagonist, droperidol evokes extrapyramidal reactions in about 1% of patients (do not administer to patients being treated for Parkinson's disease).

Acute dystonia (laryngospasm) is a rate complication. Diphenhydramine administered intravenously is an effective treatment for droperidol-induced extrapyramidal reactions.

Cardiovascular Effects

Droperidol can decrease systemic blood pressure as a result of action in the CNS and by peripheral α-adrenergic blockade. Hypertension may occur after the administration of droperidol to patients with pheochromocytoma. Droperidol is a cardiac antidysrhythmic and protects against epinephrine-induced dysrhythmias.

Prolonged QTc Interval

Droperidol, like many drugs administered during anesthesia (thiopental, propofol, isoflurane, sevoflurane, succinylcholine, neostigmine, atropine, glycopyrrolate, metoclopramide, SSRIs, 5HT3 receptor antagonists) produces dose-dependent prolongation of the QTc interval on the ECG in some patients. Many confounding factors make it difficult to establish a cause and effect relationship between droperidol administration and adverse cardiac events (torsade de pointes). Of note, since droperidol was approved in 1970, not a a single case report has surfaced in which droperidol in doses used for the management of postoperative nausea and vomiting has been associated with QTc prolongation, cardiac dysrhythmias, or cardiac arrest. A "black box" warning accompanies the package insert for droperidol.

Ventilation

Resting ventilation and the ventilatory response to carbon dioxide are not altered by droperidol.

Clinical Uses

Neuroleptanalgesia

Neuroleptanalgesia (using droperidol combined with fentanyl in a 50:1 ratio) is characterized by trance-like (cataleptic) immobility in an outwardly tranquil patient who is dissociated and indifferent to the external surroundings. Analgesia is intense.

Antiemetic

Droperidol (0.625 to 1.25 mg IV) is a powerful antiemetic, as a result of the inhibition of dopamine-2 receptors in the chemoreceptor trigger zone of the medulla. Despite the black box warning in the package insert (related to a potential for droperidol to prolong the QTc interval) droperidol is widely accepted as a safe, cost-effective first-line therapy for the management of postoperative nausea and vomiting.

Prostaglandins

20

Prostaglandins are among the most prevalent of the naturally occurring, physiologically active endogenous substances (autocoids) (Stoelting RK, Hillier SC. Prostaglandins. In: *Pharmacology and Physiology in Anesthetic Practice,* 4th ed. Philadelphia: Lippincott Williams & Wilkins, 2006: 420–428). They have been detected in almost every tissue and body fluid. Indeed, the cellular mechanisms responsible for the formation of prostaglandins are present in all organs of the body. No other autocoids (histamine, serotonin, angiotensin II, plasma kinins) show more numerous and diverse effects than do the prostaglandins.

NOMENCLATURE AND STRUCTURE–ACTIVITY RELATIONSHIPS

The generic term *eicosanoids* refers to the 20-carbon, hairpin-shaped fatty acid chain that includes a cyclopentane ring, characteristic of prostaglandins (Fig. 20-1). The letters PG denote the word prostaglandin. A subscript that follows the third letter denotes the number of double bonds in the structure as well as the fatty acid precursor of the prostaglandin (subscript 2 indicates two double bonds and arachidonic acid as the fatty acid precursor). Prostaglandins with two double bonds are referred to as *dienoic prostaglandins.* An α or β after the subscript indicates the orientation of the hydroxyl group at the number 9 carbon atom to the plane of the cyclopentane ring.

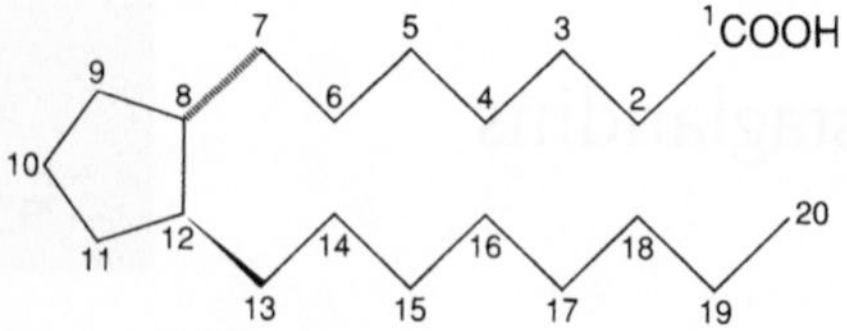

Figure 20-1. A 20-carbon hairpin-shaped fatty acid chain is characteristic of prostaglandins.

SYNTHESIS

The principal precursor of dienoic prostaglandins in mammalian cells is the polyunsaturated 20-carbon essential fatty acid, arachidonic acid; it is an ubiquitous component of cell membranes and is released by the action of phospholipase C and phospholipase A2. Once cleaved from the cell membranes, arachidonic acid becomes available to serve as a substrate for the production of prostaglandins via either the cyclooxygenase (COX) or the lipoxygenase pathway (Fig. 20-2).

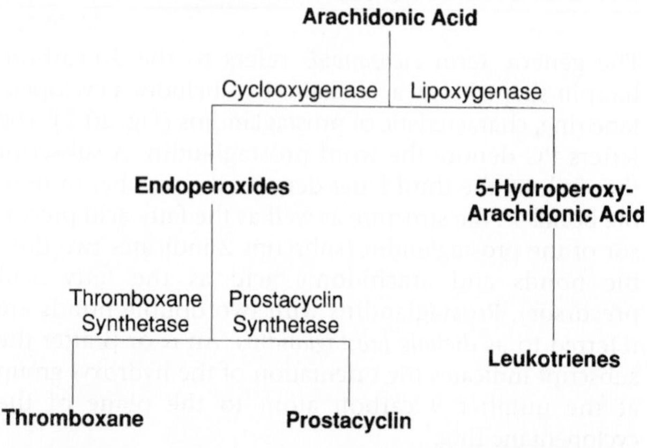

Figure 20-2. Synthesis of prostaglandins from arachidonic acid occurs via a cyclooxygenase pathway and a lipoxygenase pathway.

Cyclooxygenase

COX is a widely distributed complex of microsomal enzymes necessary for the initial synthesis (oxidation) of prostaglandins (PGE2 and PGH2), known as *endoperoxides* (see Fig. 20-2). Two distinct isoforms of COX exist—COX-1 and COX-2—that are encoded by two different genes and differentially expressed in a variety of tissues. In particular, COX-1 is expressed in platelets and gastric mucosa. COX-2 is expressed in inflamed tissues (in response to mitogenic stimuli and inflammatory cytokines, such as interleukin-1 and tumor necrosis factor) and the brain and spinal cord.

Lipoxygenase Enzymes

Lipoxygenase enzymes are localized principally in platelets, vascular endothelium, the lungs, and leukocytes (see Fig. 20-2). Compounds formed by the enzyme-induced lipoxygenation of arachidonic acid are termed *leukotrienes*.

Leukotriene D (formerly designated as slow-reacting substance of anaphylaxis) has preferential effects on peripheral airways and is a more potent bronchoconstrictor than histamine.

MECHANISM OF ACTION

In many tissues, prostaglandins act on specific cell membrane receptors to activate adenylate cyclase, with a resulting increase in intracellular concentrations of cyclic 3′5′-adenosine monophosphate (cAMP). cAMP activates protein kinase A to express its effects, including a decreased free intracellular calcium in vascular smooth muscle that results in vascular relaxation. Prostaglandins are produced during inflammation by the action of COX, which increases the sensitivity of nociceptors and nociceptive neurons to other pain-producing stimuli such as histamine, bradykinin, and thermal changes.

METABOLISM

The metabolism of prostaglandins to inactive substances is rapid and catalyzed by specific enzymes that are widely distributed in the body in such organs as the lungs (act as filters to protect the cardiovascular system and other organs from prolonged effects due to recirculation of these substances), kidneys, and liver and in the gastrointestinal tract. *Thromboxane* is hydrolyzed rapidly (elimination half-time 30 seconds) to an inactive product, thus largely limiting its actions to the microenvironment of its release. *Prostacyclin,* with an elimination half-time of about 3 minutes, is nonenzymatically converted to 6-keto-PGF1α; the measurement of this metabolite serves as an indicator of prostacyclin release or lack of release, as occurs in the presence of known inhibitors (aspirin, ibuprofen) or H1 receptor antagonists (diphenhydramine).

PROSTACYCLIN

Prostacyclin (PGI2, epoprostenol) is a vasodilator and the most potent known inhibitor of platelet aggregation. The endothelial release of nitric oxide is stimulated by prostacyclin. Intravenous administration of prostacyclin has the significant disadvantage of not being a selective pulmonary vasodilator, thus producing parallel decreases in pulmonary and systemic vascular resistance and increasing intrapulmonary shunting.

ILOPROST

Iloprost is a stable and long-acting (elimination half-time 20 to 30 minutes) derivative of prostacyclin that is a potent inhibitor of platelet aggregation (immediate effect). Iloprost causes vasodilation, but it is associated with less hypotension than prostacyclin.

EFFECTS ON ORGAN SYSTEMS (TABLE 20-1)

Hematologic System

Thromboxane, the principal COX product of arachidonic acid in platelets, acts as an intense stimulus for platelet aggregation, presumably reflecting the inhibition of adenylate cyclase and subsequent decreased cAMP synthesis in platelets. Conversely, prostacyclin is the most potent endogenous inhibitor of platelet aggregation. A normal thromboxane-to-prostacyclin ratio is important in maintaining platelet activity and coagulation. An increase in this ratio, as may occur when atherosclerotic plaques release substances that inhibit the synthesis of prostacyclin, results in a predominance of thromboxane activity, manifesting as platelet aggregation and vasoconstriction.

A similar imbalance in the thromboxane-to-prostacyclin ratio in the venous circulation could lead to venous thromboembolism. Bleeding disorders are likely in the presence of thromboxane depletion or excess prostacyclin. Thromboxane production in platelets is inhibited by small doses of aspirin, whereas large doses of aspirin inhibit both thromboxane and prostacyclin production. If a patient is being treated with low doses of aspirin, thromboxane is no longer present to opposed prostacyclin, and platelet aggregation does not occur.

Cardiovascular System

Prostaglandins play an important role in cardiovascular homeostasis by promoting vasodilation and enhancing sodium excretion. The intravenous administration of prostacyclin causes a decrease in systemic blood pressure that results from a decrease in systemic vascular resistance and reflects vasodilation in several vascular beds, including coronary, renal, mesenteric, and skeletal muscle circulation. The activity of vascular smooth muscle in

TABLE 20-1.
COMPARATIVE EFFECTS OF PROSTAGLANDINS

	Platelet Aggregation	Systemic Vascular Resistance	Airway Resistance	Uterine Muscle Tone	Gastric Acid Secretion
Thromboxane (TXAX2)	I	I	I		
Prostacyclin (PGI2)	D	D	?I		
Iloprost	D	D	D		
Alprostadil (PGE1)	D	D	I	I	
Misoprostol		NC		I	D
Carboprost				I	
Dinoprost (PGF2α)		I,D	I	I	
Dinoprostone (PGE2)		I			

I, increased; D, decreased; NC, no change.

various vascular beds may be modulated by the relative magnitude of vasoconstriction and vasodilation produced by thromboxane and prostacyclin, respectively. For example, events leading to coronary artery spasm and thrombosis may arise from a deficiency of prostacyclin-induced vasodilation relative to thromboxane-induced vasoconstriction.

Alprostadil

Alprostadil (PGE1, Prostin VR Pediatric) has a variety of pharmacologic effects, the most important of which are vasodilation, inhibition of platelet aggregation, and stimulation of gastrointestinal and uterine smooth muscle.

Clinical Uses

The clinical uses of alprostadil include maintenance of patent ductus arteriosus in infants with congenital heart disease (pulmonary atresia, tetralogy of Fallot) and the treatment of pulmonary hypertension (mitral valve disease, acute respiratory distress syndrome, following heart transplantation).

Metabolism

Alprostadil is metabolized so rapidly that it must be administered as a continuous infusion. Nearly 70% of circulating alprostadil is metabolized in one passage through the lungs, and the metabolites are excreted by the kidneys.

Pulmonary Circulation

Pulmonary vasoconstriction may be related to increased circulating concentrations of thromboxane, PGE2, and PGE2α. The pulmonary vasoconstriction, pulmonary hypertension, and bronchoconstriction that, on rare occasions, are associated with the administration of protamine may reflect protamine-induced production of the prostaglandin vasoconstrictor thromboxane. Prostacyclin is an ubiquitous and potent vasodilator.

Prostacyclin

Prostacyclin has a brief half-time (about 3 minutes), thus necessitating its administration by the intravenous route. Intravenous prostacyclin has an established role in the long-term management of primary pulmonary hypertension. Inhaled (aerosolized) prostacyclin has been shown to produce greater decreases in pulmonary vascular resistance than nitric oxide. Inhaled prostacyclin, in common with nitric oxide, has no effect on pulmonary vascular resistance in patients with normal pulmonary vasculature. Inhaled prostacyclin has some potential advantages over inhaled nitric oxide. For example, the lack of toxicity of prostacyclin (unlike nitric oxide, methemoglobin formation is not a risk of prostacyclin therapy) or its metabolites suggests that accurate measurement of the concentrations of delivered drug and its metabolites in inspiratory and expiratory gases is not necessary, unlike inhaled nitric oxide. Furthermore, in contrast to inhaled nitric oxide, the apparatus for delivery of prostacyclin is inexpensive and readily available. Inhaled prostacyclin is useful for the treatment of patients with pulmonary hypertension and acute right ventricular failure after cardiac surgery.

Side Effects

Prostacyclin is a potent vasodilator, and side effects to inhaled prostacyclin include anxiety, flushing, dizziness, nausea, and vomiting. As with nitric oxide, the abrupt withdrawal of intravenous infusions of prostacyclin may result in severe rebound pulmonary hypertension and cardiogenic shock.

Iloprost

Iloprost, when inhaled, has comparable pulmonary hemodynamic effects to inhaled nitric oxide and prostacyclin. Compared with prostacyclin, iloprost is soluble in saline, thus obviating the need for an alkaline buffer; is less viscous, which aids in nebulization; and significantly longer-acting, thus permitting intermittent rather than continuous nebulization. Inhaled iloprost appears to have comparable hemodynamic effects to inhaled nitric oxide.

Uniprost

Uniprost is an analog of prostacyclin that is administered subcutaneously through a portable pump, similar to that used for the infusion of insulin.

Beraprost

Beraprost is a chemically stable analog of prostacyclin that is effective when administered orally.

Lungs

The lungs are a major site of prostaglandin synthesis. Prostaglandins may produce bronchoconstriction or bronchodilation. Indeed, an imbalance between the production of thromboxane and prostacyclin in the lungs might contribute to symptoms of bronchial asthma. Leukotrienes are several thousand times more potent as constrictors of bronchial smooth muscle than is histamine. A predominant role of leukotrienes in asthma-induced bronchoconstriction in individual patients is suggested by the ineffectiveness of antihistamines. Aspirin-induced asthma may reflect an inhibition of the COX pathway by the drug, leading to increased availability of arachidonic acid to the lipoxygenase pathway to form leukotrienes (see Fig. 20-2).

Kidneys

The intrarenal release of prostaglandins may be an important mechanism for modulating renal blood flow and glomerular filtration rate. Inhibition of the COX system with nonsteroidal anti-inflammatory drugs (NSAIDs) and aspirin does not have clinically significant effects on renal hemodynamics in patients with normal kidneys. Conversely, when renal vasoconstrictor systems have been activated, inhibition of the production of vasodilator prostaglandins (prostacyclin) by NSAIDs may interfere with normal renal prostaglandin protective mechanisms and accentuate catecholamine-induced renal vasoconstriction.

Misoprostol

Misoprostol is a PGE1 analogue with oral bioavailability that improves renal function and decreases the incidence of acute rejection in renal transplant patients treated concurrently with cyclosporine and prednisone. Misoprostol inhibits the secretion of gastric acid by a direct action on parietal cells and maintains or increases mucosal blood flow in response to gastric irritants; it may increase secretion of mucus and bicarbonate by the gastric and duodenal mucosa. For these reasons, misoprostol is recommended for the prevention of NSAID-induced gastric ulcers in patients at high risk. An important side effect of misoprostol is increased uterine contraction, which can provoke abortion.

Gastrointestinal Tract

Certain prostaglandins inhibit gastric acid secretion. Nevertheless, prostaglandin therapy is not considered a preferred alternative to H2 receptor antagonists in the management of patients with peptic ulcer disease.

Uterus

The nongravid and gravid uterus is predictably contracted by PGE2 and PGF2α. In contrast to oxytocin, this effect of prostaglandins is observed at all stages of pregnancy, accounting for the usefulness of certain prostaglandins for inducing labor as well as abortion. The increased synthesis of prostaglandins in the endometrium is speculated to be a cause of dysmenorrhea. Indeed, inhibitors of prostaglandin synthesis, such as aspirin or indomethacin, decrease the pain associated with dysmenorrhea.

Carboprost

Carboprost is a synthetic analog of naturally occurring PGF2α. Drug-induced uterine contractions are similar to those that accompany labor. Carboprost is successful in inducing uterine contractions in >90% of patients between 12 and 20 weeks of gestation. Mean time to abortion is 16 hours after an intramuscular injection of carboprost. Vomiting and diarrhea occur in >60% of patients. Body temperature increases of 1 °C to 2 °C occur in nearly 10% of patients and must be differentiated from fever due to endometriosis.

Dinoprost

Dinoprost is PGF2α that is administered intra-amniotically to induce uterine contractions. The mean time to abortion is about 20 hours. Generalized tonic-clonic (grand mal) seizures are possible in patients prone to epilepsy.

Dinoprostone

Dinoprostone is PGE2 and produces physiologic-like uterine contractions by activating adenylate cyclase and thus increasing intracellular concentrations of calcium ions. A vaginal suppository is used to induce elective abortion.

Immune System

Prostaglandins, such as prostacyclin, contribute to the signs and symptoms of inflammation, accentuating the pain and edema produced by bradykinin.

LEUKOTRIENE ANTAGONISTS

The inhibitors of the leukotriene pathway are useful drugs in the management of patients with bronchial asthma.

Zileuton

Zileuton is a 5-lipoxygenase inhibitor that impairs the conversion of arachidonic acid to leukotriene A4, thus inhibiting the generation of leukotrienes involved in asthma and inflammation. This drug is not recommended for administration to patients with hepatic dysfunction.

Montelukast and Zafirlukast

Montelukast and zafirlukast are cysteinyl-leukotriene-1 antagonists that competitively block the ability of leukotrienes to bind to the cysteinyl-1-leukotriene receptors. Bronchospasm, vasoconstriction, and eosinophil recruitment are in part mediated by leukotriene binding to these receptors. Side effects may include an elevation of the plasma concentrations of liver transaminase enzymes.

21

Histamine and Histamine Receptor Antagonists

HISTAMINE

Histamine is a low-molecular weight, naturally occurring hydrophilic endogenous amine (autocoid) that produces a variety of physiologic and pathologic responses in different tissues and cells through G protein–coupled membrane receptors (Stoelting RK, Hillier SC. Histamine and histamine receptor antagonists. In: *Pharmacology and Physiology in Anesthetic Practice,* 4th ed. Philadelphia: Lippincott Williams & Wilkins, 2006:429–443). Histamine is also an important chemical mediator of inflammation in allergic disease. *Mast cells* located in the skin, lungs, and gastrointestinal tract, as well as circulating *basophils* contain large amounts of histamine. Histamine does not easily cross the blood-brain barrier, and central nervous system (CNS) effects are usually not evident.

Synthesis

The synthesis of histamine in tissues is through the decarboxylation of histidine. Histamine is stored in vesicles in a complex with heparin. Stored histamine is subsequently released in response to antigen–antibody reactions or in response to certain drugs.

Metabolism

Two pathways of histamine metabolism exist in humans. The most important pathway involves metabolism catalyzed by histamine-*N*-methyltransferase, which is further degraded by monoamine oxidase. In the other pathway, histamine undergoes oxidative deamination catalyzed by diamine oxidase (histaminase), which is a nonspecific enzyme widely distributed in body tissues. The resulting metabolites are pharmacologically inactive.

Receptors

The effects of histamine are mediated via histamine receptors (H_1, H_2, H_3) (Table 21-1). All three receptor subtypes are found in varying degrees in the heart. Histamine-induced effects mediated by the activation of H_1 receptors are suppressed by specific H_1 receptor antagonists (Table 21-2).

Effects on Organ Systems

Histamine exerts profound effects on the cardiovascular system, airways, and gastric hydrogen ion secretion. Histamine in large doses stimulates ganglion cells and chromaffin cells in the adrenal medulla, evoking the release of catecholamines.

Cardiovascular System

The predominant cardiovascular effects of histamine are due to the dilation of arterioles and capillaries (flushing, decreased peripheral vascular resistance, decreases in systemic blood pressure, decreased capillary permeability). Vascular dilatation results from a direct effect of histamine on the blood vessels, mediated by H_1 and H_2 receptors, independent of autonomic nervous system innervation.

Flushing, although generalized, is most obvious in the skin of the face and upper part of the body (blush area). Increased capillary permeability is due to a histamine-induced contraction of capillary endothelial cells. In

TABLE 21-1.
EFFECTS MEDIATED BY ACTIVATION OF HISTAMINE RECEPTORS

	Receptor Subtype Activated
Increased intracellular cyclic guanosine monophosphate	H_1
Mediate release of prostacyclin	H_1
Slowed conduction of cardiac impulses through the atrioventricular node	H_1
Coronary artery vasoconstriction	H_1
Bronchoconstriction	H_1
Increased intracellular cyclic adenosine monophosphate	H_2
Central nervous system stimulation	H_2
Cardiac dysrhythmias	H_2
Increased myocardial contractility	H_2
Increased heart rate	H_2
Coronary artery vasodilation	H_2
Bronchodilation	H_2
Increased secretion of hydrogen ions by gastric parietal cells	H_2
Increased capillary permeability	H_1, H_2
Peripheral vascular vasodilation	H_1, H_2
Inhibit synthesis and release of histamine	H_3

addition to peripheral vasodilation, histamine can produce inotropic (H_2), chronotropic (H_2), and antidromic effects (slowed conduction of cardiac impulses through the atrioventricular node is due to histamine activation of H_1 receptors). Coronary artery vasoconstriction is mediated by H_1 receptors, whereas coronary artery vasodilation is mediated by H_2 receptors.

Airways

Histamine activates H_1 receptors to constrict bronchial smooth muscles, whereas the stimulation of H_2 receptors

TABLE 21-2.
CLASSIFICATION OF HISTAMINE RECEPTOR ANTAGONISTS

	Sedative Effects	Anticholinergic Activity	Antiemetic Effects	Duration of Action (hrs)	Adult Dose (mg)
H_1 antagonists (first generation)					
Diphenhydramine	Marked	Marked	Moderate	3–6	50
Pyrilamine	Mild	None	None	3–6	25–50
Chlorpheniramine	Mild	Mild	None	4–12	2–4
Promethazine	Moderate	Marked	Marked	4–24	25–50
Hydroxyzine	—	—	—	—	—
H_1 antagonists (second generation)					
Fexofenadine	Absent	None	None	12	20–40
Loratadine	Absent	None	None	24	10
Levocabastine	Absent	None	None	—	—
H_2 antagonists					
Cimetidine	Mild*	None	None	5–7	300
Ranitidine	None	None	None	8–12	150
Famotidine	None	None	None	12	20–40
Nizatidine	None	None	None	8–12	150

*Manifests as confusion and agitation.

relaxes bronchial smooth muscles. Patients with obstructive airway disease, such as asthma or bronchitis, are more likely to develop increasers in airway resistance in response to histamine.

Gastric Hydrogen Ion Secretion

Histamine evokes a copious secretion of gastric fluid containing high concentrations of hydrogen ions. Histamine activates a membrane enzyme pump (hydrogen-potassium-ATPase) that extrudes protons.

Allergic Reactions

During allergic reactions, histamine is only one of several chemical mediators released, and its relative importance in producing symptoms is greatly dependent on the species studied. In humans, histamine receptor antagonists (antihistamines) are effective in preventing edema formation and pruritus. Hypotension is attenuated, but not totally blocked, whereas bronchoconstriction often is not prevented, thus emphasizing the predominant role of leukotrienes in this response in humans.

Clinical Uses

Histamine has been used to assess the ability of gastric parietal cells to secrete hydrogen ions and to determine parietal cell mass. Anacidity or the hyposecretion of hydrogen ions in response to histamine may reflect pernicious anemia, atrophic gastritis, or gastric carcinoma. The fact that intradermal histamine causes a flare that is mediated by axon reflexes allows a test for the integrity of sensory nerves that may be of value in the diagnosis of certain neurologic conditions.

HISTAMINE RECEPTOR ANTAGONISTS

H_1 and H_2 receptor antagonists are presumed to act by occupying receptors on effector cell membranes, to the exclusion of agonist molecules, without themselves initiating a response. It is important to recognize that H_1 and H_2 receptor antagonists do not inhibit the release of histamine but rather attach to receptors and prevent responses mediated by histamine.

H_1 RECEPTOR ANTAGONISTS (TABLE 21-2)

Pharmacokinetics (Table 21-3)

Side Effects

First-generation H_1 antagonists often have adverse effects on the CNS, including somnolence (present in nonprescription sleeping aids) and impairment of cognitive function. Second-generation H_1 antagonists are unlikely to produce CNS side effects such as somnolence, unless the recommended doses are exceeded. Enhancement of the effects of diazepam or alcohol are unlikely by second-generation drugs. Fexofenadine, a metabolite of terfenadine, does not prolong the QTc. Antihistamine intoxication is similar to anticholinergic poisoning and also may be associated with seizures and cardiac conduction abnormalities resembling tricyclic antidepressant overdose. Older nonsedating antihistamine drugs (terfenadine, astemizole) were associated with prolongation of the QTc interval and atypical (torsade de pointes) ventricular tachycardia.

Clinical Uses (Table 21-4)

H_2 Receptor Antagonists

Despite the presence of H_2 receptors throughout the body, the inhibition of histamine binding to the receptors on gastric parietal cells is the major beneficial effect of H_2 receptor antagonists (cimetidine, ranitidine, famotidine, nizatidine).

Mechanism of Action

H_2 receptor antagonists competitively and selectively inhibit the binding of histamine to H_2 receptors, thereby

TABLE 21-3.
PHARMACOKINETICS OF H_1 RECEPTOR ANTAGONISTS

	Time to Peak Plasma Level (hrs)	Elimination Half-Time (hrs)	Clearance Rate (ml/kg/min)
First-generation receptor antagonists			
Chlorpheniramine	2.8	27.9	1.8
Diphenhydramine	1.7	9.2	23.3
Hydralazine	2.1	20.0	98
Second-generation receptor antagonists			
Loratadine	1.0	11.0	202
Acrivastine	0.85–1.4	1.4–2.1	4.56
Azelastine	5.3	22	8.5

TABLE 21-4.
CLINICAL USES OF H_1 RECEPTOR ANTAGONISTS

Allergic rhinoconjunctivitis (first-generation H_1 receptor antagonists are being replaced by second generation drugs)
Chronic urticaria
Sedative (diphenhydramine)
Antipruritic (diphenhydramine)
Antiemetic (diphenhydramine)
Anaphylactic reactions
Prophylaxis prior to administration of radiocontrast dyes
Motion sickness (dimenhydrinate)

decreasing the intracellular concentrations of cAMP and the subsequent secretion of hydrogen ions by parietal cells. The relative potencies of the four H_2 receptor antagonists for the inhibition of secretion of gastric hydrogen ions varies from 20- to 50-fold, with cimetidine as the least potent and famotidine the most potent (Table 21-5).

Pharmacokinetics (Table 21-5)

The renal clearance of all four H_2 receptor antagonists is typically two to three times greater than creatinine clearance, reflecting extensive renal tubular secretion. Renal failure increases the elimination half-time of all four drugs, with the greatest effect on nizatidine and famotidine. Decreases in the doses of all four drugs are recommended for patients with renal dysfunction. Hepatic dysfunction does not seem to significantly alter the pharmacokinetics of H_2 receptor antagonists.

Clinical Uses

H_2 receptor antagonists are most commonly administered for the treatment of duodenal ulcer disease associated with hypersecretion of gastric hydrogen ions. In the preoperative period, H_2 receptor antagonists have been administered as chemoprophylaxis to increase the pH level of gastric fluid before the induction of anesthesia. The ability of

TABLE 21-5.

PHARMACOKINETICS OF H_2 RECEPTOR ANTAGONISTS

	Cimetidine	Ranitidine	Famotidine	Nizatidine
Potency	1	4–10	20–50	4–10
EC50 (μg/mL)*	250–500	60–165	10–13	154–180
Bioavailability (%)	60	50	43	98
Time to peak plasma concentration (hrs)	1–2	1–3	1.0–3.5	1–3
Volume of distribution (L/kg)	0.8–1.2	1.2–1.9	1.1–1.4	1.2–1.6
Plasma protein binding (%)	13–26	15	16	26–35
Cerebrospinal fluid: plasma	0.18	0.06–0.17	0.05–0.09	Unknown
Clearance (mL/min)	450–650	568–709	417–483	667–850
Hepatic clearance (%)				
Oral	60	73	50–80	22
Intravenous	25–40	30	25–30	25

(*continued*)

TABLE 21-5.
(continued)

	Cimetidine	Ranitidine	Famotidine	Nizatidine
Renal clearance (%)				
Oral	40	27	25–30	57–65
Intravenous	50–80	50	65–80	75
Elimination half-time (hrs)	1.5–2.3	1.6–2.4	2.5–4	1.1–1.6
Decrease dose in presence of				
Renal dysfunction	Yes	Yes	Yes	Yes
Hepatic dysfunction	No	No	No	No
Interfere with drug metabolism by cytochrome P-450 enzymes	Yes	Minimal	No	No

*EC50 denotes the plasma concentration of the drug necessary to inhibit the pentagastrin-stimulated secretion of hydrogen ions by 50%.

H_2 receptor antagonists to decrease gastric fluid volume is unpredictable. Furthermore, H_2 receptor antagonists, in contrast to antacids, have no influence on the pH level of gastric fluid that is already present in the stomach. The preoperative preparation of patients with allergic histories or patients undergoing procedures associated with an increased likelihood of allergic reactions (radiographic contrast dye administration) may include the prophylactic oral administration of an H_1 receptor antagonist (diphenhydramine, 0.5 to 1.0 mg/kg) and an H_2 receptor antagonist (cimetidine, 4 mg/kg) every 6 hours in the 12 to 24 hours preceding the possible triggering event. Pretreatment with an H_1 receptor antagonist (diphenhydramine) or H_2 receptor antagonist (cimetidine) alone is not effective in preventing the cardiovascular effects of histamine that is released in response to rapid intravenous administration of certain drugs (morphine, atracurium, mivacurium, protamine), thus emphasizing the role of both H_1 and H_2 receptors in these responses.

Side Effects (Table 21-6)

Drug Interactions (Table 21-7)

PROTON PUMP INHIBITORS

Proton pump inhibitors are the drugs of choice in the treatment of moderate to severe gastroesophageal reflux disease, hypersecretory disorders, and peptic ulcer disease (Table 21-8).

Omeprazole

Omeprazole is a substituted benzimidazole that acts as a prodrug that becomes a proton pump inhibitor. Daily administration results in about 66% inhibition of gastric acid secretion after 5 days. Likewise, discontinuation of omeprazole is not followed immediately by return of gastric acid secretion. Omeprazole is superior to H_2 receptor

TABLE 21-6.
SIDE EFFECTS OF H_2 RECEPTOR ANTAGONISTS

Interaction with cerebral H_2 receptors (headache, somnolence, confusion)
Interaction with cardiac H_2 receptors (bradycardia, hypotension, heart block)
Hyperprolactinemia
Acute pancreatitis
Increased hepatic transaminases
Alcohol dehydrogenase dehydration
Thrombocytopenia
Agranulocytosis
Interstitial nephritis
Interfere with drug metabolism by cytochrome P-450

antagonists for the treatment of reflux esophagitis and is the best pharmacologic treatment of Zollinger-Ellison syndrome.

Preoperative Medication

As a preoperative medication, omeprazole effectively increases gastric fluid pH levels and decreases gastric fluid volume. In this regard, the onset of the gastric antisecretory effect of omeprazole after a single dose (20 mg orally) occurs within 2 to 6 hours. The duration of action is prolonged (>24 hour), because the drug is concentrated selectively in the acidic environment of gastric parietal cells. Omeprazole, 20 mg orally administered the night before surgery increases gastric fluid pH level, whereas administration on the day of surgery (up to 3 hours before induction of anesthesia) fails to improve the environment of the gastric fluid. This suggests that omeprazole should be administered >3 hours before anticipated induction of anesthesia to ensure adequate chemoprophylaxis.

Side Effects

Omeprazole crosses the blood-brain barrier and may cause headache, agitation, and confusion. There is no

TABLE 21-7.
DRUG INTERACTIONS WITH CIMETIDINE

Drug	Effect of Cimetidine on Plasma Concentration	Clearance of Drug (% Decrease)	Mechanism
Ketoconazole	Decreased	No change	Decreased absorption due to increased gastric fluid pH that slows dissolution
Warfarin*	Increased	23–36	Decreased hydroxylation of dextrorotatory isomer
Theophylline*	Increased	12–34	Decreased methylation
Phenytoin*	Increased	21–24	Decreased hydroxylation (?)
Propranolol	Increased	20–27	Decreased hydroxylation
Nifedipine	Increased	38	Unknown
Lidocaine	Increased	14–30	Decreased *N*-dealkylation
Quinidine	Increased	25–37	Decreased 3-hydroxylation (?)
Imipramine	Increased	40	Decreased *N*-demethylation
Desipramine	Increased	36	Decreased hydroxylation in rapid metabolizers
Triazolam	Increased	27	Decreased hydroxylation
Meperidine	Increased	22	Decreased oxidation
Procainamide*	Increased	28	Competition for renal tubular secretion

*Lesser drug interactions also occur with ranitidine.

TABLE 21-8.
PHARMACOKINETICS OF PROTON PUMP INHIBITORS

	Bioavailability	Time to Peak Plasma	Protein Binding	Elimination Half-Time (hrs)	Hepatic Metabolism	Interfere with Cytochrome P-450
Omeprazole	60%	2–4	>90%	0.5–1.0	Yes	Minimal
Esomeprazole	60%	2–4	>90%	0.5–1.0	Yes	Minimal
Lasoprazole	85%	1.5–3.0	97%	1.5	Yes	Minimal
Pantoprazole	77%	2.5	98%	1.9	Yes	No
Rabeprazole	85%	2.9–3.8	96%	1	Yes	No

need to decrease the dose of proton pump inhibitors in the presence of renal or hepatic dysfunction.

Esomeprazole

Esomeprazole is the levorotatory isomer of omeprazole.

Pantoprazole

Pantoprazole is a potent and fast-acting proton pump inhibitor. Administration of pantoprazole (40 mgIV) and ranitidine (50 mgIV) 1 hour before the induction of anesthesia is effective in decreasing gastric fluid volume and pH level.

CROMOLYN

Cromolyn inhibits the antigen-induced release of histamine and other autocoids, including leukotrienes, from pulmonary mast cells as well as from mast cells at other sites during antibody-mediated allergic responses. The principal use of cromolyn is in the prophylactic treatment of bronchial asthma. Given before an antigenic challenge, cromolyn inhibits bronchoconstriction and prevents signs of an acute asthmatic attack. This protective effect lasts for several hours.

Serotonin, Plasma Kinins, and Renin

22

SEROTONIN

Serotonin (5-hydroxytryptamine, 5-HT) is a widely distributed endogenous vasoactive substance that evokes complex changes in the cardiovascular system (cerebral, coronary, and pulmonary vascular vasoconstriction) and functions as an important neurotransmitter in emesis and pain transmission (Stoelting RK, Hillier SC. Serotonin, plasma kinins, and renin. In: *Pharmacology and Physiology in Anesthetic Practice*, 4th ed. Philadelphia: Lippincott Williams & Wilkins, 2006:444–455). About 90% of the body's stores of serotonin are present in the enterochromaffin cells of the gastrointestinal tract.

Mechanism of Action

Serotonin receptors are classified as 5-HT1 through 5-HT4 (Table 22-1). Physiologically, serotonin acts as a cerebral stimulant ("waking neurotransmitter"), and it is likely that all 5-HT receptors are involved in the etiology of anxiety.

Synthesis and Metabolism

Serotonin is synthesized in cells from the amino acid precursor tryptophan, which is derived from dietary sources (Fig. 22-1). Carcinoid tumors that synthesize serotonin may divert so much tryptophan from protein synthesis to produce serotonin that hypoalbuminemia and pellagra result.

TABLE 22-1.
SEROTONIN RECEPTORS AND ASSOCIATED RESPONSES

5-HT1	Cerebral vasoconstriction (agonist drugs used to treat migraine headache)
5-HT2	Coronary artery and pulmonary artery vasoconstriction, bronchoconstriction
5-HT3	Emesis, appetite, addiction, pain, anxiety
5-HT4	Gastrokinetic effects (metoclopramide)

The metabolism of serotonin occurs mainly by oxidative deamination mechanisms (monoamine oxidase enzymes) and is similar to the breakdown of other amines, such as catecholamines. The principal metabolite of serotonin deamination is 5-hydroxyindolacetic acid, and its urinary excretion is an indicator of the endogenous metabolism of serotonin.

Serotonin Agonists

Sumatriptan

Sumatriptan is a 5-HT1 receptor agonist that is useful in the treatment of migraine headache and cluster headache. It has cerebral vasoconstrictive effects that are useful in treating these headaches; however, because the same vasoconstriction also may so occur in the coronary arteries, it may be prudent to avoid the use of sumatriptan in patients with known coronary artery disease.

Fenfluramine and Dexfenfluramine

Fenfluramine, and its isomer, dexfenfluramine, are sympathomimetic amines whose central nervous system (CNS) effects, when combined, tend to cancel each other: Thus, most patients experience weight loss, due to appetite suppression that reflects serotonin release and the inhibition of its cellular uptake and metabolism, without mood

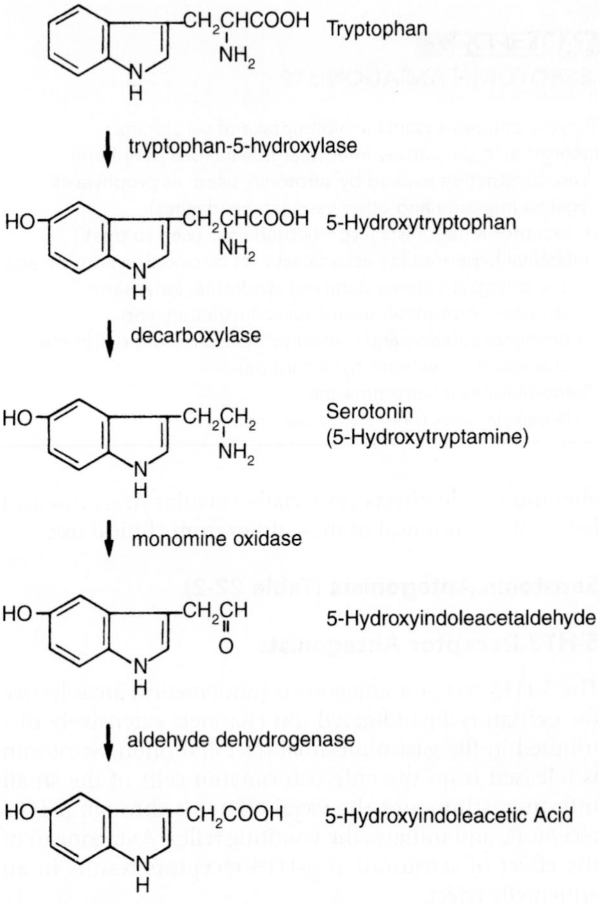

Tryptophan ($CH_2CHCOOH$, NH_2)

↓ tryptophan-5-hydroxylase

5-Hydroxytryptophan (HO–, $CH_2CHCOOH$, NH_2)

↓ decarboxylase

Serotonin (5-Hydroxytryptamine) (HO–, CH_2CH_2, NH_2)

↓ monomine oxidase

5-Hydroxyindoleacetaldehyde (HO–, CH_2CH, O)

↓ aldehyde dehydrogenase

5-Hydroxyindoleacetic Acid (HO–, CH_2COOH)

Figure 22-1. Synthesis and metabolism of serotonin.

TABLE 22-2.
SEROTONIN ANTAGONISTS

Tricyclic antidepressants (inhibit uptake of serotonin)
Lysergic acid derivatives (methysergide inhibits peripheral vasoconstriction evoked by serotonin; used as prophylaxis against migraine and other vascular headaches)
H_1 receptor antagonists (cyproheptadine is used to treat intestinal hypermotility associated with carcinoid syndrome and in the postgastrectomy dumping syndrome; ketanserin attenuates serotonin-induced vasoconstriction and bronchoconstriction and is used to treat carcinoid syndrome and associated systemic hypertension)
Phenothiazines (chlorpromazine)
β-Haloalkylamines (phenoxybenzamine)

alteration. Side effects (especially valvular heart disease) led to the withdrawal of these drugs from clinical use.

Serotonin Antagonists (Table 22-2)

5-HT3 Receptor Antagonists

The 5-HT3 receptor antagonists (antiemetics) are selective for excitatory ligand-gated ion channels extensively distributed in the gastrointestinal tract and brain. Serotonin is released from the enterochromaffin cells of the small intestine, stimulates the vagal efferents through 5-HT3 receptors, and initiates the vomiting reflex. Antagonism of the effect of serotonin at 5-HT3 receptors results in an antiemetic effect.

Clinical Uses

The 5-HT3 receptor antagonists are highly specific antiemetics having minimal side effects. As such, they are useful in the prophylaxis and treatment of chemotherapy, radiation, and postoperative nausea and vomiting. These drugs are not effective for the treatment of motion-induced nausea and vomiting and nausea and vomiting due to vestibular stimulation. Unlike the prevention and treatment of chemotherapy-induced emesis, which is guided by evidence-based consensus guidelines, the recommendations regarding the timing of prophylactic antiemetic therapy (with the preanesthetic medication, near the completion of surgery) cannot be made on the basis of scientific data. However, if patients experience breakthrough postoperative nausea and vomiting despite prophylaxis, they should be treated with an antiemetic from a different class than that used for prophylaxis.

The cost–benefit ratio does not support the use of 5-HT3 receptor antagonists for routine antiemetic prophylaxis.

Pharmacokinetics

The 5-HT3 receptor antagonists are readily absorbed after oral administration and readily cross the blood-brain barrier. Metabolites undergo principally renal excretion.

Ondansetron

Ondansetron is a carbazolone derivative that is structurally related to serotonin and possesses specific 5-HT3 subtype receptor antagonist properties, without altering dopamine, histamine, adrenergic, or cholinergic receptor activity. Cardiac dysrhythmias and conduction disturbances (atrioventricular heart block) have been reported after the intravenous administration of ondansetron and metoclopramide. Ondansetron and other 5-HT3 receptor antagonists can cause slight prolongation of the QTc interval on the electrocardiogram of treated patients, but this has not created the same level of concern as that ascribed to droperidol. It is estimated that for every 100 patients who receive ondansetron for the prevention of postoperative nausea and vomiting, 20 patients will not vomit who would have vomited without treatment ("number needed to treat"), and three of these 100 patients will develop headache who would not have had this adverse effect without the drug ("number needed to harm"). Ondansetron, 4 to 8 mg IV (administered over 2 to 5 minutes immediately before the induction of anesthesia) is highly effective in decreasing the incidence of postoperative nausea and vomiting in a susceptible patient population (ambulatory gynecologic surgery, middle ear surgery). The most significant feature of ondansetron prophylaxis and treatment is the relative freedom from side effects, compared with previously used classes of drugs.

Tropisetron

Tropisetron is a highly selective 5-HT3 receptor antagonist that resembles ondansetron but has a longer elimination half-time.

Granisetron

Granisetron is a more selective and longer acting 5-HT3 receptor antagonist than ondansetron.

Dolasetron

Dolasetron is a potent and selective 5-HT3 receptor antagonist.

PLASMA KININS

Plasma kinins are polypeptides that include kallidin and bradykinin. Plasma kinins are the most potent known endogenous vasodilators. Vasodilation results in marked decreases in systolic and diastolic blood pressure. Plasma kinins may increase airway resistance in patients with reactive airway disease, such as bronchial asthma.

Mechanism of Action

Specific kinin receptors are postulated, whereas some responses to kinins may be mediated by the production of prostaglandins.

Pharmacokinetics

The elimination half-time of plasma kinins is <15 s, with $>90\%$ metabolized (peptidyl dipeptidase converting enzyme, which is identical to the enzyme necessary for the conversion of angiotensin I to angiotensin II) during a single passage through the lungs.

Bradykinin

Bradykinin is formed from kininogen by the action of the enzyme kallikrein, which circulates as the inactive form known as prekallikrein. The factors that activate prekallikrein are involved in factor VIII-initiated coagulation and fibrinolysis. Hereditary angioedema is associated with the absence of C1 esterase inhibitor of the complement system, which is also an inhibitor of kallikrein.

Aprotinin

Aprotinin is a naturally occurring serine protease inhibitor that decreases the activation of plasminogen and the activity of plasmin. Decreased bleeding is thought to reflect an inhibition of fibrinolysis (plasmin inhibition), reduction of thrombin generation, and preservation of platelet function. The enzymatic activity of aprotinin is generally expressed in kallikrein inactivator units (KIU).

Side Effects (Table 22-3)

Pharmacokinetics

Plasma aprotinin concentrations decrease rapidly after intravenous administration because of redistribution to peripheral tissues (approximately 80% of an injected dose of aprotinin can be localized in the proximal renal tubular epithelial cells).

Clinical Uses

Cardiac Surgery

Aprotinin can decrease perioperative blood loss and transfusion requirements in cardiac surgical patients undergoing cardiopulmonary bypass (Table 22-4).

TABLE 22-3.
SIDE EFFECTS OF APROTININ

Tubular overloading (spilling of normally filtered proteins due to accumulation of aprotinin in renal tubular cells)
Renal vasoconstriction (avoid use in presence of radiocontrast dye or nonsteroidal anti-inflammatory drugs)
Allergic reactions (reflects antigenic properties as a protein derived from bovine lungs; test dose is recommended before intravenous administration)
Thrombotic events (theoretical concern based on antifibrinolytic effects; incidence of deep vein thrombosis is not increased)

Total Hip Replacement

The use of aprotinin during total hip replacement results in decreases in total blood loss and the amount of blood transfused.

RENIN

Renin is a proteolytic enzyme that is synthesized and stored by juxtaglomerular cells present in the walls of renal afferent arterioles (Table 22-5).

TABLE 22-4.
INFUSION PROTOCOL DESIGNED TO MAINTAIN THE PLASMA APROTININ CONCENTRATION AT APPROXIMATELY 250 KIU/ML

	Infusion rate
Induction to skin incision (0 to 30 mins)	52,000 KIU/min
Skin incision to 60 mins	26,000 KIU/min
60 mins to end of surgery	10,400 KIU/min
Add to prime of cardiopulmonary bypass circuit	500,000 KIU/min

KIU, kallikrein inhibitor units.

TABLE 22-5.
STIMULI FOR RELEASE OF RENIN

Decrease in renal perfusion pressure
Hemorrhage
Dehydration
Chronic sodium ion depletion
Renal artery stenosis
Sympathetic nervous system stimulation

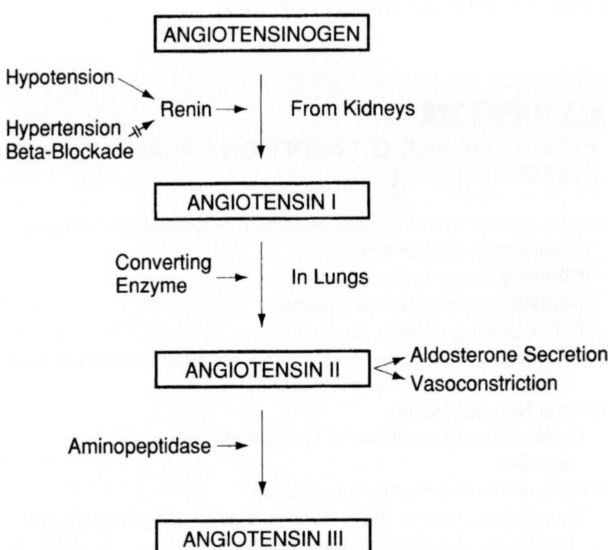

Figure 22-2. Schematic diagram of the renin-angiotensin-aldosterone system.

Formation of Angiotensins

The release of renin initiates the formation of active hormones knows as *angiotensins* (Fig. 22-2).

Effects on Organ Systems

Vasoconstriction and stimulation of the synthesis and secretion of aldosterone by the adrenal cortex are the principal physiologic effects of angiotensin II (Table 22-6). Aldosterone causes renal conservation of sodium, retention of water, and loss of potassium and hydrogen ions.

Factors Altering Plasma Renin Activity

The institution of positive end-expiratory pressure results in significant increases in plasma renin activity and circulating levels of antidiuretic hormone.

TABLE 22-6.
EFFECTS OF ANGIOTENSIN II ON ORGAN SYSTEMS

Cardiovascular System (vasoconstriction of arterioles > venules)
- Renal artery vasoconstriction
- Coronary artery vasoconstriction
- Increased systemic blood pressure
- Reflex slowing of heart rate
- Decreases intravascular fluid volume (separation of endothelial cells increases vascular permeability)

Central Nervous System
- Enhanced central outflow of sympathetic nervous system impulses

Peripheral Autonomic Nervous System
- Stimulation of sympathetic nervous system ganglion cells and facilitation of ganglionic transmission

Adrenal Cortex
- Stimulates synthesis and secretion of aldosterone

Exogenous Infusion

The exogenous infusion of angiotensin II produces intense vasoconstriction and increases in systemic blood pressure. Compared with norepinephrine, angiotensin is a more potent vasoconstrictor, produces a more sustained effect, infrequently causes cardiac dysrhythmias, and is less likely to be associated with hypotension when a chronic infusion is abruptly discontinued.

Antagonists of the Renin-Angiotensin-Aldosterone System

Antagonists of the renin-angiotensin-aldosterone system act by blocking those receptors responsive to angiotensin II (losartan) and by inhibiting the activity of the converting enzyme necessary for converting angiotensin I to angiotensin II (captopril).

Hormones as Drugs

23

Preparations that contain synthetic hormones identical to those secreted endogenously by endocrine glands may be administered as drugs (Stoelting RK, Hillier SC. Hormones as drugs. In: *Pharmacology and Physiology in Anesthetic Practice,* 4th ed. Philadelphia: Lippincott Williams & Wilkins, 2006:456–476). These hormones are created using recombinant DNA technology to produce pure hormones devoid of allergic properties. Typically, the clinical application of these drugs is for hormone replacement to provide a physiologic effect. In certain patients, however, large does of synthetic hormones are used to exert pharmacologic effects.

ANTERIOR PITUITARY HORMONES (TABLE 23-1)

The perioperative replacement of anterior pituitary hormones may be necessary for patients receiving exogenous hormones because of a prior hypophysectomy (cortisol must be provided continuously, whereas thyroid stimulating hormone [TSH] has a long elimination half-time and can be omitted for several days).

Growth Hormone

Growth hormone is used to treat hypopituitary dwarfism, based on documentation that the plasma concentration of the hormone is inadequate.

Octreotide

Octreotide is a somatostatin analog that inhibits the release of growth hormone, making it an effective treatment in

TABLE 23-1.
ANTERIOR PITUITARY HORMONES

Growth hormone
Prolactin
Gonadotropins
Luteinizing hormone
Follicle-stimulating hormone
Adrenocorticotrophins hormone (ACTH)
Thyroid stimulating hormone (TSH)

patients with acromegaly. Because somatostatin analogs inhibit the secretion of insulin, decreased glucose tolerance and even overt hyperglycemia might be expected to occur during treatment with octreotide.

Gonadotropins

Gonadotropins are used most often for the treatment of infertility and cryptorchism.

Adrenocorticotrophic Hormone

The physiologic and pharmacologic effects of adrenocorticotrophic hormone (ACTH) result from this hormone's stimulation of corticosteroid secretion from the adrenal cortex, principally cortisol.

Treatment of disease states with ACTH is not physiologically equivalent to the administration of a specific hormone, because ACTH exposes the tissues to a mixture of glucocorticoids, mineralocorticoids, and androgens. Maximal stimulation of the adrenal cortex is produced by ACTH, 25 U.

THYROID GLAND HORMONES

The thyroid gland is the source of triiodothyronine (T3), thyroxine (T4), and calcitonin. The effectiveness of treatment of hypothyroidism using commercial preparations of T3 and T4 is judged by the return of the plasma concentration of thyroid stimulating hormone (TSH) to normal.

Levothyroxine

Levothyroxine is the most frequently administered drug for the treatment of diseases requiring thyroid hormone replacement.

Liothyronine

Liothyronine is the levorotatory isomer of T3 and is 2.5 to 3.0 times more potent than levothyroxine.

Calcitonin

The endogenous release of calcitonin decreases plasma calcium concentrations as a reflection of decreased osteoclast activity and bone resorption.

DRUGS THAT INHIBIT THYROID HORMONE SYNTHESIS

Antithyroid Drugs

Antithyroid drugs, such as propylthiouracil and methimazole, inhibit the formation of thyroid hormone by interfering with the incorporation of iodine into tyrosine residues of thyroglobulin. Drug-induced decreases in excessive thyroid activity usually require several days because preformed hormone must be depleted before symptoms begin to wane.

Side Effects (Table 23-2)

Inhibitors of Iodide Transport

The inhibitors of iodide transport mechanisms (thiocyanate, perchlorate) interfere with the uptake of iodide

TABLE 23-2.
SIDE EFFECTS OF ANTITHYROID DRUGS

Urticarial or papular skin rash
Granulocytopenia
Agranulocytosis (fever, pharyngitis)

ions by the thyroid gland. Thiocyanate may result from the metabolism of sodium nitroprusside

Iodide

Iodide provides a paradoxical treatment for hyperthyroidism, which reflects the ability of iodide to antagonize the ability of TSH and cyclic adenosine monophosphate (cAMP) to stimulate hormone release. Allergic reactions (angioedema, laryngeal edema) may accompany the administration of iodide or organic preparations that contain iodide.

Radioactive Iodine

In the treatment of hyperthyroidism in elderly patients, radioactive iodine (^{131}I) is rapidly trapped by thyroid gland cells, and the subsequent emission of destructive β-rays destroys these cells. Iatrogenic hypothyroidism must be considered preoperatively in any patient who has been previously treated with ^{131}I. Most thyroid cancers, except for follicular cancer, accumulate little radioactive iodine, so that effectiveness of ^{131}I for the treatment of cancer is limited.

OVARIAN HORMONES

Estrogens

Estrogens are effective in treating the unpleasant side effects of menopause, and they protect against osteoporosis. An important use of estrogens is in combination with progestins as oral contraceptives.

Route of Administration

Oral absorption is prompt and nearly complete, but metabolism in the liver limits effectiveness.

Side Effects

Large doses of estrogen may cause retention of sodium and water, which is particularly undesirable in patients with cardiac or renal disease.

Antiestrogens

Antiestrogens, such as clomiphene and tamoxifen, act by binding to estrogen receptors. Tamoxifen is administered for a period of 5 years to postmenopausal women with breast cancer that was characterized by estrogen-responsive receptors. An increased incidence of temperature disturbances ("hot flashes") may accompany treatment with tamoxifen.

Tissue-Specific Estrogens

Raloxifene is a nonsteroidal benzothiophene that acts as a selective estrogen-receptor modulator. It prevents bone loss without endometrial stimulation.

Progesterone

Orally active derivatives of progesterone (progestins) are often combined with estrogens as oral contraceptives.

Antiprogestins

Antiprogestins inhibit the hormonal effects of progesterone and are the most effective and safest means of medical abortion.

Oral Contraceptives

Oral contraceptives are most often a combination of estrogen and a progestin that results in the inhibition of ovulation.

Side Effects

Estrogens in combined preparations are believed to be responsible for most, if not all, the side effects of oral contraceptives, including thromboembolism.

ANDROGENS

Androgens are most often administered to males to stimulate the development and maintenance of secondary sexual characteristics. Androgens enhance erythropoiesis by stimulating the renal production of erythropoietin.

Route of Administration

Testosterone administered orally is metabolized so extensively by the liver that therapeutic effects do not occur (alkylation of androgens at the 17 position retards hepatic metabolism).

Side Effects

Dose-related cholestatic hepatitis and jaundice are particularly likely to accompany androgen therapy used for the palliation of neoplastic disease.

Danazol

The low androgen activity of danazol makes it the preferred androgen for treatment of hereditary angioedema.

Finasteride

Finasteride is a competitive 5-α-reductase inhibitor that does not bind to the androgen receptor, so that dihydrotestosterone production does not occur. Because androgen effects on the prostate do not occur, this accounts for the use of this drug in treating benign prostatic hyperplasia.

CORTICOSTEROIDS

Corticosteroids are classified according to the potencies of these compounds to evoke the distal renal tubular reabsorption of sodium in exchange for potassium (mineralocorticoid effect) or to produce an anti-inflammatory response (glucocorticoid effect). Naturally occurring corticosteroids are cortisol (hydrocortisone), cortisone, corticosterone, desoxycorticosterone, and aldosterone (Fig. 23-1). Although it is possible to separate mineralocorticoid and glucocorticoid effects, it has not been possible to separate the various components of glucocorticoid effects. All synthetic corticosteroids used in pharmaco-

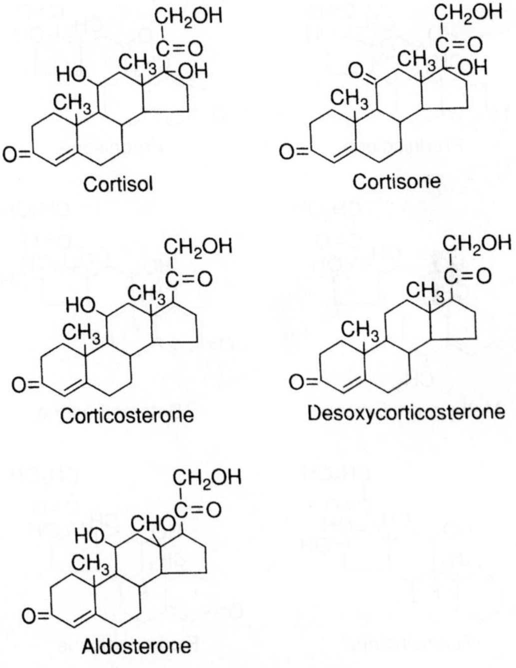

Cortisol

Cortisone

Corticosterone

Desoxycorticosterone

Aldosterone

Figure 23-1. Endogenous corticosteroids.

logic doses for their anti-inflammatory effects also produce less desirable effects, such as suppression of the hypothalamic-pituitary-adrenal (HPA) axis, weight gain, and skeletal muscle wasting (Fig. 23-2).

Structure–Activity Relationships

Modifications of structure, such as the introduction of a double bond in prednisolone and prednisone, have resulted in synthetic corticosteroids with more potent glucocorticoid effects than the two closely related natural hormones, cortisol and cortisone, respectively (Table 23-3).

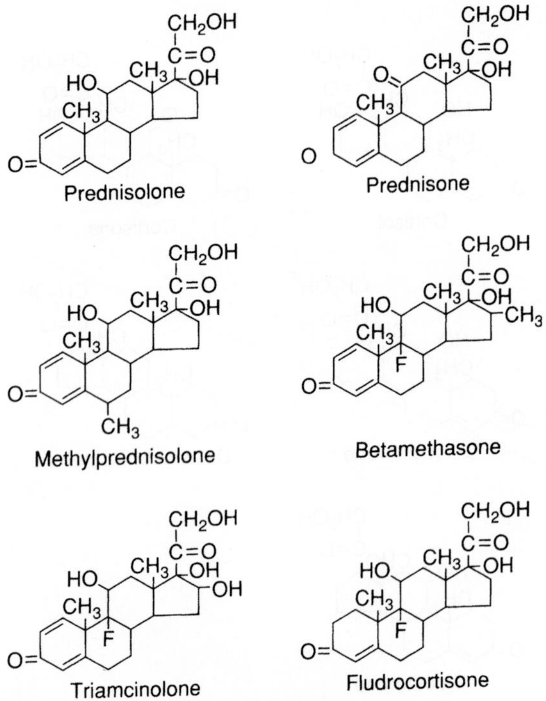

Figure 23-2. Synthetic corticosteroids.

TABLE 23-3.
COMPARATIVE PHARMACOLOGY OF ENDOGENOUS AND SYNTHETIC CORTICOSTEROIDS

	Anti-Inflammatory Potency	Sodium-Retaining Potency	Equivalent Dose (mg)	Elimination Half-Time (hrs)	Duration of Action (hrs)	Route of Administration
Cortisol	1	1	20	1.5–3.0	8–12	Oral, Topical, IV, IM, IA
Cortisone	0.8	0.8	25	0.5	8–36	Oral, Topical, IV, IM, IA
Prednisolone	4	0.8	5	2–4	12–36	Oral, Topical, IV, IM, IA
Prednisone	4	0.8	5	2–4	12–36	Oral
Methylprednisolone	5	0.5	4	2–4	12–36	Oral, Topical, IV, IM, IA, Epidural
Betamethasone	25	0	0.75	5	36–54	Oral, Topical, IV, IM, IA
Dexamethasone	25	0	0.75	3.5–5.0	36–54	Oral, Topical, IV, IM, IA
Triamcinolone	5	0	4	3.5	12–36	Oral, Topical, IV, IM, Epidural
Fludrocortisone	10	250	2	—	24	Oral, Topical, IV, IM
Aldosterone	0	3,000				

IV, intravenous; IM, intramuscular; IA, intraarticular.

Mechanism of Action

Glucocorticoids attach to cytoplasmic receptors to stimulate changes in the transcription of deoxyribonucleic acid (DNA) and thus the synthesis of proteins. Mineralocorticoid receptors are present in high concentrations in distal renal tubules and the hippocampus. Glucocorticoid receptors are more widely distributed and do not bind aldosterone. The concentration of glucocorticoid receptors may fluctuate and thus influence responsiveness to glucocorticoids.

Maintenance of Homeostasis

The permissive and protective effects of glucocorticoids are critical for the maintenance of homeostasis during severe stress. The permissive actions of glucocorticoids occur at low physiologic steroid concentrations and serve to prepare the individual to respond to stress. The protective actions of glucocorticoids occur when high plasma concentrations of steroids exert anti-inflammatory and immunosuppressive effects.

Pharmacokinetics

Cortisol is released from the adrenal glands in an episodic manner, and the frequency of pulses follows a circadian rhythm that is linked to the sleep–wake cycle (maximal plasma concentrations occur just before awakening and the lowest levels 8 to 10 hours later).

Synthetic Corticosteroids (See Table 23-1)

Prednisolone

Prednisolone is an analog of cortisol that is available as an oral or parenteral preparation. The anti-inflammatory effect of 5 mg of prednisolone is equivalent to 20 mg of cortisol.

Prednisone

Prednisone is an analog of cortisone that is rapidly converted to prednisolone after its absorption from the gastrointestinal tract.

Methylprednisolone

Methylprednisolone is the methyl derivative of prednisolone. The anti-inflammatory effect of 4 mg of methylprednisolone is equivalent to that of 20 mg of cortisol.

Betamethasone

Betamethasone is a fluorinated derivative of prednisolone. The anti-inflammatory effect of 0.75 mg is equivalent to 20 mg of cortisol.

Dexamethasone

Dexamethasone is a fluorinated derivative of prednisolone and an isomer of betamethasone. The anti-inflammatory effect of 0.75 mg is equivalent to 20 mg of cortisol.

Triamcinolone

Triamcinolone is a fluorinated derivative of prednisolone. The anti-inflammatory effect of 4 mg of triamcinolone is equivalent to that of 20 mg of cortisol.

Clinical Uses (Table 23-4)

Side Effects (Table 23-5)

Systemic corticosteroids used for short periods (<7 days) even at high doses are unlikely to cause adverse side effects. Inhaled corticosteroids are unlikely to evoke adverse systemic effects.

Suppression of the Hypothalamic-Pituitary-Adrenal Axis

It is not possible to define the precise dose of corticosteroid or duration of therapy that will produce a suppression of the HPA axis (the larger the dose and the longer the therapy, the greater is the likelihood of suppression). A dose of corticosteroid administered every other day is less likely to suppress the anterior pituitary release of ACTH. Inhaled glucocorticoids, as used to treat asthma, are not likely to suppress the HPA axis.

TABLE 23-4.
CLINICAL USES OF CORTICOSTEROIDS

Replacement therapy for deficiency states (acute replacement 100 mg IV followed by 100 mg IV every 8 hours)
Palliative effect for inflammatory disease states (prednisolone or prednisone recommended because of low mineralocorticoid effects)
Allergic therapy (topical corticosteroids)
Asthma (inhaled glucocorticoids often recommended as first-line therapy, oropharyngeal side effects include dysphonia and candidiasis)
Antiemetic effects (dexamethasone 4 mg IV administered at beginning of surgery, antiemetic effects may persist for 24 hours, safe and inexpensive, reserve more expensive serotonin antagonists for rescue therapy)
Postoperative analgesia (inhibit phospholipase enzyme necessary for production of inflammatory prostaglandins)
Cerebral edema (dexamethasone)
Aspiration pneumonitis (value unproven)
Lumbar disc disease (epidural injection of 25 to 50 mg of triamcinolone or 40 to 80 mg of methylprednisolone, may decrease inflammation and edema of the compressed nerve root, may result in suppression of the HPA axis, need for surgery is not decreased)
Immunosuppression (organ transplantation)
Arthritis (progressive disability associated with rheumatoid arthritis)
Collagen diseases
Ocular inflammation (topical corticosteroids effective for treatment of uveitis and iritis but may increase intraocular pressure)
Cutaneous disorders
Postintubation laryngeal edema (dexamethasone 0.1 to 0.2 mg/kg IV, efficacy unproven)
Ulcerative colitis
Myasthenia gravis
Respiratory distress syndrome (administer 24 hours before delivery of neonates between 24 and 36 weeks)
Leukemia
Cardiac arrest (no proven value and not recommended)

HPA, hypothalamic-pituitary-adrenal axis.

TABLE 23-5.
SIDE EFFECTS OF CORTICOSTEROIDS

Suppression of the HPA axis
Electrolyte and metabolic changes
Osteoporosis
Peptic ulcer disease
Skeletal muscle myopathy (weakness of proximal musculature)
Central nervous system dysfunction (neuroses and psychoses)
Peripheral blood changes (acute lymphocytopenia)
Inhibition of normal growth

Corticosteroid Supplementation

Corticosteroid administration should be increased whenever the patient being treated for chronic hypoadrenocorticism undergoes a surgical procedure, based on the concern these patients are susceptible to cardiovascular collapse because they cannot release additional endogenous cortisol in response to the stress of surgery. More controversial is the management of patients who may manifest suppression of the HPA axis because of current or previous administration of corticosteroids for treatment of a disease unrelated to pituitary or adrenal function. A rational regimen for corticosteroid supplementation in the perioperative period is the administration of cortisol, 25 mgIV, at the induction of anesthesia, followed by a continuous infusion of cortisol, 100 mg during the following 24 hours. In those instances in which events such as burns or sepsis could exaggerate the need for exogenous corticosteroid supplementation, the continuous infusion of cortisol, 100 mg every 12 hours should be sufficient.

No objective evidence supports increasing the maintenance dose of corticosteroid preoperatively.

Electrolyte and Metabolic Changes

Hypokalemic metabolic alkalosis reflects the mineralocorticoid effect of corticosteroids on distal renal tubules, leading to enhanced absorption of sodium and loss of potassium.

A redistribution of body fat occurs, characterized by the deposition of fat in the back of the neck and moon facies.

Inhibitors of Corticosteroid Synthesis

Metyrapone

Metyrapone decreases cortisol secretion by inhibition of the 11-β-hydroxylation, resulting in an accumulation of 11-deoxycortisol.

Aminoglutethimide

Aminoglutethimide inhibits the conversion of cholesterol to 20-α-hydroxycholesterol, which interrupts production of both cortisol and aldosterone.

NONSTEROIDAL DRUGS PRODUCING IMMUNOSUPPRESSION

Nonsteroidal drugs that produce immunosuppression are commonly administered to decrease the immune response and associated rejection of newly transplanted organs.

Cyclosporine

Cyclosporine selectively inhibits helper T-lymphocyte–mediated immune responses by blocking the transcription of cytokine genes while not affecting B-lymphocytes. The use of this immunosuppressive drug in combination with corticosteroids has greatly increased the success of organ transplantation. Cyclosporine must be administered before T-lymphocytes undergo proliferation as a result of exposure to specific antigens presented by organ transplantation.

Pharmacokinetics

Cyclosporine has a narrow therapeutic range, thus the monitoring of blood concentrations is important. Drugs inhibiting (rifampicin, anticonvulsants) or inducing

TABLE 23-6.
SIDE EFFECTS OF CYCLOSPORINE

Nephrotoxicity (avoid nonsteroidal anti-inflammatory drugs)
Systemic hypertension
Seizures
Cholestasis (hyperbilirubinemia, increased liver transaminases)
Allergic reactions
Gingival hyperplasia
Hyperglycemia

(ketoconazole, diltiazem) P-450 activity may alter cyclosporine blood levels.

Side Effects (Table 23-6)

Tacrolimus

Tacrolimus is a more potent immunosuppressant than cyclosporine and shares the ability to produce nephrotoxicity, although systemic hypertension is less.

Disease-Modifying Antirheumatic Drugs

Methotrexate remains the most commonly used disease-modifying antirheumatic drug, but newer drugs may serve as useful alternatives (Table 23-7).

Leflunomide

Leflunomide inhibits pyrimidine synthesis (pyrimidines are responsible for the proliferative effects associated with rheumatoid arthritis) by acting as a competitive enzyme inhibitor.

Side Effects (Table 23-8)

Tumor Necrosis Factor Antagonists (Etanercept, Adalimumab, Infliximab)

Adverse events that accompany these drugs include infections (tuberculosis, *Pneumocystitis carinii* pneumonia),

TABLE 23-7.
DISEASE-MODIFYING ANTIRHEUMATIC DRUGS

Drug	Mechanism of Action	Route of Administration	Elimination Half-Time	Monitoring Recommendations
Leflunomide	Inhibits pyrimidine synthesis	Oral	14 days	Baseline blood count and enzymes and then monthly until stable and then every 2 to 3 months
Etanercept	Binds tumor necrosis factor	Subcutaneous	96 hours	Be alert for infections (tuberculosis, histoplasmosis)
Adalimumab	Human anti-tumor	Subcutaneous	14 days	As for etanercept
Infliximab	Chimeric anti-tumor necrosis factor antibody		9 days	As for etanercept
Anakinra	Interleukin-1 receptor antagonist	Subcutaneous	6 hours	Baseline blood count and then monthly for 3 months and every 3 months thereafter

TABLE 23-8.
SIDE EFFECTS OF LEFLUNOMIDE

Inhibition of cytochrome P-450 (increases anticoagulant effects of warfarin)
Hepatic dysfunction
Systemic hypertension
Reversible alopecia
Peripheral neuropathy
Pancytopenia
Interstitial pneumonitis
Teratogenic in animals

cancer, multiple-sclerosis–like demyelinating diseases, liver dysfunction, aplastic anemia, and allergic reactions.

Anakinra

Anakinra is a recombinant form of human interleukin-1-receptor antagonist (interleukin-1 concentrations are increased in the inflamed joints associated with rheumatoid arthritis).

MELATONIN

Melatonin is the principal substance secreted by the pineal gland, and its physiologic effects include the regulation of circadian rhythms, sleep, and mood. In humans, the circadian rhythm for the release of melatonin from the pineal gland is closely synchronized with the habitual hours of sleep. It is unclear whether the beneficial effect of exogenous melatonin on symptoms of jet lag are due to a hypnotic effect or resynchronization of the circadian rhythm.

POSTERIOR PITUITARY HORMONES

Arginine vasopressin (AVP) (formerly known as antidiuretic hormone, ADH) and oxytocin are the two principal hormones secreted by the posterior pituitary. Target sites for AVP are the renal collecting ducts (water is passively reabsorbed) and peripheral vasculature (arterial vasoconstriction). Oxytocin elicits contractions of the uterus.

Arginine Vasopressin

AVP and its congeners (desmopressin, lypressin) are useful in the treatment of diabetes insipidus that results from inadequate secretion of the hormone from the posterior pituitary (manifests as polyuria and hypernatremia).

Trauma and surgery in the region of the posterior pituitary may cause diabetes insipidus. Nephrogenic diabetes insipidus resulting from an inability of the renal tubules to respond to AVP does not respond to the exogenous administration of this hormone.

Vasopressin

Vasopressin is the exogenous preparation of AVP that is used clinically for a variety of indications (Table 23-9).

Side Effects (Table 23-10)

Desmopressin

Desmopressin (DDAVP) is a synthetic analog of AVP, having an intense antidiuretic effect and the ability to evoke

TABLE 23-9.
CLINICAL USES OF VASOPRESSIN

Diabetes insipidus
Esophageal varices
Refractory cardiac arrest (40 units IV more effective than epinephrine in management of asystole; needs to be administered only once during cardiopulmonary resuscitation, because it lasts 10–20 minutes)
Hemorrhage and septic shock (effective in reversing hypotension in catecholamine-resistant septic shock)

TABLE 23-10.
SIDE EFFECTS OF VASOPRESSIN

Vasoconstriction and increased systemic blood pressure (higher doses than needed to treat diabetes insipidus)
Selective vasoconstriction of coronary arteries and accompanying cardiac dysrhythmias (small doses)
Stimulation of gastrointestinal and uterine smooth muscle
Decreased platelet count
Allergic reactions

the release of von Willebrand factor. Administered intranasally, DDAVP is the treatment of choice for nephrogenic diabetes insipidus.

Lypressin

Lypressin is a synthetic analog of AVP having a short duration of action.

Oxytocin

Oxytocin produces selective stimulation of uterine smooth muscle.

Clinical Uses

The principal clinical uses of oxytocin are to induce labor at term and to counter uterine hypotonicity and decrease hemorrhage in the postpartum or postabortion period.

Side Effects

High doses of oxytocin produce a direct relaxant effect on vascular smooth muscles (hypotension, flushing, reflex tachycardia).

CHYMOPAPAIN

Chymopapain is a proteolytic enzyme used in the treatment of herniated lumbar intervertebral disc disease, where it dissolves the proteoglycan portion of the nucleus pulposus.

Side Effects

An injection of chymopapain into the intervertebral disc space has been associated with fatal allergic reactions (known allergy to papaya is a contraindication to injection of chymopapain). Pretreatment with a corticosteroid and an H_1- and H_2-receptor antagonist as a single dose in the preoperative medication may decrease the incidence and severity of allergic reactions.

Insulin and Oral Hypoglycemics

24

Insulin administered exogenously is the only effective treatment for type 1 diabetes (formerly known as insulin-dependent diabetes mellitus) (Stoelting RK, Hillier SC. Insulin and oral hypoglycemics. In: *Pharmacology and Physiology in Anesthetic Practice*, 4th ed. Philadelphia: Lippincott Williams & Wilkins, 2006:477–485). Oral hypoglycemic drugs may serve as alternatives to the exogenous administration of insulin to patients with type 2 diabetes (formerly known as non-insulin-dependent diabetes mellitus).

INSULIN

Insulin is synthesized in the β-cells of the islets of Langerhans as a single polypeptide, proinsulin, which is the precursor molecule to insulin.

Mechanism of Action

The cellular actions of insulin begin with its binding to plasma membrane insulin receptors. An important effect of insulin-stimulated cascades is translocation of glucose (Glut-4) transporters to plasma membranes, where they facilitate glucose diffusion into cells and shift intracellular glucose metabolism toward storage as glycogen by activating glycogen synthetase.

Insulin receptors become fully saturated with low circulating concentrations of insulin (1 to 2 U/hour). Obesity and insulin-dependent diabetes mellitus appear to be associated with a decrease in the number of insulin receptors.

Pharmacokinetics

The elimination half-time of insulin injected intravenously is 5 to 10 minutes. Insulin is metabolized in the kidneys and liver, and approximately 50% of the insulin that reaches the liver by way of the portal vein is metabolized in a single passage through the liver. Nevertheless, renal dysfunction alters the disappearance rate of circulating insulin to a greater extent than does hepatic disease; unexpectedly prolonged effects of insulin may occur in patients with renal disease. The total daily secretion of insulin is approximately 40 U. The sympathetic and parasympathetic nervous systems innervate the insulin-producing islet cells (α-adrenergic stimulation decreases and β-adrenergic stimulation increases the basal secretion of insulin). The insulin response to glucose is greater for oral ingestion than for intravenous infusion.

Insulin Preparations and Delivery

Human insulin manufactured using recombinant DNA technology has replaced insulin extracted from beef and pork pancreas (Table 24-1). The basic principle of insulin replacement is to provide a slow, long-acting, continuous supply of insulin that mimics the nocturnal and interprandial basal secretion of normal pancreatic β-cells. In addition, a rapid and relatively short-acting form of insulin delivered before meals mimics the normal meal-stimulated release of insulin. A total daily exogenous dose of insulin for the treatment of diabetes mellitus is usually in the range of 20 to 60 U. Continuous subcutaneous insulin infusion (CSII) utilizing an external pump provides basal delivery of insulin (0.5 to 1 U/hour) and more predictable acute increases in plasma insulin before meals by delivering bolus doses of insulin. There is no advantage to giving insulin by intravenous infusion bolus rather than as a continuous intravenous infusion. Now, it is accepted that intensive insulin treatment regimens to maintain

TABLE 24-1.
CLASSIFICATION OF INSULIN PREPARATIONS

	Hours After Subcutaneous Administration*		
Insulin Preparation	**Onset**	**Peak**	**Duration**
Rapid acting			
Regular crystalline zinc (CZI)	0.5–1.0	2–3	6–8
Very rapid acting			
Lispro	0.25–0.5	0.5–1.5	4–6
Insulin aspart	0.25–0.5	0.5–1.5	4–6
Intermediate acting			
Lente (NPH)	1	4–8	10–14
Long acting			
Ultralente	1	10–14	18–24
Glargine	1.5	none	30

*Approximate.

near normoglycemia are the preferred therapy of patients with diabetes mellitus. The long-term metabolic control of diabetes is best monitored by measuring glycosylated hemoglobin (HbA1c), which reflects glycemia over the previous 8 weeks (value <7.5% best decreases the risk for microvascular complications).

Lispro

Lispro is an insulin analog designed to provide a pharmacokinetic profile that more closely parallels physiologic insulin secretion and needs. When injected subcutaneously, it begins to act within 15 minutes; the peak effect is reached in 1 to 2 hours, and the duration of action is only 4 to 6 hours.

Insulin Aspart

Insulin aspart is a synthetic rapid-acting analog having a profile of action and therapeutic benefits similar to lispro.

Glargine

Glargine is a long-acting insulin analog that is used as a basal insulin replacement.

Regular Insulin

Regular insulin (crystalline zinc insulin) is a fast-acting preparation and is the only one that can be administered intravenously as well as subcutaneously. The administration of regular insulin is preferred for treating the abrupt onset of hyperglycemia or the appearance of ketoacidosis (1 to 5 U or IV 0.5 to 2 U/hour IV).

Isophane

Isophane protamine insulin (NPH) is an intermediate-acting preparation whose absorption from its subcutaneous injection site is delayed because the insulin is conjugated with protamine (0.005 mg/U of protamine).

Ultralente

Ultralente insulin is a long-acting insulin preparation that lacks protamine but has limited clinical usefulness because of its slow onset and prolonged duration of action.

Side Effects

Hypoglycemia

Hypoglycemia is the most serious side effect of insulin therapy (especially in patients who continue to receive exogenous insulin in the absence of carbohydrate intake, as may occur in the preoperative period) (Table 24-2). The diagnosis of hypoglycemia during general anesthesia is difficult, because the classic signs of sympathetic nervous system stimulation are likely to be masked by anesthetic drugs and, if they do occur, may be confused with responses evoked by painful stimulation. Severe hypoglycemia is treated with the intravenous administration of 50 to 100 ml of 50% glucose solutions. In the absence of central nervous system (CNS) depression, carbohydrates may be administered orally.

TABLE 24-2. SYMPTOMS OF HYPOGLYCEMIA
Compensatory effects of increased epinephrine secretion
Diaphoresis
Tachycardia
Hypertension
Mental confusion (may progress to seizures and coma)

Allergic Reactions

The use of human insulin preparations has eliminated the problem of systemic allergic reactions that could result from the administration of animal-derived insulins. Local allergic reactions to insulin are common and likely are due to noninsulin materials in the insulin preparations. Chronic exposure to low doses of protamine or NPH insulin may serve as an antigenic stimulus for the production of antibodies against protamine. These patients remain asymptomatic until a relatively large dose of intravenous protamine is administered to antagonize the anticoagulant effects of heparin.

Lipodystrophy

Lipodystrophy reflects the atrophy of fat at sites of subcutaneous insulin injection; this may be prevented by rotating injection sites.

Insulin Resistance

The use of human insulins has eliminated the problem of immunoresistance that could accompany the administration of animal insulins. Acute insulin resistance is associated with trauma, as produced by surgery and infection.

Drug Interactions

Hormones may counter the hypoglycemic effects of insulin (adrenocorticotropic hormone, estrogens, glucagon). Epinephrine inhibits the secretion of insulin and stimulates glycolysis.

ORAL HYPOGLYCEMICS

Oral hypoglycemics representing different mechanisms of action are available for controlling plasma glucose concentrations in patients with type 2 diabetes mellitus (Table 24-3). None of these drugs will adequately control hyperglycemia indefinitely (use combinations).

Sulfonylureas

Sulfonylureas are capable of lowering blood glucose to hypoglycemic levels. Although sulfonylureas are derivatives

TABLE 24-3.
ORAL DRUGS FOR TREATMENT OF TYPE 2 DIABETES MELLITUS

Sulfonylureas (stimulate insulin secretion; hypoglycemia a risk)
- Glyburide
- Glipizide
- Glimepiride
- Tolbutamide
- Chlorpropamide
- Acetohexamide

Meglitinides (stimulate insulin secretion; hypoglycemia a risk)
- Repaglinide
- Nateglinide

Biguanides (inhibit glucose production by the liver; hypoglycemia not a risk)
- Metformin

Thiazolidinediones (increase sensitivity to insulin for glucose uptake by skeletal muscles and adipose tissues; hypoglycemia not a risk)
- Rosiglitazone
- Pioglitazone

α-Glucosidase inhibitors (slows digestion and absorption of carbohydrates from the diet; hypoglycemia not a risk)
- Acarbose
- Miglitol

of sulfonamides, they have no antibacterial actions. These drugs should not be administered to patients with known allergies to sulfa drugs.

Mechanism of Action

Sulfonylureas act on pancreatic β-cells to inhibit adenosine triphosphate–sensitive potassium ion channels. As a result, an influx of calcium and the stimulation of exocytosis (release) of insulin storage granules occurs.

Pharmacokinetics (Table 24-4)

Side Effects (Table 24-5)

Although hypoglycemia secondary to sulfonylureas may be infrequent, it is often more prolonged and more dangerous than hypoglycemia secondary to insulin (Table 25-6).

Clinically Useful Sulfonylureas

Glyburide

Glyburide stimulates insulin secretion over a 24-hour period. Metabolism is in the liver (one active metabolite is produced), and a mild diuretic effect accompanies the use of this drug.

Glipizide

Glipizide stimulates insulin secretion over a 12-hour period. Metabolism is in the liver to an inactive metabolite, and a mild diuretic effect accompanies the use of this drug.

Glimepiride

Glimepiride decreases blood glucose concentrations by stimulating the release of insulin from the pancreas and may also decrease hepatic glucose production.

TABLE 24-4.

CLASSIFICATION AND PHARMACOKINETICS OF SULFONYLUREA ORAL HYPOGLYCEMICS

	Relative Potency	Daily Dose Range (mg)	Doses/Day	Duration of Action (hrs)	Elimination Half-Time (hrs)*
Glyburide	150	2.5–20	1–2	18–24	4.6–12
Glipizide	100	5–40	1–2	12–24	4–7
Tolbutamide	1	500–1,000	2–3	6–12	4–8
Acetohexamide	2.5	250–1,500	2	12–18	1.3–6
Chlorpropamide	6	100–750	1	36	30–36

*Approximate.

TABLE 24-5.
SIDE EFFECTS OF SULFONYLUREA ORAL HYPOGLYCEMICS

	Overall Incidence of Side Effects (%)	Incidence of Hypoglycemia (%)	Antidiuretic	Diuretic
Glyburide	7	4–6	No	Yes
Glipizide	6	2–4	No	Yes
Tolbutamide	3	<1	Yes	Yes
Acetohexamide	4	1	No	Yes
Chlorpropamide	9	4–6	Yes	No

TABLE 24-6.
COMPARISON OF SULFONYLUREA THERAPY WITH INSULIN THERAPY

Sulfonylurea	Insulin
Failed initial response in 10% to 15% of patients	No maximum dose
Secondary failure rate each year among treated patients is about 10%	
Hypoglycemia may be more severe	Hypoglycemia may be more frequent
Associated cardiac complications	Lipid levels lowered
Patients may prefer oral medication	Patients may resist injections

Tolbutamide

Tolbutamide is the shortest-acting and least potent sulfonylurea. Side effects are few but may include hypoglycemia and hyponatremia.

Acetohexamide

Acetohexamide differs from other sulfonylureas in that most of its hypoglycemic action is due to its principal metabolite, hydroxyhexamide. This drug is not recommended for patients with renal disease, because its active metabolite is excreted by the kidneys. This is the only sulfonylurea with uricosuric properties, making it an appropriate drug for the diabetic patient with gout.

Chlorpropamide

Chlorpropamide is the longest acting sulfonylurea, with a duration of action that may approach 72 hours (elimination half-time 33 hours). Because 20% of the drug is excreted unchanged, impaired renal function can lead to chlorpropamide accumulation. Approximately 5% of patients treated with chlorpropamide develop serum sodium concentrations <129 mEq/L (usually asymptomatic). Risk factors for the development of hyponatremia include age >60 years, female gender, and the concomitant administration of thiazide diuretics.

Meglitinides

Meglitinides exert effects on β-cells similar to sulfonylurea drugs, but these drugs have a prompt effect (about 1 hour) and a shorter duration of action (about 4 hours). These drugs are administered 15 to 30 minutes before a meal and should never be ingested while fasting.

α-Glucosidase Inhibitors

α-Glucosidase inhibitors (acarbose, miglitol) decrease carbohydrate digestion and absorption of disaccharides by interfering with intestinal glucosidase activity. This action results in a slow release of glucose from food and therefore slow absorption from the gastrointestinal tract; this is useful only as monotherapy when postprandial hyperglycemia is the main problem. Although hypoglycemia does not occur with monotherapy, it can occur when α-glucosidase inhibitors are added to sulfonylureas or insulin.

Biguanides

Biguanides decrease blood glucose concentrations and have a low risk of hypoglycemia, but with the introduction of sulfonylureas, their use was largely abandoned because of the risk of severe lactic acidosis.

Metformin

Metformin produces satisfactory results in approximately 50% of cases in which sulfonylureas have failed. Hypoglycemia does not occur, and the risk of lactic acidosis is remote (but possible). If metformin cannot be omitted before surgery, it is prudent to monitor for the development of lactic acidosis (arterial blood gases).

Pharmacokinetics

In contrast to sulfonylureas, metformin is not bound to proteins and does not undergo metabolism. It is eliminated by the kidneys; therefore it should be used with caution, if at all, in patients with renal dysfunction.

Mechanism of Action

Metformin acts primarily by decreasing excessive hepatic and renal glucose production, most likely through inhibiting gluconeogenesis. Endogenous insulin secretion is not stimulated.

Side Effects

The most serious, although rare, side effect of metformin therapy is lactic acidosis (greatest risk exists in the presence of hepatic dysfunction). The management of lactic acidosis is symptomatic because the underlying pathologic change (blockade of the mitochondrial respiratory chain) cannot be treated.

Thiazolidinediones

Thiazolidinediones (TZDs) act principally on skeletal muscles and adipose tissue to decrease insulin resistance that is present in nearly all type 2 diabetics. Like metformin, TZDs require the presence of insulin and are especially effective in obese patients. TZDs can cause weight gain (partly extracellular fluid), which presents as edema; this is undesirable in the presence of concurrent congestive heart failure.

The possibility of drug-induced liver dysfunction is the reason to periodically measure plasma concentrations of hepatic transaminases.

Combination Therapy

In patients with persistent hyperglycemia, none of the oral hypoglycemic drugs reliably normalizes HbA1c when used as monotherapy. Combination therapy supports the logic of targeting two or more different causes of hyperglycemia simultaneously.

Diuretics

25

Diuretics are among the most frequently prescribed drugs, with the classic pharmacologic response being diuresis (Stoelting RK, Hillier SC. Diuretics. In: *Pharmacology and Physiology in Anesthetic Practice*, 4th ed. Philadelphia, Lippincott Williams & Wilkins, 2006:486–495). These drugs may be classified according to their site of action on renal tubules and the mechanism by which they alter the excretion of solute (Tables 25-1 and 25-2 and Fig. 25-1). All diuretics may cause hypovolemia and azotemia but these complications are most likely to occur with loop diuretics (Table 25-3).

THIAZIDE DIURETICS

Thiazide diuretics are most often administered for the maintenance of treatment of essential hypertension in which the combination of diuresis, natriuresis and vasodilation are synergistic.

Mechanism of Action

Thiazide diuretics produce diuresis by inhibiting the reabsorption of sodium and chloride ions, principally in the cortical portions of the ascending loops of Henle and, to a lesser extent, in the proximal and distal renal tubules. Thiazide diuretics, by inhibiting sodium reabsorption, lead to the delivery of higher concentrations of sodium to the distal renal tubules and the subsequent enhancement of potassium secretion into the renal tubules.

TABLE 25-1.
CLASSIFICATION OF DIURETICS

	Clinical Uses
Thiazide Diuretics	
Chlorothiazide	Essential hypertension, edema due to congestive heart failure, renal failure, hepatic failure
Hydrochlorothiazide	Same as chlorothiazide
Bendroflumethiazide	Same as chlorothiazide
Hydroflumethiazide	Same as chlorothiazide
Methyclothiazide	Same as chlorothiazide
Polythiazide	Same as chlorothiazide
Trichlormethiazide	Same as chlorothiazide
Indapamide	Same as chlorothiazide
Loop Diuretics	
Furosemide	Severe essential hypertension, edema due to congestive heart failure, renal failure, hepatic failure
Ethacrynic acid	
Bumetanide	Same as furosemide
Torsemide	Same as furosemide
Osmotic Diuretics	
Mannitol	Intracranial hypertension, prophylaxis against or treatment of the oliguric phase of acute renal failure
Urea	
Potassium-Sparing Diuretics	
Triamterene	Edema associated with congestive heart failure, renal failure, hepatic failure
Amiloride	Essential hypertension, or edema due to congestive heart failure, often in combination with thiazide or loop diuretics
Aldosterone Antagonists (Potassium-Sparing)	
Spironolactone	Edema associated with congestive heart failure, renal failure, hepatic failure

TABLE 25-1.
(continued)

Carbonic Anhydrase Inhibitors	
Acetazolamide	Glaucoma, altitude sickness, persistent metabolic alkalosis
Dopamine Receptor Agonists	
Dopamine	Not recommended as prophylaxis against oliguric phase of acute renal failure
Fenoldopam	

Antihypertensive Effect

The antihypertensive effect of thiazide diuretics is due initially to a decrease in extracellular fluid volume. The sustained antihypertensive effect of thiazide diuretics, however, is due to peripheral vasodilation, which requires several weeks to develop.

Side Effects

Thiazide diuretic–induced hypokalemic, hypochloremic, metabolic acidosis is a common side effect when these drugs are administered chronically for the treatment of essential hypertension (see Table 25-3). Intravascular fluid volume should be considered in all patients treated with thiazide diuretics and scheduled for surgery; the presence of orthostatic hypotension should arouse suspicion—laboratory evidence includes hemoconcentration manifesting as an increased hematocrit and increased blood urea nitrogen concentration.

LOOP DIURETICS

The loop diuretics (ethacrynic acid, bumetanide, furosemide) inhibit the reabsorption of sodium and chloride primarily in the medullary portions of the ascending limbs

TABLE 25-2.
SITES OF ACTION OF DIURETICS

	Thiazide Diuretics	Loop Diuretics	Osmotic Diuretics	Potassium Sparing	Aldosterone Antagonists	Carbonic Anhydrase
Early proximal convoluted tubule		+	+			
Proximal convoluted tubule	+	+				+++
Medullary portion of ascending loop of Henle		+++	+++			
Cortical portion of ascending loop of Henle	+++	+	+			
Distal convoluted tubule	+	+	+	+++		+
Collecting duct					+++	

+, minor site of action; +++, major site of action.

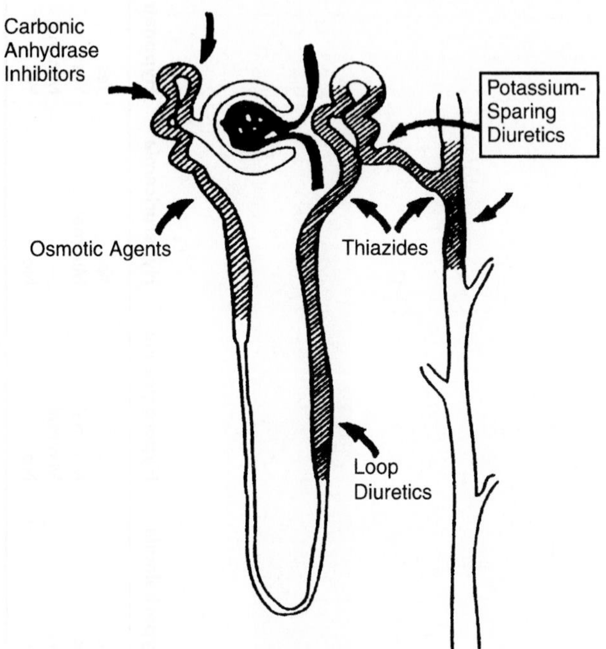

Figure 25-1. Sites of action of diuretics.

of the loops of Henle ("loop diuretics") (see Table 25-2). These are the most potent saluretic drugs available. Furosemide-induced increases in renal blood flow are inhibited by nonsteroidal antiinflammatory drugs, manifesting as an attenuated diuretic effect.

Pharmacokinetics

Ethacrynic Acid

Ethacrynic acid is excreted by the kidneys as unchanged drug and an unstable metabolite.

TABLE 25-3.
SIDE EFFECTS OF DIURETICS

	Hypokalemic, Hyperchloremic, Metabolic Alkalosis	Hyperkalemia	Hyperglycemia	Hyperuricemia	Hyponatremia
Thiazide diuretics	Yes	No	Yes	Yes	Yes
Loop diuretics	Yes	No	Minimal	Minimal	Yes
Potassium-sparing	No	Yes	Minimal	—	Minimal
Aldosterone	No	Yes	No	No	Yes

TABLE 25-4.
CLINICAL USES OF LOOP DIURETICS (FUROSEMIDE)

Mobilization of edema fluid due to renal, hepatic or cardiac dysfunction (furosemide 0.1 to 1 mg/kg IV)
Treatment of increased intracranial pressure (furosemide 0.5 to 1.0 mg/kg IV)
Differential diagnosis of acute oliguria (furosemide 0.1 mg/kg IV will stimulate diuresis in the presence of excessive arginine vasopressin; do not administer to treat acute oliguria due to decreased intravascular fluid volume, the use to treat acute renal failure is controversial)

Furosemide

Furosemide undergoes renal tubular secretion, as well as metabolism and excretion in the bile. The elimination half-time of furosemide is <1 hour, thus accounting for the short duration of action.

Clinical Uses (Table 25-4)

Side Effects (See Table 25-3 and 25-5)

TABLE 25-5.
SIDE EFFECTS OF LOOP DIURETICS (FUROSEMIDE)

Hypokalemia (increases likelihood of digitalis toxicity)
Acute tolerance (treatment is extracellular volume repletion)
Hyperuricemia
Hyperglycemia (less likely than with thiazide diuretics)
Enhances nephrotoxic effects of aminoglycosides
Allergic interstitial nephritis (similar to that produced by penicillin)
Cross-sensitivity with sulfonamides
Deafness (dose-dependent)

OSMOTIC DIURETICS

Osmotic diuretics (mannitol, urea) are freely filterable at the glomerulus, undergo limited reabsorption from renal tubules, resist metabolism, and are pharmacologically inert.

Mannitol

Mannitol is a six-carbon sugar that does not undergo metabolism. It must be administered intravenously, because it is not absorbed from the gastrointestinal tract.

Mechanism of Action

Mannitol is completely filtered at the glomeruli, and none of the filtered drug is subsequently reabsorbed from the renal tubules. Therefore, mannitol increases the osmolarity of renal tubular fluid and prevents the reabsorption of water. As a result of this osmotic effect in the renal tubular fluid, an osmotic diuretic effect occurs with the urinary excretion of water, sodium, chloride, and bicarbonate ions. In addition to causing renal tubule effects, the intravenous administration of mannitol also increases plasma osmolarity, thus drawing fluid from intracellular to extracellular spaces. This increased plasma osmolarity may result in an acute expansion of intravascular fluid volume. A redistribution of fluid from intracellular sites decreases brain bulk and may preferentially increase renal blood flow to the medulla.

Clinical Uses (Table 25-6)

Side Effects

In patients with oliguria secondary to cardiac failure, acute mannitol-induced increases in intravascular fluid volume may precipitate pulmonary edema (furosemide may be the preferred drug for the treatment of increased intracranial pressure in patients with left ventricular dysfunction). Prolonged use of mannitol may cause hypovolemia and

TABLE 25-6.
CLINICAL USES OF MANNITOL

Prophylaxis against acute renal failure (predictable diuresis but evidence of a renal protective effect is lacking)
Differential diagnosis of acute oliguria (increases urine output when cause is decreased intravascular fluid volume but not when glomerular or renal tubular function are compromised)
Treatment of increased intracranial pressure (0.25 to 1.0 mg/kg IV infused over 10 minutes draws water from tissues, including the brain, along an osmotic gradient; works within 10 to 15 minutes; administer in conjunction with corticosteroids and hyperventilation of the lungs)
Reduction of intraocular pressure

electrolyte disturbances. Diuresis secondary to mannitol does not alter the elimination rate of long-acting nondepolarizing neuromuscular-blocking drugs (predictable as mannitol does not alter the glomerular filtration rate).

Urea

Urea is an effective osmotic diuretic, but unlike mannitol, it undergoes reabsorption from the renal tubules and eventually penetrates cells and crosses the blood-brain barrier (causing a rebound increase in intracranial pressure). Another disadvantage of urea is the high incidence of venous thrombosis.

POTASSIUM-SPARING DIURETICS

Potassium-sparing diuretics (triamterene, amiloride) act directly on renal tubular transport mechanisms in the distal convoluted tubules, independent of aldosterone to produce diuresis. Diuresis is accompanied by no increase or a decrease in potassium excretion in the urine (reflects inhibition of potassium secretion into distal renal tubules).

Pharmacokinetics

The metabolism of triamterene is extensive, and some of its metabolites have diuretic activity. The half-time of triamterene is 3 to 5 hours and, for amiloride, is about 18 hours.

Clinical Uses

Potassium-sparing diuretics are most often used in combination with loop diuretics or thiazide diuretics to augment diuresis and limit the renal loss of potassium.

Side Effects

Hyperkalemia is the principal side effect of therapy using potassium-sparing diuretics (see Table 25-3).

ALDOSTERONE ANTAGONISTS

Mechanism of Action

Spironolactone binds to cytoplasmic mineralocorticoid receptors (inhibits gene expression) on collecting ducts and acts as a competitive antagonist to aldosterone. Normally, aldosterone augments the renal tubular reabsorption of sodium and chloride ions and increases the excretion of potassium ions. The effects of spironolactone on aldosterone transport last 48 to 72 hours after spironolactone is discontinued, thus emphasizing the risk of hyperkalemic, hyperchloremic acidosis in patients receiving this drug and who develop acute renal failure.

Pharmacokinetics

Spironolactone undergoes extensive hepatic first-pass metabolism, binding to plasma proteins is extensive, and virtually no unchanged drug appears in the urine.

Clinical Uses

Spironolactone is often prescribed for the treatment of refractory edematous states due to congestive heart failure and cirrhosis of the liver, on the assumption that decreased hepatic function and metabolism lead to increased plasma concentrations of aldosterone.

Side Effects

Hyperkalemia, especially in the presence of renal dysfunction, is the most serious side effect of treatment with spironolactone (see Table 25-3).

CARBONIC ANHYDRASE INHIBITORS

Acetazolamide is the prototype of this class of sulfonamide drugs that binds avidly to carbonic anhydrase enzyme, producing a noncompetitive inhibition of enzyme activity principally in the proximal renal tubules. As a result of this enzyme inhibition, the excretion of hydrogen ions is diminished and loss of bicarbonate ions is increased. Chloride is retained by the kidneys to offset the loss of bicarbonate ions. Decreased availability of hydrogen ions in the distal renal tubules results in excretion of potassium in exchange for sodium. The net effect of all these changes is excretion of an alkaline urine in the presence of hyperchloremic metabolic acidosis.

Clinical Uses (Table 25-7)

DOPAMINE RECEPTOR AGONISTS (SEE TABLE 25-1)

In the renal vasculature, dopamine-1 receptors mediate vasodilation and increase renal blood flow and glomerular

TABLE 25-7.
CLINICAL USES OF ACETAZOLAMIDE

Treat altitude sickness
Decrease intraocular pressure (inhibits formation of aqueous humor)
Inhibit seizure activity (presumably by producing metabolic acidosis)
Treat familial period paralysis (metabolic acidosis increases the local concentration of potassium in skeletal muscles)
Stimulate ventilation in patients who are hypoventilating as a compensatory response to metabolic alkalosis

filtration rate. In renal tubules, the stimulation of dopamine-1 receptors inhibits sodium reabsorption and promotes natriuresis.

Dopamine

Dopamine could provide renoprotective effects by inhibiting the sodium pump and decreasing renal tubule oxygen consumption. Nevertheless, data confirming a prophylactic renal protective effect of low-dose dopamine are lacking, and the routine use of dopamine for this purpose cannot be recommended.

Fenoldopam

Fenoldopam is a selective dopamine-1 receptor agonist that lacks dopamine-2, α-, and β-agonist effects. The principal use of fenoldopam is as an intravenous antihypertensive drug (unlike sodium nitroprusside, it does not decrease renal blood flow). A renoprotective effect of fenoldopam has not been established.

Antacids and Gastrointestinal Prokinetics

26

ANTACIDS

Antacids are drugs that neutralize or remove acid from gastric contents (Stoelting RK, Hillier SC. Antacids and gastrointestinal prokinetics. In: *Pharmacology and Physiology in Anesthetic Practice*, 4th ed. Philadelphia: Lippincott Williams & Wilkins, 2006:496–504). Clinically useful antacids are aluminum, calcium, and magnesium salts that react with hydrochloric acid to form neutral, less acidic, or poorly soluble salts. Antacids produce a beneficial effect on the rate of duodenal ulcer healing that is similar to H_2-receptor antagonists. Although antacids are commonly prescribed with nonsteroidal antiinflammatory drugs for prophylaxis against drug-induced gastroduodenal mucosa injury, little evidence supports the efficacy of this practice.

Commercial Antacid Preparations (Table 26-1)

Sodium Bicarbonate

Sodium bicarbonate results in a prompt and rapid antacid action, but the effect is brief and systemic alkalosis is possible. Sodium bicarbonate is useful if the goal is to alkalinize the urine.

TABLE 26-1.
CONTENTS (mg per 5 mL) OF PARTICULATE ANTACIDS

	Aluminum Hydroxide	Magnesium Hydroxide	Calcium Carbonate	Sodium
Aludrox	307	103		1.1
Amphojel	320			6.9
Di-Gel	282	85		10.6
Gelusil	200	200		0.7
Maalox	225	200		1.35
Mylanta	200	200		0.68
Riopan	480			0.3
Tums			500	<3
Win Gel	180	160		<2.5

Magnesium Hydroxide

Magnesium hydroxide (milk of magnesia) produces a prompt neutralization of gastric acid, and an osmotic diarrhea (laxative effect) is characteristic. The systemic absorption of magnesium may be sufficient to cause neurologic, neuromuscular, and cardiovascular impairment in patients with renal dysfunction.

Calcium Carbonate

Calcium carbonate produces a prompt and effective neutralization of gastric acid; chronic therapy may be associated with the development of metabolic alkalosis. Clinically, dangerous hypercalcemia may occur in patients with renal disease. The administration of calcium-carbonate—containing antacids may be accompanied by hypophosphatemia.

Aluminum Hydroxide

Aluminum hydroxide may produce excessive plasma and tissue concentrations of aluminum in patients with renal disease. Hypophosphatemia may occur, and increased

TABLE 26-2.
COMPLICATIONS OF ANTACID THERAPY

Acid rebound (caused only by calcium-containing antacids)
Milk-alkali syndrome (hypercalcemia, increased blood urea nitrogen, systemic alkalosis)
Phosphorus depletion (aluminum salts bind phosphate ions, may be therapeutic in patients with renal disease)
Drug interactions (hasten delivery of drugs to small intestine, deceases bioavailability if complexes with antacids are formed)

absorption of calcium ions sometimes causes hypercalcuria and nephrolithiasis.

Complications of Antacid Therapy (Table 26-2)

Antacid Selection

Considerable variation exists in the acid-neutralizing effects of different antacids. Selection must be based on mechanism of action, desired effect, and the side effect profile.

Preoperative Administration of Antacids

The potential value of the preoperative administration of antacids is based on the unproved presumption that drug-induced increases in the gastric fluid pH would decrease the likelihood of the development of severe acid pneumonitis should inhalation (aspiration) of acidic gastric fluid occur. Antacids or other prophylactic drugs administered to alter gastric fluid pH or volume (H_2-antagonists, metoclopramide) do not influence the incidence of regurgitation and aspiration. In selected patients, it seems logical to administer an antacid as a single dose approximately 30 minutes before the anticipated induction of anesthesia (repeated doses of antacid may increase gastric fluid volume).

Particulate Antacids

The occasional failure of particulate antacids to increase gastric fluid pH levels may reflect an inadequate mixing with stomach contents or an unusually large volume of gastric fluid. Layering is also common with particulate antacids. The associated pneumonitis may reflect a foreign body reaction to inhaled particulate antacid particles.

Nonparticulate Antacids

Nonparticulate or clear antacids (sodium citrate 15 to 30 mL) are less likely to cause a foreign body reaction if aspirated, and their mixing with gastric fluid is more complete than is that of particulate antacids. The onset of effect is more rapid with sodium citrate than with particulate antacids that require a longer time for adequate mixing with gastric fluid. The pH of sodium citrate is 8.4, accounting for its unpleasant taste and frequent need to add a flavoring material to improve its palatability. Bicitra and Polycitra are more palatable than sodium citrate.

SUCRALFATE

Sucralfate is a complex salt of sucrose sulfate and aluminum hydroxide that forms a viscous suspension that binds to normal and defective mucosa; it lacks an antacid action. Aluminum absorption is a consideration in patients with renal disease. Sucralfate interferes with the absorption and bioavailability of several drugs.

GASTROINTESTINAL PROKINETICS

Metoclopramide (methoxychloroprocainamide) is a dopamine antagonist that is structurally similar to procainamide but lacks local anesthetic activity. This drug acts as a gastrointestinal prokinetic (accelerated gastric clearance and shortened transit time through the small intestine) that increases lower esophageal sphincter tone.

Mechanism of Action

Metoclopramide produces selective cholinergic stimulation of the gastrointestinal tract, which is largely restricted to smooth muscles of the proximal gastrointestinal tract. This may be offset by the concomitant administration of atropine in the preoperative medication. Dopamine-induced inhibition of gastrointestinal motility is not considered to be clinically significant. In the central nervous system (CNS), metoclopramide blocks dopamine receptors (may produce extrapyramidal effects).

Pharmacokinetics

Extensive first-pass hepatic metabolism limits the bioavailability of metoclopramide.

Clinical Uses (Table 26-3)

Side Effects (Table 26-4)

Cisapride

Cisapride is a gastrointestinal prokinetic drug that stimulates gastric emptying, increases lower esophageal sphincter tone, and enhances motility in the small and large intestine by enhancing the release of acetylcholine from nerve endings in the myenteric plexus of the gastrointestinal mucosa. Opioid-induced gastric stasis, which is an important cause of postoperative nausea and vomiting, is reversed by cisapride.

Domperidone

Domperidone is a benzimidazole derivative that, like metoclopramide, acts as a specific dopamine antagonist

TABLE 26-3.
CLINICAL USES OF METOCLOPRAMIDE

Preoperative decrease of gastric fluid volume (10 to 20 mg IV over 3 to 5 minutes 15 to 30 minutes before induction of anesthesia; do not administer if known or suspected obstruction to gastric emptying)
Recent ingestion of solid food
Diabetes mellitus and gastroparesis
Trauma
Obese
Parturients
Antiemetic (antagonism of dopamine at the chemoreceptor trigger zone, reverses gastric stasis produced by morphine)
Treatment of gastroparesis
Treatment of gastroesophageal reflux

TABLE 26-4.
SIDE EFFECTS OF METOCLOPRAMIDE

Abdominal cramping
Hypotension, tachycardia, cardiac dysrhythmias (following IV administration)
Sedation
Dysphoria
Breast enlargement (galactorrhea)
Dystonic extrapyramidal reactions (oculogyric crises, opisthotonus, trismus, torticollis)
Akathisia
Inhibition of plasma cholinesterase activity (prolonged responses to succinylcholine and mivacurium, slowed metabolism of ester local anesthetics)
Drug interactions (monoamine oxidase inhibitors, tricyclic antidepressants)

that stimulates peristalsis in the gastrointestinal tract, speeds gastric emptying, and increases lower esophageal sphincter tone. Unlike, metoclopramide, domperidone does not easily cross the blood-brain barrier (lacks extrapyramidal effects) and does not appear to have any anticholinergic activity.

Erythromycin

Erythromycin increases lower esophageal sphincter tone, enhances intraduodenal coordination, and promotes the emptying of gastric liquids and solids. These prokinetic properties are attributed to cholinergic stimulatory properties.

Anticoagulants

27

Anticoagulants (heparin, enoxaparin, coumadin compounds) are drugs that delay or prevent the clotting of blood by their direct or indirect actions on the coagulation system (Stoelting RK, Hillier SC. Anticoagulants. In: *Pharmacology and Physiology in Anesthetic Practice*. 4th ed. Philadelphia, Lippincott Williams & Wilkins, 2006:505–520). Antithrombotic drugs (aspirin) usually influence the formation of thrombus by interfering with the normal adhesive and aggregation activity of platelets. Thrombolytic drugs are those that possess inherent fibrinolytic effects or enhance the body's fibrinolytic system.

HEPARIN

Heparin is composed of a mixture of highly sulfated glycosaminoglycans that produce their anticoagulant effects by binding to antithrombin, which is normally present as a naturally circulating anticoagulant (binding with heparin enhances by about 1,000 times the ability of antithrombin to inactivate a number of coagulation enzymes).

Commercial Preparations

Commercial preparations of heparin are most commonly prepared from bovine lung and bovine or porcine gastrointestinal mucosa. The designation *heparin* emphasizes the abundance of this substance in the liver. The standardization of heparin potency is based on in vitro comparison with a known standard.

Pharmacokinetics

Heparin is poorly lipid-soluble and cannot cross lipid barriers in significant amounts; it is poorly absorbed from the gastrointestinal tract and is usually administered by intravenous or subcutaneous injection. Heparin does not cross the placenta and can be administered to the mother without producing anticoagulation in the fetus.

Laboratory Evaluation of Coagulation

The anticoagulant response to heparin varies widely among patients with thromboembolic disease, possibly because of variations in the plasma concentrations of heparin-binding proteins.

Activated Plasma Thromboplastin Time

Heparin treatment is usually monitored to maintain the ratio of the activated plasma thromboplastin (APTT) within a defined range of approximately 1.5 to 2.5 times the predrug value, which is typically 30 to 35 seconds. An excessively prolonged APTT (>120 seconds) is readily shortened by omitting a dose, because heparin has a brief elimination half-time.

Activated Coagulation Time

Heparin's effect and its antagonism by protamine are commonly monitored in patients undergoing surgical procedures by measuring the activated coagulation time (ACT). During cardiopulmonary bypass, the anticoagulant effect of heparin is often considered adequate if the ACT is >300 seconds (normal 90 to 120 seconds).

Clinical Uses (Table 27-1)

Side Effects (Table 27-2)

Reversal of Heparin-Induced Anticoagulation

TABLE 27-1.
CLINICAL USES OF HEPARIN

Prophylaxis against venous thromboembolism (enoxaparin especially in patients undergoing hip surgery)
Treatment of venous thromboembolism (IV heparin to maintain activated plasma thromboplastin time 1.5 to 2.5 times normal; anticoagulation is maintained for 3 to 6 months)
Treatment of unstable angina and acute myocardial infarction (IV heparin followed by a continuous infusion)

Protamine

Protamine is the specific antagonist of heparin's anticoagulant effect; the positively charged alkaline protamine combines with the negatively charged heparin to form a stable complex that is devoid of anticoagulant activity. The clearance of protamine by the reticuloendothelial system (20 minutes) is more rapid than heparin clearance, which may

TABLE 27-2.
SIDE EFFECTS OF HEPARIN

Hemorrhage (epidural hematoma)
Thrombocytopenia
- Mild (drug-induced platelet aggregation, platelet counts <100,000 cells/mm^3, typically manifests between 3 and 15 days)
- Severe (platelet counts <50,000 cells^3, resistance to heparin effect, typically develops after 6 to 10 days, probably due to formation of heparin-dependent antiplatelet antibodies that trigger platelet aggregation)

Allergic reactions
Cardiovascular changes (decreased systemic vascular resistance and decreases in mean arterial pressure)
Altered protein binding (displaces alkaline drugs)
Altered cell morphology
Decreased antithrombin concentrations

explain, in part, the phenomenon of heparin rebound. The dose of protamine required to antagonize heparin is typically 1 mg for every 100 U of heparin predicted to still be circulating (more specific dose of protamine is calculated by in vitro titration of the patient's blood with protamine).

Hypotension

The rapid intravenous injection of protamine may be associated with histamine release (reflects the alkaline characteristics of protamine) that causes facial flushing, tachycardia, and hypotension.

Pulmonary Hypertension

In rare cases, protamine neutralization can result in the secretion of thromboxane and 5-hydroxytryptamine (serotonin), manifesting as pulmonary vasoconstriction, pulmonary hypertension, and bronchoconstriction. Arterial hypoxemia reflects ventilation–perfusion mismatching due to pulmonary edema secondary to pulmonary hypertension. These responses do not occur in patients manifesting systemic blood pressure changes traditionally attributed to histamine release.

Allergic Reactions

Allergic reactions to protamine have been described most often in patients receiving protamine-containing insulin preparations; the chronic exposure results in the formation of antibodies that result in an allergic reaction when a large dose of protamine is administered to antagonize heparin. Patients who are allergic to fish may also be at increased risk for the development of allergic reactions to protamine.

Platelet Factor 4

Platelet factor 4 is an endogenous polypeptide released during platelet aggregation that may be an alternative to protamine for the reversal of heparin anticoagulation.

Heparinase-I

Heparinase-I is a specific heparin degrading enzyme that may represent an alternative to protamine.

LOW MOLECULAR WEIGHT HEPARINS

Low molecular weight heparins (enoxaparin, dalteparin) are derived from standard commercial-grade unfractionated heparin by chemical depolymerization to yield fragments approximately one-third the size of heparin. The pharmacokinetics of these heparins is consistent between patients, so that bioavailability is greater at low doses and anticoagulant responses are more predictable. The elimination half-time is longer, thus permitting once daily dosing. Therapeutic doses do not usually affect the prothrombin time and APTT. The risk of bleeding from therapeutic doses of low-molecular weight heparin approaches that of unfractionated heparin.

Spinal and Epidural Hematoma

The incidence of spontaneous spinal and epidural hematomas is increased in the presence of low-molecular weight heparin. This increased risk of hematoma formation is a consideration when selecting regional anesthesia in patients being treated with low-molecular weight heparin.

DANAPAROID

Danaparoid is low-molecular weight heparinoid compound that attenuates fibrin formation principally by binding of antithrombin. The elimination of danaparoid is predominantly through the kidneys.

FONDAPARINUX

Fondaparinux is a synthetic anticoagulant that complexes with antithrombin and inhibits factor Xa. Dosing is once daily, and elimination is through the kidneys.

ORAL ANTICOAGULANTS

Oral anticoagulants are derivatives of 4-hydroxycoumarin (coumarin) (Table 27-3). Disadvantages of oral anticoagulants include a delayed onset of action (8 to 12 hours and peak effects in 36 to 72 hours), the need for regular laboratory monitoring, difficulty in reversal should a surgical procedure create concern about bleeding, and the need to be administered orally should gastrointestinal dysfunction be present.

Mechanism of Action

Warfarin inhibits vitamin K epoxide reductase and thus blocks the conversion of vitamin K epoxide to vitamin K. The subsequent depletion of vitamin K results in the production of hemostatically defective vitamin K–dependent coagulation proteins (prothrombin, factors VII, IX, and X). Platelet activity is not altered by oral anticoagulants.

Pharmacokinetics

Warfarin is rapidly and completely absorbed, and protein binding (97%) contributes to its negligible renal excretion and long elimination half-time (24 to 36 hours). Warfarin crosses the placenta and produces exaggerated effects in the fetus, which has limited ability to synthesize clotting factors.

Laboratory Evaluation

Treatment with oral anticoagulants is best guided by measurement of the prothrombin time. For most indications, a moderate anticoagulant effect with a targeted international normalized ratio (INR) of 2.0 to 3.0 is appropriate. An excessively prolonged prothrombin time is not readily shortened by omitting a dose because of the long elimination half-time of oral anticoagulants. Preexisting liver disease and advanced age are associated with enhanced effects of oral anticoagulants.

TABLE 27-3.
COMPARATIVE PHARMACOLOGY OF ORAL ANTICOAGULANTS

	Time to Peak Effect (hrs)	Duration After Discontinuation (days)	Initial Adult Dose (mg)	Maintenance Adult Dose (mg)
Warfarin	36–72	2–5	15 first day 10 second day 10 third day	2.5–10
Dicumarol	36–48	2–6	200–300 first day	25–200
Phenindione	18–24	1–2	300 first day 200 second day	25–200

TABLE 27-4.
CLINICAL USES OF ORAL ANTICOAGULANTS

Prevention of venous thromboembolism (maintain INR 2.0 to 3.0 following hip surgery; continue for up to 3 months after an initial course of heparin in patients with proximal deep vein thrombosis)
Prevention of systemic embolization
  Prosthetic heart valves
  Atrial fibrillation
Prevention of stroke and recurrent myocardial infarction in patients with acute myocardial infarction

Clinical Uses (Table 27-4)

Management before Elective Surgery

Relatively minor surgical procedures can be performed safely in patients receiving oral anticoagulants. For major surgery, discontinuation of oral anticoagulants 1 to 3 days preoperatively is recommended to permit the prothrombin time to return to within 20% of its normal range. If immediate reversal is needed, the administration of recombinant factor VIIa, 1 to 2 units of fresh frozen plasma, or a prothrombin complex concentrate is effective.

Drug Interactions (Table 27-5)

Side Effects

Bleeding is the main complication of oral anticoagulant therapy; this risk is increased by the intensity of anticoagulant therapy, the patient's underlying disorder (neoplasm, peptic ulcer), and the concomitant use of aspirin. Treatment of mild hemorrhage is with administration of vitamin K, 10 to 20 mg orally or 1 to 5 mg IV at a rate of 1 mg/min, which will usually return the prothrombin time to normal in 4 to 24 hours. Oral anticoagulants cross the

TABLE 27-5.
DRUG INTERACTIONS THAT INCREASE PLASMA WARFARIN LEVELS

Phenylbutazone
Amiodarone
Cimetidine
Omeprazole
Cephalosporins
Heparin
Aspirin
Nonsteroidal anti-inflammatory drugs

placenta and can produce a characteristic embryopathy and central nervous system damage.

THROMBOLYTIC DRUGS

Thrombolytic drugs act as plasminogen activators to convert the endogenous proenzyme plasminogen to the fibrinolytic enzyme plasmin (fibrinolysis) (Table 27-6).

The goal of thrombolytic therapy is to restore circulation through a previously occluded artery or vein, most often a coronary artery, within 12 hours after onset of symptoms (Table 27-7). Aspirin should also be started promptly in all patients with suspected acute coronary syndrome or unstable angina. Spontaneous bleeding, such as intracranial hemorrhage, is the principal risk of thrombolytic drug therapy, especially in patients who have recently experienced trauma or undergone surgery or invasive diagnostic procedures.

Streptokinase

Streptokinase is a protein produced by β-hemolytic streptococci that binds to plasminogen and ultimately results in plasmin. Laboratory monitoring of streptokinase can

TABLE 27-6.
COMPARISON OF THROMBOLYTIC DRUGS

	Streptokinase	Alteplase	Antistreplase
Dose (intravenous)	1.5 million units infused over 1 hour	100 mg (1.25 mg/kg infused over 3 hours)	30 units infused over 2–5 minutes
Clinical uses	ACS, PE	ACS, PE	ACS, PE
Site of action	Plasminogen	Plasminogen	Plasminogen
Elimination half-time	23 minutes	<5 minutes	<5 minutes
Clearance	Hepatic	Hepatic	Hepatic
Reperfusion success rate	50% to 70%	60% to 80%	60% to 80%
Antidote	Antifibrinolytics	Antifibrinolytics	Antifibrinolytics
Hypotensive effect	Moderate	Minimal	Minimal
Allergic reactions	Yes	No	No
Stop before surgery	3 hours	1 hour	1 hour
Prolongation of PT/PTT	Yes/Yes	Yes/Yes	Yes/Yes
Cost	Expensive	Very expensive	Very expensive

ACS, acute coronary syndrome; PE, pulmonary embolism; PT, prothrombin time; PTT, activated plasma thromboplastin time.

TABLE 27-7.
SELECTION OF PATIENTS TO RECEIVE THROMBOLYTIC DRUGS

Relative Contraindications
- Trauma or surgery more than 14 days previously
- Chronic and severe hypertension
- Active peptic ulcer disease
- Treatment with anticoagulants
- Known bleeding diathesis
- Significant liver dysfunction
- Prior exposure to streptokinase or anistreplase (not a problem with urokinase or alteplase)

Absolute Contraindications
- Active internal bleeding
- Trauma or surgery in the last 14 days
- Recent head trauma or known intracranial aneurysm
- History of hemorrhagic cerebrovascular accident
- Systemic blood pressure >200/120 mm Hg
- Previous allergic reaction (applicable only for streptokinase and anistreplase)
- Traumatic cardiopulmonary resuscitation
- Suspected aortic dissection
- Diabetic hemorrhagic retinopathy
- Pregnancy

be limited to thrombin time, which is used as a marker for an effective lytic state.

Alteplase

Alteplase (recombinant tissue plasminogen activator) is a fibrin-specific thrombolytic drug that is synthesized by endothelial cells.

Anistreplase

Anistreplase (anisoylated plasminogen streptokinase activator complex) has a longer duration of action and can be administered as a single intravenous injection.

DIRECT THROMBIN INHIBITORS

Direct thrombin inhibitors suppress platelet function and are used for the treatment of arterial and venous thrombotic disease (Table 27-8). The antithrombotic drugs include hirudin, aspirin, dipyridamole, and dextran.

Recombinant Hirudin

Recombinant hirudin (desirudin, lepirudin) is a antithrombotic drug that produces anticoagulation through the direct inhibition of thrombin. The risk of spontaneous bleeding is not increased in patients treated with hirudin, compared with heparin. Hirudin is an alternative to heparin in patients who require anticoagulation for surgery but who have developed heparin resistance or heparin-induced thrombocytopenia. Administered intravenously, the onset of action is rapid and the peak effect occurs in about 4 hours.

Ximelagatran

Ximelagatran is an orally effective direct thrombin inhibitor that may be effective prophylaxis against and treatment of thromboembolism. Monitoring of coagulation or dose adjustments is not necessary.

Argatroban

Argatroban is an arginine derivative that is a highly specific thrombin inhibitor. Argatroban is an alternative to heparin for anticoagulation in patients requiring cardiopulmonary bypass.

ADENOSINE DIPHOSPHATE INHIBITORS

Adenosine diphosphate inhibitors are used principally for the prevention of arterial thrombosis, and these drugs act by inhibiting platelet aggregation through different mechanisms (Table 27-9).

TABLE 27-8.

PROPERTIES OF DIRECT THROMBIN INHIBITORS

Drug	Route of Administration	Excretion	Clinical Uses	Stop Before Surgery (hrs)	Prolong PT/PTT	Antidote
Hirudin	Intravenous	Renal	Heparin-induced thrombocytopenia	8	Yes/Yes	Hemodialysis
Ximelagatran	Oral	Renal	Thromboprophylaxis Treatment of deep vein thrombosis	24	Yes/Yes	None
Argatroban	Intravenous	Hepatic	Heparin-induced thrombocytopenia	4–6	Yes/Yes	None
Bivalirudin	Intravenous	Hepatic	Coronary interventions	2–3	Yes/Yes	None

TABLE 27-9.

PROPERTIES OF ADENOSINE DIPHOSPHATE INHIBITORS

	Site of Action	Route of Adminis-tration	Elimination Half-Time	Clearance	Antidote	Stop Before Surgery	Prolong PT/PTT	Clinical Uses
Aspirin	COX	Oral	20 minutes	Hepatic	None	7 days	No/No	ACS Stroke
Dipyridamole	Aden-osine	Oral	40 minutes	Hepatic	None	24 hrs	No/No	PVD
Clopidogrel	ADP	Oral	7 hours	Hepatic	None	7 days	No/No	CAD PVD
Ticlopidine	ADP	Oral	4 days		None	4 days	No/No	CAD PVD

Aspirin

Aspirin inhibits thromboxane synthesis by interfering with the activity of cyclooxygenase I and 2 enzymes and the subsequent release of adenosine diphosphate by platelets and their aggregation.

Clopidogrel and Ticlopidine

Clopidogrel and ticlopidine are prodrugs that are converted to active metabolites in the liver. These metabolites block adenosine diphosphate (ADP) receptors on platelet surfaces, thus inhibiting platelet activation, aggregation, and degranulation. Side effects of these ADP receptor antagonists include neutropenia, hepatic dysfunction, and hemorrhage (intracranial, gastrointestinal).

Dipyridamole

Dipyridamole is most often administered in combination with warfarin to patients with prosthetic heart valves, because it inhibits platelet aggregation.

Dextran

Dextran may be of value in the prevention of postoperative thromboembolic disease.

PLATELET GLYCOPROTEIN IIb/IIIa ANTAGONISTS

Platelet glycoprotein IIb /IIIa antagonists act at the corresponding fibrinogen receptor that is important for platelet aggregation (Table 27-10).

Clinical Uses

Glycoprotein IIb/IIIa antagonists are indicated for acute coronary syndromes and in patients undergoing

TABLE 27-10.

PROPERTIES OF GLYCOPROTEIN IIb/IIIa ANTAGONISTS

Drug	Structure	Route of Adminis-tration	Elimination Half-Time (hrs)	Excretion	Clinical Uses	Stop Before Surgery (hrs)	Prolong PT/PTT	Antidote
Abciximab	Monoclonal antibodies	Intravenous	12–24	Plasma proteases	ACS	72	No/No	None
					PCI	24	No/No	None
Eptifibatide	Peptide	Intravenous	2–4	Renal	ACS			
Tirofiban	Nonpeptide	Intravenous	2–4	Renal (30–60%)	ACS	24	No/No	None
				Biliary (40–70%)	ACS	24	No/No	Hemodialysis

ACS, acute coronary syndrome; PCI, percutaneous coronary interventions.

interventional cardiology procedures. In the presence of acute coronary syndromes, thrombus formation initiated by platelets is important in the pathogenesis of unstable angina, myocardial infarction, and angioplasty failure.

Monitoring

It is recommended to maintain the ACT between 200 and 400 seconds in patients being treated with glycoprotein IIb/IIIa antagonists. Platelet counts should be monitored and therapy discontinued if thrombocytopenia (platelet count $<100{,}000$ cells/mm^3) develops.

Anesthetic Considerations

Avoiding regional anesthesia and delaying surgery may be reasonable, although evidence that bleeding is increased in these patients is equivocal.

Antimicrobials

28

The therapeutic value and associated dangers of antimicrobials are particularly relevant to the care of patients in the perioperative period and intensive care unit who are at risk for hospital-acquired infections (Table 28-1) (Stoelting RK, Hillier SC. Antimicrobials. In: *Pharmacology and Physiology in Anesthetic Practice*. 4th ed. Philadelphia, Lippincott Williams & Wilkins, 2006:521–550). The essential feature of effective chemotherapeutic drugs for the treatment of microbial diseases is the ability to inhibit microorganisms at concentrations that are tolerated by the host. The most successful antimicrobials are those that target anatomic structures or biosynthetic functions unique to specific microorganisms (Table 28-2). The choice of an antimicrobial is determined by both the properties of the individual drug and the nature of the infectious organism, as confirmed by bacteriologic investigation (Tables 28-3 and 28-4). In seriously ill or immunocompromised patients, the selection of bactericidal rather than bacteriostatic antimicrobials is often recommended (Table 28-5). Narrow-spectrum antimicrobials should be considered before broad-spectrum antimicrobials or combination therapy is prescribed, to preserve the patient's normal flora (Table 28-6).

ANTIMICROBIAL PROPHYLAXIS FOR SURGICAL PROCEDURES

The use of antimicrobial prophylaxis in surgery involves a risk-to-benefit evaluation that varies depending on the nature of the operative procedure (Table 28-7). It is generally believed that prophylactic antimicrobials should be administered intravenously shortly before the surgical

TABLE 28-1.
CLASSIFICATION OF ANTIMICROBIALS

Class of Drug	Specific Drugs
Penicillinase-susceptible	Penicillin G Penicillin V
Penicillinase-resistant	Methicillin Oxacillin Nafcillin Cloxacillin Dicloxacillin
Penicillinase-susceptible with activity against gram-negative bacilli	Ampicillin Amoxicillin Carbenicillin Mezlocillin Piperacillin Azlocillin
Penicillins with β-lactamase inhibitors	Amoxicillin-clavulanic acid Ampicillin-sulbactam
Cephalosporins	See Table 28-10
Carbapenems	Imipenem
Monobactams	Aztreonam
Aminoglycosides	Streptomycin Kanamycin Gentamicin Tobramycin Amikacin Neomycin
Tetracyclines	Tetracycline Doxycycline
Macrolides	Erythromycin Clarithromycin Azithromycin
Lincomycins	Clindamycin
Dichloroacetic acid derivative	Chloramphenicol
Glycopeptide derivative	Vancomycin
Streptogramins	Quinupristin-dalfopristin
Oxazolidinones	Linezolid
Polymyxins	Polymyxin B Colistimethate

TABLE 28-1.
(continued)

Class of Drug	Specific Drugs
Polypeptide derivative	Bacitracin
Sulfonamides	Sulfisoxazole Sulfamethoxazole Sulfasalazine Sulfacetamide
Pyrimidine derivative	Trimethoprim
Miscellaneous	Metronidazole
Fluoroquinolones	Norfloxacin Ciprofloxacin Ofloxacin Lomefloxacin
Urinary tract disinfectants	Nitrofurantoin Fosfomycin
Antifungal drugs	Amphotericin B Nystatin Miconazole

incision (no more than 2 hours before the incision), with the infusion completed before the induction of anesthesia. Nevertheless, the size of the bacterial inoculum may be more important than the precise timing of the prophylactic antimicrobial administration. Because of their broad antimicrobial spectrum and low incidence of allergic reactions, cephalosporins are the antimicrobials of choice for surgical procedures in which skin flora and normal flora of the gastrointestinal and genitourinary tracts are the most likely pathogens. Vancomycin is a useful prophylactic antimicrobial for patients undergoing the placement of cardiovascular or joint prostheses.

ANTIMICROBIAL SELECTION

The prompt identification of the causative organism is essential for the selection of appropriate antimicrobial

TABLE 28-2.
MECHANISM OF ACTION OF ANTIMICROBIAL DRUGS

	Anatomic Site of Biosynthetic Function Targeted by Antimicrobial Drug
Penicillins Cephalosporins Vancomycin	Interfere with synthesis of the mucopeptide layer of the bacterial cell wall, which is absent in host cells
Polymyxins	Alter permeability of bacterial cell membrane, allowing leakage of cell contents
Aminoglycosides Tetracyclines	Act on the 30S subunit of the bacterial ribosome so as to inhibit bacterial protein synthesis at the translational level
Chloramphenicol Erythromycin Clindamycin	Act on the 50S subunit of the bacterial ribosome so as to inhibit bacterial protein synthesis at the translational level
Sulfonamides	Inhibit microbial synthesis of folic acid
Quinolones	Inhibit bacterial DNA gyrase, which is the enzyme responsible for maintaining the helical structure of DNA
Rifampin	Selectively inhibits the bacterial DNA-dependent RNA polymerase but does not affect this enzyme in host cells

drugs. The efficacy of antimicrobial therapy depends on drug delivery to the site of infection (cross blood-brain barrier, remove infected prosthesis, remove obstruction to a bronchus associated with pneumonia). The indiscriminate use of broad-spectrum antimicrobials is an

TABLE 28-3.
CONSIDERATIONS IN THE SELECTION OF AN ANTIMICROBIAL DRUG

Identification of the infecting organism (Gram's stain, culture)
Determination of the antimicrobial susceptibility of the offending microorganism
Need for a bactericidal or bacteriostatic drug
Site of infection (need to cross the blood-brain barrier)
Host factors (immunosuppression, allergy, renal or hepatic dysfunction)
Need for combinations of antimicrobials
Route of administration
Duration of treatment
Risk of development of resistant strains in certain environments (hospital)
Cost (efficacy and toxicity may influence selection of more expensive drug)

important factor in the increased incidence of resistance to antimicrobials.

Nosocomial Infections

Intravascular access catheters (colonized hub or lumen reflecting skin flora) are the most common causes of bacteremia or fungemia in hospitalized patients. Initial therapy of suspected intravascular catheter infection usually includes vancomycin because of the high incidence of methicillin-resistant *Streptococcus aureus* and *epidermidis*.

Adverse Reactions

Adverse reactions to antimicrobials can be characterized as hypersensitivity reactions (independent of dose), direct drug toxicity (dose-related), and microbial superinfection (Table 28-8).

TABLE 28-4.
ANTIMICROBIAL DRUGS OF CHOICE FOR TREATMENT OF VARIOUS INFECTIONS

Infection	Drug of Choice
Gram-positive cocci	
Staphylococcus aureus	
Methicillin-resistant	Vancomycin
Non–penicillinase-producing	Penicillin G
Penicillinase-producing	Methicillin
Staphylococcus epidermidis	Vancomycin or a cephalosporin
Streptococcus	Penicillin G, penicillin V, or ampicillin
Pneumococcus	Penicillin G or penicillin V
Gram-negative cocci	
Neisseria gonorrhoeae	Ceftriaxone
Bacterial meningitis	Penicillin G
Enteric Gram-negative bacilli	
Respiratory tract strains	Penicillin G
Escherichia coli	Ampicillin or a cephalosporin
Klebsiella	Cephalosporin
Proteus mirabilis	Ampicillin
Other Gram-negative bacilli	
Haemophilus influenzae	
Bronchitis	Trimethoprim with sulfamethoxazole
Meningitis or epiglottitis	Cefotaxime or ceftriaxone
Legionnaires' disease	Erythromycin
Pseudomonas aeruginosa	
Urinary tract infections	Quinolone antimicrobial
Other infections	Gentamicin or tobramycin
Acid-fast bacilli	
Mycobacterium tuberculosis	Isoniazid plus rifampin plus pyrazinamide
Fungi	Amphotericin B
Mycoplasma	Erythromycin
Rickettsia	Tetracycline

TABLE 28-4.
(continued)

Infection	Drug of Choice
Viruses	
Herpes simplex	Acyclovir
Cytomegalovirus	Ganciclovir
Influenza	Amantadine or rimantadine
Respiratory syncytial virus	Ribavirin
Varicella-zoster	Acyclovir
Human immunodeficiency virus	Combinations of antiretroviral drugs

Parturients

The immature fetal liver may lack the enzymes necessary to metabolize certain drugs, so that pharmacokinetics and toxicities in the fetus are often different from those in older children and adults (Table 28-9).

TABLE 28-5.
EXAMPLES OF BACTERICIDAL AND BACTERIOSTATIC ANTIMICROBIALS

Bactericidal	Bacteriostatic
Penicillins	Tetracyclines
Cephalosporins	Chloramphenicol
Aminoglycosides	Erythromycin
Vancomycin	Clindamycin
Quinolones	Sulfonamides
Aztreonam	Trimethoprim
Imipenem	Linezolid (staphylococci and enterococci)
Bacitracin	
Polymyxins	
Linezolid (streptococci)	

TABLE 28-6.
EXAMPLES OF NARROW-SPECTRUM AND BROAD-SPECTRUM ANTIMICROBIALS

Narrow-Spectrum Antimicrobials	Broad-Spectrum Antimicrobials
Penicillin G	Ampicillin
Erythromycin	Cephalosporins
Clindamycin	Aminoglycosides
	Tetracyclines
	Chloramphenicol
	Quinolones

Elderly Patients

Physiologic changes that occur with increasing age can alter the oral absorption (decreased gastric acidity, reduced gastrointestinal motility), distribution (increased body fat, decreased plasma albumin concentrations), metabolism (decreased hepatic blood flow), and excretion (decreased glomerular filtration rate) of antimicrobials.

PENICILLINS

The bactericidal action of penicillin reflects the ability of these antimicrobials to interfere with the synthesis of peptidoglycan, which is an essential component of the cell wall of susceptible bacteria.

Penicillin G and Penicillin V

Penicillin G and penicillin V are highly active against Gram-positive bacteria (streptococci). Both of these penicillins are readily hydrolyzed by bacteria-produced enzymes (β-lactamases), rendering them ineffective against most strains of *Staphylococcus aureus*.

TABLE 28-7.
EXAMPLES OF SURGICAL PROCEDURES THAT MAY BENEFIT FROM PROPHYLACTIC ANTIMICROBIALS

Gynecologic surgery
- Cesarean section
- Hysterectomy (abdominal or vaginal)

Orthopedic surgery
- Arthroplasty of joints, including replacement
- Open reduction of fractures

General surgery
- Cholecystectomy
- Colon surgery
- Appendectomy
- Gastric resection
- Penetrating abdominal trauma

Urologic surgery

Oropharyngeal surgery

Cardiothoracic and vascular surgery
- Coronary artery bypass graft
- Valve annuloplasty or replacement
- Pacemaker insertion
- Thoracotomy
- Peripheral vascular surgery (possible exception: carotid endarterectomy)

Neurosurgery
- Shunt procedures
- Craniotomy

Clinical Indications

Penicillin is the drug of choice for the treatment of pneumococcal, streptococcal, and meningococcal infections. The administration of high intravenous doses of penicillin G may result in hyperkalemia in patients with renal dysfunction (10 million U of penicillin G contains 16 mEq of potassium).

Excretion

The renal excretion of penicillin is rapid, principally through renal tubular secretion.

TABLE 28-8.
DIRECT DRUG TOXICITY ASSOCIATED WITH ADMINISTRATION OF ANTIMICROBIALS

Toxicity	Antimicrobial
Allergic reactions	All antimicrobials but most often with β-lactam derivatives
Nephrotoxicity	Aminoglycosides Polymyxins Amphotericin B
Neutropenia	Penicillins Cephalosporins Vancomycin
Inhibition of platelet aggregation	Penicillins (high doses)
Prolonged prothrombin time	Cephalosporins
Bone marrow suppression (aplastic anemia, pancytopenia)	Chloramphenicol Flucytosine Linezolid (reversible)
Hemolytic anemia	Chloramphenicol Sulfonamides Nitrofurantoin Primaquine
Agranulocytosis	Macrolides Trimethoprim-sulfamethoxazole
Leukopenia and thrombocytopenia (folate deficiency)	Trimethoprim
Normocytic normochromic anemia	Amphotericin B
Ototoxicity	Aminoglycosides Vancomycin (auditory neurotoxicity) Minocycline (vestibular toxicity)
Seizures	Penicillins and other β-lactams (high doses, azotemic patients, history of epilepsy) Metronidazole

TABLE 28-8.
(continued)

Toxicity	Antimicrobial
Neuromuscular blockade	Aminoglycosides
Peripheral neuropathy	Nitrofurantoin (renal failure) Isoniazid (prevent with pyridoxine) Metronidazole
Benign intracranial hypertension	Tetracyclines
Optic neuritis	Ethambutol
Hepatotoxicity	Isoniazid Rifampin Tetracyclines (high doses) β-Lactam antimicrobials (high doses) Nitrofurantoin Erythromycin Sulfonamides
Increased plasma bilirubin concentrations	Quinupristin-dalfopristin
Gastrointestinal irritation	Erythromycin Tetracyclines
Prolongation of QTc interval	Erythromycin Fluoroquinolones
Exaggerated sympathomimetic effects in patients receiving monoamine oxidase inhibitors	Linezolid
Hyperkalemia	Trimethoprim-sulfamethoxazole
Tendinitis	Fluoroquinolones
Arthralgias and myalgias	Quinupristin-dalfopristin
Photosensitivity	Sulfonamides Tetracyclines Fluoroquinolones
Teratogenicity	Tetracyclines Metronidazole Rifampin Trimethoprim Fluoroquinolones

TABLE 28-9.
ANTIMICROBIALS IN PREGNANCY

Drug	Maternal Toxicity	Fetal Toxicity	Excreted in Colostrum
Considered Safe			
Penicillins	Allergic reactions	None known	Trace
Cephalosporins	Allergic reactions	None known	Trace
Erythromycin base	Allergic reactions Gastrointestinal irritation	None known	Yes
Use Cautiously			
Aminoglycosides	Ototoxicity Nephrotoxicity	Ototoxicity	Yes
Clindamycin	Allergic reactions Colitis	None known	Trace
Ethambutol	Optic neuritis	None known	Unknown
Isoniazid	Allergic reactions Hepatotoxicity	Neuropathy Seizures	Yes
Rifampin	Allergic reactions Hepatotoxicity	None known	Yes
Sulfonamides	Allergic reactions	Kernicterus (at term) Hemolysis (G6PD deficiency)	Yes

TABLE 28-9.
(Continued)

Drug	Maternal Toxicity	Fetal Toxicity	Excreted in Colostrum
Avoid			
Metronidazole	Allergic reactions Alcohol intolerance Peripheral neuropathy	None known (teratogenic in animals)	Yes
Contraindicated			
Chloramphenicol	Bone marrow depression	Gray syndrome	Yes
Erythromycin estolate	Hepatotoxicity	None known	Yes
Nalidixic acid	Gastrointestinal irritation	Increased intracranial pressure	Unknown
Fluoroquinolones	Gastrointestinal irritation	Arthropathies (animals)	Unknown
Nitrofurantoin	Allergic reactions Peripheral neuropathy Gastrointestinal irritation	Hemolysis (G6PD deficiency)	Trace
Tetracyclines	Hepatotoxicity Nephrotoxicity	Tooth discoloration and dysplasia Impaired bone growth	Yes
Trimethoprim	Allergic reactions	Teratogenicity	Yes

Duration of Action

Probenecid blocks the renal tubular secretion of penicillin, and the addition of the local anesthetic procaine delays absorption, resulting in a increased duration of action.

Penicillinase-Resistant Penicillins

Penicillinase-resistant penicillins (methicillin, oxacillin, nafcillin, cloxacillin, and dicloxacillin) are not susceptible to hydrolysis by staphylococcal penicillinases that would otherwise render the antimicrobial inactive. The renal excretion of methicillin, oxacillin, and cloxacillin is extensive.

Penicillinase-Susceptible Broad-Spectrum Penicillins

Penicillinase-susceptible broad-spectrum penicillins (second-generation penicillins such as ampicillin, amoxicillin, and carbenicillin) are bactericidal against Gram-positive and Gram-negative bacteria.

Ampicillin

Ampicillin is well absorbed after oral administration and undergoes extensive renal excretion. Among the penicillins, ampicillin is associated with the highest incidence of skin rash.

Amoxicillin

Amoxicillin has a spectrum of activity similar to ampicillin, but it is more efficiently absorbed from the gastrointestinal tract.

Extended-Spectrum Carboxypenicillins (Third-Generation Penicillins)

Carbenicillin

Carbenicillin is effective in the treatment of infections caused by *Pseudomonas aeruginosa* and certain *Proteus* strains that are resistant to ampicillin. Carbenicillin interferes with normal platelet aggregation so that bleeding time is prolonged but platelet count remains normal.

Extended-Spectrum Acylaminopenicillins (Fourth-Generation Penicillins)

These drugs are ineffective against penicillinase-producing strains of *S. aureus* and have not been demonstrated to be superior to carboxypenicillins.

Penicillin β-Lactamase Inhibitor Combinations

These compounds (clavulanic acid) have little intrinsic antimicrobial activity but bind reversibly to β-lactamase enzymes, thus rendering organisms sensitive to β-lactamase–susceptible penicillins (clavulanic acid combined with amoxicillin and ampicillin).

Allergy to Penicillins

Allergic reactions are noted in 1% to 10% of patients treated with penicillins, making these antimicrobials the most allergenic of all drugs. Most often, the allergic response is a delayed reaction characterized by a maculopapular rash and/or fever. Less often occurring, but more serious, is immediate hypersensitivity (laryngeal edema, bronchospasm, cardiovascular collapse) that is mediated by immunoglobulin E antibodies.

Cross-Reactivity

The presence of a common nucleus (β-lactam ring) in the structure of all penicillins means that allergy to one penicillin increases the likelihood of an allergic reaction to another penicillin. The administration of cephalosporins to patients with a history of allergy to penicillin (hypotension, bronchospasm, laryngeal edema) confirmed by a positive skin test is not recommended.

CEPHALOSPORINS

Cephalosporins, like the penicillins, are bactericidal antimicrobials that inhibit cell wall synthesis and have a low intrinsic toxicity. The intravenous administration of any of the cephalosporins may cause thrombophlebitis. The excretion of cephalosporins is principally through glomerular filtration and renal tubular secretion. Life-threatening anaphylaxis is rare, but patients who are allergic to one cephalosporin are likely to be allergic to others. The possibility of cross-reactivity between cephalosporins and penicillins seems to be very infrequent.

Classification (Table 28-10)

First-generation cephalosporins (inexpensive, low toxicity) are commonly selected for antimicrobial prophylaxis in patients undergoing at-risk surgical procedures.

First-Generation Cephalosporins

Cephalothin is the prototype of first-generation cephalosporins; it is excreted largely unchanged by the kidneys, administered intravenously, and does not easily cross the blood-brain barrier.

Cefazolin has a similar antimicrobial spectrum but achieves higher blood levels and is viewed as the drug of choice for antimicrobial prophylaxis in the perioperative period.

Second-Generation Cephalosporins

Cefoxitin and *cefamandole* possess extended activity against Gram-negative bacteria. Cefoxitin is resistant to cephalosporinases. Both drugs are excreted predominantly by the kidneys.

Third-Generation Cephalosporins

Third-generation cephalosporins have an enhanced ability to resist hydrolysis by the β-lactamases of many Gram-negative bacilli, including those causing meningitis.

TABLE 28-10.
CLASSIFICATION OF CEPHALOSPORINS

	First-Generation Cephalosporins	Second-Generation Cephalosporins	Third-Generation Cephalosporins
Oral	Cefadroxil Cephalexin Cephradine	Cefaclor Cefuroxime Cefprozil Cefditoren Loracarbef	Cefixime Cefdinir Cefpodoxime Ceftibuten
Parenteral	Cefazolin Cephapirin Cephradine Cefoperazone	Cefoxitin Cefamandole Cefonicid Cefuroxime	Cefotaxime Ceftizoxime Ceftriaxone

Ceftizoxime differs from *cefotaxime* in that it depends solely on renal clearance. *Cefoperazone* is unique among cephalosporins in depending primarily on hepatic elimination for its clearance.

OTHER B-LACTAM ANTIMICROBIALS

Imipenem

Imipenem is a bactericidal antimicrobial with the broadest antibacterial spectrum of any β-lactam antimicrobial. Clearance is through glomerular filtration, and the potential exists for cross-reactivity with other β-lactam antimicrobials.

Aztreonam

Aztreonam is effective only against Gram-negative bacteria. A unique advantage is the absence of any cross-reactivity between aztreonam and circulating antibodies of penicillin- or cephalosporin-allergic patients.

AMINOGLYCOSIDE ANTIMICROBIALS

Aminoglycoside antimicrobials are poorly lipid soluble antimicrobials that are rapidly bactericidal for aerobic Gram-negative bacteria. These drugs undergo extensive renal excretion, and the elimination half-time of aminoglycosides is prolonged 20- to 40-fold in the presence of renal failure. Determination of the plasma concentration of aminoglycosides is an essential guide to the safe administration of these antimicrobials.

Side Effects (Table 28-11)

TETRACYCLINES

Tetracyclines are the drugs of choice in the treatment of rickettsial diseases and are useful in the treatment of mycoplasma pneumonia. Tetracyclines are used as adjuvant therapy in the treatment of severe cystic acne.

TABLE 28-11.
SIDE EFFECTS OF AMINOGLYCOSIDES

Ototoxicity (vestibular dysfunction, auditory dysfunction)
Nephrotoxicity (acute tubular necrosis)
Skeletal muscle weakness (inhibition of the prejunctional release of acetylcholine)
Potentiation of nondepolarizing neuromuscular blocking drugs (exceptions are penicillins, cephalosporins, tetracyclines, erythromycin)

MACROLIDES

Erythromycin

Erythromycin has a spectrum of activity that includes most Gram-positive bacteria, and it is the preferred drug for the treatment of atypical pneumonia. In patients who cannot tolerate penicillins or cephalosporins, erythromycin is an effective alternative for the treatment of streptococcal pharyngitis, bronchitis, and pneumonia. Erythromycin is excreted to a large extent in bile and only to a minor degree in urine; thus, the dosage need not be altered in the presence of renal failure.

Effects on Gastric Emptying

Erythromycin in subtherapeutic doses (up to 200 mg) exhibits cholinergic stimulatory properties manifesting as increased lower esophageal sphincter tone, enhanced antroduodenal coordination, and intermittent gastric contractions resulting in accelerated gastric emptying of solids and liquids. These prokinetic properties of erythromycin may be beneficial in the preparation of patients considered at risk for pulmonary aspiration before the induction of anesthesia.

Clarithromycin

Clarithromycin has a similar antimicrobial spectrum to erythromycin but a longer elimination half-time.

Azithromycin

Azithromycin resembles erythromycin in its antimicrobial spectrum, but an extraordinarily prolonged elimination half-time permits once-a-day dosing.

CLINDAMYCIN

Clindamycin resembles erythromycin in antimicrobial activity, but it is more active against many anaerobes. Because severe pseudomembranous colitis can be a complication of clindamycin therapy, this drug should be used only to treat infections that cannot be adequately treated by less toxic antimicrobials.

Side Effects

Clindamycin produces prejunctional and postjunctional effects at the neuromuscular junction, and these effects cannot be readily antagonized with calcium or anticholinesterase drugs.

CHLORAMPHENICOL

Chloramphenicol may rarely be associated with aplastic anemia. Chloramphenicol is inactivated principally in the liver by glucuronyl transferase.

VANCOMYCIN

Vancomycin is a bactericidal glycopeptide antimicrobial that impairs the cell wall synthesis of Gram-positive bacteria. Vancomycin is the drug of choice in the treatment of infections caused by methicillin-resistant *S. aureus*. Likewise, vancomycin is a useful prophylactic antimicrobial in patients undergoing cardiac and orthopedic surgical procedures that involve the placement of a prosthetic device. When vancomycin is administered intravenously, the recommendation is to infuse the calculated dose (10 to 15 mg/kg) over 60 minutes; this produces a sustained plasma concentration for up to 12 hours and minimizes the occurrence of drug-induced histamine release and hypotension. Vancomycin is principally excreted by the kidneys, with 90% of a dose being recovered unchanged in the urine.

Side Effects

Rapid infusion (<30 minutes) of vancomycin has been associated with profound hypotension and cardiac arrest. Hypotension is often accompanied by signs of histamine release characterized by intense facial and truncal erythema ("red neck syndrome"). The red neck syndrome may occur even with a slow infusion of vancomycin and is not always associated with hypotension.

Cardiovascular side effects most likely reflect nonimmunologic histamine release induced by vancomycin. Plasma tryptase concentrations are not increased following vancomycin-induced anaphylactoid reactions (distinguishes it from anaphylactic reactions). Oral H_1 (diphenhydramine 1 mg/kg) and H_2 (cimetidine 4 mg/kg) administered 1 hour before the induction of anesthesia decreased histamine-related side effects of rapid vancomycin infusion (1 g over 10 minutes).

STREPTOGRAMINS

Streptogramin such as quinupristin and dalfopristin are used for the treatment of vancomycin-resistant infections; they are administered intravenously via a central line to avoid phlebitis.

The use of these drugs may increase plasma concentrations of drugs (such as fentanyl) that depend on CYP3A4 for hepatic metabolism.

OXAZOLIDIONES

Oxazolidiones (linezolid) inhibit protein synthesis by preventing the formation of the initiation complex that is required for ribosomal function. Linezolid is active against nearly all aerobic Gram-positive cocci. Nonrenal mechanisms account for 65% of the drug's clearance.

Side Effects

Reversible bone marrow suppression (thrombocytopenia, leukopenia, anemia) is a rare side effect. Because linezolid is a reversible inhibitor of monoamine oxidase (MAO), patients taking this drug may experience an exaggerated hypertensive response to sympathomimetic drugs. Patients being treated with linezolid should avoid foods and beverages with high tyramine contents.

POLYMYXIN B AND COLISTIMETHATE

Polymyxin B and colistimethate are effective against Gram-negative bacteria (severe urinary tract infections and in the topical treatment of *P. aeruginosa* corneal ulcers).

Side Effects

The polymyxins are the most potent of all the antimicrobials in their actions at the neuromuscular junction, producing skeletal muscle weakness and the potentiation of nondepolarizing neuromuscular-blocking drugs. Neostigmine or calcium does not reliably antagonize this drug-induced effect at the neuromuscular junction, which contrasts with the ability of these drugs to reverse aminoglycoside-induced skeletal muscle weakness. Nephrotoxicity is a significant risk of treatment with these drugs, and alternative antimicrobials are likely to be selected for patients with known renal dysfunction.

BACITRACINS

Bacitracins are effective against a variety of Gram-positive bacteria; their use is limited to topical application in ophthalmologic and dermatologic ointments.

SULFONAMIDES

Sulfonamides are used principally to treat uncomplicated urinary tract infections caused by *Escherichia coli*.

Mechanism of Action

The antimicrobial activity of sulfonamides is due to the ability of these drugs to prevent normal use of paraaminobenzoic acid by bacteria to synthesize folic acid. Ester local anesthetics that are hydrolyzed to paraaminobenzoic acid could theoretically antagonize the antimicrobial effects of sulfonamides.

Pharmacokinetics

These antimicrobials are rapidly and extensively absorbed, primarily from the small intestine, and readily enter tissues and cross the blood-brain barrier and placenta. The metabolism of sulfonamides is predominantly by acetylation in the liver to pharmacologically inactive compounds.

Side Effects (Table 28-12)

Clinically Useful Sulfonamides (Table 28-13)

METRONIDAZOLE

Metronidazole is bactericidal against most anaerobic Gram-negative bacilli and *Clostridium* species.

TABLE 28-12.
SIDE EFFECTS OF SULFONAMIDES

Allergic reactions
Drug fever
Hepatotoxicity
Acute hemolytic anemia (glucose-6-phosphate deficiency)
Increased effect of oral anticoagulants and hypoglycemic drugs
Jaundice (premature infants)

FLUOROQUINOLONES

Fluoroquinolones are broad-spectrum antimicrobials that are bactericidal against most enteric Gram-negative bacilli. They are rapidly absorbed from the gastrointestinal tract, and penetration into body fluids and tissues is excellent. The principal route of excretion is via the kidneys. There are several conditions in which these antimi-

TABLE 28-13.
CLINICALLY USEFUL SULFONAMIDES

Sulfisoxazole (rapid oral absorption, high water solubility minimizes risk of renal toxicity, used for treatment of urinary tract infections)
Sulfamethoxazole (crystalluria is a risk)
Sulfasalazine (poorly absorbed from the gastrointestinal tract, used for treatment of ulcerative colitis and regional enteritis)
Sulfacetamide (topical use for ophthalmic infections)
Trimethoprim (initial treatment of uncomplicated urinary tract infections)
Trimethoprim-Sulfamethoxazole (synergistic antimicrobial activity; treatment of choice for *Pneumocystis carinii* pneumonia, most common side effects are skin rashes, glossitis, and stomatitis)

TABLE 28-14.
CONDITIONS IN WHICH QUINOLONE ANTIMICROBIALS MAY BE THE PREFERRED TREATMENT

Complicated urinary tract infections
Bacterial gastroenteritis
Chronic *Salmonella* carrier state
Respiratory infections related to cystic fibrosis
Osteomyelitis due to Gram-negative bacteria
Invasive external otitis
Mycobacterial infections (as part of multidrug regimens)

crobials may be preferable to other currently available drugs (Table 28-14).

Norfloxacin

Norfloxacin is highly effective in the treatment of urinary tract infections (*E. coli*) in women.

Ciprofloxacin

Ciprofloxacin achieves high blood concentrations and tissue penetration when administered intravenously. This antimicrobial is useful for the treatment of upper and lower respiratory tract infections, bone and joint infections, and most strains of *Mycobacterium tuberculosis* are susceptible to ciprofloxacin.

Ofloxacin

Ofloxacin has an antimicrobial spectrum that resembles ciprofloxacin but is more active against *Chlamydia*.

Lomefloxacin

Lomefloxacin resembles other fluoroquinolones, but its longer elimination half-time permits once-daily dosing.

NITROFURANTOIN

Nitrofurantoin is rapidly absorbed and excreted, so that therapeutic blood levels are not achieved in the blood. The therapeutic utility of this antimicrobial is in the treatment of uncomplicated, mild urinary tract infections.

FOSFOMYCIN

Fosfomycin is a broad-spectrum antibiotic that inhibits cell-wall synthesis in *E. coli* and many other urinary tract pathogens.

DRUGS FOR TREATMENT OF TUBERCULOSIS

Patients with active tuberculosis, in the absence of drug susceptibility data, are treated with daily administration of isoniazid, rifampin, pyrazinamide, and either ethambutol or streptomycin. Patients with pulmonary tuberculosis who have positive sputum cultures should be treated in an isolation environment until three consecutive sputum samples collected on separate days are negative. As little as 2 weeks of antituberculous chemotherapy greatly decreases the infectivness of pulmonary tuberculosis.

Treatment of HIV Infected-Patients

HIV-infected patients who do not require antiretroviral therapy can receive standard antituberculous chemotherapy. Rifampin is a potent CYP450 inducer, whereas protease inhibitors are potent CYP450 inhibitors and can result in toxic plasma concentrations of rifamycin (rifampin is contraindicated in patients receiving protease inhibitors).

Antituberculous Drugs

Isoniazid

Isoniazid is considered the primary drug for the chemotherapy of tuberculosis and is the only medication proved to be efficacious for the prevention of tuberculosis.

Excretion

The rate of isoniazid acetylation is genetically determined, with plasma concentrations of isoniazid being 30 to 50 times less in rapid acetylators. The clearance of isoniazid depends to only a small degree on the status of renal function, but patients who are slow acetylators may be susceptible to an accumulation of toxic concentrations if renal function is impaired.

Side Effects (Table 28-15)

The side effects due to isoniazid can be minimized by prophylactic therapy with pyridoxine.

Rifampin

Rifampin is bactericidal for most mycobacteria; however, resistance develops rapidly, so it must not be used alone.

TABLE 28-15.
SIDE EFFECTS OF ISONIAZID

Precipitate seizures in patients with epilepsy
Optic neuritis
Peripheral neuropathy
Mental changes (euphoria, impairment of memory)
Sedation (slow acetylators)
Hepatic injury (resembles halothane hepatitis, rapid acetylators are more vulnerable; increased incidence in patients >50 years of age)
Increased defluoridation of volatile anesthetics (induces microsomal enzymes)
Drug interactions (increased plasma concentrations of phenytoin and barbiturates)

It is the drug of choice for prophylaxis against meningococcal disease in household contacts of patients with such infections.

Route of Administration

Rifampin may be administered orally or intravenously. This drug imparts a red color to the urine and saliva.

Excretion

Rifampin undergoes hepatic deacetylation, and the resulting metabolite has antibacterial activity similar to that of the parent compound.

Side Effects (Table 28-16)

Rifabutin

Rifabutin possesses an antituberculous spectrum similar to that of rifampin but is a less potent inducer of CYP450; thus it is acceptable to administer rifabutin to patients being treated with antiretroviral drugs.

TABLE 28-16. SIDE EFFECTS OF RIFAMPIN

Thrombocytopenia and anemia (high doses)
Hepatitis with jaundice (elderly patients with a history of alcohol abuse)
Potent inducer of hepatic CYP450 oxidative enzymes (accelerated metabolism of opioids—may precipitate opioid withdrawal syndrome in patients being treated with methadone, warfarin, oral contraceptives, glucocorticoids)
Fatigue and skeletal muscle weakness
Competes for biliary excretion of contrast media
Hypothyroidism (accelerated clearance of thyroxine)
Contraindicated in patients being treated with antiretroviral drugs

Rifapentine

Rifapentine is a long-acting analog of rifampin. It is administered once a week during the continuation phase of treatment of rifampin.

Pyrazinamide

Pyrazinamide is a derivative of nicotinic acid that exhibits bactericidal activity against mycobacteria.

Ethambutol

Ethambutol is useful in combination with isoniazid for the treatment of active tuberculosis, because it readily penetrates tissues, including the central nervous system (CNS).

Excretion

Approximately 50% of an ingested dose of ethambutol is excreted unchanged by the kidneys within 24 hours.

Side Effects

The most important side effect of therapy with ethambutol is optic neuritis.

ANTIFUNGAL DRUGS

Nystatin

Nystatin is both fungistatic and fungicidal but lacks effects on bacteria. This drug is used primarily to treat *Candida* infections (common in patients on immunosuppressive therapy).

Amphotericin B

Amphotericin B is the most effective antifungal drug for managing infections due to yeasts and fungi. Cryptococcal infections, histoplasmosis, coccidioidomycosis, blastomycosis, sporotrichosis, and disseminated candidiasis are treated with amphotericin B. This drug must be administered intravenously, and it does not penetrate into cerebrospinal fluid (intrathecal injection may be necessary) or vitreous humor.

Side Effects

Renal function is impaired in >80% of treated patients; thus, it is vital to monitor plasma creatinine concentrations. Hypokalemia and hypomagnesemia may occur.

Flucytosine

Flucytosine is converted to fluorouracil exclusively in fungal cells. Approximately 80% of flucytosine is excreted unchanged by the kidneys.

Griseofulvin

Griseofulvin is effective in the treatment of fungal infections of the skin, hair, and nails. Headache is common, and peripheral neuritis, fatigue, blurred vision, and syncope may occur.

ANTIVIRAL DRUGS

Some host cell surface receptors and enzymes are unique for viruses, thus providing a mechanism for the development of antiviral drugs with selective activity (Table 28-17).

Idoxuridine

Idoxuridine possesses antiviral activity that is mainly limited to DNA viruses, especially herpes simplex group; it is used as a topical treatment.

Amantadine

Amantadine inhibits the replication of strains of influenza A virus. This drug accumulates in patients with impaired renal function, and excessive plasma concentrations are associated with CNS toxicity, including seizures and coma.

TABLE 28-17.
CLASSIFICATION OF VIRUSES AND ASSOCIATED DISEASES

RNA viruses
- Picornaviruses: poliomyelitis, encephalitis, common cold
- Reoviruses: diarrhea
- Togaviruses: encephalitis, rubella
- Orthomyxoviruses: influenza
- Paramyxoviruses: croup, bronchitis, mumps, measles
- Retroviruses: acquired immunodeficiency syndrome, Leukemia

DNA viruses
- Papovaviruses: warts
- Adenoviruses: acute respiratory distress, keratitis
- Herpes viruses: cold sores, keratitis, genital lesions, varicella, shingles, cytomegalic inclusion disease, infectious mononucleosis

Vidarabine

Vidarabine is effective in the treatment of herpes simplex encephalitis and keratoconjunctivitis. Because vidarabine is poorly soluble in aqueous solutions, large volumes of water (2.5 liters) are needed to dissolve the drug for infusion in the treatment of encephalitis.

Zanamivir

Zanamivir administered intranasally decreases peak viral titers and the frequency of febrile illness associated with influenza A or B virus infections.

Acyclovir

Acyclovir has an antiviral spectrum that is limited to herpes viruses (recurrent genital herpes). Excretion is by the kidneys, principally of unchanged drug (increases in plasma creatinine concentrations may occur). Thrombophlebitis may develop at the site of intravenous administration.

Famciclovir

Famciclovir is administered orally for the treatment of acute herpes zoster. The most frequent side effects of treatment with famciclovir are headache, nausea, and fatigue.

Ganciclovir

Ganciclovir is effective in the treatment of cytomegalovirus disease. Side effects include granulocytopenia (prevented by the concomitant administration of recombinant granulocyte colony-stimulating factor), thrombocytopenia, azoospermia, and an increase in plasma creatinine concentrations.

Interferon

Interferon is a general term used to designate those glycoproteins produced in response to viral infection. In addition to having antiviral effects, interferons inhibit cell proliferation and enhances the tumoricidal activities of macrophages. Treatment with interferons may be associated with influenza-like symptoms, hematologic toxicity, neurologic symptoms, and immune system disorders (development of autoantibodies or thyroid disease).

Lamivudine

Lamivudine is effective in the treatment of chronic hepatitis B and may serve as a bridge to liver transplantation for patients with decompensated cirrhosis.

Antiretroviral Drugs Effective in the Management of Patients with AIDS (Table 28-18)

Initiation of Therapy

Antiretroviral therapy (combination of three or more drugs) is recommended for patients with acute HIV syndrome, those in whom HIV infection has been diagnosed with 6 months of seroconversion, and those with severe HIV-related symptoms or AIDS.

Side Effects (See Table 28-18)

Hypersensivity

Abacavir hypersensitivity syndrome (fever, rash, nausea, oral lesions, cough) occurs in approximately 2% to 3% of treated patients, developing in the first 3 to 4 weeks of therapy.

Lactic Acidosis

Lactic acidosis, reflected by mildly elevated serum lactate concentrations, occurs in 10% to 20% of patients receiving antiretroviral therapy.

Increased Insulin Resistance

Increased insulin resistance is associated with protease-inhibitor antiretroviral treatment.

Hypercholesterolemia

Hypercholesterolemia is associated with protease-inhibitor antiretroviral treatment. In addition, ritonavir has been associated with increases in plasma triglyceride concentrations. It is unclear if these changes predispose treated patients to cardiovascular disease.

Lipodystrophy

Lipodystrophy or fat redistribution syndrome presents as central fat distribution (abdomen, breasts, neck) or as peripheral fat wasting (face, buttocks, limbs). Insulin resistance likely is important in the etiology of this lipodystrophy.

Monitoring Treatment

Measuring $CD4^{+}T$ cell counts reflects the impact of antiretroviral therapy on immune function. Reservoirs of HIV make it impossible to completely eradicate the infection using antiretroviral treatment.

TABLE 28-18.
ANTIRETROVIRAL DRUGS USED IN TREATMENT OF HIV

Drug	Side Effects
Nucleoside Reverse Transcriptase Inhibitors	
Abacavir (ABC)	Hypersensitivity reactions (may be fatal) Lactic acidosis (rare)
Didanosine (ddI)	Peripheral neuropathy Pancreatitis Nausea Lactic acidosis (rare)
Lamivudine (3TC)	Lactic acidosis (rare)
Stavudine (d4T)	Peripheral neuropathy Lactic acidosis (rare)
Zalcitabine (ddC)	Peripheral neuropathy Stomatitis Lactic acidosis (rare)
Zidovudine (AZT)	Anemia Neutropenia Gastrointestinal irritation Headache Lactic acidosis (rare)
Nonnucleoside Reverse Transcriptase Inhibitors	
Delavirdine	Rash Increased plasma transaminase concentrations Headache
Efavirenz	Rash Confusion, agitation
Nevirapine	Rash Increased plasma transaminase concentrations (hepatitis can be fatal)
Protease Inhibitors	
Amprenavir	Gastrointestinal irritation Lipid abnormalities Perioral paresthesias

TABLE 28-18.
(continued)

Drug	Side Effects
	Lipodystrophy
Indinavir	Gastrointestinal irritation Nephrolithiasis Increased indirect serum bilirubin concentrations Headache Lipid abnormalities Lipodystrophy
Lopinavir + ritonavir	Gastrointestinal irritation Lipid abnormalities (including hypertriglyceridemia) Lipodystrophy
Nelfinavir	Diarrhea Lipid abnormalities Lipodystrophy
Ritonavir	Gastrointestinal irritation Peroral paresthesias Taste perversions Hepatitis Lipid abnormalities (including hypertriglyceridemia) Lipodystrophy
Saquinavir	Gastrointestinal irritation Headache Lipid abnormalities Lipodystrophy

Drug Interactions

Most of the protease inhibitors are also inhibitors of the cytochrome P-450 (CYP) 3A4 enzyme (ritonavir is the most potent), which is responsible for the metabolism of several drugs (fentanyl, anticoagulants, anticonvulsants, corticosteroids) thus increasing the risk of pharmacokinetic drug interactions.

Zidovudine

Zidovudine (AZT) delays the progression of AIDS, as manifested by the onset of opportunistic infections, neurologic disease, and tumors. The transmission of HIV from the mother to the infant is impaired by zidovudine. After glucuronidation in the liver, zidovudine is primarily eliminated by the kidneys.

Didanosine

Didanosine acts as a prodrug for the active intracellular moiety dideoxyadenosine triphosphate.

Zalcitabine

Zalcitabine is a prodrug that is most often administered in combination with zidovudine.

Protease Inhibitors

Protease inhibitors are useful in the treatment of individuals with HIV infection (HIV-1 protease activity is critical for the terminal maturation of infectious virions). The development of resistance and the subsequent loss of drug efficacy is the primary barrier to the long-term use of HIV-1 protease inhibitors.

Chemotherapeutic Drugs

29

Chemotherapy is the best available therapeutic approach for the eradication of malignant cells that can occur anywhere in the body (Stoelting RK, Hillier SC. Chemotherapeutic drugs. In: *Pharmacology and Physiology in Anesthetic Practice.* 4th ed. Philadelphia, Lippincott Williams & Wilkins, 2006: 551–568). The effectiveness of chemotherapy requires that there be complete destruction (total cell-kill) of all cancer cells, because a single surviving clonogenic cell can give rise to sufficient progeny to ultimately kill the host. The recognition for the need of total cell-kill leads to the use of several chemotherapeutic (antineoplastic) drugs concurrently or in planned sequence. Using a combination of chemotherapeutic drugs with different mechanisms of action also decreases the chances that drug-resistant tumor cell populations will emerge. Malignant cells are often characterized by rapid division and synthesis of DNA. Rapidly dividing normal cells (bone marrow, gastrointestinal tract, hair follicles) are vulnerable to the toxic effects of chemotherapeutic drugs, and it is predictable that clinical manifestations of toxicity may include myelosuppression, nausea, vomiting, diarrhea, mucosal ulceration, dermatitis, and alopecia. Drug-induced myelosuppression is usually reversible upon the discontinuation of the chemotherapeutic drug.

DRUG RESISTANCE

Drug resistance describes the clinical circumstance in which a tumor is no longer susceptible to several chemotherapeutic drugs.

CLASSIFICATION

Chemotherapeutic drugs are classified according to their mechanism of action (Table 29-1). Knowledge of drug-induced adverse effects and an evaluation of appropriate laboratory tests (hemoglobin, platelet count, white blood count, coagulation profile, arterial blood gases, blood glucose, electrolytes, liver and renal function tests, electrocardiogram [ECG], chest radiograph) are useful in the preoperative evaluation of patients being treated with chemotherapeutic drugs. Attention to asepsis is essential, because immunosuppression makes these patients susceptible to iatrogenic infection. The existence of mucositis makes the placement of pharyngeal airways, laryngeal mask airways, and esophageal catheters questionable. The response to inhaled and injected drugs may be altered by drug-induced cardiac, hepatic, or renal dysfunction. The response to nondepolarizing neuromuscular-blocking drugs may be altered by impaired renal function.

TOXICITIES (TABLE 29-1)

DNA ALKYLATING DRUGS

DNA alkylating drugs damage DNA and are more likely to kill malignant cells than nonmalignant cells because the rates of proliferation are greater for the cancer cells.

Side Effects

Bone marrow suppression is the most important dose-limiting factor in the clinical use of alkylating drugs.

Nitrogen Mustards

Mechlorethamine

Mechlorethamine is a rapidly acting nitrogen mustard administered intravenously. This drug, like other nitrogen

TABLE 29-1.
CLASSIFICATION OF CHEMOTHERAPEUTIC DRUGS AND ASSOCIATED SIDE EFFECTS

Group and Class	Therapeutic Uses	Side Effects (Other than Nausea and Vomiting)
Alkylating Drugs		
Nitrogen Mustards		
Mechlorethamine	Hodgkin disease Non-Hodgkin lymphoma	Myelosuppression Mucositis Alopecia
Cyclophosphamide	Acute lymphocytic leukemia Chronic lymphocytic leukemia Lymphomas Myeloma Neuroblastoma Breast, ovarian, cervical, and testicular cancer Lung cancer Wilms tumor Sarcoma	Myelosuppression Mucositis Alopecia Hemorrhagic cystitis Skin pigmentation Seizures Renal failure Cardiac failure Inappropriate secretion of vasopressin (AVP)
Melphalan	Myeloma Breast cancer	Myelosuppression
Chlorambucil	Hodgkin disease Non-Hodgkin lymphoma Macroglobulinemia	Myelosuppression Secondary leukemias
Ethyleneimines		
Hexamethylmelamine	Ovarian cancer	Myelosuppression
Thiotepa	Bladder, breast and ovarian cancer	
Alkyl Sulfonates		
Busulfan	Acute myelogenous leukemia Chronic myelogenous leukemia	Myelosuppression Thrombocytopenia
Nitrosoureas		
Carmustine (BCNU)	Hodgkin disease	Myelosuppression

(continued)

TABLE 29-1.
(continued)

Group and Class	Therapeutic Uses	Side Effects (Other than Nausea and Vomiting)
	Non-Hodgkin lymphoma Astrocytoma Myeloma Melanoma	Hepatitis Interstitial pulmonary fibrosis Renal failure Flushing
Lomustine (CCNU)	Hodgkin disease Non-Hodgkin lymphoma Astrocytoma Small cell lung cancer	Myelosuppression
Semustine (methyl-CCNU)	Colon cancer	Myelosuppression
Streptozotocin	Insulinoma Carcinoid tumor	Myelosuppression Hepatitis Renal failure
Triazines		
Dacarbazine (DTIC)	Hodgkin disease Melanoma Sarcomas	Myelosuppression Flulike syndrome
Temozolomide	Astrocytoma Melanoma	Hepatic toxicity Hyperglycemia Anemia Thrombocytopenia Lymphocytopenia
Bioreductive Alkylating Drugs		
Mitomycin-C	Head and neck, breast, lung, gastric, colon, rectal, and cervical cancer	Myelosuppression Mucositis Cardiac failure Interstitial fibrosis Hemolytic-uremic syndrome
Platinating Agents		
Platinum Compounds		
Cisplatin	Head and neck, thyroid, lung, ovarian,	Myelosuppression Peripheral neuropathy

TABLE 29-1.
(continued)

	endometrial, cervical and testicular cancer Neuroblastoma Osteogenic sarcoma	Allergic reactions Renal toxicity Electrolyte abnormalities (hypocalcemia, hypomagnesemia, hypophosphatemia)
Carboplatin	as for Cisplatin	Myelosuppression
Oxaliplatin	Colon cancer	Myelosuppression Peripheral neuropathy
Nucleic Acid Synthetase Inhibitors		
Folate Analogs		
Methotrexate	Head and neck, breast, and lung cancer Acute lymphocytic leukemia Non-Hodgkin lymphoma Osteogenic sarcoma	Myelosuppression Mucositis Pneumonitis Hepatic fibrosis
Pyrimidine Analogues		
Fluorouracil (5-FU)	Head and neck, breast, gastric, pancreatic, bladder, ovarian, cervical and prostate cancer Hepatoma	Myelosuppression Mucositis Alopecia Pigmentation Chest pain
Cytarabine	Acute lymphocytic leukemia Acute myeloid leukemia Non-Hodgkin lymphoma	Myelosuppression Mucositis Hepatitis
Gemcitabine	Breast, lung, pancreatic, and bladder cancer	Myelosuppression Flulike syndrome
Purine Analogues		
Mercaptopurine	Acute lymphocytic leukemia Acute myeloid leukemia	Myelosuppression Anorexia Jaundice

(*continued*)

TABLE 29-1.
(continued)

Group and Class	Therapeutic Uses	Side Effects (Other than Nausea and Vomiting)
	Chronic myeloid leukemia	
Thioguanine	As for Mercaptopurine	Myelosuppression Anorexia
Fludarabine	Chronic lymphocytic leukemia Non-Hodgkin lymphoma	Myelosuppression Optic neuritis Peripheral neuropathy Seizures Coma Depletion of CD4 cells
Pentostatin	Chronic lymphocytic leukemia Cutaneous T-cell lymphoma Hairy cell leukemia	Myelosuppression Depletion of T cells Hepatitis
Cladribine	Chronic lymphocytic leukemia Cutaneous T-cell lymphoma Hairy cell leukemia Waldenstrom macroglobulinemia	Myelosuppression Tumor lysis syndrome Asthenia
Hydroxyurea	Chronic myeloid leukemia Polycythemia vera Thrombocytopenia Melanoma	Myelosuppression Dermatologic changes
DNA Topoisomerase Inhibitors		
Anthracyclines		
Doxorubicin	Hodgkin disease Non-Hodgkin lymphoma Acute lymphocytic leukemia Neuroblastoma	Myelosuppression Cardiomyopathy Mucositis

TABLE 29-1. (continued)

	Thyroid, breast, lung, and gastric cancer	
Daunomycin	Acute myeloid leukemia Acute lymphocytic leukemia	
Idarubicin	As for Daunomycin	
Epirubicin	Hodgkin disease Non-Hodgkin lymphoma Acute lymphocytic leukemia Breast, lung, gastric, and bladder cancer	Myelosuppression Cardiomyopathy Alopecia Phlebitis
Anthracenediones		
Mitoxantrone	Acute myeloid leukemia Breast cancer	Myelosuppression Mucositis
Epipodophyllotoxins		
Etoposide	Hodgkin disease Non-Hodgkin lymphoma Acute myeloid leukemia Kaposi sarcoma Breast, lung, and testicular cancer	Myelosuppression Systemic hypotension Hepatitis Mucositis
Teniposide	Acute lymphocytic leukemia (children) Acute myeloid leukemia (children)	Myelosuppression Systemic hypotension
Dactinomycin	Wilms tumor Rhabdomyosarcoma Choriocarcinoma Kaposi sarcoma Ewing sarcoma Testicular cancer	Myelosuppression Mucositis Cheilitis Glossitis Alopecia Cutaneous erythema
Camptothecins		
Irinotecan	Colon cancer Ovarian cancer	Myelosuppression Alopecia
Topotecan	Lung cancer Ovarian cancer	As for Irinotecan

(*continued*)

TABLE 29-1. (continued)

Group and Class	Therapeutic Uses	Side Effects (Other than Nausea and Vomiting)
Other DNA-Damaging Drugs		
Antibiotic		
Bleomycin	Hodgkin disease Non-Hodgkin lymphoma Head and neck cancer Testicular cancer	Interstitial pulmonary fibrosis Allergic reactions Skin pigmentation
Antimicrotubule Drugs		
Vinca Alkaloids		
Vinblastine	Hodgkin disease Non-Hodgkin lymphoma Breast cancer Testicular cancer	Myelosuppression Peripheral neuropathy
Vincristine	Hodgkin disease Non-Hodgkin lymphoma Small cell lung cancer Neuroblastoma Wilms tumor Rhabdomyosarcoma Acute lymphocytic leukemia	Myelosuppression Peripheral neuropathy
Vinorelbine	Breast cancer Lung cancer	Myelosuppression Peripheral neuropathy
Taxanes		
Paclitaxel	Breast, lung, bladder, and ovarian cancer	Myelosuppression Peripheral neuropathy Allergic reactions Alopecia totalis
Docetaxel	Breast, lung, bladder, and ovarian cancer	Myelosuppression Peripheral neuropathy Allergic reactions Alopecia totalis

TABLE 29-1.
(continued)

		Cardiac dysrhythmias Capillary leakage
Signal Transduction Modulators		
Antiestrogens		
Tamoxifen	Breast cancer	Venous thrombosis Weight gain Amenorrhea Hypercalcemia Endometrial cancer Hot flashes
Toremifene	Breast cancer	Venous thrombosis Hot flashes
Raloxifene	Breast cancer	Venous thrombosis Hot flashes
Antiandrogens		
Flutamide	Prostate cancer	Gynecomastia Hot flashes
Bicalutamide	Prostate cancer	Gynecomastia Hot flashes
Nilutamide	Prostate cancer	Gynecomastia Hot flashes Delayed visual adaptation to dark
Monoclonal Antibodies		
Rituximab	Chronic lymphocytic leukemia Non-Hodgkin lymphoma	Infusion-related chills, rash, and fever Non-infusion related myalgias, angioedema, bronchospasm, cardiac dysrhythmias Myelosuppression
Trastuzumab	Breast cancer	Fever and chills
Aromatase Inhibitors		
Aminoglutethimide	Breast cancer	Orthostatic hypotension Glucocorticoid deficiency Cutaneous rash

(*continued*)

TABLE 29-1.
(continued)

Group and Class	Therapeutic Uses	Side Effects (Other than Nausea and Vomiting)
Anastrazole	Breast cancer	Asthenia Headache Hot flashes
Letrozole	Breast cancer	Headache Heartburn
Gonadotropin-Releasing Drugs		
Leuprolide	Breast cancer Prostate cancer	Impotence Hot flashes Pain at sites of bony metastases (tumor flare)
Buserelin	Breast cancer Prostate cancer	As for Leuprolide
Progestin		
Megestrol acetate	Breast cancer Endometrial cancer	Weight gain

mustards, is a vesicant, requiring that gloves be worn by personnel handling the drug.

Clinical Uses

Mechlorethamine produces beneficial effects in the treatment of Hodgkin's disease and less predictably, in other lymphomas.

Side Effects

Leukopenia and thrombocytopenia limit the amount of drug that may be administered. Herpes zoster is frequently associated with nitrogen mustard therapy. Thrombophlebitis is a potential complication.

Cyclophosphamide

Cyclophosphamide is converted to an active form in the liver following oral administration.

Clinical Uses

Cyclophosphamide is one of the most frequently used chemotherapeutic drugs, because it is effective orally and parenterally for a wide range of cancers.

Side Effects

Hypersensitivity reactions and fibrosing pneumonitis may occur, and large doses of cyclophosphamide are associated with a high incidence of pericarditis and pericardial effusion. Thrombocytopenia is less frequent than with other nitrogen mustards. Hemorrhagic cystitis presumably reflects the chemical irritation produced by reactive metabolites of cyclophosphamide. Water intoxication may reflect the inappropriate secretion of arginine vasopressin hormone.

Melphalan

Melphalan is a phenylalanine derivative of nitrogen mustard with a wide range of activity. Unlike other nitrogen mustards, it is not a vesicant.

Side Effects

Side effects of melphalan are primarily hematologic and are similar to those of other alkylating drugs. Nausea and vomiting are not common, and changes in renal or hepatic function are unlikely.

Chlorambucil

Chlorambucil is the treatment of choice in chronic lymphocytic leukemia and in primary (Waldenström's) macroglobulinemia.

Side Effects

Side effects on the bone marrow, lymphoid organs, and epithelial cells are similar to those observed with other alkylating drugs.

Alkyl Sulfonates

Busulfan

Busulfan is eliminated by the kidneys as methane sulfonic acid. Busulfan produces remissions in up to 90% of patients with chronic myelogenous leukemia.

Side Effects

Busulfan can produce progressive pulmonary fibrosis and prognosis is poor once clinical symptoms appear. Enhanced toxicity with supplemental oxygen has been noted. Allopurinol is recommended to minimize renal complications from hyperuricemia (purine catabolism from rapid cellular destruction).

Nitrosoureas

Nitrosoureas possess a wide spectrum of activity for human malignancies, including intracranial tumors, melanomas, and gastrointestinal and hematologic malignancies. With the exception of streptozocin, the clinical use of nitrosoureas is limited by profound drug-induced myelosuppression.

Carmustine

Carmustine is capable of inhibiting the synthesis of both RNA and DNA. Because of its ability to cross the blood-brain barrier, carmustine is used to treat meningeal leukemia and primary as well as metastatic brain tumors.

Side Effects

Carmustine has been associated with interstitial pneumonitis, as is bleomycin (cumulative dose is the major risk factor). A unique side effect of carmustine is a delayed onset (after approximately 6 weeks of treatment) of leukopenia and thrombocytopenia.

Lomustine and Semustine

Lomustine and semustine possess clinical toxicity similar to carmustine.

Streptozocin

Streptozocin has a unique affinity for β-cells of the islets of Langerhans. Approximately 70% of patients receiving this drug develop hepatic or renal toxicity. Myelosuppression is not produced by this drug.

Mitomycin

Mitomycin inhibits the synthesis of DNA and is of value in the palliative treatment of gastric adenocarcinoma.

Side Effects

Myelosuppression is a prominent side effect of mitomycin. Mitomycin is capable of inducing pulmonary fibrosis (like bleomycin, it appears to act synergistically with thoracic radiation and oxygen therapy; it is prudent to avoid hyperoxia in patients treated with mitomycin).

PLATINATING DRUGS

Cisplatin

Cisplatin must be administered intravenously, and high concentrations are found in the kidneys, liver, intestines, and testes with only poor penetration into the CNS.

Side Effects

Renal toxicity is the dose-limiting toxic effect of cisplatin. Hypomagnesemia associated with cisplatin's renal tubular injury may predispose patients to cardiac dysrhythmias and decrease the dose requirements for neuromuscular-blocking drugs. Peripheral sensory neuropathies are common but usually reversible.

NUCLEIC ACID SYNTHESIS INHIBITORS

Nucleic acid synthesis inhibitors (antimetabolites) are particularly effective in destroying cells during the S phase of the cell cycle when DNA is synthesized.

Folate Analogs

Methotrexate

Methotrexate inhibits dihydrofolate reductase, which is the enzyme that uses reduced folate as a methyl donor in the synthesis of pyrimidine and purine nucleosides (1-carbon transfer reactions necessary for the synthesis of DNA and RNA cease). Significant metabolism of methotrexate does not seem to occur, with more than 50% of the drug appearing in urine; thus, toxic concentrations may develop in patients with renal insufficiency.

Clinical Uses

Methotrexate is widely used in the treatment of malignant (choriocarcinoma) and nonmalignant disorders (psoriasis, rheumatoid arthritis). Methotrexate is poorly transported across the blood-brain barrier and acquired resistance may develop (reflects increased concentrations of intracellular dihydrofolate reductase).

Side Effects

The most important side effects of methotrexate occur in the gastrointestinal tract (hemorrhagic enteritis) and bone marrow (leukopenia and thrombocytopenia). Pulmonary toxicity and renal toxicity are possible. Hepatic dysfunction is usually reversible but may sometimes lead to cirrhosis; it may be useful to measure liver function tests preoperatively.

Pyrimidine Analogs

Fluorouracil

Fluorouracil is converted to it 5′-monophosphate nucleotide, which blocks the production of thymine nucleotides by inhibiting thymidylate synthase.

Clinical Uses

Fluorouracil may be of palliative value in breast and gastrointestinal tract cancers and is often used for topical treatment of premalignant keratoses of the skin and superficial basal cell carcinomas.

Side Effects

The side effects of fluorouracil are difficult to anticipate because of their delayed appearance (myocardial infarction, especially in patients with underlying heart disease; myelosuppression).

Capecitabine

Capecitabine is metabolized to fluorouracil after its oral absorption.

Pemetrexal

Pemetrexal is a folate antagonist that is effective in the treatment of mesothelioma and lung cancer.

Cytarabine

Cytarabine is activated by conversion to 5′-monophosphate nucleotide before inhibition of DNA synthesis can occur.

Clinical Uses

This drug is particularly effective in treating acute leukemia in children and adults.

Side Effects

Cytarabine is a potent myelosuppressive drug. Thrombophlebitis at the site of infusion is common.

Gemcitabine

Gemcitabine is active in several nonhematologic cancers, whereas *cytarabine* is not effective.

Purine Analogues

Mercaptopurine

Mercaptopurine is incorporated into DNA or RNA strands and either blocks further strand synthesis or causes structural alterations that damage DNA. Allopurinol, as an inhibitor of xanthine oxidase, prevents the conversion of mercaptopurine to 6-thiouric acid and thus increases the exposure of cells to mercaptopurine.

Side Effects

The principal side effect of mercaptopurine is a gradual development of bone marrow depression manifesting as thrombocytopenia, granulocytopenia, or anemia several weeks after the initiation of therapy. Jaundice occurs in approximately one-third of patients and is associated with bile stasis and occasional hepatic necrosis.

Thioguanine

Thioguanine is of particular value in the treatment of acute granulocytic leukemia. Minimal amounts of 6-thiouric acid are formed, and thioguanine can be administered concurrently with allopurinol without a reduction in dosage (in contrast to mercaptopurine).

Pentostatin and Cladribine

Pentostatin and cladribine act by irreversibly binding to adenosine deaminase (pentostatin) or by chemical modification of the enzyme substrate, thus rendering it resistant to the action of adenosine deaminase (cladribine). The minimal toxicity of cladribine makes it an attractive choice for the treatment of hairy-cell leukemia.

Hydroxyurea

Hydroxyurea acts on the enzyme ribonucleoside diphosphate reductase to interfere with the synthesis of DNA. The primary use of hydroxyurea is in the treatment of chronic granulocytic leukemia.

Side Effects

Myelosuppression manifesting as leukopenia, megaloblastic anemia, and occasionally thrombocytopenia is the major side effect produced by hydroxyurea.

DNA TOPOISOMERASE INHIBITORS

Topoisomerases are enzymes that correct those alterations in DNA that occur during replication and transcription. Because cancer cells possess more topoisomerase activity than normal cells, more drug-induced DNA damage occurs, resulting in cell death. These drugs exhibit a broad spectrum of chemotherapeutic activity, being useful in the treatment of leukemia, lung, colon, and ovarian cancer.

Doxorubicin and Daunorubicin

Doxorubicin and daunorubicin are anthracycline antibiotics that most likely act by binding to DNA, which results in changes in the DNA helix. Drug-induced free radicals may overwhelm the heart's antioxidant defenses and lead to cardiotoxicity. These drugs do not cross the blood-brain barrier to any significant extent. The urine may become red for 1 to 2 days after administration of these drugs. Ultimately, approximately 40% of the drugs are metabolized (clinical toxicity may result in patients with hepatic dysfunction).

Clinical Uses

Doxorubicin is one of the most widely used single drugs for treating solid tumors (adenocarcinoma of the breast, carcinoma of the bladder, bronchogenic carcinoma, osteogenic carcinoma)

Side Effects

Cardiomyopathy and myelosuppression are side effects of the chemotherapeutic antibiotics.

Cardiomyopathy

Cardiomyopathy manifesting as congestive heart failure is a unique dose-related and often irreversible side effect of the anthracycline antibiotics, (increased plasma concentrations of troponin T). Previous treatment with anthracycline antibiotics may enhance the myocardial depressant effects of anesthetics, even in patients with normal resting cardiac function. Two types of cardiomyopathy may occur (Table 29-2). Dexrazoxane is a free radical scavenger that protects the heart from doxorubicin-associated damage.

Dactinomycin

Dactinomycin (actinomycin D) is an antibiotic with chemotherapeutic activity resulting from its ability to bind to DNA and block the transcription of DNA. Hepatic metabolism does not occur, and this drug does not cross the blood-brain barrier.

TABLE 29-2.
TYPES OF CARDIOMYOPATHY IN PATIENTS TREATED WITH ANTHRACYCLINE ANTIBIOTICS

Acute cardiomyopathy (occurs approximately 10% of patients, reversible)
- Benign changes on the electrocardiogram
  - Nonspecific ST-T changes
  - Decreased QRS voltage (diffuse myocardial damage)
- Cardiac dysrhythmias
  - Premature ventricular contractions
  - Supraventricular tachycardia

Insidious onset of cardiomyopathy
- Dry nonproductive cough followed rapidly by congestive heart failure that is not responsive to inotropic drugs
- High mortality

Clinical Uses

The most important clinical use of dactinomycin is the treatment of Wilms' tumor in children and of rhabdomyosarcoma.

Side Effects

Myelosuppression manifesting as pancytopenia may occur 1 to 7 days after completion of therapy.

Bleomycin

Bleomycin produces free radicals that create DNA breaks. Excretion is primarily by the kidneys, and excessive concentrations of the drug occur if usual doses are administered to patients with impaired renal function.

Clinical Uses

Bleomycin is effective in the treatment of testicular carcinoma, particularly if administered in combination with vinblastine.

Side Effects

The most common side effects of bleomycin are mucocutaneous reactions (stomatitis, pruritus, hyperpigmentation). In contrast to other chemotherapeutic drugs, bleomycin causes minimal myelosuppression.

Pulmonary Toxicity (Table 29-3)

Pulmonary toxicity is the most serious dose-related side effect. Bleomycin is concentrated preferentially in the lungs and is inactivated by hydrolase enzyme, which is relatively deficient in lung tissue. Initially, bleomycin produces pulmonary capillary damage, and interstitial fibrosis may progress to involve the entire lung. The first signs of pulmonary toxicity are cough and dyspnea, which may progress in one of two directions. A mild form of pulmonary toxicity is characterized by exertional dyspnea and normal resting PaO_2. A more severe form of pulmonary toxicity is associated with arterial hypoxemia at rest and radiographic findings of interstitial pneumonitis and fibrosis. Pulmonary function studies have been of no greater value than clinical signs in detecting the onset of pulmonary toxicity. Patients with prior exposure to bleomycin

TABLE 29-3.
RISK FACTORS FOR DEVELOPMENT OF CHEMOTHERAPY-INDUCED PULMONARY TOXICITY

Total drug dose
Age
Concurrent or prior chest radiation
Oxygen therapy
Combination chemotherapy
Preexisting pulmonary disease
Genetic predisposition
Cigarette smoking (?)

but no risk factors appear to be at minimum risk from hyperoxia. In contrast, those patients with one or more major risk factors (preexisting pulmonary damage from bleomycin, renal dysfunction, exposure to bleomycin within a 1- to 2-month period) may be at higher risk for bleomycin-induced hyperoxic pulmonary injury in the operating room. It may be prudent to maintain these patients on the minimum inspired oxygen concentration that can be used safely in the operating room to provide oxygen saturations >90%. An additional consideration is the replacement of fluids with colloids rather than crystalloids to decrease or prevent pulmonary interstitial edema in bleomycin-treated patients undergoing surgery.

ANTIMICROTUBULE DRUGS

Vinca alkaloids and taxanes are examples of antimitotic chemotherapeutic drugs that disrupt the normal function of microtubules (subcellular structures that form the architecture to maintain cell shape) leading to cell death.

Vinca Alkaloids

Vinca alkaloids represent the active medicinal ingredients from the periwinkle plant.

Side Effects

Myelosuppression, manifesting as leukopenia, thrombocytopenia, and anemia, is the most prominent side effect of vinca alkaloids, manifesting 7 to 10 days after initiation of treatment. Symmetric peripheral sensory-motor neuropathy often occurs and may become the dose-limiting side effect (may require months to resolve following discontinuation of the drug). Autonomic neuropathy with orthostatic hypotension and cranial nerve involvement (laryngeal nerve paralysis with hoarseness) is present in about 10% of treated patients. Hyponatremia associated with high urinary sodium and inappropriate secretion of arginine vasopressin hormone may occur.

Taxanes

Taxanes provide a broad spectrum of chemotherapeutic activity against breast, lung, ovarian, and bladder cancer. Taxanes block the function of the mitotic apparatus by impeding the normal function of microtubules. Hepatic metabolism and biliary excretion appears to be responsible for most of the plasma clearance.

Side Effects

Taxanes are associated with myelosuppression, peripheral neuropathy (sensory symptoms in a glove-and-stocking distribution), and alopecia. Severe neurotoxicity precludes the administration of high doses of taxanes. Fluid retention may be decreased by pretreatment with dexamethasone. Hypersensitivity reactions (flushing, bronchospasm, dyspnea, systemic hypotension), caused by the direct release of histamine or other chemical mediators, may occur in 25% to 30% of patients treated with taxanes.

Estramustine

Estramustine inhibits microtubule assembly and exhibits high binding to prostate tissue, thus making it possibly useful as part of combination therapy in hormone-refractory prostate cancer.

SIGNAL TRANSDUCTION MODULATORS

Signal transduction modulators (hormones) used as chemotherapeutic drugs produce a disruption of growth factor receptor interactions.

Progestins

Progestins are useful in the management of patients with endometrial carcinoma.

Estrogens and Androgens

Malignant changes in the breast and prostate often depend on hormones for their continued growth. Hypercalcemia may be associated with androgen and estrogen therapy, requiring adequate hydration in an attempt to facilitate the renal excretion of calcium.

Antiestrogens

Antiestrogens (tamoxifen) are useful in the treatment of breast cancer that expresses estrogen or progesterone receptors. Tamoxifen is antiestrogenic in breast and ovarian tissue but is estrogenic in the uterus, liver, and bone. As a result, tamoxifen is effective in the prevention and treatment of breast cancer but produces undesired estrogen side effects including deep vein thrombosis and early menopausal symptoms (hot flashes).

Antiandrogens

Antiandrogens (flutamide) are competitive antagonists of the interactions between androstenedione and androgen receptors. Flutamide is an effective treatment for hormone-dependent prostate cancer; however, it produces a male menopause state characterized by gynecomastia, hot flashes, loss of facial hair, skeletal muscle weakness, and osteoporosis. Methemoglobinemia can be induced by flutamide.

Monoclonal Antibodies

Monoclonal antibodies that target specific antigen sites on cancer cells are available.

Aromatase Inhibitors

Inhibition of aromatase enzyme blocks the conversion of androgens to estrone in peripheral tissues including breast tissue.

Antiepileptic Drugs

30

It is estimated that 50 million people (1 to 2% of the population) worldwide have epilepsy (recurrent seizures) (Table 30-1) (Stoelting RK, Hillier SC. Antiepileptic drugs. In: *Pharmacology and Physiology in Anesthetic Practice.* 4th ed. Philadelphia, Lippincott Williams & Wilkins, 2006:569–579). About 30% of patients with seizures have an identifiable neurologic or systemic disorder, and the remainder have idiopathic epilepsy. Approximately 70% of patients with epilepsy will become seizure-free utilizing a single antiepileptic drug (Table 30-2). Dose-related side effects are common and frequently limit the use of antiepileptic drugs (Table 30-3).

PHARMACOKINETICS (TABLE 30-4)

Antiepileptic drugs induce or inhibit drug metabolism (except gabapentin, levetiracetam, vigabatrin) and may be associated with pharmacokinetic drug interactions in which plasma drug concentrations and the resulting pharmacologic effects of concomitantly administered drugs may be altered.

Drug Interactions Related to Protein Binding

Medications (salicylates) that compete for protein-binding sites of highly bound antiepileptic drugs (phenytoin, valproate, carbamazepine) can displace the bound drug and lead to increases in the plasma concentration of pharmacologically active antiepileptic drug. Hypoalbuminemia, as may accompany renal or hepatic disease, malnutrition, or

TABLE 30-1.
CLASSIFICATION OF EPILEPTIC SEIZURES

Partial seizures (beginning locally)
- Simple partial seizures (consciousness not impaired)
- Complex partial seizures (consciousness impaired)
- Partial seizures evolving into secondary generalized seizures

Generalized seizures (convulsive or nonconvulsive)
- Absence seizures (petit mal)
- Myoclonic seizures
- Clonic seizures
- Tonic seizures
- Tonic-clonic seizures

Unclassified seizures

pregnancy, can result in increased plasma concentrations of unbound antiepileptic drugs and result in toxicity despite therapeutic plasma concentrations.

Drug Interactions Related to Accelerated Metabolism

The enzyme-inducing (P-450 activity) antiepileptic drugs that accelerate metabolism (carbamazepine, oxcarbazepine, phenobarbital, phenytoin, topiramate) may render oral contraceptives ineffective at usual doses. Patients being treated with antiepileptic drugs have increased dose requirements for thiopental, propofol, midazolam, opioids, and nondepolarizing neuromuscular-blocking drugs.

PRINCIPLES OF DOSING

An effective dose is one at which seizures cease but side effects do not appear (see Table 30-3).

TABLE 30-2.

ANTIEPILEPTIC DRUGS USED TO TREAT EPILEPSY

Drug	Principal Mechanism of Action	Targeted Seizure Type	Dosage
Carbamazepine	Sodium ion channel blockade	Partial seizures	10–40 mg/kg/day in 3–4 divided doses
Ethosuximide	T–type calcium ion channel	Generalized seizures	15–40 mg/kg/day in 2–3 divided doses
Felbamate	Sodium ion channel blockade Glutamate antagonism Calcium ion channel blockade	Partial seizures Generalized seizures	15–45 mg/kg/day in 2–3 divided doses
Gabapentin	Unknown (? Increases GABA release)	Partial seizures Generalized seizures	10–60 mg/kg/day
Lamotrigine	Sodium ion channel blockade Calcium ion channel blockade	Partial seizures Generalized seizures	200–500 mg/day in 2 divided doses
Levetiracetam	Unknown (? potassium and calcium ion channel blockade)	Partial seizures Generalized seizures	1,000–3,000 mg/day in 2 divided doses
Oxcarbazepine	Sodium ion channel blockade	Partial seizures Generalized seizures	900–2, 400 mg/day in 2 divided doses

(*continued*)

TABLE 30-2.
(continued)

Drug	Principal Mechanism of Action	Seizure Type	Targeted Dosage
Phenobarbital	Chloride ion channels	Partial seizures Generalized seizures	2–5 mg/kg/day every day or in 2 divided doses
Phenytoin	Sodium ion channel blockade Calcium ion channels NMDA receptors	Partial seizures Generalized seizures	3–7 mg/kg/day in 3 divided doses
Primidone	Chloride ion channels GABA uptake	Partial seizures Generalized seizures	500–1500 mg/day in 2–3 divided doses
Tiagabine	Enhanced GABA activity Carbonic anhydrase inhibition	Partial seizures Generalized seizures	32–56 mg/kg/day in 2–4 divided doses
Topiramate	Sodium ion channel blockade Enhanced GABA activity Glutamate antagonism Calcium ion channel blockade	Partial seizures Generalized seizures	500–3,000 mg/day in 2–4 divided doses
Valproate	Sodium ion channel blockade Calcium ion channels	Partial seizures Generalized seizures	500–3,000 mg/day in 2–4 divided doses
Zonisamide	Sodium ion channel blockade Calcium ion channel blockade	Partial seizures Generalized seizures	200–600 mg/day in 2–4 divided doses
Fosphenytoin	Sodium ion channel blockade	Status epilepticus	10–20 mg/kg IV loading dose

TABLE 30-3.

SIDE EFFECTS OF ANTIEPILEPTIC DRUGS CORRECT

	Dose-related	Idiosyncratic
Carbamazepine	Diplopia Vertigo Neutropenia Nausea Drowsiness Hyponatremia	Agranulocytosis Aplastic anemia Allergic dermatitis (rash) Stevens-Johnson syndrome Hepatotoxic effects Pancreatitis Teratogenicity
Ethosuximide	Nausea Anorexia Vomiting Agitation Headache Drowsiness	Agranulocytosis Aplastic anemia Allergic dermatitis (rash) Stevens-Johnson syndrome Lupus-like syndrome
Clonazepam	Sedation Vertigo Hyperactivity (children)	Allergic dermatitis (rash) Thrombocytopenia
Felbamate	Insomnia Anorexia	Aplastic anemia Hepatotoxic effects

(*continued*)

TABLE 30-3. (continued)

	Dose-related	Idiosyncratic
Gabapentin	Nausea Headache Irritability Sedation Ataxia Vertigo Gastrointestinal disturbances	
Lamotrigine	Tremor Vertigo Diplopia Ataxia Headache Gastrointestinal disturbances	Stevens-Johnson syndrome
Levetiracetam	Sedation Anxiety Headache	Allergic dermatitis (rash)
Oxcarbazepine		Allergic dermatitis (rash)
Phenobarbital	Sedation Depression	Agranulocytosis Allergic dermatitis (rash)

TABLE 30-3.
(continued)

	Dose-related	**Idiosyncratic**
	Hyperactivity (children)	Stevens-Johnson syndrome Arthritic changes Hepatotoxic effects Teratogenicity
Phenytoin	Nystagmus Ataxia Nausea and vomiting Gingival hyperplasia Depression Megaloblastic anemia Drowsiness	Agranulocytosis Aplastic anemia Allergic dermatitis (rash) Stevens-Johnson syndrome Hepatotoxic effects Pancreatitis Acne Coarse facies Hirsutism Teratogenicity Dupuytren's contracture
Primidone	Sedation	Rash Thrombocytopenia Agranulocytosis Lupus-like syndrome Teratogenicity

(*continued*)

TABLE 30-3.
(continued)

	Dose-related	Idiosyncratic
Tiagabine	Dizziness Aphasia Tremor	Allergic dermatitis (rash)
Topiramate	Sedation Ataxia Dizziness	Allergic dermatitis (rash)
Valproic acid	Tremor Weight gain Dyspepsia Nausea and vomiting Alopecia Peripheral edema Encephalopathy Teratogenicity	Agranulocytosis Aplastic anemia Allergic dermatitis (rash) Stevens-Johnson syndrome Hepatotoxic effects Pancreatitis
Zonisamide	Sedation Dizziness Ataxia Nephrolithiasis Hyperactivity (children) Mania (adults)	Allergic dermatitis (rash)

TABLE 30-4.
PHARMACOKINETICS OF ANTIEPILEPTIC DRUGS

	Plasma Therapeutic Concentration (μg/mL)	Protein Binding (%)	Elimination Half–Time (hrs)	Route of Elimination
Carbamazepine	6–12	70–80	8–24	Hepatic metabolism (active metabolite)
Clonazepam	0.02–0.08	80–90	30–40	Hepatic metabolism
Diazepam		95	20–35	Hepatic metabolism (active metabolites)
Ethosuximide	40–100	0	20–60	Hepatic metabolism (25% excreted unchanged)
Felbamate		22–25	20–23	Renal excretion
Gabapentin	2–20	0	6	Renal excretion
Lamotrigine		54	25	Hepatic metabolism
Lorazepam		80	14	Hepatic metabolism
Oxcarbazepine		40	8–10	Renal excretion
Phenobarbital	10–40	48–54	72–144	Hepatic metabolism (25% excreted unchanged)

(*continued*)

TABLE 30-4.
(continued)

	Plasma Therapeutic Concentration (μg/mL)	Protein Binding (%)	Elimination Half–Time (hrs)	Route of Elimination
Phenytoin	10–20	90–93	9–40	Saturable hepatic metabolism
Primidone	5–12	20–30	4–12	Hepatic metabolism to active metabolites of which 40% are excreted unchanged
Tiagabine		95	5–8	Hepatic metabolism
Topiramate		10	8–15	Renal excretion and hepatic metabolism
Valproic acid	50–100	88–92	7–17	Hepatic metabolism (active metabolites)
Zonisamide		50	50–70	Hepatic metabolism

PLASMA CONCENTRATIONS AND LABORATORY TESTING

The titration to clinical efficacy is recommended for guiding the dosages of all antiepileptic drugs. If a patient does not respond to a particular drug as expected, checking the plasma drug concentration may aid in determining compliance and identifying potential pharmacokinetic interactions. Because many antiepileptic drugs are associated with rare but potentially life-threatening bone marrow suppression as well as hepatotoxicity, baseline as well as routine monitoring of hematological and liver functions may be recommended.

MECHANISM OF SEIZURE ACTIVITY

Seizure activity in most patients with epilepsy has a localized or focal origin (local biochemical changes, ischemia, infections, head trauma). The spread of seizure activity to neighboring normal cells is presumably restrained by normal inhibitory mechanisms (changes in blood glucose concentrations, PaO_2, $PaCO_2$, pH levels, electrolytes balance, stress, and fatigue may result in the spread of a seizure focus into areas of normal brain). If the spread is sufficiently extensive, the entire brain is activated and a tonic-clonic seizure with unconsciousness ensues.

MECHANISM OF DRUG ACTION

It is commonly presumed that antiepileptic drugs control seizures by decreasing neuronal excitability or enhancing the inhibition of neurotransmission. This is achieved by altering intrinsic membrane ion currents (sodium, potassium, calcium) or by affecting the activity of inhibitory neurotransmitters (γ-aminobutyric acid [GABA]).

MAJOR ANTIEPILEPTIC DRUGS (SEE TABLE 30-1 AND 30-2)

Adverse Side Effects (See Table 30-3)

Maternal epilepsy is associated with the risk of fetal malformations (such as ventricular septal defects and cleft palate and lip), and treatment with antiepileptic drugs increases this risk.

Carbamazepine

Carbamazepine is effective for the suppression of nonconvulsive and convulsive partial seizures and may be useful in the management of patients with trigeminal neuralgia and glossopharyngeal neuralgia.

Pharmacokinetics

This drug is available only as an oral preparation, and its active metabolite may be responsible for many of its dose-limiting side effects. Carbamazepine induces its own metabolism, and many patients require a dosage increase in 2 to 4 weeks after the initiation of therapy.

Side Effects

The toxicity of carbamazepine is similar to that produced by phenytoin (see Table 30-3). Aplastic anemia, thrombocytopenia, hepatocellular and cholestatic jaundice, oliguria, hypertension, and cardiac dysrhythmias are rare but potential life-threatening complications.

At high plasma concentrations, carbamazepine has an arginine vasopressin hormone-like action that may result in hyponatremia.

Ethosuximide

Ethosuximide is the drug of choice for the suppression of absence (petit mal) epilepsy in patients who do not also have tonic-clonic seizures.

Pharmacokinetics

This drug is available only as an oral preparation. Approximately 25% of the drug is excreted unchanged in the urine, and the remainder is metabolized to inactive metabolites by hepatic microsomal enzymes.

Side Effects

The toxicity of ethosuximide is low, although bone marrow suppression is a rare possibility.

Felbamate

Because of its potential to produce life-threatening side effects, felbamate is not used as a first-line drug for the treatment of seizures but rather is reserved for patients with intractable epilepsy.

Pharmacokinetics

Oral absorption is prompt, and hepatic metabolism is minimal, with most of the drug being excreted unchanged by the kidneys.

Side Effects

Serious side effects include aplastic anemia and hepatotoxicity (see Table 30-3). Monitoring of treated patients with complete blood counts and liver function tests is indicated. Felbamate is a potent inhibitor of P-450 enzymes and can slow the metabolism of phenytoin, phenobarbital, and valproic acid.

Gabapentin

Gabapentin is an effective antiepileptic drug and has been effective in a number of chronic pain syndromes. The drug's mechanism of action is poorly understood but most likely reflects an increase in the synthesis of GABA. Structurally, gabapentin resembles GABA, but the inclusion of a carbon ring greatly enhances its lipid solubility and ability to cross the blood-brain barrier.

Excretion is by the kidneys and the dose should be decreased in patients with renal dysfunction. Pharmacokinetic drug interactions with other drugs do not seem to occur, reflecting the absence of protein binding and any effect on the metabolism of other drugs.

Lamotrigine

Lamotrigine most likely acts by stabilizing voltage-sensitive sodium ion channels thus preventing the release of aspartate and glutamate.

Levetiracetam

Levetiracetam is effective in the management of partial-onset seizures in adults, and side effects are minor.

Oxcarbazepine

Oxcarbazepine is a keto-analog of carbamazepine that provides equivalent seizure control but with fewer adverse side effects.

Phenobarbital

Phenobarbital is effective against all seizure types except nonconvulsive primary generalized seizures. Because of side effects (cognitive and behavioral) phenobarbital is considered a second-line drug in the treatment of epilepsy.

Phenobarbital appears to exert its antiepileptic properties partly through the modulation of the postsynaptic inhibitory actions of GABA and of the excitatory postsynaptic actions of glutamate. These drug-induced effects prolong the duration of chloride channel opening and thus limit the spread of seizure activity and increase the seizure threshold.

Pharmacokinetics

The oral absorption of phenobarbital is slow but nearly complete and approximately 25% of phenobarbital is eliminated by pH-dependent renal excretion, with the remainder inactivated by hepatic microsomal enzymes. The development of tolerance to the drug's CNS effects makes the toxic threshold imprecise.

Side Effects (See Table 30-3)

Sedation in adults and children and irritability and hyperactivity in children are the most troublesome side effects when this drug is used to treat epilepsy. Interactions between phenobarbital and other drugs usually involve the induction of hepatic microsomal enzymes by phenobarbital; phenobarbital is a classic example of a hepatic microsomal enzyme inducer that can accelerate the metabolism of many lipid-soluble drugs.

Phenytoin

Phenytoin is effective for the treatment of partial and generalized seizures (oral or intravenous administration).

Mechanism of Action

Phenytoin regulates neuronal excitability (providing a stabilizing effect) and thus controls the spread of seizure activity from a seizure focus by regulating sodium and possibly calcium transport across neuronal membranes.

Pharmacokinetics

Phenytoin is a weak acid that is maintained in aqueous solutions as a sodium salt; it precipitates in solutions with a pH of <7.8.

Plasma Concentrations

The control of seizures is usually obtained when plasma concentrations are 10 to 20 μg/mL (8 to 16 μg/mL is usually sufficient to suppress cardiac dysrhythmias). Adverse side effects of phenytoin, such as nystagmus and ataxia, are likely when the plasma concentration of drug is more than 20 μg/mL.

Metabolism

The metabolism of phenytoin to inactive metabolites is through hepatic microsomal enzymes that are susceptible to stimulation or inhibition by other drugs. An estimated 98% of phenytoin is metabolized to the inactive derivative parahydroxyphenyl.

Side Effects

The side effects of phenytoin include CNS toxicity (nystagmus, ataxia) and peripheral neuropathy. Gingival hyperplasia occurs in approximately 20% of chronically treated patients. Hyperglycemia and glycosuria may reflect phenytoin-induced inhibition of insulin secretion. Phenytoin-induced hepatotoxicity, although rare, may occur in genetically susceptible patients who lack the enzyme phenytoin epoxide. Phenytoin can induce the oxidative metabolism of many lipid-soluble drugs. Patients receiving phenytoin chronically have higher dose requirements for nondepolarizing neuromuscular-blocking drugs such as vecuronium; this reflects an induction of hepatic enzymes and up-regulation of acetylcholine receptors.

Primidone

Primidone is metabolized to phenobarbital; the efficacy of this drug resembles that of phenobarbital but it is less well tolerated.

Tiagabine

Tiagabine is a potent inhibitor of GABA uptake. Drug interactions are unlikely, because tiagabine has no effect on hepatic enzymes.

Topiramate

Topiramate is a broad-spectrum antiepileptic drug that is also effective in the treatment of other neurologic and psychiatric disorders (bulimia, migraine headache, essential tremor). This drug is a weak inhibitor of carbonic anhydrase and does not affect hepatic P-450 enzymes.

Valproic Acid

Valproic acid is a branched chain carboxylic acid that is effective in the treatment of all primary generalized epilepsies and all convulsive epilepsies. This drug acts by limiting sustained repetitive neuronal firing through voltage-dependent sodium channels.

Pharmacokinetics

After oral administration, absorption is prompt, and more than 70% of the drug can recovered as inactive glucuronide conjugates.

Side Effects

Weight gain is common, and distal tremor and thrombocytopenia may occur. The most serious side effect of valproic acid is hepatotoxicity (incidence decreases dramatically after 2 years of age). Approximately 20% of treated patients have hyperammonemia without hepatic damage. Because valproic acid is eliminated as a ketone-containing metabolite, the urine ketone test may show false-positive results. Valproic acid is an enzyme inhibitor that slows the metabolism of phenytoin and phenobarbital.

Zonisamide

Zonisamide is a broad-spectrum antiepileptic drug that has an effect on voltage-dependent calcium ion channels and enhances GABA-mediated neuronal inhibition. Nephrolithiasis may occur in 3% of treated patients. Pharmacokinetic drug interactions are unlikely, because zonisamide does not displace other drugs from protein binding sites, and its effects on the metabolism of other drugs is minimal.

Benzodiazepines

Benzodiazepines bind to $GABA_A$ receptors and potentiate GABA-mediated neuronal inhibition, causing an increased chloride ion permeability that results in cellular hyperpolarization and the inhibition of neuronal firing.

Clonazepam

Clonazepam is first-line drug therapy only for myoclonic seizures.

Pharmacokinetics

Intravenous clonazepam results in rapid CNS effects. Clonazepam is extensively metabolized to inactive products, with >2% of an injected dose appearing unchanged in the urine.

Side Effects

Sedation is present in approximately 50% of patients, but tends to subside with chronic administration (see Table 30-3). Skeletal muscle incoordination and ataxia occur in approximately 30% of patients. Generalized seizure activity may be precipitated if the drug is discontinued abruptly. Hypotension and depression of ventilation have been observed after the intravenous administration of clonazepam.

Diazepam

Diazepam is a mainstay for the treatment of status epilepticus and local anesthetic-induced seizures (0.1 mg/kg IV every 10 to 15 minutes until seizure activity has been suppressed or a maximum dose of 30 mg has been administered).

Lorazepam

Lorazepam has a shorter elimination half-time than diazepam but a longer duration of action because it is not rapidly redistributed. Lorazepam is metabolized in the liver and has no active metabolites.

STATUS EPILEPTICUS

Status epilepticus is defined as continuous seizures or two or more seizures occurring in sequence without recovery of consciousness between seizures.

Treatment (Table 30-5)

TABLE 30-5.
TREATMENT OF STATUS EPILEPTICUS

Life support (patent upper airway that may require tracheal intubation and mechanical ventilation of the patient's lungs)

Intravenous access

Treat empirically with IV glucose (50 mL of 50% glucose for adults and 2 mL/kg of 25% glucose for children

Benzodiazepine (diazepam)

Long-acting antiepileptic drug (fosphenytoin up to 150 mg/min IV; hypotension and prolongation of the QTc interval on the electrocardiogram may necessitate slowing of the infusion)

31

Drugs Used for Treatment of Parkinson's Disease

The goal of treating Parkinson's disease is to enhance the inhibitory effect of dopamine or to decrease the excitatory effect of acetylcholine through the administration of centrally acting drugs (Stoelting RK, Hillier SC. Drugs used for treatment of Parkinson's disease. In: *Pharmacology and Physiology in Anesthetic Practice*. 4th ed. Philadelphia, Lippincott Williams & Wilkins, 2006:580–584). In patients with Parkinson's disease, the basal ganglia content of dopamine is only approximately 10% of normal. As a result, an excess of excitatory cholinergic activity occurs, manifesting as progressive tremor, skeletal muscle rigidity, bradykinesia, and disturbances of posture.

LEVODOPA

Levodopa crosses the blood-brain barrier (dopamine does not readily cross) and is converted to dopamine by aromatic-L-amino-acid decarboxylase (a dopa decarboxylase enzyme); this acts to replenish dopamine stores in the basal ganglia. The beneficial therapeutic response to levodopa typically diminishes after 2 to 5 years of treatment, presumably reflecting a progression of the disease process and continuing loss of nigrostriatal neurons with a capacity to store dopamine. Levodopa should be continued throughout the perioperative period, being included in the preoperative medication. An abrupt discontinuation of levodopa may result in a precipitous return of symptoms of Parkinson's disease, and this has been associated with a neuroleptic malignant-like syndrome.

Metabolism

Approximately 95% of orally administered levodopa is rapidly decarboxylated to dopamine during the initial passage through the liver (resulting dopamine cannot easily cross the blood-brain barrier). In this regard, the inhibition of the peripheral activity of decarboxylase enzyme greatly increases the fraction of administered levodopa that remains intact to cross the blood-brain barrier. Most metabolites of dopamine are excreted by the kidneys.

Side Effects (Table 31-1)

TABLE 31-1.
SIDE EFFECTS ASSOCIATED WITH THE ADMINISTRATION OF LEVODOPA

Gastrointestinal dysfunction
- Nausea and vomiting (antiemetic drugs that interfere with dopamine are not recommended; treat with domperidone 10 to 20 mg orally, which does not cross the blood-brain barrier)

Cardiovascular changes (reflect α- and β-adrenergic effects of dopamine)
- Orthostatic hypotension
- Cardiac dysrhythmias (sinus tachycardia, atrial and ventricular premature contractions, atrial fibrillation, ventricular tachycardia; propranolol an effective treatment)

Abnormal involuntary movements (tics, grimacing, rocking movements of arms, legs, and trunk are the most common side effects of chronic levodopa therapy)

Psychiatric disturbances (elderly most vulnerable; treatment with neuroleptic drugs not recommended)

Endocrine changes
- Inhibition of prolactin secretion
- Increased plasma levels of aldosterone (hypokalemia)

Laboratory Measurements

The urinary metabolites of levodopa causes false-positive tests for ketoacidosis. These metabolites also color the urine red and then black upon exposure to air. Increased liver transaminases concentrations occasionally occur.

Drug Interactions (Table 31-2)

PERIPHERAL DECARBOXYLASE INHIBITORS

Levodopa is usually administered with a peripheral noncompetitive decarboxylase inhibitor such as carbidopa or benserazide; neither cross the blood-brain barrier, and they are pharmacologically inactive when administered alone. As a result, more levodopa escapes metabolism to dopamine in the peripheral circulation and is available to enter the central nervous system (CNS). Furthermore, the side effects related to high systemic concentrations of dopamine are decreased when levodopa is administered with a peripheral decarboxylase inhibitor.

TABLE 31-2.
DRUG INTERACTIONS IN PATIENTS BEING TREATED WITH LEVODOPA

Antipsychotic drugs (butyrophenones and phenothiazines can antagonize the effects of dopamine, droperidol has resulted in acute skeletal muscle rigidity and pulmonary edema)
Monoamine oxidase inhibitors (interfere with inactivation of dopamine and can result in hypertension and hyperthermia)
Anticholinergic drugs (act synergistically with levodopa)
Pyridoxine (dose present in multivitamin preparations can abolish the therapeutic efficacy of levodopa by enhancing the activity of pyridoxine-dependent dopa decarboxylase)

Catechol-O-Methyltransferase (COMT) Inhibitors

Catechol-O-methyltransferase (COMT) is partially responsible for the peripheral breakdown of levodopa. Blocking COMT enzyme activity with tolcapone or entacapone slows the elimination of carbidopa-levodopa.

Side Effects (Table 31-3)

SYNTHETIC DOPAMINE AGONISTS

Synthetic dopamine agonists (bromocriptine, pergolide) act directly on postsynaptic dopamine receptors. The effectiveness of bromocriptine in the treatment of acromegaly reflects the paradoxical inhibitory effect of dopamine agonists on the secretion of growth hormone. Bromocriptine also suppresses the excess prolactin secretion that often is associated with growth hormone secretion.

Side Effects (Table 31-4)

ANTICHOLINERGIC DRUGS

Anticholinergic drugs (trihexyphenidyl, benztropine) blunt the effects of the excitatory neurotransmitter acetyl-

TABLE 31-3.
SIDE EFFECTS OF CATECHOL-O-METHYLTRANSFERASE INHIBITORS

Worsen levodopa dyskinesias
Nausea and vomiting
Hepatotoxicity (monitor liver function tests)
Rhabdomyolysis
Orange urine
Piloerection

TABLE 31-4.
SIDE EFFECTS OF SYNTHETIC DOPAMINE AGONISTS

Visual and auditory hallucinations
Hypotension
Dyskinesia
Pleuropulmonary fibrosis (pleural effusions)
Erythromelalgia (red edematous tender extremities)
Increases in plasma concentrations of serum transaminases and alkaline phosphatase (asymptomatic)
Vertigo
Nausea

choline, thus correcting the balance between dopamine and acetylcholine that is disturbed in the direction of cholinergic dominance. Although the peripheral and CNS actions of synthetic anticholinergic drugs are less prominent than those of atropine, side effects including memory disturbances (especially in elderly patients), sedation, mydriasis, cycloplegia, adynamic ileus, and urinary retention may still occur.

AMANTADINE

Amantadine is an antiviral drug used for prophylaxis against influenza A that also produces symptomatic improvement in patients with Parkinson's disease by unknown mechanisms. More than 90% of the drug is excreted unchanged by the kidneys, necessitating dosage adjustments in patients with renal dysfunction.

SELEGILINE

Selegiline is a highly selective and irreversible inhibitor of monoamine oxidase type B enzyme that has a weak antiparkinsonian effect when used alone and a moderate effect when used as an adjunct to carbidopa-levodopa. The metabolism of norepinephrine in peripheral nerve endings is not altered by selegiline, which minimizes the likelihood of adverse responses during anesthesia in response to sympathomimetics. Insomnia is a significant side effect of selegiline.

NONPHARMACOLOGIC TREATMENT

The transplantation of fetal mesencephalic tissue and posteroventral pallidotomy represent surgical approaches to the treatment of patients with Parkinson's disease.

Drug Treatment of Lipid Disorders

32

Increased plasma concentrations of total cholesterol and low-density lipoproteins (LDL) and low plasma concentrations of high-density lipoproteins (HDL) are associated with an increased risk of atherosclerotic heart disease (Stoelting RK, Hillier SC. Drug treatment of lipid disorders. In: *Pharmacology and Physiology in Anesthetic Practice.* 4th ed. Philadelphia, Lippincott Williams & Wilkins, 2006:585–590). A high plasma HDL cholesterol concentration is a powerful protective factor against the development of coronary artery disease because HDLs are essential for the retrieval of cholesterol from cells and tissues. Guidelines for the treatment of patients with increased plasma concentrations of cholesterol focus on interventions to decrease LDL cholesterol (Table 32-1). The choice of drug or drugs to treat lipid disorders is guided by the patient's triglyceride levels (Table 32-2).

DRUGS TO TREAT INCREASED PLASMA LOW-DENSITY LIPOPROTEIN CHOLESTEROL CONCENTRATIONS

Drugs for treatment of increased plasma LDL cholesterol concentrations act by a variety of mechanisms.

Bile Acid–Binding Resins

Bile acid–binding resins (sequestrants) are effective for the treatment of lipid disorders in which the primary abnormality is an increased plasma LDL concentration

TABLE 32-1.
DRUGS AVAILABLE FOR TREATMENT OF LIPID DISORDERS

Bile Acid–Binding Resins
Cholestyramine
Colestipol
Statins (HMG-CoA reductase inhibitors)
Atorvastatin
Fluvastatin
Lovastatin
Pravastatin
Simvastatin
Niacin
Fibrates
Gemfibrozil
Ω-3 fatty acids

with a normal or near normal triglyceride level. These drugs have a low toxicity but are only available as powders that must be hydrated before ingestion. No systemic absorption of these resins occurs

Cholestyramine
Cholestyramine is the chloride salt of an ion exchange resin that binds bile acids in the intestine; this results in the increased production of hepatic LDL receptors, which increases the uptake of LDL cholesterol from blood and lowers plasma concentrations of LDL cholesterol.

Colestipol
Colestipol is a bile-sequestering drug with pharmacologic effects similar to those of cholestyramine.

Statins
Statins are drugs that act as inhibitors of HMG-CoA reductase (a rate-limiting enzyme that catalyzes the conversion of substrate HMG-CoA to mevalonate); this is an

TABLE 32-2.

CHOICE OF DRUGS FOR TREATMENT OF LIPID DISORDERS

Lipid/Lipoprotein Abnormality	Single Drug	Drug Combination
Increased low density lipoproteins Triglycerides <200 mg/dL	Statin Resin Niacin	Statin and Resin Resin and Niacin Statin and Niacin
Increased low density lipoproteins Triglycerides 200–400 mg/dL	Statin Niacin	Statin and Niacin Statin and Gemfibrozil Niacin and Resin Niacin and Gemfibrozil
Triglycerides >1,000 mg/dL	Niacin Gemfibrozil Ω-3 fatty acids	Niacin and Gemfibrozil

TABLE 32-3.
SIDE EFFECTS OF CHOLESTYRAMINE

Poor palatability
Constipation (minimize with high fluid intake)
Transient increases in plasma transaminases and alkaline phosphatase
Hyperchloremic acidosis
Hypoprothrombinemia (theoretical risk as interferes with absorption of fat soluble vitamins)
Bind other drugs (thiazides, warfarin, digitalis, β-blockers)

early and rate-limiting step in the biosynthesis of cholesterol. The resulting inhibition of the endogenous synthesis of cholesterol is accompanied by decreases (as much as 60%) in the plasma concentrations of LDL cholesterol.

Statins are commonly the first choice when pharmacologic intervention is used to lower plasma concentrations of LDL cholesterol. Statins lower cardiac events in patients with or without atherosclerosis and are recommended early following an acute myocardial infarction.

Side Effects

Statins are usually well tolerated. Rare but potential side effects of statin therapy include hepatic dysfunction and myopathy.

Hepatic Dysfunction

Discontinuation of the drug is recommended if plasma aminotransferase concentrations increase to more than three times normal.

Myopathy

Myopathy is characterized by proximal muscle weakness, myalgia, increases in plasma concentrations of creatine phosphokinase and myopathic changes on the electromyogram. Because cholesterol is the principal sterol constituent of skeletal muscle membranes, decreases of the normal cholesterol pool available for membrane synthesis can increase membrane fluidity, leading to unstable sarcolemma, myotonic discharges and. in advanced but rare situations, rhabdomyolysis and acute renal failure. Drugs likely to be administered during anesthesia have not been shown to increase the incidence of statin-induced myopathy.

Origin and Chemical Structure

Lovastatin is a naturally occurring product isolated from the strain of *Aspergillus terreus. Simvastatin* is derived synthetically from a fermentation product of the same fungus. *Atorvastatin* and *fluvastatin* are synthetic drugs.

Pharmacokinetics

Statins are variably absorbed from the gastrointestinal tract following oral ingestion. Lovastatin and simvastatin are prodrugs. Except for pravastatin, all the statins undergo extensive metabolism by hepatic P-450 enzymes (large volumes of grapefruit juice may inhibit cytochrome P-450 activity). Despite the short elimination half-times, the duration of pharmacodynamic effects is about 24 hours (a consideration in the preoperative period). Atorvastatin and fluvastatin undergo minimal renal excretion, whereas dosages of pravastatin, lovastatin, and simvastatin may need to be adjusted in patients with renal insufficiency.

Niacin

Niacin (nicotinic acid) is a water soluble B-complex vitamin that inhibits the synthesis of very low-density lipoproteins (VLDLs) in the liver. In addition, niacin inhibits the release of free fatty acids from adipose tissue and increases the activity of lipoprotein lipase. The result is a decrease in LDL cholesterol, a decrease in triglycerides, and an increase in HDL.

Pharmacokinetics

Niacin is readily absorbed from the gastrointestinal tract and undergoes extensive hepatic first-pass metabolism.

TABLE 32-4.
SIDE EFFECTS OF NIACIN

Intense cutaneous flushing (prostaglandin induced)
Abdominal pain
Nausea and vomiting
Hepatic dysfunction (likely a direct toxic effect and administration of niacin to patients with liver disease is not recommended)
Hyperglycemia
Increased plasma concentrations of uric acid (gouty arthritis)
Orthostatic hypotension (exaggerated peripheral vasodilation in patients being treated with antihypertensive drugs)
Reactivation of peptic ulcer disease
Increased risk of myopathy in combination with statins

Side Effects

Niacin, unlike the resins and statins, has many side effects that may limit its usefulness (Table 32-4).

FIBRATES

Fibrates are derivatives of fibric acid and are the most effective drugs for decreasing plasma concentrations of triglycerides. In the postoperative period, treatment with fibrates is restarted when the patient is well hydrated and able to ingest oral medications.

Gemfibrozil

Gemfibrozil is the best tolerated drug for the treatment of patients with increased plasma concentrations of triglycerides, with or without a concomitant increase in plasma LDL cholesterol concentrations. Drug-induced increases in the activity of lipoprotein lipase is the likely mechanism for the triglyceride-lowering effects of gemfibrozil.

Pharmacokinetics

Gemfibrozil is well absorbed from the gastrointestinal tract, and an estimated 70% of the drug appears unchanged in the urine (a consideration when administering to patients with renal dysfunction).

Side Effects (Table 32-5)

Fenofibrate

Fenofibrate is a prodrug that is hydrolyzed by esterases to the active metabolite, fenofibric acid. Metabolism is by conjugation, and renal excretion is extensive. Increased plasma concentrations of liver transaminase enzymes are more likely to occur with fenofibrate than with the other fibrates.

Clofibrate

Clofibrate is an option in patients with severe hypertriglyceridemia who do not tolerate or respond to niacin and/or gemfibrozil.

TABLE 32-5.
SIDE EFFECTS OF GEMFIBROZIL

Abdominal pain
Nausea
Increased formation of gallstones (increases cholesterol content of bile)
Skeletal muscle myopathy in combination with statins
Potentiation of anticoagulant effect of warfarin
Increase in plasma transaminase enzymes

Ω-3 FATTY ACIDS

Ω-3 fatty acids (fish oil) are highly unsaturated fats present in marine fish oils. The primary effect of this fatty acid is to decrease the plasma concentrations of triglycerides, whereas the effect on LDL cholesterol concentrations is variable.

33

Central Nervous System Stimulants and Muscle Relaxants

CENTRAL NERVOUS SYSTEM STIMULANTS

Drugs that stimulate the central nervous system (CNS) as their primary action are classified as analeptics or convulsants (Stoelting RK, Hillier SC. Central nervous system stimulants. In: *Pharmacology and Physiology in Anesthetic Practice.* 4th ed. Philadelphia, Lippincott Williams & Wilkins, 2006:591–598). Analeptics were previously used in the treatment of generalized CNS depression accompanying deliberate drug overdoses. This practice, however, has been abandoned because these drugs lack specific antagonist properties and their margin of safety is narrow.

Doxapram

Doxapram is a centrally acting analeptic that selectively increases minute ventilation by activating the carotid bodies. The stimulus to ventilation produced by the administration of doxapram, 1 mg/kg IV, is similar to that produced by a PaO_2 of 38 mm Hg acting on the carotid bodies. Doxapram has a large margin of safety, as reflected by a 20- to 40-fold difference between the dose that stimulates ventilation and the dose that produces seizures. Nevertheless, continuous infusion of doxapram, as required to produce a sustained effect on ventilation, often results in evidence of subconvulsive CNS stimulation (hypertension, tachycardia, cardiac dysrhythmias, vomiting, increased body temperature). Doxapram is extensively metabolized, with <5% of an IV dose being excreted unchanged in urine. A single IV dose produces an effect on ventilation that lasts only 5 to 10 minutes.

Clinical Uses

Doxapram administered as a continuous infusion (2 to 3 mg/min) has been used as a temporary measure to maintain ventilation during the administration of supplemental oxygen to patients with chronic obstructive airway disease, who otherwise depend on a hypoxic drive to maintain an adequate minute ventilation. Because controlled ventilation of the lungs and standard supportive therapy are effective in managing ventilatory failure, doxapram should not be used in patients with drug-induced coma or exacerbation of chronic lung disease. More specific tests (peripheral nerve stimulation, airway pressures, head lift) render the diagnostic use of doxapram in postanesthetic apnea or hypoventilation of minimal clinical value. Arousal from the residual effects of inhaled anesthetics follows the administration of doxapram, but the effect is transient, nonselective, and not recommended.

Amphetamine and Methamphetamine

Amphetamine and methamphetamine are powerful CNS stimulants. These drugs cause the release and inhibit the reuptake of stimulatory neurotransmitters in the cerebral cortex, motor nuclei, and the reticular activating system. The chronic administration of amphetamines may lower systemic blood pressure, owing to the metabolism of amphetamine and methamphetamine to false neurotransmitters.

Toxicity (Table 33-1)

The treatment of acute amphetamine intoxication includes acidification of the urine to enhance renal excretion of the drug and administration of medications to treat cardiovascular side effects. Dantrolene is indicated if hyperpyrexia is present.

TABLE 33-1.
SIGNS AND SYMPTOMS OF AMPHETAMINE TOXICITY

Restlessness
Aggressive behavior
Paranoid delusions
Tachycardia and hypertension (may be followed by convulsions and circulatory collapse as fatal terminal events)
Hyperpyrexia
Disseminated intravascular coagulation

Methylphenidate

Methylphenidate is a mild CNS stimulant, with more prominent effects on mental than on motor activities. The abuse potential of methylphenidate is the same as that of amphetamine.

Clinical Uses

Methylphenidate is useful in the treatment of hyperkinetic syndromes in children. Methylphenidate may also be effective in the treatment of narcolepsy, either alone or in combination with tricyclic antidepressants.

Methylxanthines

Methylxanthines (such as caffeine, theophylline, and theobromine) stimulate the CNS, produce diuresis, increase myocardial contractility, and relax smooth muscle, especially that in the airways.

Mechanism of Action

Methylxanthines antagonize the receptor-mediated actions of adenosine, thus facilitating the release of catecholamines. Unlike adults, premature infants metabolize theophylline in part to caffeine. Furthermore, the clearance of methylxanthines is greatly prolonged in the neonate, compared with that in the adult.

Clinical Uses

The slowed metabolism of methylxanthines in neonates compared to adults is a consideration when using theophylline to stimulate ventilation in neonates. Selective β-2-adrenergic agonists delivered by inhalation have largely replaced theophylline preparations in the treatment of bronchospasm associated with asthma. The administration of theophylline during the maintenance of anesthesia appears to have no added bronchodilator effect over that of the volatile anesthetic alone. Methylxanthines decrease systemic vascular resistance but increase cerebral vascular resistance; the associated vasoconstriction may be responsible for the relief of postdural puncture headaches.

Toxicity

A single oral dose of theophylline, 5 mg/kg, will produce a peak plasma concentration of 10 μg/mL in adults within 1 to 2 hours following ingestion. Theophylline plasma concentrations only slightly greater than the recommended therapeutic range (10 to 20 μg/kg) can produce evidence of CNS stimulation (nervousness, tremors), and at higher concentrations, seizures are a possibility. Tachycardia and cardiac dysrhythmias may appear, most likely due to the drug-induced release of catecholamines from the adrenal medulla.

Drug Interactions (Table 33-2)

Caffeine

Caffeine is a methylxanthine-derived phosphodiesterase inhibitor that is present in a variety of beverages and nonprescription medications (Table 33-3). In addition, this substance acts as a cerebral vasoconstrictor and may cause the secretion of acidic gastric fluid. The pharmacologic uses of caffeine include its administration to neonates experiencing apnea of prematurity. Postdural puncture headache may respond to administration of caffeine, 300 mg orally (presumably reflects a cerebral vasoconstrictor effect). Caffeine

TABLE 33-2.
DRUG INTERACTIONS IN PATIENTS BEING TREATED WITH THEOPHYLLINE

Enhanced metabolism of theophylline (cimetidine, erythromycin)
Decreased metabolism of theophylline (carbamazepine, rifampin)
Increased dose requirements for benzodiazepines
Increased seizure threshold in presence of ketamine
Antagonism of effects of nondepolarizing neuromuscular blocking-drugs

may be included in common cold remedies in an attempt to offset the sedating effects of certain antihistamines.

Nicotine

Nicotine has no therapeutic action, but its toxicity and presence in tobacco have created medical importance for

TABLE 33-3.
CAFFEINE CONTENT OF COMMON SUBSTANCES

Substance	Caffeine (mg)
Coffee (150 ml)	
Freeze dried	66
Percolator	107
Drip grind	142
Tea (150 mL)	15–47
Cocoa (150 mL)	13
Coca-Cola (360 ml)	65
Pepsi-Cola (360 ml)	43
Dr. Pepper (360 ml)	61
Mountain Dew (360 ml)	55
Jolt Cola	71
Candy bar (1.2 oz)	5
No-Doze	100

this compound. Smoking is the single most important preventable cause of death, being responsible for more than one in every six fatalities. The highly addictive nature of nicotine results in a withdrawal syndrome that presents a major barrier to the successful cessation of tobacco use. A principal metabolite is cotinine, which has approximately one-fifth the pharmacologic activity of nicotine. Cigarette smoking alters the activity of many drugs, presumably reflecting the induction of liver microsomal enzymes by polycyclic hydrocarbons in cigarette smoke. Enzyme activity remains increased for up to 6 months after cessation of cigarette smoking.

Effects on Organ Systems

The primary action of nicotine is an initial CNS stimulation, quickly followed by persistent depression of autonomic ganglia. Nicotine characteristically increases heart rate and systemic blood pressure and evokes peripheral vasoconstriction. In contrast to the effects on the cardiovascular system, the effects of nicotine on the gastrointestinal tract are largely due to parasympathetic nervous system stimulation, leading to vomiting and diarrhea.

Overdose

Overdose from nicotine may occur from the ingestion of insecticide sprays containing nicotine or from ingestion of tobacco products. The fatal dose of nicotine in adults is approximately 60 mg. Individual cigarettes deliver up to 2.5 mg of nicotine. The onset of symptoms of nicotine overdose is rapid (Table 33-4).

Almitrine

Almitrine is a peripheral chemoreceptor agonist that increases PaO_2 and decreases $PaCO_2$ in patients with chronic respiratory failure associated with obstructive pulmonary disease. The side effects of prolonged oral almitrine therapy include dyspnea and peripheral neuropathy. It is presumed

TABLE 33-4.
SYMPTOMS OF NICOTINE OVERDOSE

Nausea, salivation, and abdominal cramps
Mental confusion
Skeletal muscle weakness
Hypotension
Dyspnea (paralysis of intercostal muscles)
Tachycardia
Terminal seizures

that this improvement in gas exchange is due to an enhancement of hypoxic pulmonary vasoconstriction.

CENTRALLY ACTING MUSCLE RELAXANTS

Centrally acting muscle relaxants act in the CNS or directly on skeletal muscles to relieve spasticity.

Mephenesin

The relative efficacy of centrally acting muscle relaxants that are related to mephenesin has not been determined. These drugs produce skeletal muscle relaxation by an unknown mechanism in the CNS.

Benzodiazepines

Benzodiazepines are widely used as centrally acting skeletal muscle relaxants. Sedation may limit the efficacy of diazepam as a muscle relaxant.

Baclofen

Baclofen is the chlorophenol derivative of γ-aminobutyric acid (GABA). It acts as an agonist at GABA receptors and is often administered for the treatment of spastic hypertonia of cerebral and spinal cord origin, resulting from diseases or injury of the spinal cord. Baclofen is particularly effective in the treatment of flexor spasms and skeletal muscle rigidity associated with spinal cord injury or multiple sclerosis. The intrathecal administration of baclofen may be an effective treatment of spinal spasticity that has not responded to oral administration of the drug. The use of baclofen is limited by its side effects (Table 33-5).

Cyclobenzaprine

Cyclobenzaprine is related structurally and pharmacologically to tricyclic antidepressants. Its anticholinergic effects are similar to those of tricyclic antidepressants and can include dry mouth, tachycardia, blurred vision, and sedation. Cyclobenzaprine must not be administered in the presence of monoamine oxidase inhibitors.

Dantrolene

Dantrolene produces skeletal muscle relaxation by inhibiting calcium release from the endoplasmic reticulum (intracellular storage site of dischargeable calcium in neurons) through ryanodine receptors and inositol 1,4,5-triphosphate receptor channels into cytosol.

TABLE 33-5.
SIDE EFFECTS OF BACLOFEN

Skeletal muscle weakness
Confusion and sedation
Withdrawal reactions (multiple organ system failure, tachycardia, auditory and visual hallucinations)
Vocal cord spasm
Coma
Depression of ventilation
Seizures (threshold may be lowered in patients with epilepsy)

Pharmacokinetics

Absorption of dantrolene from the gastrointestinal tract, as well as intravenous injection, provides sustained dose-related concentrations of drug in the plasma. The IV preparation of dantrolene is alkaline (pH 9.5), and phlebitis may follow its injection. Extravasation of dantrolene may result in tissue necrosis. Diuresis may accompany IV administration, reflecting the addition of mannitol to the dantrolene powder to make the solution isotonic. For this reason, it is recommended that patients receiving IV dantrolene also have a urinary catheter in place. Dantrolene is metabolized in the liver, principally to 5-hydroxydantrolene, which is 30% to 50% as effective in depressing the twitch response. Less than 1% of dantrolene appears unchanged in urine. The minimal effective blood level of dantrolene is not known, although plasma concentrations of 2.8 µg/mL or greater in animals are associated with near-maximal depression of skeletal muscle contractile activity. For this reason, it seems prudent to maintain blood levels of dantrolene of at least 2.8 µg/mL when the drug is being administered for prophylaxis against or treatment of malignant hyperthermia.

TABLE 33-6.
CLINICAL USES OF DANTROLENE

Management of spasticity due to upper motor neuron lesions
Prevention and treatment of malignant hyperthermia
Prophylaxis
- Oral administration of 5 mg/kg in three or four divided doses every 6 hours with the last dose 4 hours preoperatively, should result in plasma levels of dantrolene >2.8 µg/mL at the time of induction of anesthesia
- Administer 2.4 mg/kg IV over 10 to 30 minutes just before induction of anesthesia and repeat 1.2 mg/kg in 6 hours

Treatment
- Administer 2 mg/kg IV with repeated doses until symptoms subside or a cumulative dose of 10 mg/kg is reached

TABLE 33-7.
SIDE EFFECTS OF DANTROLENE

Skeletal muscle weakness (may be sufficient to interfere with adequate ventilation and airway protection from aspiration)
Nausea
Uterine atony
Hyperkalemia (when administered with verapamil in an animal model)
Hepatitis (monitor hepatic function when dantrolene therapy is continued for >45 days)

Clinical Uses (Table 33-6)

Side Effects (Table 33-7)

Breast feeding can be expected to be safe for the newborn 48 hours after the discontinuation of intravenous dantrolene administration to the mother.

34 Vitamins, Dietary Supplements, and Herbal Remedies

VITAMINS

Vitamins are a group of structurally diverse organic substances (water soluble or fat soluble) that must be provided in small amounts in the diet for subsequent synthesis of cofactors that are essential for various metabolic reactions (Table 34-1) (Stoelting RK, Hillier SC. Vitamins, dietary supplements and herbal remedies. In: *Pharmacology and Physiology in Anesthetic Practice*. 4th ed. Philadelphia, Lippincott Williams & Wilkins, 2006:599–610). Many otherwise healthy individuals take supplemental vitamins, despite the absence of scientific evidence that these substances are necessary or useful (healthy adults require no vitamin supplementation except during pregnancy and lactation). The excessive intake of fat-soluble vitamins, particularly vitamins A and D, is more likely to cause toxicity than is the intake of water-soluble vitamins. The use of dietary supplements is medically indicated in situations associated with inadequate intake, malabsorption, increased tissue needs, or inborn errors of metabolism. Disturbances of vitamin absorption may occur in diseases of the liver and biliary tract, diarrhea, hyperthyroidism, small-bowel bypass surgery for treatment of obesity, and alcoholism. Antibiotic therapy may alter the usual bacterial flora of the gastrointestinal tract necessary for synthesis of vitamin K.

TABLE 34-1.
VITAMINS

	Function	Deficiency	Toxic Effects	Sources
Thiamine (B_1)	Metabolism of carbohydrates, alcohol, amino acids	Beriberi Wernicke-Korsakoff syndrome	None	Grains Legumes Poultry Meat
Riboflavin (B_2)	Cellular oxidation-reduction reactions	Stomatitis Dermatitis Anemia	None	Grains Dairy products Meat Eggs Green vegetables
Nicotinic acid (niacin, B_3)	Oxidative metabolism Decreases LDL cholesterol Increases HDL cholesterol	Pellagra	Flushing Headaches Pruritus Hyperglycemia Hyperuricemia	Meat Poultry Fish Grains Peanuts Tryptophan in foods
Pyridoxine (B_6)	Amino acid metabolism Heme synthesis	Anemia Cheilosis	Neurotoxicity	Liver Poultry

TABLE 34-1.
(continued)

	Function	Deficiency	Toxic Effects	Sources
	Neuronal excitability Decreases blood homocysteine levels	Dermatitis		Fish Grains Bananas
Pantothenic acid	Metabolic processes	Rare	None	Many foods
B_{12} (cobalamin, cyanocobalamin)	DNA synthesis Myelin synthesis Decreases blood homocysteine levels	Megaloblastic anemia Peripheral neuropathies	None	Liver Poultry Fish Dairy products
Folic acid	DNA synthesis Decreases blood homocysteine levels	Megaloblastic anemia Birth defects	None	Legumes Grains Fruit Poultry Meat
Ascorbic acid (vitamin C)	Collagen synthesis Possible protection against certain cancers	Scurvy	Nephrolithiasis Diarrhea	Fruits Green vegetables Potatoes Cereals

(*continued*)

TABLE 34-1.
(continued)

	Function	Deficiency	Toxic Effects	Sources
Vitamin A (retinol, retinoic acid)	Vision Epithelial integrity Possible protection	Night blindness Susceptibility to infection	Teratogenicity Hepatotoxicity Cerebral edema	Liver Dairy products Green vegetables
Vitamin D (calciferol)	Intestinal calcium Absorption	Osteomalacia Rickets	Hypercalcemia	Dairy products Fish Eggs Liver
Vitamin E (tocophberol)	Decreases peroxidation of fatty acids Possible protection against atherosclerosis	Rare	Antagonism of vitamin K Headaches	Vegetable oils Wheat germ Nuts
Vitamin K	Synthesis of clotting factors (VII, IX, X)	Hemorrhagic diathesis	None	Green vegetables Intestinal bacteria

Water-Soluble Vitamins

Thiamine

Thiamine (vitamin B_1) is essential for the decarboxylation of α-keto acids, such as pyruvate, and in the use of pentose in the hexose-monophosphate shunt pathway (increased plasma concentrations of pyruvate are a diagnostic sign of thiamine deficiency).

Causes of Deficiency

The need for thiamine is greatest when carbohydrate is the source of energy (patients on hyperalimentation should receive supplemental amounts of thiamine). Thiamine requirements are also increased during pregnancy and lactation.

Symptoms of Deficiency

Symptoms of deficiency (beriberi) include loss of appetite, skeletal muscle weakness, a tendency to develop peripheral edema, decreased systemic blood pressure, and low body temperature. Severe thiamine deficiency (Korsakoff's syndrome), which may occur in alcoholics, is associated with peripheral polyneuritis, impairment of memory, and encephalopathy. High-output cardiac failure with extensive peripheral edema reflecting hypoproteinemia is often prominent.

Treatment of Deficiency

Severe thiamine deficiency is treated with the intravenous (IV) administration of the vitamin.

Riboflavin

Riboflavin (vitamin B_2) is converted in the body to one of two physiologically active coenzymes: flavin mononucleotide or flavin adenine dinucleotide. These coenzymes primarily influence hydrogen ion transport in oxidative enzyme systems, including cytochrome C reductase, succinic dehydrogenase, and xanthine oxidase.

Symptoms of Deficiency

Pharyngitis and angular stomatitis are typically the first signs of riboflavin deficiency. Later glossitis, red denuded lips, seborrheic dermatitis of the face, and dermatitis over the trunk and extremities occur. Anemia and peripheral neuropathy may be prominent.

Nicotinic Acid

Nicotinic Acid (Niacin, Vitamin B_3) is converted to the physiologically active coenzyme nicotinamide adenine dinucleotide (NAD) and nicotinamide adenine dinucleotide phosphate (NADP).

Symptoms of Deficiency

Pellagra is the all-inclusive term for the symptoms of nicotinic acid deficiency (dermatitis, diarrhea, and dementia). The tongue becomes very red and swollen. The relationship between nicotinic acid requirements and the intake of tryptophan explains the association of pellagra with tryptophan-deficient corn diets. Carcinoid syndrome is associated with the diversion of tryptophan from the synthesis of nicotinic acid to the production of serotonin (5-hydroxytryptamine), leading to symptoms of pellagra. Isoniazid inhibits the incorporation of nicotinic acid into NAD and may produce pellagra. Pellagra is uncommon in the United States, reflecting the supplementation of flour with nicotinic acid. The toxic effects of nicotinic acid include flushing, pruritus, hepatotoxicity, hyperuricemia, and activation of peptic ulcer disease. Nicotinic acid has also been prescribed to decrease the plasma concentrations of cholesterol.

Pyridoxine

Pyridoxine (vitamin B_6) is converted to its physiologically active form, pyridoxal phosphate, which serves an important role in metabolism as a coenzyme for the conversion of tryptophan to serotonin and methionine to cysteine.

Symptoms of Deficiency

Pyridoxine deficiency is frequent in alcoholics (estimated incidence 30%), manifesting as dermatitis, central nervous system dysfunction, and anemia. Seizures accompanying deficiency of pyridoxine and peripheral neuritis, such as carpal tunnel syndrome, are common. The lowered seizure threshold may reflect decreased concentrations of the inhibitory neurotransmitter γ-aminobutyric acid (GABA), the synthesis of which requires a pyridoxal phosphate-requiring enzyme.

Drug Interactions

Isoniazid and hydralazine act as potent inhibitors of pyridoxal kinase, thus preventing the synthesis of the active coenzyme form of the vitamin. Pyridoxine enhances the peripheral decarboxylation of levodopa and decreases its effectiveness for the treatment of Parkinson's disease.

Pantothenic Acid

Pantothenic acid is converted to its physiologically active form, coenzyme A, which serves as a cofactor for enzyme-catalyzed reactions involving transfer of two carbon (acetyl groups). Such reactions are important in the oxidative metabolism of carbohydrates, gluconeogenesis, and the synthesis and degradation of fatty acids.

Biotin

Biotin is an organic acid that functions as a coenzyme for enzyme-catalyzed carboxylation reactions and fatty acid synthesis. In adults, a deficiency of biotin manifests as glossitis, anorexia, dermatitis, and mental depression.

Cyanocobalamin

Cyanocobalamin (cobalamin, Vitamin B_{12}) in the presence of hydrogen ions in the stomach is released from proteins and subsequently binds to a glycoprotein intrinsic factor.

Causes of Deficiency

Gastric achlorhydria and decreased gastric secretion of intrinsic factor are more likely causes of vitamin B_{12} deficiency in adults. Surgical resection or disease of the ileum predictably interferes with the absorption of vitamin B_{12}. Nitrous oxide irreversibly oxidizes the cobalt atom of vitamin B_{12}, so that the activity of two vitamin B_{12}–dependent enzymes, methionine synthetase and thymidylate synthetase, is decreased.

Diagnosis of Deficiency

The plasma concentration of vitamin B_{12} (cobalamin) is <200 pg/mL when there is a deficiency state.

Symptoms of Deficiency

A deficiency of vitamin B_{12} results in defective synthesis of DNA, especially in tissues with the greatest rate of cell turnover (hematopoietic and nervous systems). Clinically, the earliest sign of vitamin B_{12} deficiency is megaloblastic (pernicious) anemia. Encephalopathy is a well-recognized complication of vitamin B_{12} deficiency, manifesting as myelopathy, optic neuropathy, and peripheral neuropathy (paresthesias of the hands and feet and diminution of sensation of vibration and proprioception with resultant unsteadiness of gait), either alone or in any combination. Folic acid therapy corrects the hematopoietic, but not nervous system, effects produced by vitamin B_{12} deficiency.

Treatment of Deficiency

In the presence of clinically apparent vitamin B_{12} deficiency, oral absorption is not reliable; the preparation of choice is cyanocobalamin administered intramuscularly. Folic acid as monotherapy masks the anemia and fails to prevent the neurological complications. Platelet counts can be expected to reach normal levels within days of initiating treatment; the granulocyte count requires a longer period to normalize. Memory and sense of well-being may improve within 24 hours after initiation of therapy.

Neurologic signs and symptoms that have been present for prolonged periods, however, often regress slowly and may never return to completely normal function. Once initiated, vitamin B_{12} therapy must be continued indefinitely at monthly intervals. It is important to monitor plasma concentrations of vitamin B_{12} and examine the peripheral blood cells every 3 to 6 months to confirm the adequacy of treatment.

Folic Acid

Folic acid is transported and stored as 5-methylhydrofolate after its absorption from the small intestine, principally the jejunum. Conversion to the metabolically active form, tetrahydrofolate, is dependent on the activity of vitamin B_{12}. Virtually all foods contain folic acid, but protracted cooking can destroy up to 90% of the vitamin.

Causes of Deficiency

Folic acid deficiency is a common complication of diseases of the small intestine. Alcoholism is the most common cause of folic acid deficiency, with decreases in the plasma concentrations of folic acid manifesting within 24 to 48 hours of continuous alcohol ingestion.

Symptoms of Deficiency

Megaloblastic anemia is the most common manifestation of folic acid deficiency. The rapid onset of megaloblastic anemia produced by folic acid deficiency (1 to 4 weeks) reflects the limited in vivo stores of this vitamin and contrasts with the slower onset (2 to 3 years) of symptoms of vitamin B_{12} deficiency.

Treatment of Deficiency

Folic acid is available as an oral preparation alone or in combination with other vitamins and as a parenteral injection (pregnancy increases folic acid requirements).

Folate Therapy

No evidence suggests that vitamin therapy (using a combination of folic acid, vitamin B_6, and vitamin B_{12}) alters the risk of restenosis after coronary angioplasty.

Leucovorin

Leucovorin (citrovorum factor) is a metabolically active, reduced form of folic acid. After treatment with folic acid antagonists, such as methotrexate, patients may receive leucovorin (rescue therapy), which serves as a source of the tetrahydrofolate that cannot be formed due to the drug-induced inhibition of dihydrofolate reductase.

Ascorbic Acid

Ascorbic acid (vitamin C) is necessary for the synthesis of collagen, carnitine, and corticosteroids. Ascorbic acid is readily absorbed from the gastrointestinal tract, and many foods, such as orange juice and lemon juice, have a high content of ascorbic acid. Apart from its role in nutrition, ascorbic acid is commonly used as an antioxidant to protect the natural flavor and color of many foods. Controlled studies do not support the efficacy of even large doses of ascorbic acid in treating cancer of the colon or viral respiratory tract infections. A risk of large doses of ascorbic acid is the formation of kidney stones resulting from the excessive secretion of oxalate. Excessive ascorbic acid doses can also enhance the absorption of iron and interfere with anticoagulant therapy.

Symptoms of Deficiency

Humans, in contrast to many other mammals, are unable to synthesize ascorbic acid, thus emphasizing the need for dietary sources of the vitamin to prevent scurvy. Scurvy is encountered among the elderly, alcoholics, and drug addicts. Ascorbic acid requirements are increased during pregnancy, lactation, and stresses such as infection or after surgery. Infants receiving formula diets with inadequate concentrations of ascorbic acid can develop scurvy. Patients receiving hyperalimentation should receive supplemental ascorbic acid.

Fat-Soluble Vitamins

The fat-soluble vitamins (A, D, E, and K) are absorbed from the gastrointestinal tract by a complex process that parallels the absorption of fat. Thus, any condition that causes the malabsorption of fat, such as obstructive jaundice, may result in deficiency of one or all these vitamins. Because these vitamins are metabolized very slowly, overdose may produce toxic effects. Vitamin D, despite its name, functions as a hormone.

Vitamin A

Vitamin A (retinol, retinoic acid) is important in the function of the retina, integrity of mucosal and epithelial surfaces, bone development and growth, reproduction, and embryonic development. Sufficient vitamin A is stored in the liver of well-nourished persons to satisfy requirements for several months. Plasma concentrations of vitamin A are maintained at the expense of hepatic reserves and thus do not always reflect a person's vitamin A status.

Symptoms of Deficiency

Plasma concentrations of vitamin A of <20 μg/dL indicate the risk of deficiency. Skin lesions such as follicular hyperkeratosis and infections are often the earliest signs of deficiency. The most recognizable manifestation of vitamin A deficiency is night blindness (nyctalopia).

Hypervitaminosis A

Hypervitaminosis A is the toxic syndrome that results from the excessive ingestion of vitamin A, particularly in children. Plasma concentrations of vitamin A of >300 μg/dL are diagnostic of hypervitaminosis A (Table 34-2). Treatment consists of withdrawal of the vitamin source, which is usually followed within 7 days by a

TABLE 34-2.
SYMPTOMS OF VITAMIN A INTOXICATION

Psychiatric disturbances (mimics mental depression or schizophrenia)
Fatigue
Myalgia
Diplopia
Nystagmus
Gingivitis
Hepatosplenomegaly (portal vein hypertension and ascites)
Increased intracranial pressure (pseudotumor cerebri)
Increased plasma alkaline phosphatase concentrations (hypercalcemia may accompany osteoblastic activity)

disappearance of the manifestations of excess vitamin A activity.

Vitamin D

Vitamin D (calciferol) is the generic designation for several sterols and their metabolites that act as hormones to maintain plasma calcium concentrations and phosphate ions in an optimal range for neuromuscular function, mineralization of bones, and other calcium-dependent functions. This regulation of the plasma concentrations of calcium and phosphate reflects the ability of vitamin D to facilitate the absorption of these ions from the gastrointestinal tract and enhance the mobilization of calcium from bones.

Symptoms of Deficiency

A deficiency of vitamin D results in decreased plasma concentrations of calcium and phosphate ions, with the subsequent stimulation of parathyroid hormone secretion. Parathyroid hormone acts to restore plasma calcium concentrations at the expense of bone calcium (rickets in infants and children and osteomalacia in adults).

Hypervitaminosis D

Hypervitaminosis D manifests as hypercalcemia, skeletal muscle weakness, fatigue, headache, and vomiting. Early impairment of renal function from hypercalcemia manifests as polyuria, polydipsia, proteinuria, and decreased urine-concentrating ability. In addition to the withdrawal of the vitamin, treatment includes increased fluid intake and the administration of corticosteroids.

Vitamin E

Vitamin E (α-tocopherol) is a group of fat-soluble substances occurring in plants. α-Tocopherol is the most abundant and important of the eight naturally occurring tocopherols that constitute vitamin E. An important chemical feature of the tocopherols is that they are antioxidants. In acting as an antioxidant, vitamin E presumably prevents the oxidation of essential cellular constituents or prevents the formation of toxic oxidation products. Epidemiologic studies have provided evidence of an inverse relation between coronary artery disease and antioxidant intake, and vitamin E supplementation in particular. This association has been explained on the basis of the antioxidants' ability to prevent the oxidation of lipids in low-density lipoproteins.

Vitamin K

Vitamin K is a lipid-soluble dietary compound that is essential for the biosynthesis of several factors required for normal blood clotting. Phytonadione (vitamin K_1) is present in a variety of foods and is the only natural form of vitamin K available for therapeutic use. Vitamin K_2 represents a series of compounds that are synthesized by Gram-positive bacteria in the gastrointestinal tract. Vitamin K is absorbed from the gastrointestinal tract only in the presence of adequate quantities of bile salts. Despite its lipid solubility, significant amounts are not stored in the body for prolonged periods of time.

Mechanism of Action

Vitamin K functions as an essential cofactor for the hepatic microsomal enzyme that converts glutamic acid residues to γ-carboxyglutamic acid residues in factors II (prothrombin), VII, IX, and X. If vitamin K deficiency occurs, the plasma concentrations of these coagulation factors decrease and a hemorrhagic disorder develops (ecchymoses, epistaxis, hematuria, gastrointestinal bleeding, postoperative hemorrhage). Prothrombin time is used to monitor vitamin K activity.

Clinical Uses

Vitamin K is administered to treat its deficiency (inadequate dietary intake, decreased bacterial synthesis due to antibiotic therapy, impaired gastrointestinal absorption resulting from obstructive biliary disease and absence of bile salts, hepatocellular disease) and attendant decreases in plasma concentrations of prothrombin and related clotting factors. Neonates have hypoprothrombinemia due to vitamin K deficiency until adequate dietary intake of the vitamin occurs and normal intestinal bacterial flora are established. Vitamin K replacement therapy is not effective when severe hepatocellular disease is responsible for the decreased production of clotting factors. In the absence of severe hepatocellular disease and the presence of adequate bile salts, the administration of oral vitamin K preparations is effective in reversing hypoprothrombinemia.

Phytonadione

Phytonadione (vitamin K_1) is the preferred drug to treat hypoprothrombinemia, particularly if large doses or prolonged therapy is necessary. A frequent indication for phytonadione is to reverse the effects of oral anticoagulants (10 to 20 mg orally or administered IV at a rate of 1 mg/min). The oral and intramuscular routes of administration are less likely than IV injections of phytonadione to cause side effects and are thus preferred for the nonemergency reversal of oral anticoagulants. Even large doses of phytonadione are ineffective against heparin-induced anticoagulation. The intravenous injection of phytonadione may cause life-threatening allergic reactions characterized by hypotension and bronchospasm. Intramuscular administration may produce local hemorrhage at the injection site in hypoprothrombinemic patients.

Menadione

Menadione has the same actions and uses as phytonadione. The water-soluble salts of menadione do not require the presence of bile salts for their systemic absorption after oral administration. This characteristic becomes important when malabsorption of vitamin K is due to biliary obstruction. The administration of large doses of menadione or phytonadione may depress liver function, particularly in the presence of preexisting liver disease.

DIETARY SUPPLEMENTS

Dietary supplements of vitamins, minerals, herbs (flowering plants, shrubs, seaweed, and algae), amino acids, and enzymes are products taken orally and intended to supplement the diet. The U.S. Food and Drug Administration (FDA) has no control over the herbal industry in terms of safety guidelines that would regulate the purity and consistency of compounds.

Adverse Effects and Drug Interactions (Tables 34-3 and 34-4)

The most serious side effects associated with these substances include cardiovascular instability; bleeding tendency, particularly in conjunction with other anticoagulants such as warfarin; and delayed awakening from anesthesia.

TABLE 34-3.

DIETARY SUPPLEMENTS AND HERBAL REMEDIES

	Suggested Uses	Potential Toxicity	Drug Interactions
Black cohosh	Menopausal symptoms	Gastrointestinal discomfort	
Chaste tree berries	Premenstrual symptoms	Pruritus	Dopamine-receptor antagonists
Cranberry	Urinary tract infections	Nephrolithiasis	
Dong quai	Menopausal symptoms	Rash	Warfarin
Echinacea	Upper respiratory Infections	Hypersensitivity reactions Hepatic inflammation	
Evening primrose	Eczema Irritable bowel syndrome Premenstrual symptoms Rheumatoid arthritis	Nausea Vomiting Diarrhea Flatulence	Antiepileptic drugs
Feverfew	Prevent migraine Arthritis Allergies	Hypersensitivity reactions Inhibits platelet activity	Warfarin
Garlic	Hypertension Hypertriglyceridemia Hypercholesterolemia	Gastrointestinal discomfort Hemorrhage	Warfarin

TABLE 34-3.
(continued)

	Suggested Uses	Potential Toxicity	Drug Interactions
Ginger	Motion sickness Vertigo		Warfarin
Ginkgo biloba	Dementia Claudication Tinnitus	Gastrointestinal discomfort Headache Dizziness Bleeding Seizures	Warfarin
Ginseng	Fatigue Diabetes	Tachycardia Hypertension	Warfarin
Goldenseal	Laxative	Hypertension Edema	
Kava kava	Anxiety	Rash Sedation Liver toxicity	Benzodiazepines Alcohol Anesthetic drugs
Kola nut	Fatigue	Irritability Insomnia	Stimulants
Licorice	Gastric ulcers	Hypertension	

(*continued*)

TABLE 34-3.
(continued)

Saw palmetto	Prostatic hyperplasia	Gastrointestinal discomfort	
St. John's wort	Depression Anxiety	Headache Insomnia Dizziness Gastrointestinal discomfort	Digoxin Oral contraceptives Serotonin antagonists Anesthetic drugs
Valerian	Insomnia	Headaches	Benzodiazepines Anesthetic drugs Antiepileptic drugs

TABLE 34-4.
NONHERBAL DIETARY SUPPLEMENTS

	Suggested Uses	Potential Toxicity	Drug Interactions
Coenzyme Q10	Congestive heart failure Hypotension	Dyspepsia Nausea Diarrhea	Warfarin
Glucosamine	Osteoarthritis	Gastrointestinal discomfort	Warfarin
Melatonin	Insomnia Jet lag	Fatigue Sedation	
S-adenosylmethionine	Osteoarthritis Depression	Nausea Gastrointestinal discomfort	Tricyclic antidepressants

Based on the risk of adverse reactions, it was concluded by the FDA that dietary supplements containing *ephedra* present an unreasonable risk of illness or injury. *Ginseng* may cause tachycardia or systemic hypertension, particularly in combinations with other cardiac stimulant drugs. In addition, ginseng may decrease the anticoagulant effects of warfarin. *Feverfew* may enhance bleeding by inhibition of platelet activity. Warfarin may also be potentiated by concomitant use of *garlic, ginkgo biloba,* and *ginger. St. John's wort,* which is alleged to be a natural antidepressant, has been shown to inhibit serotonin, dopamine, and norepinephrine reuptake and thus present the possibility of interactions with monoamine oxidase inhibitors and other serotoninergic drugs. *Valerian, kava-kava,* and possibly St. John's wort may delay awakening from anesthesia by prolonging the sedative effects of anesthetic drugs.

Minerals and Electrolytes

Many minerals function as essential constituents of enzymes and regulate a variety of physiologic functions, including the maintenance of osmotic pressure, transport of oxygen, skeletal muscle contraction, integrity of the central nervous system (CNS), growth and maintenance of tissues and bones, and hematopoiesis (Stoelting RK, Hillier SC. Minerals and electrolytes. In: *Pharmacology and Physiology in Anesthetic Practice*. 4th ed. Philadelphia, Lippincott Williams & Wilkins, 2006:611–622). Elements present in the body in large amounts include calcium, phosphorus, sodium, potassium, magnesium, sulfur, and chloride. Iron, cobalt (in vitamin B_{12}), copper, zinc, chromium, selenium, manganese, and molybdenum are present in trace amounts.

A balanced, varied diet supplies adequate amounts of trace elements, and dietary supplements containing minerals should be used only if evidence of deficiency exists or if demands are known to be increased, as during pregnancy and lactation. Mineral deficiencies may develop during prolonged hyperalimentation, emphasizing the importance of monitoring plasma concentrations of trace metals in these patients.

CALCIUM

Calcium is present in the body in greater amounts than any other mineral. The plasma concentration of calcium is maintained between 4.5 and 5.5 mEq/L (8.5 to

10.5 mg/dL) by an endocrine control system that includes vitamin D, parathyroid hormone, and calcitonin. It is the ionized fraction of calcium that produces physiologic effects (represents approximately 45% of the total plasma concentration and a normal plasma ionized calcium concentration is 2 to 2.5 mEq/L). The ionized concentration of calcium depends on arterial pH, with acidosis increasing and alkalosis decreasing the concentration. The plasma albumin concentration must be considered when interpreting plasma calcium concentrations. If the serum albumin concentration is decreased, less calcium is bound to protein. The total plasma calcium concentration can be decreased in the presence of hypoalbuminemia, but symptoms of hypocalcemia do not occur unless the ionized calcium concentration is also decreased. Accurate interpretation of the plasma concentration of calcium is not possible without knowledge of the plasma albumin concentration.

Role of Calcium (Table 35-1)

Cardiovascular Effects

Calcium is recognized as a positive inotropic drug. Increasing the plasma concentrations of ionized calcium with calcium chloride or calcium gluconate is commonly used to treat the cardiac depression that may

TABLE 35-1.
ROLE OF CALCIUM

Neuromuscular transmission
Skeletal muscle contraction
Cardiac muscle contractility
Blood coagulation
Exocytosis (necessary for release of neurotransmitters and autocoids)

accompany the administration of volatile anesthetics and transfusion of citrated blood, and following the termination of cardiopulmonary bypass. Calcium is necessary for the excitation-contraction coupling in vascular smooth muscle and may result in a vasoconstricting effect on coronary arteries that impairs coupling of coronary blood flow to augment myocardial oxygen demand.

Hypocalcemia

Hypocalcemia is defined by a plasma concentration of calcium <4.5 mEq/L (Table 35-2).

Symptoms (Table 35-3)

Treatment

The treatment of hypocalcemia is with commercially available preparations of calcium (calcium chloride, calcium gluconate, calcium gluceptate) administered IV. Administered IV over 5 to 15 minutes, equivalent doses of calcium chloride (3 to 6 mg/kg) and calcium gluconate (7 to 14 mg/kg) produce similar effects on the plasma concentration of calcium.

TABLE 35-2.
CAUSES OF HYPOCALCEMIA

Hypoalbuminemia
Hypoparathyroidism
Acute pancreatitis
Vitamin D deficiency
Chronic renal failure (associated with hyperphosphatemia)
Malabsorption states
Citrate binding (supplemental administration of calcium to adults receiving stored blood is not indicated in the absence of evidence of hypocalcemia, neonates may require supplemental calcium)

TABLE 35-3.
SYMPTOMS OF HYPOCALCEMIA

Tetany
Circumoral paresthesias
Increased neuromuscular excitability
Laryngospasm
Seizures
Hypotension (abrupt decreases in ionized calcium)
Prolonged QTc interval on the electrocardiogram (not a consistent observation)

Hypercalcemia

Cancer is the most common cause of life-threatening hypercalcemia (plasma calcium concentration >5.5 mEq/L), presumably reflecting activation of osteoclasts by various cytokines (interleukin-1, interleukin-6, tumor necrosis factor) secreted by tumor cells in the microenvironment of the bone marrow. Because hypoalbuminemia frequently accompanies malignancy, the total plasma concentration of calcium underestimates the severity of the hypercalcemia. The most common cause of mild hypercalcemia is hyperparathyroidism. Hyperparathyroidism due to chronic renal failure may persist as hypercalcemia after successful renal transplantation. Sarcoidosis is associated with hypercalcemia in approximately 20% of patients.

Symptoms (Table 35-4)

Treatment

The treatment of hypercalcemia is through the correction of dehydration (IV administration of saline, 2 to 3 L daily) combined with the administration of a bisphosphonate (disodium etidronate, 7.5 mg/kg IV for 3 days) (Heath, 1989). Furosemide-induced diuresis may contribute to the speed of renal excretion of calcium.

TABLE 35-4.
SYMPTOMS OF HYPERCALCEMIA

Sedation
Vomiting
Cardiac conduction disturbances (prolonged P-R interval, wide QRS complex and shortened QTc interval)
Renal damage

Bone Composition

Bone is composed of an organic matrix that is strengthened by deposits of calcium salts. The organic matrix is >90% collagen fibers, and the remainder is a homogenous material called *ground substance,* made up of proteoglycans that include chondroitin sulfate and hyaluronic acid. Bone is continually being deposited by osteoblasts and is constantly being absorbed where osteoclasts are active. The parathyroid controls the bone-absorptive activity of osteoclasts. Except in growing bones, the rate of bone deposition and absorption are equal, so the total mass of bone remains constant. Osteoblasts secrete large amounts of alkaline phosphatase when they are actively depositing bone matrix. New bone formation is mirrored by a measurement of the plasma concentration of alkaline phosphatase. Alkaline phosphatase concentrations are also increased by any disease process that causes destruction of bone (metastatic cancer, osteomalacia, rickets).

Exchangeable Calcium

Exchangeable calcium is that calcium in the body that is in equilibrium with calcium in the extracellular fluid. Most of this exchangeable calcium is in bone, thus providing a rapid buffering mechanism to keep the calcium concentration in the extracellular fluid from changing excessively in either direction.

Teeth

The tooth is divided into the *crown,* which is the portion that protrudes above the gum; the *root,* which protrudes into the bony sockets of the mandible and maxilla; and the *neck,* which separates the crown from the root.

Structure

Dentine is the main body of the tooth and is composed principally of hydroxyapatite crystals similar to those in bone. The outer surface of the tooth is covered by a layer of enamel that is formed by special epithelial cells before the eruption of the tooth. Once the tooth has erupted, no more enamel is formed. *Cementum* is a body substance secreted by cells that line the socket of the tooth. This substance is important in holding the tooth in place in the bony socket. The interior of each tooth is filled with pulp containing nerves, blood vessels, and lymphatics.

Dental Caries

Dental caries result from the action of bacteria, the most common of which are streptococci. The first event in the development of caries is the deposition of plaque, which is a film of precipitated products of saliva and food. Bacteria inhabit this plaque, setting the stage for the development of caries. Bacteria depend on carbohydrates for survival, explaining the association between caries and the frequent ingestion of food containing glucose. Teeth formed in children who drink fluorinated water develop enamel that is approximately three times more resistant than normal to the formation of caries.

Dental Injuries

Dental injuries attributed to excessive force applied with the laryngoscope blade during direct laryngoscopy may actually be due to involuntary postoperative biting (bruxism) on the endotracheal tube or oral airway.

Bisphosphonates in the Treatment of Bone Diseases

The main action of bisphosphonates is to induce a marked and prolonged inhibition of bone resorption by decreasing osteoclastic activity.

Clinical Uses

Bisphosphonates, because of their favorable benefit-to-risk ratio, are the preferred alternative to estrogen-replacement therapy in women with postmenopausal osteoporosis and are the treatment of choice for patients with Paget's disease, corticosteroid-induced bone loss, and hypercalcemia due to malignancy (Table 35-5). Bisphosphonates are useful as adjuvant therapy in patients with multiple myeloma and bone metastases to decrease bone pain and the risk of fractures and hypercalcemia. Monthly infusions of pamidronate may protect against skeletal muscle complications in women with metastatic breast cancer.

Side Effects

The toxicity of bisphosphonates is low, with relatively few side effects outside the skeleton. A transient acute influenza-like syndrome may accompany initial treatment with pamidronate. Venous irritation may accompany the IV administration of pamidronate. Oral bisphosphonates increase the tubular reabsorption of phosphate, which, in turn, can lead to secondary hyperparathyroidism. Calcium should be given to blunt the increase in the serum level of parathyroid hormone.

Pharmacokinetics

All bisphosphonates share some pharmacokinetic features, including poor systemic absorption after oral administration, especially in the presence of food (bioavailability 1% to 10%) (see Table 35-5). After a brief period in the circulation, most bisphosphonates are cleared rapidly entering bone (20% to 50% of an orally absorbed dose)

TABLE 35-5.

PHARMACOKINETICS AND CLINICAL USES OF BISPHOSPHONATES

	Etidronate	Clodronate	Pamidronate	Alendronate
Route of administration	Oral IV	Oral IV	IV	Oral IV
Oral bioavailability (%)	1–10	1–10	1–10	1–10
Clinical uses				
Paget's disease	++	+	+++ (IV)	+++
Osteoporosis	+++	+	++	++++

IV, intravenous; +, possible benefit.

where it is tightly bound to hydroxyapatite, whereas the remaining drug is excreted unchanged by the kidneys.

POTASSIUM

Potassium is the second most common cation in the body and the principal intracellular cation. The concentration in the extracellular fluid is about 4 mEq/L, and the intracellular concentration is 150 mEq/L, with only 2% of total body potassium being extracellular. Estimation of total body potassium concentration from serum potassium values is not accurate because of the predominance of intracellular potassium.

Role of Potassium

Potassium is involved in the function of excitable cell membranes (nerves, skeletal muscles, cardiac muscle) and is directly involved in the function of the kidneys. Disturbances of potassium homeostasis are reflected as cardiac dysrhythmias, skeletal muscle weakness, and acid–base disturbances. The kidneys are the principal organ involved in potassium homeostasis. Aldosterone acts at the collecting ducts to increase the reabsorption of sodium ions, which favors potassium secretion. Acidosis opposes and alkalosis favors potassium secretion.

Hypokalemic and Hyperkalemic Drug Effects (Table 35-6)

Hypokalemia

Failure to confirm an increased incidence of serious cardiac dysrhythmias in chronically hypokalemic patients has resulted in less acute potassium replacement therapy and a decrease in the frequency of cancellation of elective operations on the basis of arbitrary serum potassium concentrations. Active intervention with supplemental

TABLE 35-6.
DRUGS THAT ALTER PLASMA CONCENTRATIONS OF POTASSIUM

Hypokalemic Drug Effects
- Catecholamines (shift potassium intracellularly)
- β-Adrenergic agonists (treatment of asthma, premature labor)
- Insulin
- Laxatives (gastrointestinal losses)
- Thiazide diuretics
- Antibiotics (large doses of penicillin, aminoglycoside)

Hyperkalemic Drug Effects
- Succinylcholine (as much as 0.5 mEq/L increase)
- β-Adrenergic antagonists (extracellular shift)
- Nonsteroidal antiinflammatory drugs (prevents aldosterone release)
- Potassium-sparing diuretics

potassium is still recommended for select patients, including those receiving digitalis preparations or who have evidence of acute myocardial ischemia.

Symptoms

Skeletal muscle weakness, a predisposition to cardiac dysrhythmias, enhanced cardiac automaticity, and a decreased rate of myocardial repolarization that predisposes to tachydysrhythmias are recognized symptoms of clinically significant hypokalemia. There is no serum potassium value below which there is an undisputed risk of serious cardiac dysrhythmias.

Treatment

It is important to determine the cause of hypokalemia (redistribution, total body depletion) before aggressive potassium replacement is initiated. Life-threatening hypokalemia, presenting as malignant cardiac dysrhythmias, acute digitalis intoxication, or extreme neuromuscular collapse, requires supplemental IV potassium administration (common recommendation is the administration of 40 mEq/hour). If the starting serum potassium concentration is >2.5 mEq/L, the administration of 0.5 mEq/kg of potassium chloride would be expected to increase the serum potassium concentration 0.6 mEq/L. Morbidity associated with supplemental potassium therapy is not trivial. Patients with diminished internal potassium regulation, especially diabetics and renal failure patients, are at risk for accidental treatment-induced hyperkalemia. The lack of demonstrated perioperative risk from chronic hypokalemia in patients without clinical symptoms should influence the decision to treat chronic hypokalemia acutely.

Hyperkalemia

The earliest sign of hyperkalemia is usually an electrocardiographic (ECG) change, such as a peaked T-wave, which typically occurs when the serum potassium concentration reaches 6 mEq/L. As the extracellular concentration increases further, the transmembrane gradient is decreased, with a prolongation of the P-R interval and QRS widening on the ECG, thus indicating an increased risk of ventricular fibrillation or asystole due to cardiac conduction blockade.

Treatment

If ECG changes other than peaked T-waves occur, or if the serum potassium concentration is >6.5 mEq/L, the incidence of serious cardiac compromise is high, and rapid intervention is indicated (Table 35-7).

PHOSPHATE

Phosphate is important in energy metabolism and the maintenance of acid–base balance. Phosphate ions are the most abundant buffer in the distal renal tubules, allowing the excretion of large quantities of hydrogen

TABLE 35-7.
TREATMENT OF HYPERKALEMIA

Calcium chloride 10 to 20 ml IV (offsets the adverse effects of potassium on cardiac conduction and contractility)
Sodium bicarbonate 0.5 to 1.0 mEq/kg IV (shifts potassium intracellularly)
Glucose-insulin (50 ml of 50% glucose plus 10 U regular insulin IV, produces sustained transfer of potassium into cells and lowers serum potassium concentrations 1.5 to 2.5 mEq/L after approximately 30 minutes)
Epinephrine (shifts potassium intracellularly)
β-Agonists (shift potassium intracellularly)

ions. Vitamin D stimulates the systemic absorption of phosphate from the gastrointestinal tract. Profound skeletal muscle weakness sufficient to contribute to hypoventilation may be a manifestation of hypophosphatemia. Central nervous system dysfunction and peripheral neuropathy may accompany hypophosphatemia. Alcohol abuse and prolonged parenteral nutrition are causes of phosphorus deficiency.

MAGNESIUM

Magnesium is the fourth most important cation in the body and the second most important intracellular cation after potassium. Normal plasma concentrations of magnesium are achieved and maintained by absorption from the small intestine and renal excretion. Abnormalities of plasma and cellular magnesium concentrations frequently accompany other electrolyte abnormalities (correlation between hypomagnesemia and hypokalemia). Plasma magnesium concentrations may remain normal despite significant intracellular deficits because only 5% of the available magnesium pool is extracellular.

TABLE 35-8.
ROLE OF MAGNESIUM

Cardiac cell membrane ion transport (regulates intracellular calcium levels)
Enzyme activity (adenosine triphosphate)
Physiologic antagonist of calcium
Analgesic effects (antagonist of N-methyl-D-aspartate [NMDA] receptors)
Systemic and coronary vasodilation
Inhibits platelet function
Decreases reperfusion injury

Role of Magnesium (Table 35-8)

Hypomagnesemia

Hypomagnesemia (serum magnesium concentration <1.6 mEq/L) may be the most common unrecognized electrolyte deficiency. The emergency treatment of life-threatening hypomagnesemia is through the infusion of magnesium, 10 to 20 mg/kg IV, administered over 10 to 20 minutes.

Causes (Table 35-9)

Symptoms (Table 35-10)

Chronic hypomagnesemia is less likely to be symptomatic than an acute hypomagnesemia, suggesting a normalization of the intracellular to extracellular magnesium ratio with time, similar to that which occurs in chronic hypokalemia. Magnesium (1 to 2 g IV over 5 to 60 minutes, or a continuous infusion, 0.5 to 1.0 g/hour) is recommended for the treatment of torsades de pointes with QTc interval prolongation or as adjunct management for cardiac dysrhythmias in the presence of hypomagnesemia, hypokalemia, or digitalis toxicity.

TABLE 35-9.
CAUSES OF HYPOMAGNESEMIA

Chronic alcoholism (poor diet)
Hyperalimentation
Malabsorption
Dilutional effects from cardiopulmonary pump-priming solutions
Diuretic therapy
Secondary aldosteronism
Large volume infusion of nonelectrolyte solutions (organ donors)
Cyclosporine
Hypokalemia (repletion of intracellular potassium is impaired in presence of hypomagnesemia)

Hypermagnesemia

Hypermagnesemia is present when the plasma concentration of magnesium is >2.6 mEq/L. Treatment of life-threatening hypermagnesemia is with calcium gluconate, 10 to 15 mg/kg IV, followed by fluid loading and drug-induced diuresis.

Causes

The most common cause of hypermagnesemia is the parenteral administration of magnesium to treat pregnancy-induced hypertension. Patients with chronic renal

TABLE 35-10.
SYMPTOMS OF HYPOMAGNESEMIA

Neuromuscular manifestations (resemble hypocalcemia)
Chvostek's and Trousseaus' signs
Carpopedal spasm
Stridor
Skeletal muscle weakness
Ventricular dysrhythmias (may manifest during anesthesia)

TABLE 35-11.
SYMPTOMS OF HYPERMAGNESEMIA

Sedation
Myocardial depression
Suppression of peripheral neuromuscular transmission (decreased acetylcholine release from motor nerve endings)
Direct relaxant effect on skeletal muscles
Diminished deep tendon reflexes (>10 mEq/L)
Skeletal muscle paralysis (apnea) and heart block (>12 mEq/L)
Potentiation of nondepolarizing muscle relaxants (not reliably antagonized by calcium)
Skeletal muscle weakness (Eaton-Lambert syndrome, myasthenia gravis)

dysfunction are at an increased risk for developing hypermagnesemia, because the excretion of magnesium depends on glomerular filtration.

Symptoms (Table 35-11)

Clinical Uses (Table 35-12)

TABLE 35-12.
CLINICAL USES OF MAGNESIUM

Pregnancy-Induced Hypertension
Initial dose (40 to 60 mg/kg IV) and a continuous infusion (15 to 30 mg/kg/hour) to maintain serum magnesium concentrations in a therapeutic range of 4 to 6 mEq/L.
Cardiac Dysrhythmias and Hypertension
Initial dose (2 g IV) administered over 5 minutes followed by a continuous infusion, 1 to 2 g/hour
Cardioprotective Effects
Useful for patients who develop torsade de pointes-type ventricular tachycardia following acute myocardial infarction.

IRON

Iron that is present in food is absorbed from the proximal small intestine, especially the duodenum, into the circulation, where it is bound to transferrin. Approximately 80% of the iron in plasma enters the bone marrow to be incorporated into new erythrocytes. A normal range for the plasma iron concentration is 50 to 150 μg/dL. Hemoglobin synthesis is the principal determinant of the plasma iron turnover rate. When blood loss occurs, hemoglobin concentration is maintained by the mobilization of tissue iron stores. Hemoglobin concentrations become chronically decreased only after these iron reserves are depleted. For this reason, the presence of a normal hemoglobin concentration is not a sensitive indicator of tissue iron stores.

Iron Deficiency

Iron deficiency is estimated to be present in 20% to 40% of menstruating women and fewer than 5% of adult men and postmenopausal women.

Causes

The causes of iron-deficiency anemia include inadequate dietary intake of iron (nutritional) or increased iron requirements due to pregnancy, blood loss, or interference with absorption from the gastrointestinal tract.

Diagnosis

Plasma ferritin concentrations of <12 μg/dL are diagnostic of iron deficiency. Iron-deficiency anemia is present when the depletion of total body iron is associated with a recognizable decrease in the blood concentration of hemoglobin. The large physiologic variation in hemoglobin concentration, however, makes it difficult to reliably identify all individuals with iron-deficiency anemia.

Treatment

The prophylactic use of iron preparations should be reserved for individuals at high risk for developing iron deficiency, such as pregnant and lactating women, low-birth-weight infants, and women with heavy menses. The administration of medicinal iron is followed by an increased rate of erythrocyte production that manifests as an improved hemoglobin concentration within 72 hours. An increase of 2 g/dL or more in the plasma concentration of hemoglobin within 3 weeks is evidence of a positive response to iron. If a positive response does not occur within this time, the presence of continuous bleeding, an infectious process, or impaired gastrointestinal absorption of iron should be considered. No justification exists for continuing iron therapy beyond 3 weeks if a favorable response in the hemoglobin concentration has not occurred. Once a response to iron therapy is demonstrated, the medication should be continued until the hemoglobin concentration is normal.

Oral Iron

Ferrous sulfate, administered orally, is the most frequently used approach for the treatment of iron-deficiency anemia. The usual therapeutic dose of iron for adults to treat iron-deficiency anemia is 2 to 3 mg/kg (200 mg daily) in three divided doses. Nausea and upper abdominal pain are the most frequent side effects of oral iron therapy, particularly if the dosage is >200 mg daily. Hemochromatosis is unlikely to result from oral iron therapy that is administered to treat nutritional anemia. If iron overdose is suspected, a plasma concentration of >0.5 mg/dL confirms the presence of a life-threatening situation that should be treated with deferoxamine.

Parenteral Iron

Parenteral iron acts similarly to oral iron but should be used only if patients cannot tolerate or do not respond to oral therapy (continuing loss is greater than can be replaced because of limitations of oral absorption). An iron dextran injection contains 50 mg/mL of iron and is available for IM of IV use. After absorption, the iron must be split from the glucose molecule of the dextran before it becomes available to tissues. IM injection is painful, and concern exists about malignant changes at the injection site. For these reasons, the IV administration of iron is preferred over IM injection. A dose of 500 mg of iron can be infused over 5 to 10 minutes. The principal side effect of parenteral iron therapy is the rare occurrence of a severe allergic reaction, presumably due to the presence of dextran.

COPPER

Copper is present in ceruloplasmin and is a constituent of other enzymes, including dopamine β-hydroxylase and cytochrome-C oxidase. Copper deficiency is rare in the presence of an adequate diet. Supplements of copper should be given during prolonged hyperalimentation.

ZINC

Zinc is a cofactor of enzymes and is essential for cell growth and synthesis of nucleic acid, carbohydrates, and proteins. Adequate zinc is provided by a diet containing sufficient animal protein. Diets in which protein is obtained primarily from vegetable sources may not supply adequate zinc. Severe zinc deficiency occurs most often in the presence of malabsorption syndromes. The cutaneous manifestations of zinc deficiency may occur during prolonged hyperalimentation, emphasizing the need for zinc supplements in these patients. Symptoms of zinc deficiency include disturbances in taste and smell, suboptimal growth in children, hepatosplenomegaly, alopecia, cutaneous rashes, glossitis, and stomatitis.

CHROMIUM

Chromium is important in a cofactor complex with insulin and thus is involved in normal glucose use.

Deficiency has been accompanied by a diabetes-like syndrome, peripheral neuropathy, and encephalopathy.

SELENIUM

Selenium is a constituent of several metabolically important enzymes. A deficiency of selenium has been associated with cardiomyopathy, suggesting the need to add this trace element to supplements administered during prolonged hyperalimentation.

MANGANESE

Manganese is concentrated in mitochondria, especially in the liver, pancreas, kidneys, and pituitary. Deficiency is unknown clinically, but supplementation is recommended during prolonged hyperalimentation.

MOLYBDENUM

Molybdenum is an essential constituent of many enzymes. It is well absorbed from the gastrointestinal tract and is present in bones, liver, and kidneys.

Blood Components, Substitutes, and Hemostatic Drugs

36

Blood components and certain drugs are most often administered systemically to improve oxygenation and decrease bleeding due to specific coagulation defects (Stoelting RK, Hillier SC. Blood components, substitutes, and hemostatic drugs. In: *Pharmacology and Physiology in Anesthetic Practice*. 4th ed. Philadelphia, Lippincott Williams & Wilkins, 2006:623–634). The transmission of infectious diseases (hepatitis C, hepatitis B, human immunodeficiency virus [HIV], cytomegalovirus) hemolytic and nonhemolytic transfusion reactions, and immunosuppression are potential adverse sequelae of blood component therapy. The topical application of hemostatics is used to control surface bleeding and capillary oozing. Blood substitutes lack coagulation activity but are administered systemically to replace and maintain intravascular fluid volume.

BLOOD COMPONENTS

The administration of specific components is recommended in all circumstances other than acute hemorrhage. In the presence of acute hemorrhage, whole blood is indicated to replace both oxygen-carrying capacity and intravascular fluid volume. A unit of whole blood can be divided into several components (Table 36-1).

TABLE 36-1.

COMPONENTS AVAILABLE FOR WHOLE BLOOD

Component	Content	Approximate Volume (mL)	Shelf-Life
Packed erythrocytes	Erythrocytes Leukocytes Plasma clotting factors	300	35 days in CPDA-1 42 days in Adsol
Platelet concentrates	Leukocytes (limited) Plasma Erythrocytes (limited)	50	1–5 days
Fresh frozen plasma	Clotting factors	225	Frozen: 1 yr. Thawed: 6 hrs.
Cryoprecipitate	Factor VIII	Lyophilized powder	Determined by manufacturer

TABLE 36-1.
(Continued)

Component	Content	Approximate Volume (mL)	Shelf-Life
Factor IX concentrate	Factor IX Factors II, VII and X (limited)	Lyophilized powder	Determined by manufacturer
Granulocyte concentrates	Leukocytes Platelets Erythrocytes (limited)	50–300	24 hrs.
Albumin	5% albumin 25% albumin	250 or 500 50 or 100	3 yrs
Plasma protein fraction	Albumin α-Globulins β-Globulins	500	3 yrs
Immune globulins	γ-Globulin	1–2	3 yrs

Adsol, adenine-glucose-mannitol-sodium chloride; CPDA-1, citrate-phosphate dextrose preservative.

Packed Erythrocytes

Packed erythrocytes are prepared by removing most of the plasma from whole blood (resulting volume is about 300 mL, and the hematocrit is 70% to 80%.). The decreased amounts of plasma infused with packed erythrocytes decreases the likelihood of allergic transfusion reactions, compared with whole blood. The addition of adenine to the citrate-phosphate dextrose preservative (CPDA-1; CPD-A) increases storage time from 28 days to 35 days. Adenine increases erythrocyte survival by allowing cells to resynthesize the adenosine triphosphate (ATP) needed to fuel metabolic reactions. The addition of extra nutrients to citrate-phosphate-dextrose (adenine, glucose, mannitol, sodium chloride) results in Adsol and an increased storage time to 42 days. Adsol contains about 100 mL of additional saline, making the hematocrit of packed erythrocytes stored in Adsol 55% rather than 70%. Adenine-glucose-mannitol-sodium chloride (ADSOL) preservative extends the shelf life of blood to 49 days.

Clinical Uses

Packed erythrocytes are selected when the goal is to increase oxygen-carrying capacity in the absence of preexisting hypovolemia (packed erythrocytes may be used to replace blood loss that is <1,500 mL in an adult). One unit of packed erythrocytes typically increases the hematocrit 3% or hemoglobin concentration 1 g/dL in a 70-kg nonbleeding adult. Erythrocyte transfusion is rarely indicated when the hemoglobin concentration is >10 g/dL and is almost always indicated when it is <6 g/dL, especially when anemia is acute. The determination of whether intermediate hemoglobin concentrations (6 to 10 g/dL) justify or require erythrocyte transfusion should be based on the patient's risk for complications of inadequate oxygenation. The administration of packed erythrocytes is facilitated by reconstituting them with crystalloid solutions (5% glucose in 0.9% saline, 0.9% saline, Normosol) to decrease viscosity. Lactated Ringer's solution should probably not be used for this purpose because the calcium ions present could induce clotting.

Platelet Concentrates

One unit of platelet concentrate will increase the platelet count 5,000 to 10,000 cells/mL^3. The usual therapeutic dose is one platelet concentrate per 10 kg of body weight. Although platelet concentrates contain only a few erythrocytes, they do contain large amounts of plasma (leukocytes) and administration on the basis of ABO compatibility is desirable. Likewise, the small quantity of erythrocytes present can cause Rh immunization if platelets from an Rh-positive donor are administered to an Rh-negative recipient. For this reason, Rh-compatible platelets should be used in women of child-bearing age.

Clinical Uses

Surgical and obstetric patients usually require platelet transfusion if the platelet count is <50,000 cells/mL^3 and rarely require therapy if it is >100,000 cells/mL^3 With intermediate platelet counts (50,000 to 100,000 cells/mL^3), the determinant is based on the patient's risk for more significant bleeding. In nonsurgical patients, spontaneous bleeding is uncommon with platelet counts of >10,000 cells/mL^3.

Fresh Frozen Plasma

Fresh frozen plasma contains all procoagulants except platelets in a concentration of 1 unit/mL, as well as naturally occurring inhibitors. Compatibility for ABO antigens is desirable, but cross-matching is not necessary. Life-threatening allergic reactions may occur, and the transmission of diseases, including hepatitis and HIV, is possible.

Clinical Uses

The usual starting dose of fresh frozen plasma is two units (400 to 500 mL) or one plasmapheresis unit to treat active bleeding due to a congenital or acquired deficiency of coagulation factors as confirmed by a prothrombin time >1.5 times normal (usually >18 s), partial thromboplastin time >1.5 times normal (usually >55 to 60 s), or coagulation factor assay of <25% activity. Fresh frozen plasma (5 to 8 mL/kg IV) is recommended for the urgent reversal of warfarin therapy, as may be needed before emergency surgery. Fresh frozen plasma may be considered for the treatment of continued bleeding in patients receiving massive blood transfusions (>5,000 mL in an adult). Fresh frozen plasma is not recommended for the treatment of hypovolemia or hypoalbuminemia.

Cryoprecipitated Antihemophiliac Factor

Cryoprecipitated antihemophiliac factor (factor VIII) is that fraction of plasma that precipitates when fresh frozen plasma is thawed. Multiple transfusions of cryoprecipitate may result in hyperfibrinogenemia, emphasizing the substantial fibrinogen content of these preparations. Hepatitis is the most common adverse side effect of pooled plasma products, reflecting the multiple donor sources of the fibrinogen content. Hemolytic anemia may occur when cryoprecipitated antihemophiliac factor is administered to individuals with group A, B, or AB erythrocyte antigens.

Clinical Uses

Cryoprecipitate is useful for treating hemophilia A because it contains high concentrations of factor VIII (80 to 120 units) in a volume of only about 10 mL. Hemophilia A patients with factor VIII levels of >5% of normal usually do not experience spontaneous bleeding. Effective hemostasis during and after major surgery, however, requires maintenance of factor VIII levels of ≥40% of normal for 7 to 10 days. Cryoprecipitate is recommended for the treatment of bleeding patients with von Willebrand's disease and for correction of bleeding in massively transfused patients with fibrinogen concentrations of <80 to 100 mg/dL. Most cases of hypofibrinogenemia are associated with conditions that cause consumption coagulopathy and require treatment with other blood components as well. Cryoprecipitate is the only approved blood component that contains fibrinogen in a concentrated form.

Desmopressin

Desmopressin is a synthetic analog of arginine vasopressin (formerly known as antidiuretic hormone), that greatly increases factor VIII activity in patients with mild to moderate hemophilia and von Willebrand's disease. The routine administration of desmopressin to patients undergoing elective cardiac surgery does not alter blood loss after cardiopulmonary bypass. Decreases in systemic blood pressure associated with evidence of peripheral vasodilation may occur in association with the infusion of desmopressin. In contrast to blood components, desmopressin administration does not introduce the risk of transmission of viral diseases.

Factor IX Concentrate

Factor IX concentrate (prothrombin complex, plasma thromboplastin component) can be infused without typing or cross-matching. Hypervolemic reactions do not occur because of the concentrated nature of these products and the small amount of fluid needed for administration. Factor IX concentrates have significant potential to cause hepatitis because of the pooled origin of these products. In addition, a high risk of thrombotic complications is associated with infusion, presumably reflecting the high concentrations of prothrombin and factor X that result from factor IX.

Fibrin Glue

Fibrin Glue (cryoprecipitated fibrinogen) is prepared from bovine thrombin and human fibrinogen, which form a clot when combined. This glue has been used for sealing suture holes, such as those associated with vascular anastomoses.

Antifibrinolytics

Synthetic (aminocaproic acid, tranexamic acid) and natural (aprotinin) antifibrinolytics have been popularized as drugs to decrease postoperative bleeding and the need for transfusions after cardiopulmonary bypass, scoliosis surgery, and orthotopic liver transplantation and to decrease bleeding associated with lower urinary tract surgery. The antifibrinolytic effect of these drugs is due to the formation of a reversible complex with plasminogen thus preventing fibrinolysis that would normally occur with the activation of plasminogen to plasmin. As result of this inhibition, fibrin is not lysed, which allows for the formation of a more stable clot and decreased risk of recurrent bleeding. Treatment with fibrinolytic inhibitors is associated with a theoretical risk of an increased thrombotic tendency. The administration of aminocaproic acid in the presence of renal or ureteral bleeding is not recommended, because ureteral clot formation and possible obstruction may result. Indeed, unchanged aminocaproic acid is rapidly excreted by the kidneys. Aminocaproic acid does not control hemorrhage caused by thrombocytopenia or most other coagulation defects.

Granulocyte Concentrates

Granulocytes have been beneficial in patients recovering from bone marrow transplants. Fever often accompanies granulocyte transfusion and can be ameliorated by the administration of an antihistamine and an antipyretic. Granulocytes should be administered slowly to avoid the pulmonary insufficiency that may be caused by a sequestration of these cells in the pulmonary capillaries. Cytomegalovirus infections frequently are observed after granulocyte transfusions because the virus is concentrated in granulocytes.

Albumin

Albumin is obtained by fractionating human plasma that is nonreactive for hepatitis. Coagulation factors and blood group antibodies are not present. Albumin, 25 g, is equivalent osmotically to about 500 mL of plasma but contains only about one-seventh the amount of sodium present in the same volume of plasma. Hypoalbuminemia is the most frequent indication for the administration of albumin. The administration of hypertonic 25% albumin will draw 3 to 4 mL of fluid from the interstitial space into the intravascular fluid space for every 1 mL of albumin administered. Thus, 25% albumin is not recommended for administration to patients in cardiac failure or in the presence of anemia. The 5% solution of albumin is isotonic with plasma and is most often administered undiluted at a rate of 2 to 4 mL/minute. In patients in an intensive care unit, the administration of either albumin or normal saline for fluid resuscitation results in similar outcomes at 28 days.

Antioxidant Activity

Albumin possesses potential free radical scavenging characteristics and is the principal intravascular source of reduced sulfhydryl groups. These sulfhydryl groups are avid scavengers of reactive oxygen and nitrogen molecules. Antioxidants may have therapeutic value in reducing cellular damage, particularly during local and systemic inflammatory responses.

Plasma Protein Fraction

Plasma protein fraction is a 5% pooled solution of stabilized human plasma proteins in saline. The preparation is equivalent osmotically to an equal volume of plasma. Although plasma protein fraction is prepared from large pools of normal human plasma, the transmission of viral diseases is not a hazard because of heating to 60° C for 10 hours. It must be recognized that plasma protein fraction does not contain any coagulation factors and may even dilute the plasma concentration of existing coagulants.

Clinical Uses

Plasma protein fraction is administered to treat hypovolemic shock and to provide protein to patients with hypoproteinemia. It is also effective for the initial treatment of shock in infants and small children with dehydration, hemoconcentration, and electrolyte deficiency caused by diarrhea.

Immune Globulin

Immune globulin is a concentrated solution of globulins, primarily immunoglobulins, prepared from large pools of human plasma. This preparation protects against clinical manifestations of hepatitis A when administered before or within 2 weeks after exposure.

TOPICAL HEMOSTATICS

Topical hemostatics may help to control surface bleeding and capillary oozing. Although usually innocuous, the presence of bacterial contamination at the site of application of topical hemostatics may exacerbate infections.

Absorbable Gelatin Sponge

Absorbable gelatin sponge (Gelfoam) is a sterile gelatin-base surgical sponge that controls bleeding in highly vascular areas that are difficult to suture. The preparation may be left in place after closure of the surgical wound. Absorption is complete in 4 to 6 weeks, and scar formation or cellular reaction is minimal.

Absorbable Gelatin Film

Absorbable gelatin film (Gelfilm) is a sterile, thin film used primarily in neurologic and thoracic surgery for nonhemostatic purposes to repair defects in the dura and pleural membranes.

Oxidized Cellulose (Oxycel) and Oxidized Regenerated Cellulose (Surgical)

Oxycel and oxidized regenerated cellulose do not enter into the normal clotting cascade, but when exposed to blood, they expand and are converted to a reddish brown or black gelatinous mass that forms an artificial clot.

Microfibrillar Collagen Hemostat (Avitene)

When applied directly onto a bleeding surface, this water-insoluble, fibrous material attracts and entraps platelets to initiate the formation of a platelet plug and development of a natural clot. This topical hemostatic appears to retain its effectiveness in heparinized patients, in those receiving oral anticoagulants, and in the presence of moderate thrombocytopenia. Microfibrillar collagen hemostat is a useful adjunct to therapy in the oral cavity of patients with hemophilia.

Thrombin

Thrombin is applied topically as a powder or in a solution to control capillary oozing in operative procedures and to shorten effectively the duration of bleeding from puncture sites in heparinized patients.

BLOOD SUBSTITUTES

Blood substitutes may be viewed as oxygen-carrying volume expanders that, in contrast to blood products, have a prolonged shelf life and do not introduce the risk for disease transmission or need for compatibility testing. In contrast to blood, blood substitutes do not contain any coagulant factors.

Hydroxyethyl Starch

Hydroxyethyl starch (hetastarch) is a complex polysaccharide (average molecular weight 450,000 daltons) that is available in a 6% and 10% aqueous solutions for intravascular volume expansion (plasma substitute in place of 5% albumin) during the perioperative period. In addition to volume replacement, hydroxyethyl starch is useful for acute normovolemic hemodilution and to improve blood rheology by decreasing blood viscosity. Hydroxyethyl starch may produce a coagulopathy (dose-dependent decrease in factor VIII and von Willebrand factor and interference with platelet function).

Pharmacokinetics

Hydroxyethyl starch is removed from the circulation by renal excretion and redistribution. The reversible swelling of renal tubular cells may reflect a reabsorption of hydroxyethyl starch macromolecules. The duration of volume expansion approximates 24 hours, which is similar to that produced by albumin. The solution administered clinically consists of 6 g or 10 g of hydroxyethyl starch in 100 mL of saline with an osmolarity of 310 mOsm/L and a pH of 3.5 to 7.

Side Effects

Hydroxyethyl starch may interfere with coagulation and accumulate in tissues. Serum macroamylasemia may follow the transfusion of hydroxyethyl starch. For this reason, serum amylase concentrations as a diagnostic marker of pancreatic disease should not be relied on for 3 to 5 days after hydroxyethyl starch infusion. Pruritus associated with the deposition of hydroxyethyl starch in the skin may be treated with topical capsaicin.

Coagulopathy

Hydroxyethyl starch has been associated with a prolongation of the activated partial thromboplastin time and a decrease in the plasma concentrations of factor VIII, von Willebrand's factor, and fibrinogen plus decreased platelet function that appears to be independent of the dose administered.

Dextran

Dextran-70 is a water-soluble glucose polymer (polysaccharide) synthesized by certain bacteria from sucrose. This high-molecular-weight dextran is treated to yield low-molecular-weight dextran (dextran-40), having a molecular weight of about 40,000 daltons and a higher colloid osmotic pressure. Dextrans are eliminated largely through the kidneys, although small amounts are metabolized. Dextran-70 may persist in the circulation for 72 hours and interfere with platelet activation. Ultimately, dextran-70 is degraded enzymatically to glucose.

Clinical Uses

High-molecular-weight dextrans remain in the intravascular space for about 12 hours. For this reason, they may be suitable alternatives to blood or plasma for the expansion of intravascular fluid volume. For replacement of intravascular fluid volume, the recommended maximum dose during the first 24 hours is 20 mL/kg IV and then 10 mg/kg IV on subsequent days. A special solution of dextran (32% dextran-70) is used in hysteroscopy to help distend and irrigate the uterine cavity and to decrease the likelihood of tubal adhesions after reconstructive tubal surgery for infertility. Because this dextran may be absorbed, adverse reactions are the same as those encountered after IV administration. Dextran-40 remains intravascular for only 2 to 4 hours and is used most often to prevent thromboembolism by decreasing blood viscosity.

Side Effects (Table 36-2)

The potential side effects of dextran must be considered before the blood substitute is selected in lieu of safer, though more expensive, products such as albumin or plasma protein fraction.

Gelatin Solutions

Gelatin solutions (Hemaccel, Gelofusin) are inexpensive and have a relatively short intravascular half-time, although

TABLE 36-2.
SIDE EFFECTS OF DEXTRAN SOLUTIONS

Allergic reactions (less with low-molecular weight dextrans, discontinuation of the infusion is usually sufficient treatment)
Increased bleeding time (decreased platelet adhesiveness especially with high-molecular weight dextran and a dose >1,500 mL)
Rouleaux formation (interferes with subsequent cross-matching of blood)
Noncardiogenic pulmonary edema (systemic absorption)

it exceeds that of colloid solutions. Metabolism is in the liver, and the gelatin is completely eliminated via the kidneys thus resulting in an osmotic diuresis. Coagulation problems are unlikely and, when they occur, are probably related to hemodilution. Gelatin-induced histamine release has been associated with hypotension, bronchospasm, and cutaneous rashes.

Hemoglobin Solutions

Pure solutions of hemoglobin (stroma-free) provide oxygen-carrying capacity but have a limited duration of action due to their rapid clearance from the circulation.

Recombinant Human Hemoglobin

Recombinant human hemoglobin is a genetically engineered protein produced in *Escherichia coli* that yields a pure solution of hemoglobin (P50 in a normal range) without remnants of red blood cell stroma. The intravascular half-time of these products is short, and they are cleared from the circulation by the reticuloendothelial system.

Perfluorocarbons

Perfluorocarbons are inert synthetic compounds that dissolve large amounts of carbon dioxide and act as solvents for oxygen molecules (oxygen carrying colloid). The oxygen content of perfluorocarbons is directly proportional to the oxygen partial pressure. Because perfluorocarbons exchange gases by simple diffusion, they load and unload oxygen two times faster than hemoglobin. Intravascularly administered fluorocarbons are excreted intact by exhalation and are also cleared from the circulation by phagocytosis and subsequent uptake into the reticuloendothelial system, from which they are progressively excreted through the lungs. Perfluorocarbons do not affect coagulation but do appear as platelets in automated cell counters, which may result in an overestimate of platelet counts, especially in thrombocytopenic blood samples. Fluosol-DA 20% is licensed only for oxygen delivery (not as a erythrocyte substitute) during coronary angioplasty when the balloon is inflated. Perfusion of coronary arteries after percutaneous transluminal angioplasty is a current use of 20% perfluorocarbon (Fluosol-DA 20).

37 Enteral and Parenteral Nutrition

Enteral nutrition is defined as providing nourishment to a patient utilizing a liquid diet of specific composition that is delivered directly into the gastrointestinal tract, through the use of a nasogastric tube, nasointestinal tube, gastrostomy tube, or jejunostomy tube (Stoelting RK, Hillier SC. Enteral and parenteral nutrition. In: *Pharmacology and Physiology in Anesthetic Practice*. 4th ed. Philadelphia, Lippincott Williams & Wilkins, 2006: 635–639). Parenteral nutrition is defined as the delivery of nutrients directly into the venous circulation, through a peripheral or central vein. Total parenteral nutrition (TPN) is utilized when the only source of nutrient supply is via the parenteral route. TPN should be continued during the perioperative period, whereas enteral nutrition should be discontinued about 6 hours before surgery (reflecting recommendations for food ingestion prior to elective surgery) and a glucose infusion initiated to minimize the risk of hypoglycemia.

HYPERALIMENTATION

Hyperalimentation is intended to supply all the essential inorganic and organic nutritional elements necessary to maintain optimal body composition as well as positive nitrogen balance. Alimentation through the gastrointestinal tract (enteral nutrition) is preferred to intravenous alimentation (parenteral nutrition) because it avoids catheter-induced sepsis, maintains gut integrity by providing luminal nutrients (especially glutamine) and thus lessening the translocation of bacteria from the gastrointestinal tract, and maintains the absorptive activity of the small intestine. Thus, even if the patient's caloric and nitrogen requirements cannot be met with luminal nutrition, the enteral route of feeding should be used unless it is contraindicated (bowel obstruction, inadequate bowel surface area, intractable diarrhea). The enteral and parenteral routes may be used simultaneously to meet nutritional requirements. Most patients do not need nutritional support, and clear-cut benefits of this expensive intervention have been established for only a select group of patients (Table 37-1). Data suggest that preoperative nutritional support should be reserved for malnourished patients undergoing major elective surgery and should be provided for no more than 10 days. Postoperative nutritional support is indicated in patients who cannot eat by postoperative day 10 to 14. Patients not expected to resume adequate oral feedings within 7 to 10 days of surgery should begin nutritional support within 2 to 4 days postoperatively. Elderly patients, especially those

TABLE 37-1.
ESTABLISHED INDICATIONS FOR USE OF NUTRITIONAL SUPPORT

Major elective surgery in severely malnourished patients
Major trauma (blunt or penetrating injury, head injury)
Burns
Hepatic dysfunction
Renal dysfunction
Bone marrow transplant recipients undergoing intensive chemotherapy
Patients unable to eat or absorb nutrients for an indefinite period (neurologic impairment, oropharyngeal dysfunction, short bowel syndrome)
Well-nourished, minimally stressed patients unable to eat for 10 to 14 days

with weight loss, may benefit from nutritional supplementation during their hospitalization. Adequate caloric intake is essential for the efficient use of amino acids. Lipid calories from infusions of propofol may be significant and should be included when calculating caloric intake.

ENTERAL NUTRITION

A variety of enteral solutions containing various amounts of protein (amino acids), carbohydrates (glucose), fat micronutrients, and electrolytes are available. Carbohydrates are the source of up to 90% of the calories, emphasizing the increased osmolarity of these solutions. Unless the patient has maldigestion or malabsorption of fat, formulas with a normal range of fat content are preferred. In patients with hepatic cirrhosis or portocaval shunts, excessive plasma concentrations of fatty acids may act synergistically with high levels of ammonia and other toxins to exacerbate or cause hepatic encephalopathy. Low-protein formulations, however, are indicated for patients with severe renal dysfunction. Increased amounts of protein or amino acids are indicated when the nitrogen requirement is increased, as in patients with trauma, burns, or sepsis.

Enteral Tube Feeding

Enteral tube feeding may be necessary when patients are unable to consume nutritionally complete, liquefied food orally. An important consideration when utilizing enteral nutrition is the placement and positioning of the small bore (8 to 12 French) silastic delivery tube. Most often, patients receive continuous infusions of enteral nutrition through a nasoenteric tube. Dislodgement of the tip, especially in the presence of gastroparesis, can result in pulmonary aspiration. In patients likely to have gastroparesis (critically ill patients), it is common to place the tip of the feeding tube distal to the ligament of Treitz in an effort to prevent pooling of fluids in the stomach, with the attendant risk of pulmonary aspiration. The surgical placement of an esophagostomy or gastrostomy tube may be indicated for long-term feeding. For slow-drip feeding, an automated infusion pump to control the rate of administration is useful.

Side Effects (Table 37-2)

PARENTERAL NUTRITION

Parenteral nutrition is indicated for patients who are unable to ingest or digest nutrients or to absorb them from the gastrointestinal tract. Parenteral nutrition using isotonic solutions delivered through a peripheral vein is acceptable when the patient requires <2,000 calories daily and the anticipated need for nutritional support is brief. When nutritional requirements are >2,000 calories daily, or prolonged nutritional support is required, a catheter is placed in the central venous system to permit the infusion of a hypertonic (1,900 mOsm/L) nutrition solution.

TABLE 37-2.
SIDE EFFECTS OF ENTERAL NUTRITION

Gastric retention
Abdominal distension
Hypovolemia (osmotic diuresis induced by glycosuria)
Nonketotic coma (hyperosmolar dehydration from high glucose load)
Hypophosphatemia
Cutaneous rashes (fatty acid deficiency)
Pulmonary aspiration (maintain semi-sitting position during feeding and for 1 hour after feeding)
Risk of sepsis

Short-term Parenteral Therapy

Short-term parenteral therapy (3 to 5 days in patients without nutritional deficits) after uncomplicated surgical procedures is most often provided by hypocaloric, non-nitrogen glucose-electrolyte solutions (Table 37-3). These solutions provide total fluid and electrolyte needs and sufficient calories to decrease protein catabolism and prevent ketosis.

Long-term (Total) Parenteral Nutrition

Long-term (total) parenteral nutrition (intravenous hyperalimentation) is the technique of providing total nutrition needs through an infusion of amino acids combined with glucose and varying amounts of fat emulsion. These hypertonic solutions must be infused into a central vein having a high blood flow to provide rapid dilution (a catheter is often placed percutaneously into the subclavian vein and guided into the right atrium). When intermittent administration is used, the infusion must be decreased gradually during the 60 to 90 minutes preceding discontinuation to avoid hypoglycemia. The efficacy of nutritional support is reflected by body weight measurements that confirm a maintenance or increase of lean body mass. Daily weight gains of >0.5 kg, however, may signify fluid retention. Serum electrolytes, blood glucose concentrations, and blood urea nitrogen (BUN) should be measured periodically during total parenteral nutrition. Tests of hepatic and renal function are also recommended but can be performed at less frequent intervals.

Side Effects (Table 37-4)

Monitoring During Total Parenteral Nutrition

Access sites are observed for signs of infection. Additional vitamin K may be indicated, based on the measurement of prothrombin and plasma thromboplastin times. Increases

TABLE 37-3.

CONTENTS OF VARIOUS CRYSTALLOID SOLUTIONS

	Glucose (mg/dL)	Sodium (mEq/L)	Chloride (mEq/L)	Potassium (mEq/L)	Magnesium (mEq/L)	Calcium (mEq/L)	Lactate (mEq/L)	pH	Osmolarity (mOsm/L)
5% glucose in water	5,000	0	0	0	0	0	0	5.0	253
5% glucose in 0.45% sodium chloride	5,000	77	77	0	0	0	0	4.2	407
5% glucose in 0.9% sodium chloride	0	154	154	0	0	0	0	4.2	561
0.9% sodium chloride	0	154	154	0	0	0	0	5.7	308
Lactated Ringer's Solution	0	130	109	4	0	3	28	6.7	273
5% glucose in lactated Ringer's Solution	5,000	130	109	4	0	3	28	5.3	527
Normosol-R	0	140	98	5	3	0	*	7.4	295

*Contains 27 mEq/liter of acetate and 23 mEq/liter of gluconate.

TABLE 37-4.
SIDE EFFECTS ASSOCIATED WITH TOTAL PARENTERAL NUTRITION

Pneumothorax (related to catheter placement)
Thrombosis of central veins
Sepsis (spiking temperature is an indication to remove catheter and culture tip; do not to use this catheter for blood sampling)
Pneumonia
Fatty acid deficiency
Hyperglycemia (monitor during the perioperative period; elderly patients vulnerable; osmotic diuresis can lead to hypovolemia)
Nonketotic hyperosmolar hyperglycemic coma
Hypoglycemia (risk of sudden discontinuation of infusion; recommendation is to decrease over 60 to 90 minutes; reflects persistent pancreatic insulin response)
Hepatobiliary complications
Metabolic acidosis (liberation of hydrochloric acid during metabolism of amino acids)
Hypercarbia (metabolism of large quantities of glucose; may result in need to initiate mechanical ventilation or failure to wean from mechanical support)
Fluid overload
Renal dysfunction
Hepatic dysfunction

in aminotransferases and alkaline phosphatase suggest the development of hepatic steatosis. Careful maintenance of fluid intake and output is needed, because critically ill patients often experience significant fluid shifts.

Preparation of Total Parenteral Nutrition Solutions

Total parenteral nutrition solutions are prepared from commercially available solutions by mixing hypertonic glucose with an amino acid solution. Requirements for vitamins may be increased, emphasizing the need to add a multivitamin preparation to total parenteral nutrition solutions. The serum albumin concentration will usually increase in patients receiving total parenteral nutrition if adequate amino acids and calories are provided. Fat emulsions are not mixed with the total parenteral nutrition solutions. Instead, these isotonic emulsions are administered intravenously through a separate peripheral vein or by a Y-connector into the same vein. To decrease the possibility of bacterial contamination, total parenteral nutrition solutions are prepared aseptically under a laminar air-flow hood, refrigerated, and administered within 24 to 48 hours.

Immunonutrition

Immunonutrition is an attempt to enhance immunity and cellular integrity by incorporating specific additives (such as Ω-3 fatty acids, arginine to enhance lymphocyte cytotoxicity, and purine as a precursor of RNA and DNA) into enteral diets.

Crystalline Amino Acid Solutions

Mild thrombophlebitis occurs infrequently during and after infusion of amino acid solutions. Because amino acids increase the BUN concentration, they should be given cautiously to patients with impaired renal function. In patients with severe liver disease, hepatic coma may be precipitated by an accumulation of nitrogenous substances in the blood.

Intralipid

Intralipid is a fat emulsion that is used to prevent or correct essential fatty acid deficiency and to provide calories in a high-density form on a regular basis during prolonged total parenteral nutrition. Because intralipid is isotonic with plasma, it is suitable for peripheral infusion and, if sufficient calories can be provided by this method, the use of hypertonic glucose (>10%) by way of a central vein catheter may be avoided.

Side Effects

Increased plasma concentrations of triglycerides occur predictably when Intralipid is infused too rapidly or the emulsion is administered to patients with impaired fat metabolism. Hepatomegaly, altered liver function tests, decreased pulmonary diffusing capacity, thrombocytopenia, and anemia may occasionally occur. Indeed, periodic liver function tests and platelet counts should be performed during long-term total parenteral nutrition.

Liposyn

Liposyn is an intravenous fat emulsion that, like Intralipid, is used to prevent essential fatty acid deficiency and as a source of calories during total parenteral nutrition.

Travamulsion

Travamulsion is an intravenous fat emulsion that is 56% linoleic acid.

38 Antiseptics and Disinfectants

Substances that are applied topically to living tissues to kill or prevent the growth of microorganisms are antiseptics (Table 38-1) (Stoelting RK, Hillier SC. Antiseptics and disinfectants. In: *Pharmacology and Physiology in Anesthetic Practice*. 4th ed. Philadelphia, Lippincott Williams & Wilkins, 2006:640–643). A disinfectant is an agent that is applied topically to an inanimate object to destroy pathogenic microorganisms and thus prevent the transmission of infection (see Table 38-1). *Sterilization* is the complete and total destruction of all microbial life, including vegetative bacteria, spores, fungi, and viruses. Ethylene oxide is the only chemical available that is approved for the sterilization of objects that cannot be heated or sterilized by other physical methods, such as radiation.

ALCOHOLS

Alcohols are applied topically to decrease local cutaneous bacterial flora (immediate antisepsis and quick drying) before penetration of the skin with needles. On the skin, 70% ethyl alcohol kills nearly 90% of the cutaneous bacteria within 2 minutes, provided the area is kept moist. Greater than a 75% decrease in cutaneous bacterial count is unlikely with a single wipe of an ethyl alcohol. Isopropyl alcohol has a slightly greater bactericidal activity than ethyl alcohol due to its greater depression of surface tension. Neither of the alcohols, however, is fungicidal or virucidal.

TABLE 38-1.
ANTISEPTICS AND DISINFECTANTS

Antiseptics
Ethyl and isopropyl alcohols
Cationic surface-active quaternary ammonium compounds
Chlorhexidine
Iodine compounds
Hexachlorophene
Disinfectants
Formaldehyde
Glutaraldehyde
Cresol
Elemental iodine

Fire Risks

Alcohol-based preps are flammable until all the liquid has evaporated. Alcohol-based surgical prep solutions can create a fire hazard (flash fire), especially if the prep solution is allowed to pool (umbilicus) or the patient is draped before the prep is completely dry, resulting in trapped alcohol vapors being channeled to the surgical site where a heat source will be used.

QUATERNARY AMMONIUM COMPOUNDS

Quaternary ammonium compounds (benzalkonium and cetylpyridinium [mouthwash]) are bactericidal in vitro to a wide variety of Gram-positive and Gram-negative bacteria. Many fungi and viruses are also susceptible. Mycobacterium tuberculosis, however, is relatively resistant. Alcohol enhances the germicidal activity of quaternary ammonium compounds so that tinctures are more effective than aqueous solutions. Quaternary ammonium compounds have been widely used for the sterilization of instruments (endoscopes and other instruments made of polyethylene or polypropylene absorb quaternary ammonium compounds).

CHLORHEXIDINE

Chlorhexidine (Hibiclens®) is a colorless chlorophenol biguanide solution that disrupts the cell membranes of the bacterial cells and is effective against both Gram-positive and Gram-negative bacteria. Chlorhexidine is mainly used for the preoperative cutaneous preparation of the surgeon and patient; it persists on the skin to provide continued antibacterial protection. 2% chlorhexidine is superior to povidone iodine for skin preparation and the prevention of catheter-related blood stream infections due to placement of invasive intravascular catheters. Chlorhexidine solutions in an alcohol base are not appropriate for instillation into the eye (corneal injury) or middle ear (deafness).

IODINE

Iodine is a rapid-acting antiseptic that, in the absence of organic material, kills bacteria, viruses, and spores. For example, on the skin, 1% tincture of iodine will kill 90% of the bacteria in 90 seconds, whereas a 5% solution achieves this response in 60 seconds. The local toxicity of iodine is low, with cutaneous burns occurring only with concentrations of >7%. In rare instances, an individual may be allergic to iodine and react to topical application (usually manifests as fever and generalized skin eruption). The most important use of iodine is disinfection of the skin, for which it is probably superior to any other antiseptic. For this use, it is best used in the form of a tincture of iodine because the alcohol vehicle facilitates spreading and penetration.

Iodophors

Iodophors (povidone-iodine) are loose complexes of elemental iodine with an organic carrier that not only increases the solubility of iodine but also provides a reservoir for sustained release.

Clinical Uses

The iodophors have a broad antimicrobial spectrum and are widely used as hand washes, including surgical scrubs; for preparation of the skin before surgery or needle puncture; and in the treatment of minor cuts, abrasions, and burns. A standard surgical scrub with a 10% povidone-iodine solutions (Betadine®) will decrease the usual cutaneous bacterial population by >90%, with a return to normal in about 6 to 8 hours. For the disinfection of endoscopes and other instruments, povidone-iodine is superior to 3% hexachlorophene.

Corneal Toxicity

Chemical burns to the cornea may follow exposure (accidental splashes) to a variety of disinfectant solutions (chlorhexidine, hexachlorophene, iodine, alcohol, detergents containing iodine-based solutions). Povidone iodine solution without detergent appears to be least toxic to the cornea.

HEXACHLOROPHENE

Hexachlorophene (pHisoHex®) is a polychlorinated bisphenol that exhibits bacteriostatic activity especially against Gram-positive but not Gram-negative organisms. Because most of the potentially pathogenic bacteria on the skin are Gram-positive, 3% hexachlorophene is commonly used by physicians and nurses to decrease the spread of contaminants from caregiver's hands. This antiseptic is also used to cleanse the skin of patients scheduled for certain surgical procedures. Hexachlorophene may be absorbed through intact skin in sufficient amounts to produce neurotoxic effects, including cerebral irritability. Thus, the routine use of hexachlorophene by health care providers who are pregnant may be questionable.

FORMALDEHYDE

Formaldehyde is a volatile, broad-spectrum disinfectant that kills bacteria, fungi, and viruses by precipitating proteins; it is useful to disinfect inanimate objects, such as surgical instruments.

GLUTARALDEHYDE

Glutaraldehyde is superior to formaldehyde as a disinfectant because it is rapidly effective against all microorganisms, including viruses and spores. This disinfectant also possesses tuberculocidal activity. Glutaraldehyde is less volatile than formaldehyde and hence causes minimal odor and irritant fumes. As a sterilizing solution for endoscopes, glutaraldehyde is superior to iodophors and hexachlorophene.

PASTEURIZATION

Pasteurization (hot water disinfection) is a process that destroys microorganisms (all bacteria of significance in human disease as well as many fungi and viruses) in a liquid medium through the application of heat (coagulates cell proteins). Pasteurization may be a cost-effective alternative to other disinfecting solutions such as glutaraldehyde.

CRESOL

Cresol is bactericidal against common pathogenic organisms including *Mycobacterium tuberculosis*. It is widely used for disinfecting inanimate objects (burns can result from tissue contact with materials that absorb cresol).

SILVER NITRATE

Silver nitrate is used as a caustic, antiseptic, and astringent. A solid form is used for cauterizing wounds and removing granulation tissue. Silver sulfadiazine or nitrate is used in the treatment of burns. With this use, hypochloremia may occur, reflecting the combination of silver ions with chloride. Hyponatremia also may result, because the sodium ions are attracted by chloride ions into the exudate. Furthermore, absorbed nitrate can cause methemoglobinemia.

MERCURY

Organic mercurial compounds are nonirritating but lack bactericidal activity.

ETHYLENE OXIDE

Ethylene oxide is a readily diffusible gas that is noncorrosive and antimicrobial to all organisms at room temperature. This gaseous alkylating material is widely used as an alternative to heat sterilization. Special sterilizing chambers are required, because the gas must remain in contact with the objects for several hours. Adequate airing of sterilized materials, such as tracheal tubes, is essential to ensure the removal of residual ethylene oxide and thus minimize tissue irritation (ethylene oxide sensitization is most likely in the presence of latex sensitization).

Physiology

II

39

Cell Structure and Function

The basic living unit of the body is the cell; the human body consists of 100 trillion or more cells, of which 25 trillion are red blood cells (Stoelting RK, Hillier SC. Cell structure and function. In: *Pharmacology and Physiology in Anesthetic Practice*. 4th ed. Philadelphia, Lippincott Williams & Wilkins, 2006:644–655). A common characteristic of all cells is a dependence on oxygen to combine with nutrients (carbohydrates, lipids, proteins) to release the energy necessary for cellular function.

CELL ANATOMY (FIG. 39-1)

Cytoplasm

A cell's cytoplasm consists of water, electrolytes, proteins, enzymes, lipids, and carbohydrates.

Cell Membrane

The cell membrane acts as a permeability barrier, allowing the cell to maintain a cytoplasmic composition different from that of extracellular fluid (Table 39-1). The lipid bilayer of cell membranes is nearly impermeable to water and water-soluble substances, such as ions and glucose. Several types of proteins are present in the cell membrane (see Table 39-1). In addition to structural proteins (microtubules), transport proteins (sodium-potassium adenosine triphosphatase [ATPase]) are present that function as pumps, actively transporting ions across the cell membrane.

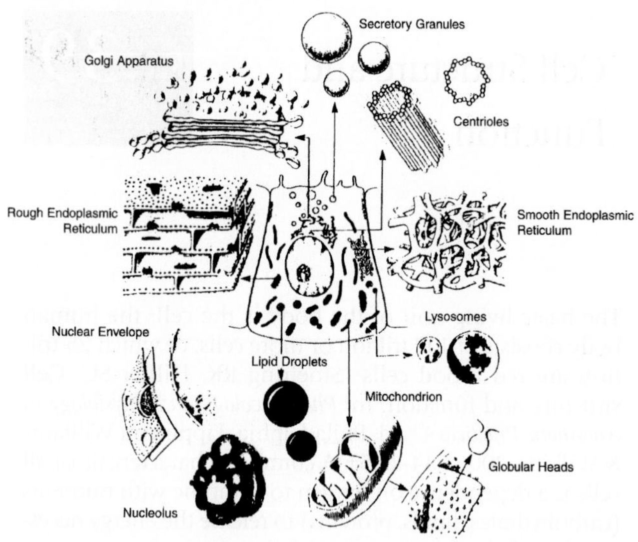

Figure 39-1. Schematic diagram of a hypothetical cell (center) and its organelles. (From Junqueira LC, Carneiro J, Kelley RO. *Basic Histology*, 7th ed. Norwalk, CT: Appleton & Lange, 1992; with permission.)

TABLE 39-1.
CELL MEMBRANE COMPOSITION

Phospholipids
- Lecithins (phosphatidylcholines)
- Sphingomyelins
- Amino phospholipids (phosphatidylethanolamine)

Proteins
- Structural proteins (microtubules)
- Transport proteins (sodium-potassium ATPase)
- Ion channels
- Receptors
- Enzymes (adenylate cyclase)

ATPase, adenosine triphosphatase.

Nucleus

The nucleus is made up of chromosomes that carry the blueprint for the heritable characteristics of the cell. Each chromosome consists of a molecule of DNA that is covered with proteins. The ultimate units of heredity are *genes* on the chromosomes, and each gene is a portion of the DNA molecule. During normal cell division by mitosis, the chromosomes duplicate themselves and then divide in such a way that each daughter cell receives a full complement (diploid number) of 46 chromosomes.

Structure and Function of DNA and RNA

Deoxyribonucleic acid (DNA) consists of two nucleotide chains containing adenine, guanine, thymine, and cytosine. The genetic message is determined by the sequence of these amino acids in the nucleotide chains. DNA determines the type of ribonucleic acid (RNA) that is formed; RNA is responsible for transferring the genetic message to the site of protein synthesis in cytoplasm (ribosomes). Cell reproduction (mitosis) is determined by the DNA-genetic system. If an insufficient number of some types of cells are present in the body, these cells will grow and reproduce rapidly until appropriate numbers are again present (liver, bone marrow, gastrointestinal epithelium). Highly differentiated cells, such as nerve and muscle cells, are not capable of reproduction to replace lost cells.

Regulation of Gene Expression

Genes may be activated by steroids and by proteins manufactured by other genes in the cell. *Oncogenes* are genes that, when activated, produce uncontrolled cell reproduction (tumors).

Organelles

Organelles are structures in the cytoplasm that have specific roles in cellular function.

Mitochondria

Mitochondria are the power-generating units of cells (oxidative phosphorylation and the synthesis of adenosine triphosphate [ATP] are localized to mitochondria).

Endoplasmic Reticulum

The endoplasmic reticulum is a complex series of tubules in the cytoplasm. The portion of the membrane containing these ribosomes is known as the *rough endoplasmic reticulum*. The part of the membrane that lacks ribosomes is the *smooth endoplasmic reticulum.*

Lysosomes

Lysosomes are scattered throughout the cytoplasm, providing an intracellular digestive system.

Golgi Apparatus

The Golgi apparatus is a collection of membrane-enclosed sacs that are responsible for storing proteins to serve specific functions.

Nucleus

The nucleus contains granules rich in RNA; it is the site of ribosomal synthesis. The specific type of RNA formed and, thus, the protein synthesized is determined by DNA, which functions as a gene.

Centrioles

Centrioles are present in the cytoplasm near the nucleus and are concerned with the movement of chromosomes during cell division.

TRANSFER OF MOLECULES ACROSS CELL MEMBRANES

The uptake of particulate matter (bacteria, damaged cells) by cells is called *phagocytosis*, whereas the uptake of materials in solution in the extracellular fluid is *pinocytosis*. The process of phagocytosis is initiated when antibodies attach to damaged tissue and foreign substances (opsonization); this results in the acquisition of a positive charge. Typically, objects that have a negative charge are repelled by cell membranes and thus are not vulnerable to phagocytosis.

TRANSFER OF MOLECULES THROUGH CELL MEMBRANES

Some molecules (oxygen, carbon dioxide, nitrogen) move through cell membranes by diffusion among the molecules that make up the membrane, whereas the passage of other molecules (glucose, amino acids) requires the presence of specific transport proteins in cell membranes.

Diffusion

Diffusion is the process whereby molecules intermingle because of their random thermal motion. Because of the slowness of diffusion over macroscopic distances, organisms have developed circulatory systems to deliver nutrients within the reasonable diffusion ranges of cells (Table 39-2).

TABLE 39-2.
PREDICTED RELATIONSHIP BETWEEN DIFFUSION DISTANCE AND TIME

Diffusion Distance (mm)	Time Required for Diffusion
0.001	0.5 ms
0.01	50 ms
0.1	5 s
1	498 s
10	14 hrs.

Lipid Bilayer

The lipid bilayer of cell membranes is the principal barrier to substances that permeate membranes by simple diffusion. Highly lipid-soluble oxygen and carbon dioxide diffuse readily.

Protein Channels

Ion channels constitute a class of proteins that is ultimately responsible for generating and orchestrating the electrical signals passing through the brain, heart, and skeletal muscles (Fig. 39-2). These ion channels are macromolecular protein tunnels that span the lipid bilayer of the cell membrane. Approximately 30% of the energy expended by cells is used to maintain the gradient of sodium and potassium ions across cell membranes. Some channels are highly specific with respect to ions allowed to pass (sodium, potassium), whereas other channels allow all ions below a certain size to pass (Table 39-3).

Aquaporins

Aquaporins are highly specific protein channels that facilitate the passage of water across cell membranes at a velocity that exceeds simple diffusion. In the absence of aquaporins, the diffusion of water may not be sufficiently rapid for many physiologic processes. Aquaporins may be contributory to numerous disorders involving fluid transport including cerebral edema, cirrhosis of the liver, congestive heart failure, and glaucoma.

Protein-Mediated Transport

Protein-mediated transport is responsible for the movement of certain substances into or out of cells by way of specific carriers or channels that are intrinsic proteins of cell membranes.

Facilitated Diffusion

Poorly lipid-soluble substances, such as glucose and amino acids, may pass through lipid bilayers by facilitated diffusion.

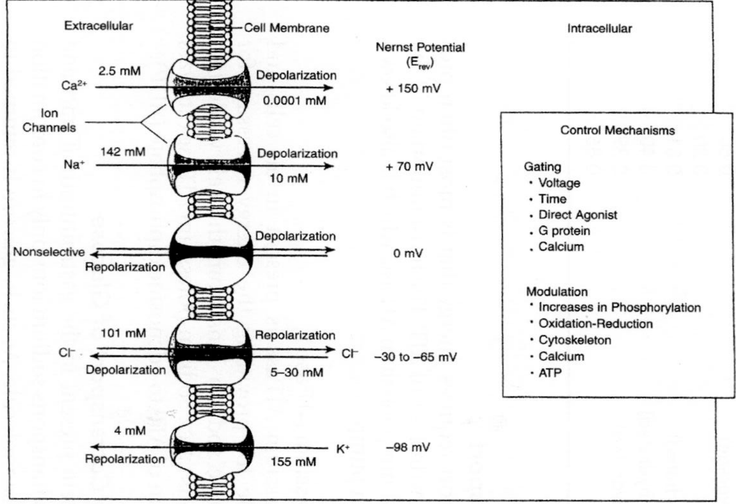

Figure 39-2. The five major types of protein ion channels are calcium, sodium, nonselective, chloride, and potassium. Flow of ions through these channels (calcium and sodium into cells and potassium outward) determines the transmembrane potential of cells. (From Ackerman MJ, Clapham DE. Ion channels—basic science and clinical disease. *N Engl J Med* 1997;336: 1575–1586; with permission.)

TABLE 39-3.
DIAMETERS OF IONS, MOLECULES, AND CHANNELS

	Diameter (nm)*
Channel (average)	0.80
Water	0.30
Sodium (hydrated)	0.51
Potassium (hydrated)	0.40
Chloride (hydrated)	0.39
Glucose	0.86

*1 nm = 10 Å.

Active Transport

Active transport requires energy that is most often provided by the hydrolysis of ATP. The most important of the ATPases is sodium-potassium ATPase, which is also known as the sodium pump.

Sodium-Potassium ATPase

Sodium-potassium ATPase is present in all cells and is responsible for providing the energy necessary for extruding three sodium ions from the cell while two potassium ions enter. Sodium-potassium ATPase catalyzes the conversion of ATP to adenosine diphosphate (ADP).

Sodium Ion Cotransport of Glucose

A carrier system present in the gastrointestinal tract and renal tubules transports sodium ions only in combination with a glucose molecule. As such, glucose is returned to the circulation, thus preventing its excretion.

Sodium Ion Cotransport of Amino Acids

Epithelial cells lining the gastrointestinal tract and renal tubules are able to reabsorb amino acids into the circulation through the sodium ion cotransport process, thus preventing their excretion.

Calcium ATPase

Calcium ATPase is present in cell membranes to maintain the large gradient between calcium ion concentrations in the cytoplasm and extracellular fluid. The activity of calcium ATPase is highly regulated by *calmodulin*, an intracellular regulatory protein that increases the affinity of this enzyme for calcium ions at the inner surface of cell membranes.

ELECTRICAL POTENTIALS ACROSS CELL MEMBRANES

The electrical potentials across cell membranes reflect the difference in transmembrane concentrations of sodium and potassium ions that is maintained by the enzyme sodium-potassium ATPase. This results in the establishment of a voltage difference across cell membranes, known as the *resting membrane potential*. The cytoplasm is usually electrically negative (about −70 mV) relative to the extracellular fluid (Fig. 39-3).

Action Potentials

The action potential is the rapid change in transmembrane potential, followed by a return to the resting membrane potential. Propagation of the action potential along the entire length of a nerve axon or muscle cell is the basis of the signal-carrying ability of nerve cells and allows muscle cells to contract simultaneously. The size and shape of the action potential varies among excitable tissues (see Fig. 39-3). An action potential is triggered when successive conductance increases to sodium and potassium ions cause a threshold potential (about −50 mV) to be reached. *Acetylcholine*, as an endogenous neurotransmitter, is the most important chemical substance that is capable of enlarging sodium ion channels and increasing the permeability of cell membranes to sodium. The initial, sudden, inward rush of sodium ions leads to a

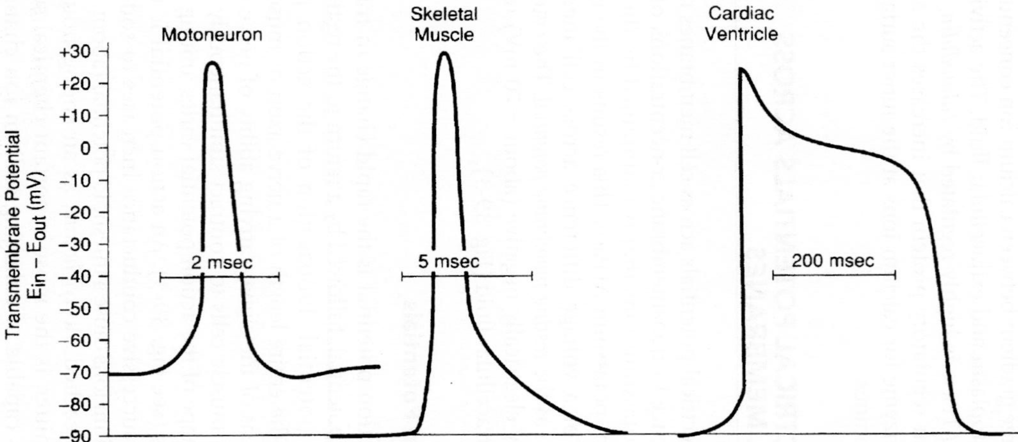

Figure 39-3. The transmembrane potential and duration of the action potential varies with the tissue site. (From Berne RM, Levy MN, Koeppen B, et al. *Physiology*, 5th ed. St. Louis: Mosby, 2004; with permission.)

positive charge inside the cell, corresponding to the phase of the action potential known as *depolarization*. Subsequent increased permeability of the cell membrane to potassium allows the loss of this positive ion, tending to return the electrical charge inside the cell toward the resting membrane potential (repolarization).

Properties of Ion Channels

Ion channels may be voltage-gated (regulated by membrane potentials) or chemically gated (regulated by binding of a neurotransmitter).

Measurement of Current

Current flowing through individual ion channels can be measured by patch-clamping electrophysiology.

Properties of Action Potentials

During much of the action potential, the cell membrane is completely refractory to further stimulation (absolute refractory period). During the last portion of the action potential, a stronger than normal stimulus can evoke a second action potential (relative refractory period). Low potassium ion concentrations in extracellular fluid increase the negativity of the resting membrane potential, resulting in hyperpolarization and decreased cell membrane excitability. Skeletal muscle weakness that accompanies hypokalemia presumably reflects the hyperpolarization of skeletal muscle membranes. Local anesthetics decrease the permeability of nerve cell membranes to sodium ions, thus preventing the achievement of a threshold potential that is necessary for the generation of an action potential. The blockage of cardiac sodium ion channels by local anesthetics may result in an altered conduction of cardiac impulses and decreases in myocardial contractility.

Conduction of Action Potentials

Action potentials are conducted along nerve or muscle fibers by local current flow that produces depolarization of adjacent areas of the cell membrane. The entire action potential usually occurs in <1 ms. Conduction velocity is greatly increased by myelination, which decreases capacitance of the axon and permits an action potential to be generated only at the nodes of Ranvier. Myelinated nerves are more efficient metabolically than nonmyelinated axons because ion exchange is restricted to the nodes of Ranvier and less ion pumping is thus required to maintain sodium and potassium ion gradients.

INTRACELLULAR COMMUNICATION

Cells communicate (transfer biologic information) with their environments in different ways that include stimulation or inhibition of cytoplasmic receptors, transmembrane receptors, and enzyme systems (Fig. 39-4). Most clinically useful drugs and endogenously secreted hormones mediate their effects via one of three types of excitable transmembrane proteins (Table 39-4). Transmembrane receptors located in lipid cell membranes interact with endogenous chemical messengers (hormones, neurotransmitters) or exogenous compounds (drugs), resulting in the initiation of a cascade of biochemical changes that lead to cellular responses (physiologic effects) (see Fig. 39-4). Chemical messengers (first messengers, ligands) generally exert their effects by increasing the concentrations of second messengers (cyclic adenosine monophosphate [cAMP], calcium ions) in target cells (Tables 39-5 and 39-6). Steroids and thyroid hormones are examples of chemical messengers that produce their effects by altering RNA in the cell's cytoplasm.

Receptors

Receptors can be classified by their cellular localization. Most signaling molecules are hydrophobic and interact with cell surface receptors that are directly or indirectly coupled to effector molecules. Three known classes of

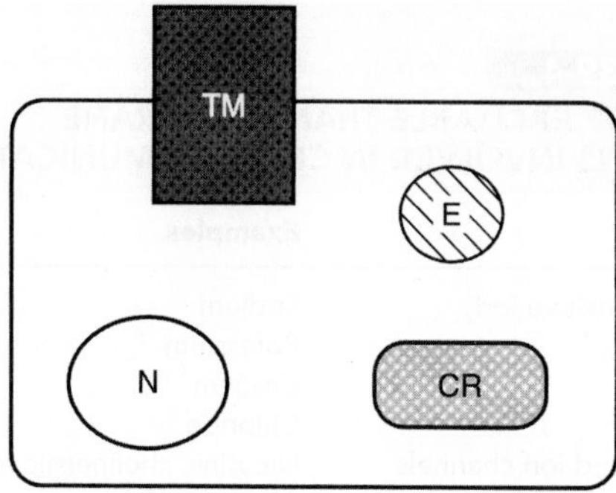

Figure 39-4. Cell communication that manifests as cellular (physiologic), and ultimately as clinical responses, occurs via cytoplasmic receptors (CR), stimulation or inhibition of enzyme systems (E), and excitable transmembrane (TM) proteins. The location of each system is illustrated schematically in relation to the cell nucleus (N) and cell membrane. Examples of CRs may be steroid receptors, whereas E may be represented by phosphodiesterase inhibitors. Most clinically useful drugs and endogenously secreted hormones mediate their effects via excitable TM proteins. (From Schwinn DA. Adrenoceptors as models for G protein–coupled receptors: structure, function, and regulation. *Br J Anaesth* 1993;71:77–85; with permission.)

cell surface receptors exist, as defined by their signal transduction mechanisms: G protein–coupled receptors, ligand-gated ion channels, and receptor-linked enzymes. Most hormones and neurotransmitters are water soluble signaling molecules that interact with G protein–coupled cell-surface receptors to translate information encoded in neurotransmitters and hormones into cellular responses (Fig. 39-5). Ligand-gated ion channels (inotropic receptors) are involved principally with fast synaptic transmission between excitable cells in which the binding of signaling molecules to receptors causes an immediate conformational change in receptor-ion channels. Specific neurotransmitters bind to these receptors and transiently open or close the associated ion channel to alter the ion permeability of plasma membranes and

TABLE 39-4.
TYPES OF EXCITABLE TRANSMEMBRANE PROTEINS INVOLVED IN CELL COMMUNICATION

	Examples
Voltage-sensitive ion channels	Sodium Potassium Calcium Chloride
Ligand-gated ion channels	Nicotinic cholinergic receptors Amino acid receptors γ-Aminobutyric acid N-methyl-D-aspartate
Transmembrane receptors (signal transduction)	Adrenoceptors (α, β) Muscarinic cholinergic Opioid Serotonin Dopamine

TABLE 39-5.
LIGANDS THAT ACT BY ALTERING INTRACELLULAR CYCLIC ADENOSINE MONOPHOSPHATE (cAMP) CONCENTRATIONS

Increase cAMP
- Adrenocorticotropic hormone
- Catecholamines (β1 and β2 receptors)
- Glucagon
- Parathyroid hormone
- Thyroid-stimulating hormone
- Follicle-stimulating hormone
- Vasopressin

Decrease cAMP
- Catecholamines (α2 receptors)
- Dopamine (dopamine2 receptors)
- Somatostatin

TABLE 39-6.
LIGANDS THAT INCREASE INTRACELLULAR CALCIUM ION CONCENTRATION

Catecholamines (α1 receptors)
Acetylcholine (muscarinic receptors)
Serotonin
Substance P
Vasopressin (V1 receptors)
Oxytocin

thereby membrane potentials. An example of an ion channel whose conductance is regulated by receptor activation is the γ-aminobutyric acid (GABA) receptor, in which chloride ion conductance through the associated ion channel is the effector mechanism (see Fig. 39-5).

Receptor Concentration

Receptors in cell membranes are not static components of cells. Excess circulating concentrations of ligand (norepinephrine due to a pheochromocytoma) result in a decrease in the density of β-adrenergic receptors in cell membranes (down-regulation). Drug-induced antagonism of β-adrenergic receptors results in an increased density of receptors in cell membranes (up-regulation) and the possibility of exaggerated sympathetic nervous system activity if the β-adrenergic antagonist drug is abruptly discontinued, as in the preoperative period. Desensitization of receptor responsiveness is the waning of a physiologic response over time, despite the presence of a constant stimulus (Fig. 39-6).

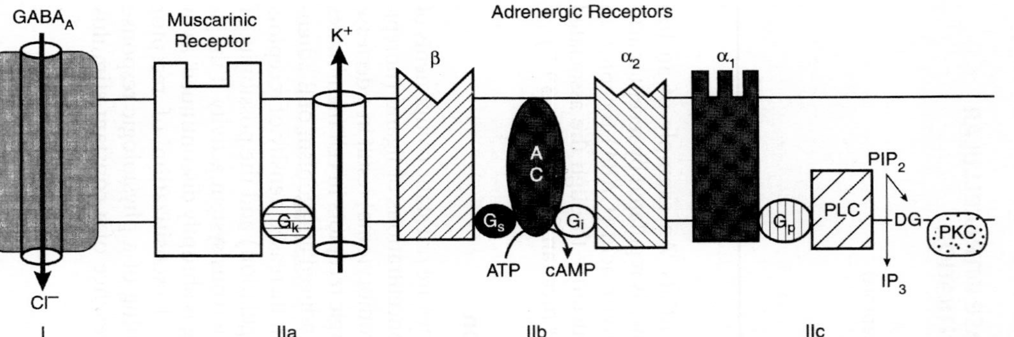

Figure 39-5. Schematic depiction of receptors on cell surfaces. Stimulation of the γ-aminobutyric acid (GABA) receptor by an agonist results in flow of chloride ions into the cell along the protein ion channel (I). Stimulation of the muscarinic receptor by an agonist (acetylcholine) causes the coupling guanine (G) protein (Gk) to facilitate conductance of potassium ions to the exterior of the cell (IIa). Adenylate cyclase (AC) activity can be enhanced via a stimulatory G protein (Gs) on activation of a β-adrenergic receptor by an agonist ligand, whereas the enzyme's activity can be attenuated via an inhibitory G protein (Gi) that is coupled with an α2-adrenergic receptor, thus controlling the conversion of adenosine triphosphate (ATP) to cyclic adenosine monophosphate (cAMP) (IIb). On stimulation of the α1-adrenergic receptor by an agonist ligand, the coupling G protein (Gp) activates phospholipase C (PLP) to hydrolyze phosphatidylinositol biphosphate (PIP2) into inositol triphosphate (IP3) and diacylglycerol (DG), which then activates protein kinase C (PKC) (IIc). (From Maze M. Transmembrane signaling and the Holy Grail of anesthesia. *Anesthesiology* 1990;72:959–961; with permission.)

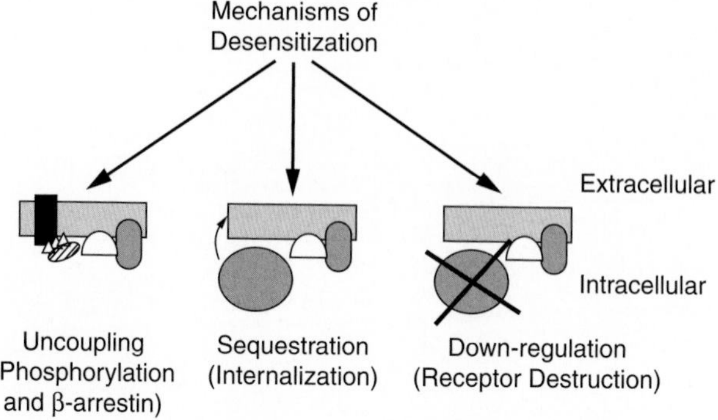

Figure 39-6. Three basic mechanisms for desensitization of receptors are uncoupling (preventing receptor interaction with G proteins), sequestration (mobilization of the receptor to intracellular vesicles over minutes to hours and recycling it back to the cell membrane surface once agonist stimulation terminates), and down-regulation (destruction of sequestered receptors over a period of hours to days). (From Schwinn DA. Adrenoceptors as models for G protein–coupled receptors: Structure, function, and regulation. *Br J Anaesth* 1993;71:77–85; with permission.)

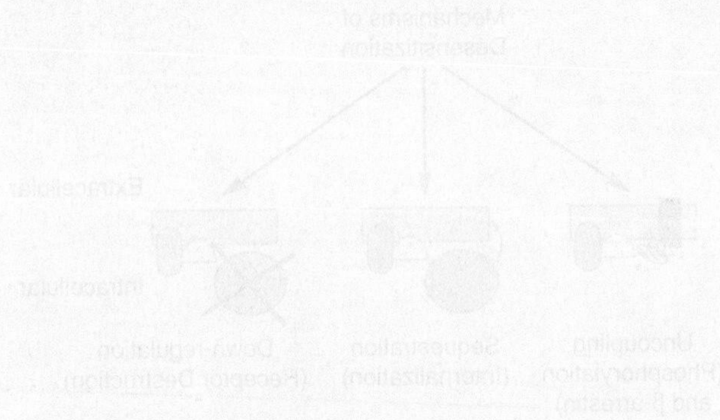

Body Fluids

40

Total body fluids can be divided into intracellular and extracellular fluid, depending on its location relative to the cell membrane (Fig. 40-1) (Stoelting RK, Hillier SC. Body fluids. In: *Pharmacology and Physiology in Anesthetic Practice*. 4th ed. Philadelphia, Lippincott Williams & Wilkins, 2006:656–660). Approximately 28 liters of the total body fluid (about 42 liters) present in an adult are contained inside the estimated 75 trillion cells of the body. The fluid in these cells, despite individual differences in constituents, is collectively designated *intracellular fluid*. The 14 liters of fluid outside the cells is referred to as *extracellular fluid*. Extracellular fluid is divided into *interstitial fluid* and *plasma* (intravascular fluid) by the capillary membrane (see Fig. 40-1). Excess amounts of fluid in the interstitial space manifest as peripheral edema. The total amount of water in a man weighing 70 kg is about 42 liters, accounting for nearly 60% of total body weight (see Fig. 40-1). Total body water is less in women and in obese individuals, reflecting the decreased water content of adipose tissue (Table 40-1). The normal daily intake of water (drink and internal product of food metabolism) by an adult averages 2.5 liters, of which about 1.5 liters is excreted as urine, 100 mL is lost in sweat, and 100 mL is present in feces. All gases that are inhaled become saturated with water vapor (47 mm Hg at 37°C). This water vapor is subsequently exhaled, accounting for an average daily water loss through the lungs of 300 to 400 mL (less in warm temperatures).

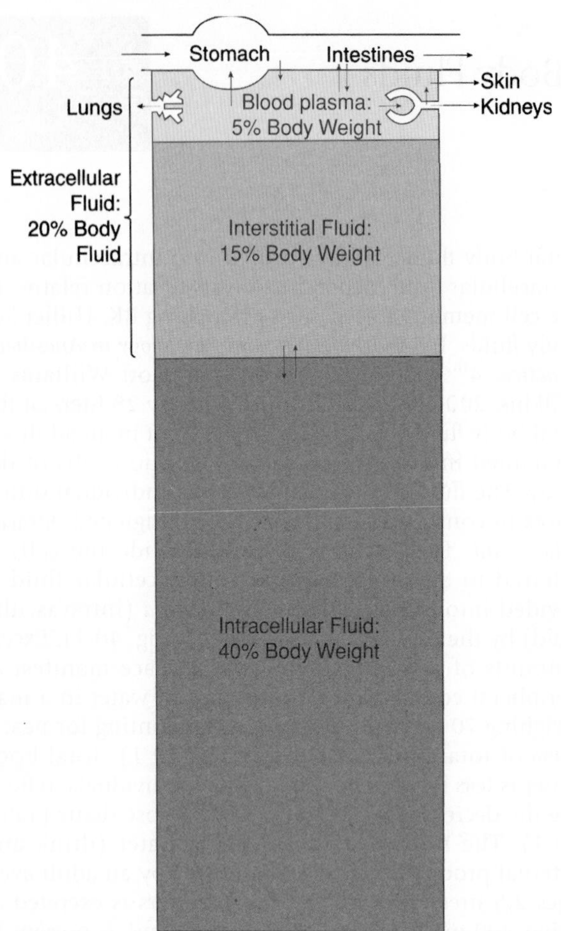

Figure 40-1. Body fluid compartments and the percentage of body weight represented by each compartment. The location relative to the capillary membrane divides extracellular fluid into plasma or interstitial fluid. Arrows represent fluid movement between compartments. (From Gamble JL. *Chemical Anatomy, Physiology, and Pathology of Extracellular Fluid*, 6th ed. Boston: Harvard University Press, 1954; with permission.)

TABLE 40-1.
TOTAL BODY WATER BY AGE AND GENDER

	Total Body Water	
Age (yrs.)	**Men (%)**	**Women (%)**
18–40	61	51
40–60	55	47
>60	52	46

BLOOD VOLUME

The main priority of the body is to maintain intravascular fluid volume. The average blood volume of an adult is 5 liters (70 mL/kg), of which about 3 liters is plasma and 2 liters is erythrocytes. The greater the ratio of fat to body weight, however, the less is the blood volume in milliliters per kilogram because adipose tissue has a decreased vascular supply.

Hematocrit

The true hematocrit is about 96% of the measured value, because 3% to 8% of plasma remains entrapped among the erythrocytes even after centrifugation. The measured hematocrit is about 40% for men and 36% for women.

MEASUREMENT OF COMPARTMENTAL FLUID VOLUMES

The volume of a fluid compartment can be measured by the indicator dilution principle, whereas interstitial fluid volume is calculated as extracellular fluid volume minus plasma volume.

Blood Volume

Substances used for measuring blood volume must be capable of dispersing throughout the blood with ease and then must remain in the circulation for a sufficient time for measurements to be completed. Using the dilution principle, the total blood volume is calculated.

CONSTITUENTS OF BODY FLUID COMPARTMENTS

The constituents of body fluid compartments are identical, but the quantity of each substance varies among the compartments (Fig. 40-2). The unequal distribution of ions results in the establishment of a potential (voltage) difference across cell membranes. Trauma is associated with progressive loss of potassium through the kidneys. For example, a patient undergoing surgery excretes about 100 mEq of potassium in the first 48 hours postoperatively and, after this period, about 25 mEq daily. Plasma potassium concentrations are not good indicators of total body potassium content because most potassium is intracellular.

OSMOSIS

Osmosis is the movement of water (solvent molecules) across a semipermeable membrane from a compartment in which the nondiffusible solute (ion) concentration is lower, to a compartment in which the solute concentration is higher (Fig. 40-3).

Osmotic Pressure

Osmotic pressure is the pressure on one side of the semipermeable membrane that is just sufficient to keep water from moving to a region of higher solute concentration (see Fig. 40-3).

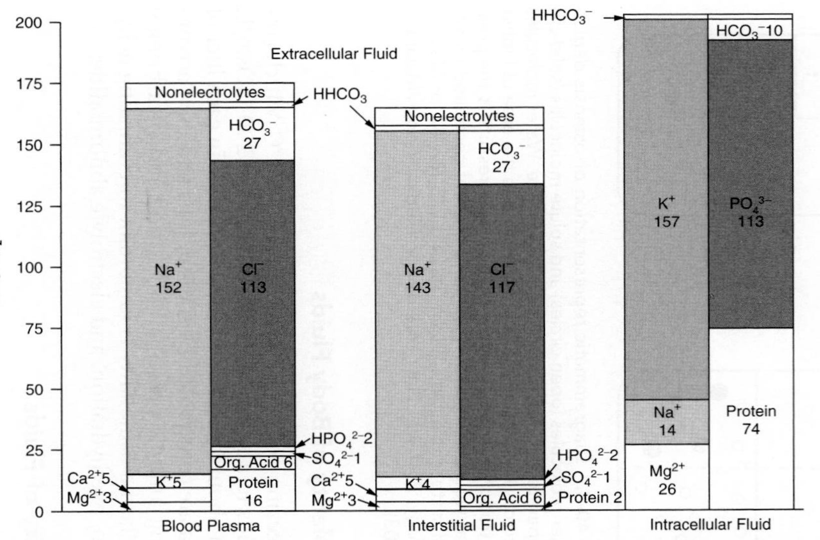

Figure 40-2. Electrolyte composition of body fluid compartments. (From Leaf A, Newburgh LH. *Significance of the Body Fluids in Clinical Medicine*, 2nd ed. Springfield, IL: Thomas, 1955; with permission.)

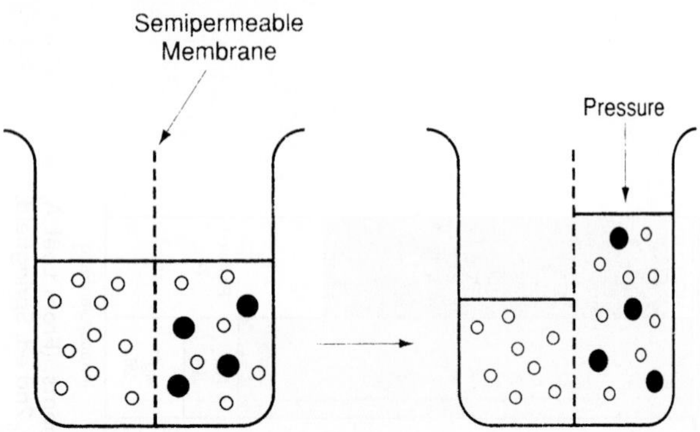

Figure 40-3. Diagrammatic representation of osmosis depicting water molecules (open circles) and solute molecules (solid circles) separated by a semipermeable membrane. Water molecules move across the semipermeable membrane to the area of higher concentration of solute molecules. Osmotic pressure is the pressure that would have to be applied to prevent continued movement of water molecules. (From Ganong WF. *Review of Medical Physiology*, 21st ed. New York: Lange Medical Books/McGraw-Hill, 2003).

Osmolarity of Body Fluids

The freezing point of plasma averages 0.54°C, which corresponds to a plasma osmolarity of about 290 mOsm/L. All but about 20 mOsm of the 290 mOsm in each liter of plasma are contributed by sodium ions and their accompanying anions, principally chloride and bicarbonate ions. Plasma osmolarity is important in evaluating dehydration, overhydration, and electrolyte abnormalities.

Tonicity of Fluids

Solutions that have the same osmolarity as plasma are said to be *isotonic* (no transfer of fluid into or out of cells occurs), those with higher osmolarity are *hypertonic* (cells shrink), and those with a lower osmolarity are *hypotonic* (cells swell). A solution of 5% glucose in water is initially isotonic when infused, but glucose is metabolized, so the net effect is that of infusing a hypotonic solution.

CHANGES IN VOLUMES OF BODY FLUID COMPARTMENTS

Intravenous Fluids

The goal of fluid management is to maintain normovolemia characterized by hemodynamic stability. Crystalloids consist of water, electrolytes, and occasionally glucose that freely distribute along a concentration gradient between the two extracellular spaces. After 20 to 30 minutes, an estimated 75% to 80% of an isotonic saline or a lactate-containing solution will have distributed outside the confines of the circulation thus limiting the efficacy of these solutions in treating hypovolemia. Intravenous fluids that do not remain in the circulation can dilute extracellular fluid, causing it to become hypotonic with respect to intracellular fluid. Within a few minutes, this water becomes distributed almost evenly among all body fluid compartments. Increased intracellular fluid volume is particularly undesirable in patients with intracranial masses or increased intracranial pressure.

Hypertonic Saline Solutions

Hypertonic saline solutions (7.5% sodium chloride) are useful for rapid intravascular fluid repletion during resuscitation, as occurs during hemorrhagic and septic shock.

Dehydration

The loss of water by gastrointestinal or renal routes or by diaphoresis is associated with an initial deficit in extracellular fluid volume. Clinical signs of dehydration are likely when about 5% to 10% (severe dehydration) of total body fluids have been lost within a brief period. Physiologic mechanisms can usually compensate for acute loss of 15% to 25% of the intravascular fluid volume, whereas a greater loss places the patient at risk for hemodynamic decompensation.

Central Nervous System

41

The activity of the central nervous system (CNS) reflects a balance between excitatory and inhibitory influences that are normally maintained within relatively narrow limits (Stoelting RK, Hillier SC. Central nervous system. In: *Pharmacology and Physiology in Anesthetic Practice*. 4th ed. Philadelphia, Lippincott Williams & Wilkins, 2006: 661–685). The three components of the CNS are the cerebral hemispheres (cerebral cortex, limbic system, thalamus, hypothalamus), brainstem (nuclei of cranial nerves, reticular activating system, cerebellum), and spinal cord (medulla oblongata to lower lumbar vertebrae).

CEREBRAL HEMISPHERES

For each area of the cerebral cortex, a corresponding and connecting area to the thalamus exists, so that stimulation of a small portion of the thalamus activates the corresponding and much larger portion of the cerebral cortex. The functional part of the cerebral cortex is comprised mainly of a 2- to 5-mm layer of neurons covering the surface of all the convolutions (estimated that the cerebral cortex contains 50 to 100 billion neurons).

Cerebral Cortex (Fig. 41-1)

Topographic Areas

Somesthetic Cortex

The area of the cerebral cortex to which the peripheral sensory signals are projected from the thalamus is desig-

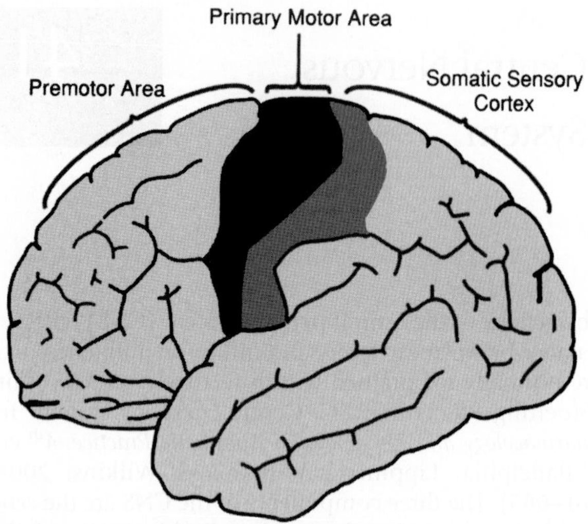

Figure 41-1. The sensorimotor cortex consists of the motor cortex, pyramidal (Betz) cells, and somatic sensory cortex. (From Guyton AC, Hall JE. *Textbook of Medical Physiology*, 10th ed. Philadelphia. Saunders, 2000; with permission.)

nated the *somesthetic cortex* (see Fig. 41-1). In the motor cortex, various topographic areas are present, from which skeletal muscles in different parts of the body can be activated.

Motor Cortex

In general, the size of the area in the motor cortex is proportional to the preciseness of the skeletal muscle movement required (digits, lips, tongue, and vocal cords have large representations in humans). The motor cortex is commonly damaged by loss of blood supply, as occurs during a stroke.

Corpus Callosum

The two hemispheres of the cerebral cortex, with the exception of the anterior portions of the temporal lobes, are connected by fibers in the corpus callosum.

Dominant versus Nondominant Hemisphere

Language

Language function and interpretation depend more on one cerebral hemisphere (dominant hemisphere) than the other, whereas spatiotemporal relationships (ability to recognize faces) depend on the other (nondominant) hemisphere.

Dominance

Based on genetic determinations, 90% of individuals are right-handed and the left hemisphere is dominant. Likewise, the left hemisphere is dominant in about 70% of persons who are left-handed.

Memory

The cerebral cortex, especially the temporal lobes, serves as a storage site for information that is often characterized as memory.

Short-Term Memory

Short-term memory may involve the presence of reverberating circuits. Evidence in favor of a reverberating theory of short-term memory is the ability of a general disturbance of brain function (fright, loud noise) to erase short-term memory immediately. An alternative explanation for short-term memory is the phenomenon of post-tetanic potentiation.

Long-Term Memory

Long-term memory does not depend on the continued activity of the nervous system, as evidenced by a total inactivation of the brain by hypothermia or anesthesia without detectable significant loss of long-term memory.

It is assumed that long-term memory results from physical or chemical alterations in the size and conductivities of the dendrites.

Maximum consolidation requires at least 1 hour, as typified by a lightly anesthetized patient who reacts purposefully to a painful stimulus but later has no recall if the depth of anesthesia is increased after the purposeful movement.

A sensory stimulus allowed to persist for 5 to 10 minutes may result in at least partial establishment of a memory trace. If the sensory stimulus is unopposed for 60 minutes, it is likely that the memory will have become fully consolidated. Rehearsal of the same information accelerates and potentiates the process of consolidation, thus converting short-term memory to long-term memory.

Awareness during Anesthesia

Awareness during anesthesia (defined as a conscious memory of events during general anesthesia) is estimated to be 0.13%. A higher incidence has been described for major trauma cases (11% to 43%). Most cases of conscious awareness during surgery can be attributed to physician error and/or equipment malfunction.

Subanesthetic Doses

Subanesthetic doses of inhaled anesthetics (0.45 to 0.6 MAC isoflurane) have powerful inhibitory effects on short-term memory, and the decrease in the transfer of information from the periphery to the cerebral cortex associated with general anesthesia prevents the recall of intraoperative events.

Recognizing Awareness

Monitoring patients during general anesthesia for the recognition of awareness is challenging: The physiologic indicators (heart rate, blood pressure) and skeletal muscle movement are often masked by anesthetic and adjuvant drugs (β-adrenergic blockers) and/or neuromuscular blocking drugs.

Methods to recognize awareness that are less affected by drugs include brain wave monitors, such as the Bispectral Index (BIS). Based on published studies, the Food and Drug Administration (FDA) has determined that the use of BIS monitoring to guide anesthetic administration may be associated with a reduction of the incidence of awareness with recall in adults during general anesthesia and sedation.

Pyramidal and Extrapyramidal Tracts

A major pathway for the transmission of motor signals from the cerebral cortex to the anterior motor neurons of the spinal cord is through the pyramidal (corticospinal) tracts (Fig. 41-2).

Function

The pyramidal tracts cause continuous facilitation and therefore a tendency to produce increases in skeletal muscle tone, whereas the extrapyramidal tracts transmit inhibitory signals through the basal ganglia with a resultant inhibition of skeletal muscle tone. Selective or predominant damage to one of these tracts manifests as spasticity or flaccidity.

Babinski Sign

A positive Babinski sign reflects damage to the pyramidal tracts and is characterized by upward extension of the first toe and outward fanning of the other toes in response to a firm tactile stimulus applied to the dorsum of the foot.

Thalamocortical System

The thalamocortical system serves as the pathway for the passage of nearly all afferent impulses from the cerebellum; basal ganglia; and visual, auditory, taste, and pain receptors as they pass through the thalamus on the way to

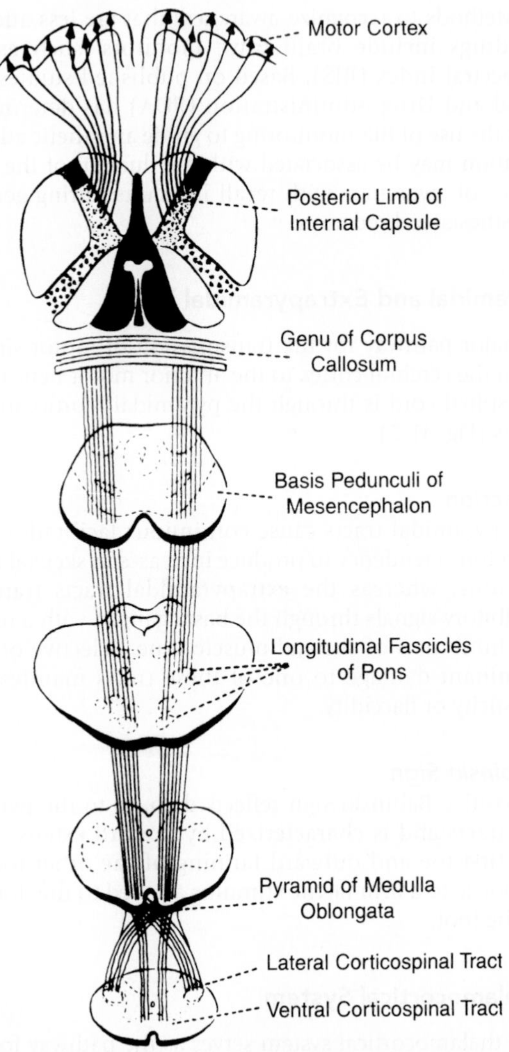

Figure 41-2. The pyramidal tracts are major pathways for transmission of motor signals from the cerebral cortex to the spinal cord. (From Guyton AC, Hall JE. *Textbook of Medical Physiology*, 10th ed. Philadelphia. Saunders, 2000; with permission.)

the cerebral cortex; this controls the activity level of the cerebral cortex.

BRAINSTEM

The subconscious activities of the body (intrinsic life processes including breathing, blood pressure) are controlled in the brainstem. The thalamus serves as a relay station for most afferent impulses before they are transmitted to the cerebral cortex.

Limbic System and Hypothalamus

Behavior associated with emotions is primarily a function of structures known as the limbic system (hippocampus, basal ganglia). The hypothalamus functions in many of the same roles as the limbic system and also controls many internal conditions of the body (core temperature, thirst, appetite).

Basal Ganglia

The basal ganglia (caudate nucleus, putamen, globus pallidus, substantia nigra, subthalamus) often provide impulses that are inhibitory (inhibitory neurotransmitters are dopamine and γ-aminobutyric acid [GABA]). Whenever destruction of the basal ganglia occurs, associated skeletal muscle rigidity occurs (chorea, Parkinson's disease).

Reticular Activating System

The reticular activating system is a polysynaptic pathway that is intimately concerned with the electrical activity of the cerebral cortex. It is likely that many of the clinically used injected and inhaled anesthetics exert depressant effects on the reticular activating system.

Sleep and Wakefulness

Sleep is a state of unconsciousness from which an individual can be aroused by sensory stimulation. The depression of the reticular activating system by anesthetics or as present in comatose individuals cannot be defined as sleep.

Slow-Wave Sleep

Most of the sleep that occurs each night is slow-wave sleep. The electroencephalogram (EEG) is characterized by the presence of high-voltage delta waves occurring at a frequency of <4 cycles/s. During slow-wave sleep, sympathetic nervous system activity decreases, parasympathetic nervous system activity increases, and skeletal muscle tone is greatly decreased. A 10% to 30% decrease occurs in systemic blood pressure, heart rate, breathing frequency, and basal metabolic rate during physiologic sleep.

Desynchronized Sleep

Desynchronized sleep (rapid eye movement sleep) is characterized by active dreaming, irregular heart rate and breathing, and a desynchronized pattern of low-voltage β-waves on the EEG, similar to those that occur during wakefulness (active cerebral cortex or rapid eye movement sleep).

Cerebellum

The cerebellum operates subconsciously to monitor and elicit corrective responses in motor activity caused by stimulation of other parts of the brain and spinal cord. The cerebellum is also important in the maintenance of equilibrium and postural adjustments of the body.

Dysfunction of the Cerebellum

In the absence of cerebellar function, a person cannot predict prospectively how far movements will go; this results in overshoot of the intended mark (past pointing). This overshoot is known as *dysmetria,* and the resulting incoordinate movements are called *ataxia.*

Dysarthria is present when rapid and orderly succession of skeletal muscle movements of the larynx, mouth, and chest do not occur.

SPINAL CORD

The spinal cord extends from the medulla oblongata to the lower border of the first and, occasionally, the second lumbar vertebra. Below the spinal cord, the vertebral canal is filled by the roots of the lumbar and sacral nerves, which are collectively known as the *cauda equina*.

Gray Matter of the Spinal Cord

The gray matter of the spinal cord is divided into anterior, lateral, and dorsal horns consisting of nine separate laminae that are H-shaped when viewed in cross-section (Fig. 41-3).

Cells of the intermediate neurons located in the portion of the dorsal horns of the spinal cord known as the substantia gelatinosa (laminae II to III) transmit afferent tactile, temperature, and pain impulses to the spinothalamic tract. The dorsal horn serves as a gate where impulses in sensory nerve fibers are translated into impulses in ascending tracts.

White Matter of the Spinal Cord

The white matter of the spinal cord is divided into dorsal, lateral, and ventral columns (see Fig. 41-3). The dorsal column of the spinal cord is composed of spinothalamic tracts that transmit touch and pain impulses to the brain.

Imaging the Nervous System

Magnetic Resonance Imaging

Comparative studies indicate that magnetic resonance imaging (MRI) is superior to computed tomography (CT) in evaluating most cerebral parenchymal lesions. Nevertheless, CT is preferable for patients with acute trauma who are accompanied by cumbersome life-support

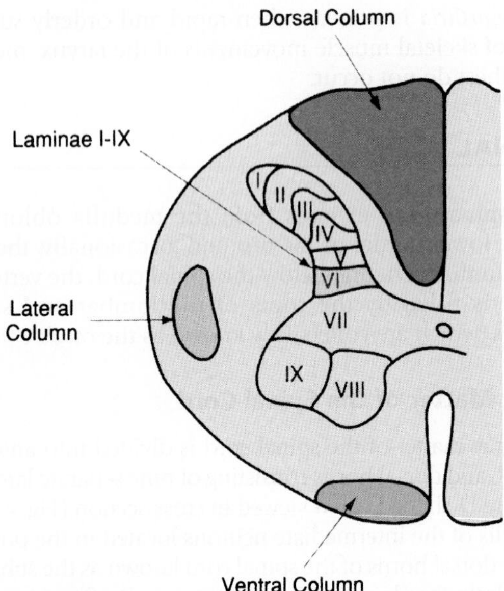

Figure 41-3. Schematic diagram of a cross-section of the spinal cord depicting anatomic laminae I to IX of the spinal cord gray matter and the ascending dorsal, lateral, and ventral sensory columns of the spinal cord white matter.

equipment or patients who cannot voluntarily remain immobile (uncooperative, movement disorders, children), as is required for MRI.

Computed Tomography

Computed tomography (CT) is the imaging procedure of choice after injuries to the head or spine because of its rapidity. CT is useful in visualizing intracranial blood that may be present in patients with subdural hematomas or cerebral hemorrhage.

Spinal Nerve

A pair of spinal nerves arises from each of 31 segments of the spinal cord. Each spinal nerve innervates a segmental area of skin designated a *dermatome* and an area of skeletal muscle known as a *myotome* (Fig. 41-4).

Covering Membranes

The spinal cord is enveloped by membranes (dura, arachnoid, pia) that are direct continuations of the corresponding membranes surrounding the brain. Drugs such as local anesthetics or opioids cannot travel cephalad in the epidural space beyond the foramen magnum.

The inner layer of the dura extends as a dural cuff that blends with the perineurium of spinal nerves. The cerebral arachnoid extends as the spinal arachnoid, ending at the second sacral vertebra. The pia is in close contact with the spinal cord.

CT demonstrates the occasional presence of a connective tissue band (dorsomedian connective tissue band or plica mediana dorsalis) that divides the epidural space at the dorsal midline; this band makes it difficult to feel loss of resistance during attempted midline identification of the epidural space. The band may also explain the occasional occurrence of unilateral analgesia after injection of local anesthetic solutions into the epidural space.

PATHWAYS FOR PERIPHERAL SENSORY IMPULSES

Sensory information from somatic segments of the body enter the gray matter of the spinal cord via the dorsal nerve roots. After entering the spinal cord, these neurons give rise to long, ascending fiber tracts that transmit sensory information to the brain (Figs. 41-5 and 41-6).

Impulses in the dorsal column pathways cross in the spinal cord to the opposite side before passing upward to the thalamus.

Synapses in the thalamus are followed by neurons that extend into the somatic sensory area of the cerebral cortex. All sensory information that enters the cerebral cortex, with the exception of the olfactory system, passes through the thalamus.

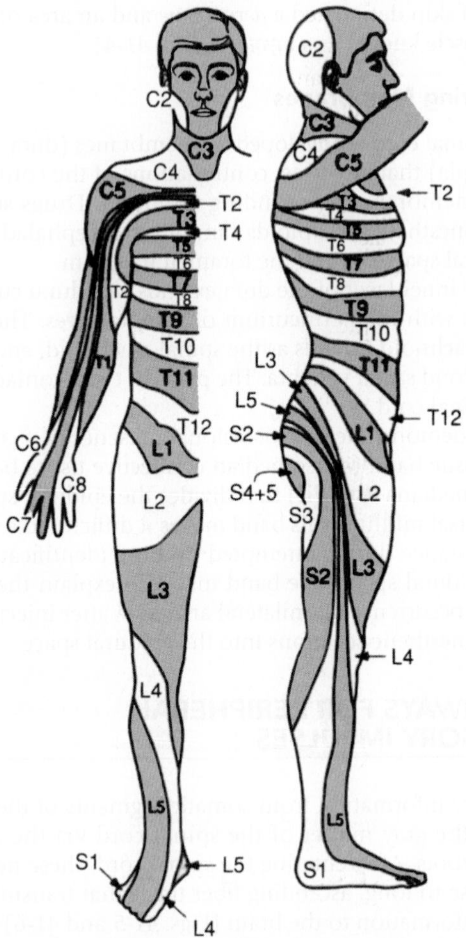

Figure 41-4. Dermatome map that may be used to evaluate the level of sensory anesthesia produced by regional anesthesia. (From Guyton AC, Hall JE. *Textbook of Medical Physiology*, 10th ed. Philadelphia. Saunders, 2000; with permission.)

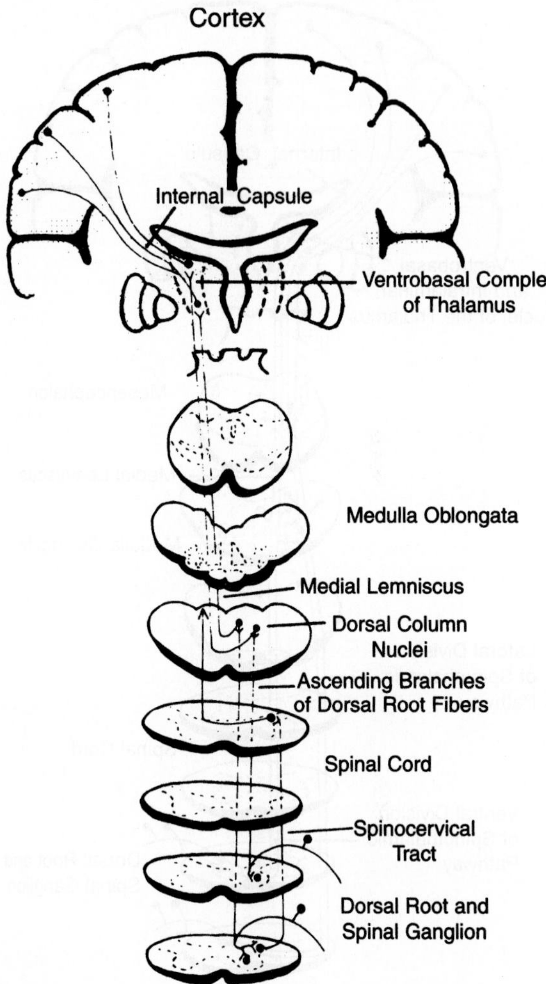

Figure 41-5. Sensory signals are transmitted to the brain by the dorsal column pathways and spinocervical tracts of the dorsal-lemniscal system. (From Guyton AC, Hall JE. *Textbook of Medical Physiology*, 10th ed. Philadelphia. Saunders, 2000; with permission.)

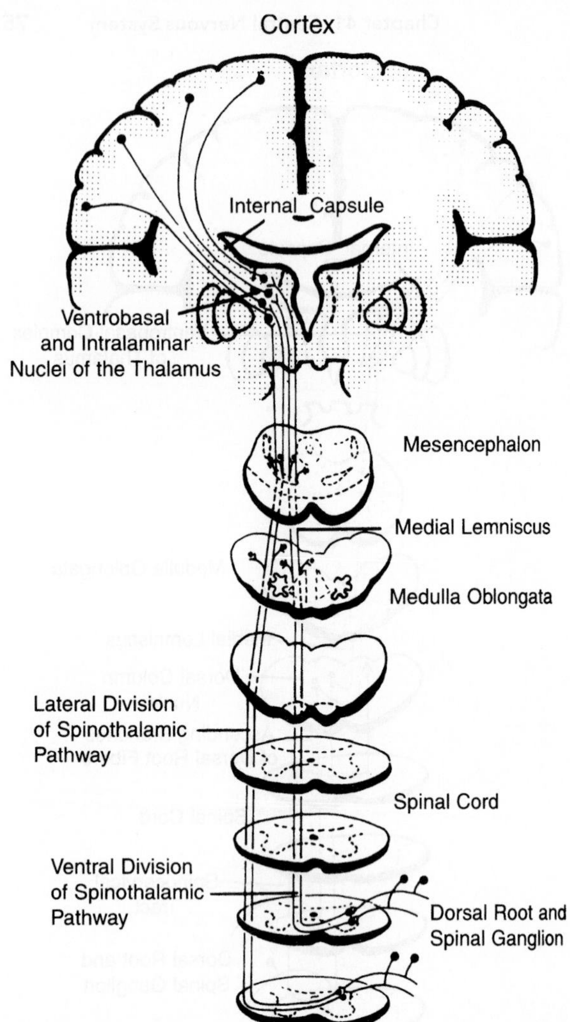

Figure 41-6. The anterolateral spinothalamic system fibers cross in the anterior commissure of the spinal cord before ascending to the brain. The fibers of this system transmit signals via ventral and lateral spinothalamic tracts. (From Guyton AC, Hall JE. *Textbook of Medical Physiology*, 10th ed. Philadelphia. Saunders, 2000; with permission.)

PATHWAYS FOR PERIPHERAL MOTOR RESPONSES

Sensory information is integrated at all levels of the nervous system and causes appropriate motor responses. Anterior motor neurons in the anterior horns of the spinal cord gray matter give rise to A-α fibers, which leave the spinal cord by way of anterior nerve roots and innervate skeletal muscles.

Upper and Lower Motor Neurons

The motor system is often divided into upper and lower motor neurons.

Lower motor neurons are those from the spinal cord that directly innervate skeletal muscles. A lower motor neuron lesion is associated with flaccid paralysis, atrophy of skeletal muscles, and absence of stretch reflex responses.

Spastic paralysis with accentuated stretch reflexes in the absence of skeletal muscle paralysis is due to destruction of upper motor neurons in the brain.

Autonomic Reflexes

Segmental autonomic reflexes occur in the spinal cord and include changes in vascular tone, diaphoresis, and evacuation reflexes from the bladder and colon.

The simultaneous excitation of all the segmental reflexes is the mass reflex (denervation hypersensitivity or autonomic hyperreflexia). The mass reflex typically occurs in the presence of spinal cord transection when a painful stimulus occurs to the skin below the level of the spinal cord transection or distention of a hollow viscus is present, such as in the bladder or gastrointestinal tract (analogous to seizures that involve the CNS).

The principal manifestation of the mass reflex is systemic hypertension due to intense peripheral vasoconstriction, reflecting an inability of vasodilating inhibitory impulses from the CNS to pass beyond the site of spinal cord transection.

Spinal Shock

Spinal shock is a manifestation of the abrupt loss of spinal cord reflexes that immediately follows transection of the spinal cord. It manifests as hypotension due to loss of vasoconstrictor tone and absence of all skeletal muscle reflexes.

ANATOMY OF NERVE FIBERS

Nerve fibers are *afferent* if they transmit impulses from peripheral receptors to the spinal cord and *efferent* if they relay signals from the spinal cord and CNS to the periphery.

Neurons

Neurons consists of a cell body or soma, dendrites, and a nerve fiber or axon (Fig. 41-7). The transmission of impulses between responsive neurons at a synapse is mediated by the presynaptic release of a chemical mediator (neurotransmitter), such as norepinephrine or acetylcholine.

Classification of Afferent Nerve Fibers (Table 41-1)

Myelin

Myelin that surrounds type A and B nerve fibers acts as an insulator that prevents flow of ions across nerve membranes. The myelin sheath is interrupted approximately every millimeter by the nodes of Ranvier. Successive excitation of nodes of Ranvier by an impulse that jumps between successive nodes is termed *saltatory excitation*. Saltatory conduction greatly increases the velocity of nerve transmission in myelinated fibers.

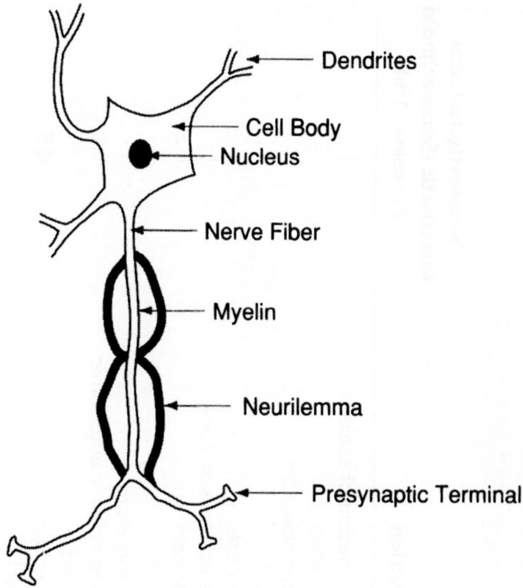

Figure 41-7. Anatomy of a neuron.

Evaluation of Peripheral Nerve Function

Peripheral nerves may be injured by ischemia of the intraneural vasa nervorum that accompanies stretch of the nerve or external compression of the nerve.

Nerve Conduction Studies

Nerve conduction studies are useful in the localization and assessment of peripheral nerve dysfunction. Focal demyelination of nerve fibers causes a slowing of conduction and decreased amplitudes of compound muscle and sensory action potentials.

Electromyography

Electromyographic studies are an adjunct to nerve conduction studies. The presence of denervation potentials

TABLE 41-1.
CLASSIFICATION OF PERIPHERAL NERVE FIBERS

	Myelinated	Fiber Diameter (mm)	Conduction Velocity (m/s)	Function	Sensitivity to Local Anesthetic (Subarachnoid Procaine, 1%)
A-α	Yes	12–20	70–120	Innervation of skeletal muscles Proprioception	1
A-β	Yes	5–12	30–70	Touch Pressure	1
A-γ	Yes	3–6	15–30	Skeletal muscle tone	1
A-δ	Yes	2–5	12–30	Fast pain Touch Temperature	0.5
B	Yes	3	3–15	Preganglionic autonomic fibers	0.25
C	No	0.4–1.2	0.5–2.0	Slow pain Touch Temperature Postganglionic sympathetic fibers	0.5

in a skeletal muscle indicates axon or anterior horn cell loss. Signs of denervation on the electromyogram after acute nerve injury require 18 to 21 days to develop.

NEUROTRANSMITTERS

Neurotransmitters are chemical mediators that are released into the synaptic cleft in response to the arrival of an action potential at the nerve ending. The release of all neurotransmitters is voltage dependent and requires the influx of calcium ions into the presynaptic terminals.

Neurotransmitters may be excitatory or inhibitory, depending on the configurational change produced in the protein receptor by its interaction with the neurotransmitter.

Types of Neurotransmitters (Table 41-2)

ELECTRICAL EVENTS DURING NEURONAL EXCITATION

Resting Transmembrane Potentials

The resting transmembrane potentials of neurons in the CNS are about −70 mV, which is less than the −90 mV in large peripheral nerve fibers and skeletal muscles.

Inhibitory Synapses

At the inhibitory synapses, a neurotransmitter increases the permeability of postsynaptic receptors to potassium and chloride ions. Receptors responding to inhibitory neurotransmitters are associated with protein channels that are too small to allow the passage of larger hydrated sodium ions.

The predominant outward diffusion of potassium ions increases the negativity of the resting transmembrane potential, and the neuron is hyperpolarized (functions as an inhibitory neuron).

TABLE 41-2.
TYPES OF NEUROTRANSMITTERS

Glutamate (major excitatory amino acid neurotransmitter in the CNS; glutamate receptors [includes N-methyl-D-aspartate receptors] are ligand-gated ion channels.)
γ-Aminobutyric acid (major inhibitory neurotransmitter in the CNS; when two molecules of GABA bind to the receptor, the chloride ion channel opens and allows chloride ions to flow into the neuron causing it to become hyperpolarized.)
Acetylcholine (excitatory neurotransmitter that interacts with muscarinic and nicotinic receptors in the CNS; contrasts with the inhibitory effects [increased potassium permeability] on the peripheral parasympathetic nervous system.)
Dopamine (high concentrations are present, especially in the basal ganglia; most likely it is an inhibitory neurotransmitter.)
Norepinephrine (neurons responding to norepinephrine send predominantly inhibitory impulses.)
Epinephrine
Glycine (principal inhibitory neurotransmitter in the spinal cord.)
Substance P (excitatory neurotransmitter presumed to be released by terminals of pain fibers that synapse in the substantia gelatinosa of the spinal cord.)
Endorphins (excitatory neurotransmitters for descending pathways that inhibit the transmission of pain.)
Serotonin (inhibitory neurotransmitter exerting profound effects on mood and behavior.)
Histamine

Permeability

The permeability changes evoked by excitatory neurotransmitters decrease the negativity of the resting transmembrane potential, bringing it nearer threshold potential. As a result, these neurons function in the excitatory mode.

Synaptic Delay

The synaptic delay is the 0.3 to 0.5 s necessary for the transmission of an impulse from the synaptic varicosity to the postsynaptic neuron.

Synaptic Fatigue

Synaptic fatigue is a decrease in the number of discharges by the postsynaptic membrane when excitatory synapses are repetitively and rapidly stimulated (stores of neurotransmitters are exhausted).

Posttetanic Facilitation

Posttetanic facilitation is an increased responsiveness of the postsynaptic neuron to stimulation after a rest period that was preceded by repetitive stimulation of an excitatory synapse.

Factors Influencing Neuron Responsiveness

Neurons are highly sensitive to changes in the pH of the surrounding interstitial fluids (alkalosis enhances and acidosis depresses neuron excitability). Inhaled anesthetics may increase cell membrane threshold for excitation and thus decrease neuron activity throughout the body.

CEREBRAL BLOOD FLOW (TABLE 41-3)

ELECTROENCEPHALOGRAM

Clinical Uses

The EEG is useful in diagnosing different types of epilepsy and for determining the seizure-causing focus in the brain (Table 41-4). Monitoring of the EEG during carotid endarterectomy, cardiopulmonary bypass, or controlled hypotension may provide an early warning of inadequate cerebral blood flow.

Brain Wave Monitors

Bispectral Index

The bispectral index (BIS) is a variable derived from the EEG that is a quantifiable measure of the sedative

TABLE 41-3.
CARBON DIOXIDE AND CEREBRAL PHYSIOLOGY

Cerebral Blood Flow (CBF)
- Changes 1–2 mL/100 g/min for each 1 mm Hg change in $Paco_2$ between 20 and 80 mm Hg
- Slope of the response depends on normocapnic CBF
- CBF returns to baseline over several hours during sustained alterations in $Paco_2$ (reflects correction of brain extracellular fluid pH)
- Response to hypocapnia not altered by aging if CBF is maintained
- Response to changes in $Paco_2$ not altered by untreated hypertension
- Hypothermia decreases normocapnic CBF and the response of CBF to changes in $Paco_2$

Cerebral Blood Volume (CBV)
- Changes 0.05 mL/100g for each 1 mm Hg change in $Paco_2$
- Returns to baseline during sustained alterations in $Paco_2$

Cerebral Autoregulation
- Modest hypercapnia impairs and marked hypercapnia abolishes
- Hypotension below the lower limit of autoregulation abolishes hypocapnic cerebral vasoconstriction

Carbon Dioxide Response and Anesthetics
- Maintained during inhaled and intravenous anesthetics
- Relative response to hypocapnia depends on normocapnic CBF (anesthetics that increase CBF enhance the reduction of CBF by hypocapnia)

Carbon Dioxide Response in Presence of Disease or Injury
- Hypercapnic response intact with hypertension
- Hypocapnic response present with brain injury (subarachnoid hemorrhage) but may be attenuated if vasospasm is present
- During temporary focal cerebral ischemia neither hypercapnia or hypocapnia improve outcome (may worsen outcome)
- Acute hyperventilation in the presence of increased intracranial pressure (ICP) may reduce ICP and improve CBF (effect on outcome is uncertain)
- Intraoperative hyperventilation useful for controlling the effects of inhaled anesthetics on ICP
- Prudent to avoid unnecessary hyperventilation

(Adapted from Brian JE. Carbon dioxide and the cerebral circulation. *Anesthesiology* 1998;88:1365–1386.)

TABLE 41-4.
CLASSIFICATION OF BRAIN WAVES ON THE ELECTROENCEPHALOGRAM

*α-Waves (typical of an awake state and disappear during sleep)
β-Waves (increased mental activity, visual stimulation)
θ-Waves (sleep, general anesthesia)
δ-Waves (sleep, general anesthesia)

and hypnotic effects of anesthetic drugs on the CNS (expressed as a dimensionless numerical index from 0 to 100). Decreasing numerical values correlate with sedation and predict the response of patients to surgical stimulation (values of <60 are associated with a low probability of recall and a high probability of unresponsiveness during surgery). BIS monitoring may serve as a useful intraoperative monitor for guiding drug administration.

Spectral Entropy

Spectral entropy represents an alternative concept to bispectral analysis for quantifying the EEG.

Epilepsy

Epilepsy is characterized by excessive activity of either a part or all of the CNS. Generalized tonic-clonic (grand mal) epilepsy is characterized by intense neuronal discharges in multiple areas of the cerebral and reticular activating system.

Status Epilepticus

Status epilepticus is present when tonic-clonic seizure activity is sustained. Diazepam, administered intravenously, is an often recommended treatment to stop seizures and permit the resumption of effective breathing.

EVOKED POTENTIALS

Evoked potentials are the electrophysiologic responses of the nervous system to sensory, motor, auditory, or visual stimulation. The amplitude and latency of evoked potentials may be influenced by a number of events, especially volatile anesthetics. Evoked potentials are used to monitor (a) spinal cord function during operations near or on the spinal cord, and (b) auditory nerve and brainstem function, as during operations on pituitary tumors or other lesions that impinge on the optic nerves or optic chiasm.

Somatosensory Evoked Potentials

Somatosensory evoked potentials are produced by the application of a low-voltage electrical current that stimulates a peripheral nerve, such as the median nerve at the wrist or the posterior tibial nerve at the ankle. The resulting evoked potentials reflect the intactness of sensory neural pathways from the peripheral nerve to the somatosensory cortex.

Inhaled anesthetics, especially volatile anesthetics, produce a dose-dependent depression of somatosensory evoked potentials.

Although less so than volatile anesthetics, morphine and fentanyl also produce depressant effects on somatosensory evoked potentials, with a low-dose continuous infusion of the opioid producing less depression than intermittent injections.

Motor Evoked Potentials

Motor evoked potentials reflect the intactness of motor neural pathways from the peripheral nerve to the motor cerebral cortex. Motor evoked potentials are extremely sensitive to depression by anesthetics, and it is not possible to monitor motor evoked potentials in the presence of significant drug-induced neuromuscular blockade.

During scoliosis surgery or other operations that place spinal cord motor function at risk, the use of motor evoked potentials obviates the need for an intraoperative wake-up test.

Auditory Evoked Potentials

Auditory evoked potentials arise from brainstem auditory pathways. Volatile anesthetics produce a dose-dependent depression of auditory evoked potentials.

Visual Evoked Potentials

Visual evoked potentials are produced by flashes from light-emitting diodes that are mounted on goggles placed over the patient's closed eyes. Volatile anesthetics produce a dose-dependent depression of visual evoked potentials.

CEREBROSPINAL FLUID

Cerebrospinal fluid (CSF) is present in the (a) ventricles of the brain, (b) cisterns around the brain, and (c) subarachnoid space around the brain and spinal cord. A major function of CSF is to cushion the brain in the cranial cavity.

Formation

The major sites of CSF formation are the choroid plexuses in the four cerebral ventricles (cauliflower-like growths of blood vessels covered by a thin layer of epithelial cells).

The pH of CSF is closely regulated and maintained at 7.32. Changes in $PaCO_2$, but not arterial pH, promptly alter CSF pH, reflecting the ability of carbon dioxide, but not hydrogen ions, to cross the blood-brain barrier easily. As a result, acute respiratory acidosis or alkalosis produces corresponding changes in CSF pH. The active transport of bicarbonate ions eventually returns the CSF pH to 7.32, despite the persistence of alterations in arterial pH.

Reabsorption

Almost all the CSF formed each day is reabsorbed into the venous circulation through special structures known as arachnoid villi or granulations.

Circulation (Fig. 41-8)

Hydrocephalus

Obstruction to the free circulation of CSF in the neonate results in hydrocephalus.

Intracranial Pressure

Normal intracranial pressure (ICP) is <15 mm Hg. Phasic variations in systemic blood pressure are transmitted as variations in ICP.

Papilledema

Anatomically, the dura of the brain extends as a sheath around the optic nerve and then connects with the sclera

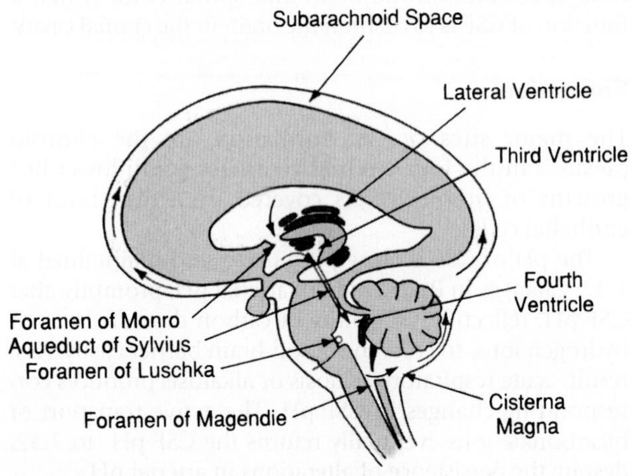

Figure 41-8. Circulation of cerebrospinal fluid.

of the eye. When ICP increases, it is also reflected in the optic nerve sheath. Swelling of the optic disc is termed papilledema.

Blood-Brain Barrier

The blood-brain barrier reflects the impermeability of capillaries in the CNS, including the choroid plexuses, to circulating substances such as electrolytes and exogenous drugs or toxins. As a result, the internal consistency of the environment to which brain neurons are exposed is maintained over a narrow limit.

An anatomic explanation for the blood-brain barrier is the tight junction between the endothelial cells of brain capillaries and the envelopment of brain capillaries by glial cells, which further decreases their permeability.

The blood-brain barrier is less developed in the neonate and tends to break down in those areas of the brain that are irradiated or infected or are the site of tumors.

VISION (FIG. 41-9)

Intraocular Fluid

Intraocular fluid lies in front and at the sides of the lens, and vitreous humor lies between the lens and retina.

Intraocular Pressure

Intraocular pressure is normally 15 to 25 mm Hg. Glaucoma is associated with increased intraocular pressure sufficient to compress retinal artery inflow to the eye, leading to ischemic pain and eventually blindness.

Retina

The retina is the light-sensitive portion of the eye containing the cones, which are responsible for color vision, and the rods, which are mainly responsible for vision in the dark. The nutrient blood supply for the retina is largely derived from the central retinal artery, which accompanies

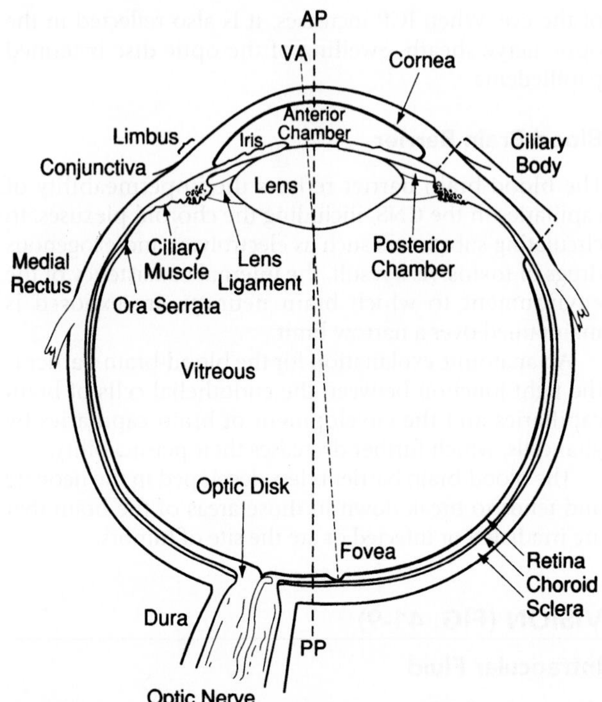

Figure 41-9. Schematic diagram of the eye. (AP, anterior pole; PP, posterior pole; VA, visual axis.) (From Ganong WF. *Review of Medical Physiology*, 21st ed. New York. Lange Medical Books/ McGraw-Hill, 2003; with permission).

the optic nerve. This independent retinal blood supply prevents rapid degeneration of the retina, should it become detached from the pigment epithelium, and allows time for surgical correction of a detached retina.

Ischemic Optic Neuropathy

Ischemic optic neuropathy (ION) results from infarction of the optic nerve and is the most frequently reported cause of vision loss following general anesthesia. ION is classified as anterior ION (nonarteritic or arteritic) and posterior ION.

Posterior Ischemic Optic Neuropathy

Posterior ION has been reported after diverse surgical procedures (prolonged spinal fusion surgery, cardiac operations requiring cardiopulmonary bypass, radical neck surgery). The etiology of posterior ION appears to be multifactorial, including intraoperative anemia and hypotension combined with at least one other factor (congenital absence of the central retinal artery, increased venous pressure owing to venous obstruction; large amounts of fluid administration; prolonged head-down position; administration of vasopressors). Prone positioning increases IOP during anesthesia and could contribute to decreases in ocular perfusion pressure (Fig. 41-10).

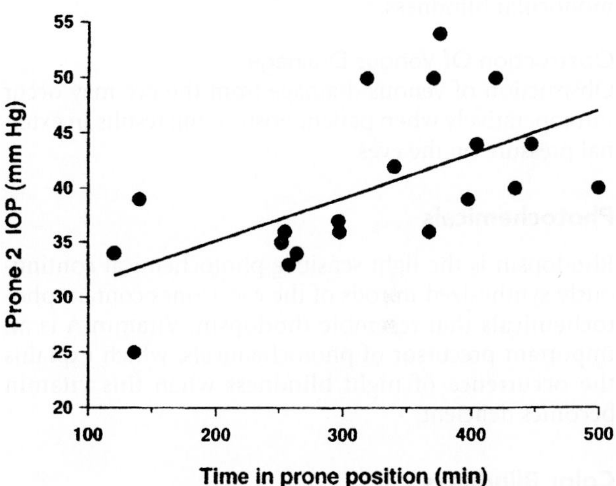

Figure 41-10. Intraocular pressure (IOP) at the conclusion of prone positioning (prone 2) is correlated with the total time spent in the prone position (minutes). (From Cheng MA, Todorov A, Tempelhoff R, et al. The effect of prone positioning on intraocular pressure in anesthetized patients. *Anesthesiology* 2001;95: 1351–1355; with permission.)

Etiology

Despite the multifactorial etiology of ION, some cases do not have any of the speculated associated factors (anemia, hypotension).

Other Causes of Postoperative Blindness

Cortical blindness, retinal occlusion, and ophthalmic venous obstruction must be excluded when postoperative blindness occurs and ION is a consideration.

Cortical Blindness

Cortical blindness is characterized by a loss of visual sensation with the retention of papillary reaction to light and normal funduscopic examination results.

Central Retinal Artery Occlusion

Central retinal artery occlusion presents as painless, monocular blindness.

Obstruction Of Venous Drainage

Obstruction of venous drainage from the eye may occur intraoperatively when patient positioning results in external pressure on the eyes.

Photochemicals

Rhodopsin is the light-sensitive photochemical continuously synthesized in rods of the eye. Cones contain photochemicals that resemble rhodopsin. Vitamin A is an important precursor of photochemicals, which explains the occurrence of night blindness when this vitamin becomes deficient.

Color Blindness

Red–green color blindness is present when red or green types of cones are absent (a sex-linked recessive trait that will not appear as long as one X chromosome carries the genes necessary for the development of color-receptor cones). About 2% of males are color blind.

Visual Pathway (Fig. 41-11)

Field of Vision

Anterior pituitary tumors may compress the optic chiasm, causing blindness in both temporal fields of vision.

Muscular Control of Eye Movements

The cerebral control system that directs the eyes toward the object to be viewed is as important as the cerebral system that interprets the visual signals. Movements of the eyes are controlled by three pairs of skeletal muscles designated as the (a) medial and lateral recti, (b) superior and inferior recti, and (c) superior and inferior obliques.

Innervation of the Eye

The eyes are innervated by the sympathetic and parasympathetic nervous system. The stimulation of the parasympathetic nervous system fibers to the eye excites the ciliary sphincter, causing miosis. Conversely, stimulation of sympathetic nervous system fibers to the eye excites the radial fibers of the iris and causes mydriasis.

Horner's Syndrome

An interruption of the superior cervical chain of the sympathetic nervous system innervation to the eye (stellate ganglion block) results in miosis, ptosis, and vasodilation with absence of sweating on the ipsilateral side of the body (Horner's syndrome).

HEARING

Ossicle System

The middle ear is an air-filled cavity containing the ossicle system that includes the malleus, incus, and stapes. The

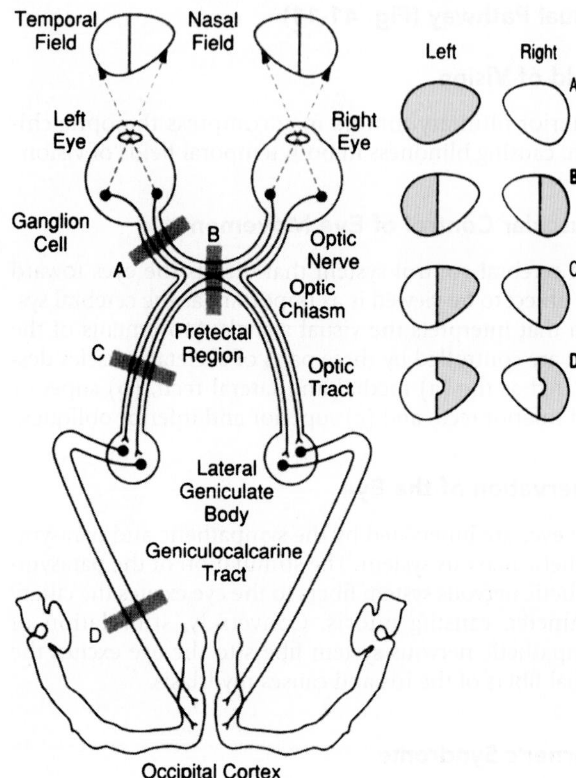

Figure 41-11. Visual impulses from the retina pass to the optic chiasm, where fibers from the nasal halves of the retina cross to the opposite side to join temporal fibers and form the optic tract. These fibers synapse in the lateral geniculate body before passing to the visual (occipital) area of the cerebral cortex. Visual field defects reflect lesions at various sites (A–D) in the nerve pathways. (From Ganong WF. *Review of Medical Physiology*, 21st ed. New York. Lange Medical Books/McGraw-Hill, 2003; with permission.)

eustachian tube allows pressures on both sides of the tympanic membrane to be equalized during chewing or swallowing (nitrous oxide may increase middle ear pressure).

Cochlea

The cochlea is a system of coiled tubes embedded in a bony cavity in the temporal bone.

Deafness

Nerve Deafness

Nerve deafness is due to an abnormality of the cochlear or auditory nerve.

Conduction Deafness

Conduction deafness is present when an abnormality exists in the middle ear mechanisms for transmitting sounds into the cochlea.

Perioperative Hearing Impairment

Perioperative hearing impairment is often subclinical and may go unnoticed unless audiometry is performed. The incidence of hearing loss after dural puncture may be as high as 50%. Unilateral hearing loss following cardiopulmonary bypass is often permanent and probably due to embolism.

EQUILIBRIUM

Utricle and Saccule

The utricle and saccule contain cilia that transmit nerve impulses to the brain necessary for maintaining orientation of the head in space.

Semicircular Canals

Separate testing of the semicircular canals is accomplished by placing ice water in the external auditory canal (selective cooling of the endolymph causes nystagmus in the presence of normally functioning semicircular canals).

CHEMICAL SENSES

Taste

Taste is mainly a function of the *taste buds*, located principally in the papillae of the tongue. Sweet, sour (acids), salty, and bitter (alkaloids) are the four primary sensations of taste. Most of what is considered taste is actually smell, thus explaining the loss of "taste" with an upper respiratory tract infection.

Smell

Olfactory hairs, or *cilia*, are believed to sense odors in the air, causing the stimulation of olfactory cells. The importance of upward air movement in smell acuity is the reason sniffing improves the sense of smell, whereas holding one's breath prevents the sensation of unpleasant odors. Olfactory receptors adapt rapidly, so that smell sensation may become extinct in about 60 seconds.

NAUSEA AND VOMITING (FIG. 41-12)

Medulla

The medullary vomiting center is located close to the fourth cerebral ventricle and receives afferents from the (a) chemoreceptor trigger zone, (b) cerebral cortex, (c) labyrinthovestibular center, and (d) neurovegetative system. Impulses from these afferents lead to nausea and vomiting.

The chemoreceptor trigger zone includes receptors for serotonin, dopamine, histamine, and opioids. Stimulation of the chemoreceptor trigger zone located on the floor of the fourth cerebral ventricle initiates vomiting independent of the vomiting center. The chemoreceptor trigger zone is not protected by the blood-brain barrier; thus, this zone

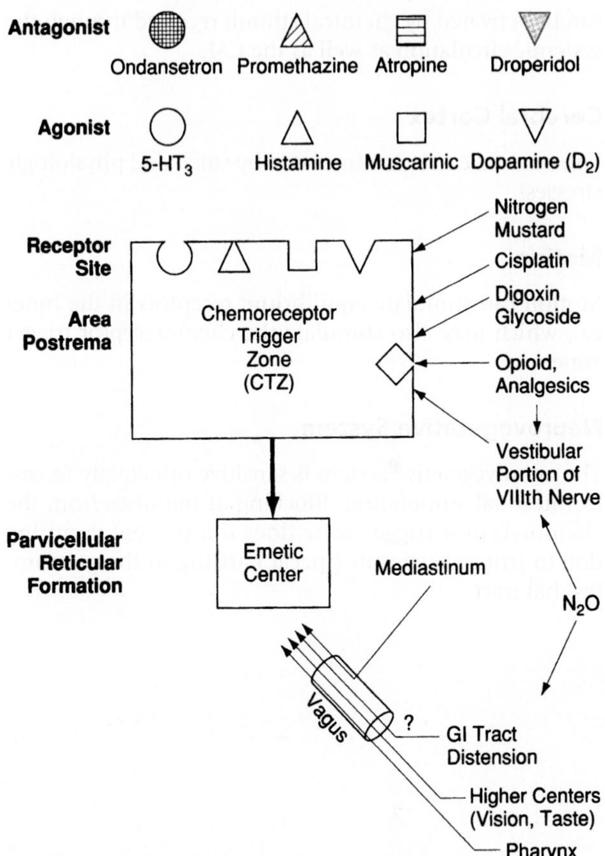

Figure 41-12. The chemoreceptor trigger zone and emetic center respond to a variety of stimuli resulting in nausea and vomiting. (5-HT3, 5-hydroxytryptamine; GI, gastrointestinal.) (From Watcha MR, White PF. Postoperative nausea and vomiting. Its etiology, treatment, and prevention. *Anesthesiology* 1992;77: 162–184; with permission.)

can be activated by chemical stimuli received through the systemic circulation as well as the CSF.

Cerebral Cortex

The cerebral cortex is stimulated by smell and physiologic stresses.

Motion

Motion can stimulate equilibrium receptors in the inner ear, which may also stimulate the chemoreceptor trigger zone.

Neurovegetative System

The neurovegetative system is sensitive principally to gastrointestinal stimulation. Blocking of impulses from the chemoreceptor trigger zone does not prevent vomiting due to irritative stimuli (ipecac) arising in the gastrointestinal tract.

Thermoregulation

42

Body temperature is determined by the relationship between heat production (product of metabolism) and heat dissipation (to the environment) (Stoelting RK, Hillier SC. Thermoregulation. In: *Pharmacology and Physiology in Anesthetic Practice.* 4th ed. Philadelphia, Lippincott Williams & Wilkins, 2006:686–693). Both heat generation and heat loss are adjusted in order to regulate body temperature within narrow limits (36 to 37.5°C); temperature is lowest in the morning and highest in the evening. This is consistent with a 10% to 15% decrease in the basal metabolic rate during physiologic sleep, presumably reflecting the decreased activity of skeletal muscles and the sympathetic nervous system.

HEAT LOSS

Heat loss from the body occurs by radiation, conduction, convection, and evaporation. Under typical circumstances most heat (~60%) is lost by radiation. Double-walled incubators are intended to reduce radiant heat loss because of the presence of warm air on both sides of the inner wall of the incubator. The conduction of heat from the body occurs by direct contact with a cooler object, for example between the patient and an adjacent mattress. Reductions in core temperature during the administration of cold intravenous fluids and blood products are attributable to conductive losses. The rate of convective loss depends on both the air temperature and its velocity (the "wind-chill" phenomenon). Evaporative heat losses are important because significant energy is required to vaporize water.

Evaporation is the only mechanism by which the body can eliminate excess heat when the temperature of the surroundings is higher than that of the skin. With continued exposure to a warm environment, sweat production may increase to 1,500 mL/hour. Evaporation accounts for two-thirds of the heat loss from the respiratory tract.

REGULATION OF BODY TEMPERATURE

Central regulation of body temperature is via feedback mechanisms that operate predominantly through the preoptic nucleus of the anterior hypothalamus. The hypothalamic thermostat detects body temperature changes and initiates autonomic, somatic, and endocrine thermoresponses when the various set points are reached. Thermoregulatory responses are graded, and each particular response is characterized by a threshold temperature at which it is initiated (vasoconstriction in response to cold occurs at 36.5°C, whereas shivering does not occur until core temperature drops to 36.2°C). In the awake individual, a narrow range of normal core temperature exists, the *interthreshold range* (36.7 to 37.1°C), within which thermoregulatory responses are not triggered. During general anesthesia, the threshold temperatures for the activation of responses to cold are decreased, and the threshold temperatures for activation of warm responses are increased (interthreshold range is significantly larger during general anesthesia). The maintenance of body temperature at a value close to the optimum for enzyme activity assures a constant rate of metabolism, optimal nervous system conduction, and skeletal muscle contraction.

Nonshivering Thermogenesis

Nonshivering thermogenesis (chemical thermogenesis) is an increase in the rate of cellular metabolism in brown adipose tissue evoked by sympathetic nervous system stimulation or by circulating catecholamines. In infants, chemical thermogenesis can increase the rate of heat production by as much as 200%.

Shivering

Shivering increases body heat production in response to decreased core temperature. The posterior hypothalamic area responsible for the response to hypothermia controls reflex shivering.

CAUSES OF INCREASED BODY TEMPERATURE (TABLE 42-1)

In hyperthermic states, the hypothalamic set-point is normal but peripheral mechanisms are unable to maintain body temperature that matches the set-point. In contrast, fever occurs when the hypothalamic set-point is increased by the action of circulating pyrogenic cytokines, causing intact peripheral mechanisms to conserve and generate heat until the body temperature increases to the elevated set-point. The treatment of hyperthermia should be directed at promoting heat dissipation, whereas the treatment of fever should be directed at the identification and eradication of pyrogens and lowering the thermoregulatory set-point with antipyretic drugs such as aspirin, acetaminophen, and other cyclooxygenase inhibitors.

Fever

Pyrogens are bacterial toxins that indirectly cause the set-point of the hypothalamic thermostat to increase. Viruses do not release pyrogens directly, but stimulate infected cells to release interferons which act as endogenous pyrogens.

Chills

A sudden resetting of the hypothalamic thermostat to a higher level, as a result of tissue destruction, pyrogens, or dehydration, results in a lag between blood temperature

TABLE 42-1. CAUSES OF HYPERTHERMIA
Disorders Associated with Excessive Heat Production
Malignant hyperthermia
Neuroleptic malignant syndrome
Thyrotoxicosis
Delirium tremens
Pheochromocytoma
Salicylate intoxication
Drug abuse (cocaine, amphetamine)
Status epilepticus
Exertional hyperthermia
Disorders Associated with Decreased Heat Loss
Autonomic nervous system dysfunction
Anticholinergics
Drug abuse (cocaine)
Dehydration
Occlusive dressings
Heat stroke
Disorders Associated with Dysfunction of the Hypothalamus
Trauma
Tumors
Idiopathic hypothalamic dysfunction
Cerebrovascular accidents
Encephalitis
Neuroleptic malignant syndrome

and the new hypothalamic set point. During this period, the person experiences chills and feels cold even though body temperature may be increased.

CUTANEOUS BLOOD FLOW

Cutaneous blood flow is a major determinant of heat loss. Nutritional requirements are so low for skin that this need does not significantly influence cutaneous blood flow. Cutaneous blood flow can decrease to as little as 50 mL/min in severe cold and may increase to as much as 2,800 mL/min in extreme heat (patients with borderline cardiac function may become symptomatic in hot environments). The cutaneous veins act as an important blood reservoir that can supply 5% to 10% of the blood volume in times of need. Inhaled anesthetics increase cutaneous blood flow, perhaps by inhibiting the temperature-regulating center of the hypothalamus.

Skin Color

The skin color in light-skinned individuals is principally due to the color of blood in the cutaneous capillaries and veins. Severe vasoconstriction of the skin forces most of this blood into the central circulation, and skin takes on the whitish hue (pallor) of underlying connective tissue, which is composed primarily of collagen fibers.

PERIOPERATIVE TEMPERATURE CHANGES (TABLE 42-2)

General anesthesia (inhaled and injected drugs) and regional anesthesia (epidural and spinal) widen the interthreshold range to 4.0°C. As a result, anesthetized patients are relatively poikilothermic, with body temperatures determined by the environment. Anesthetics inhibit

TABLE 42-2.
EVENTS THAT CONTRIBUTE TO DECREASES IN BODY TEMPERATURE DURING SURGERY

Resetting of the hypothalamic thermostat
Ambient temperature <21°C
Administration of unwarmed intravenous fluids
Drug-induced vasodilation
Basal metabolic rate decreased
Attenuated shivering response
Core compartment exposed to ambient temperature
Heat required to humidify inhaled dry gases

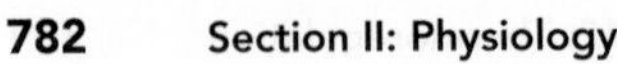

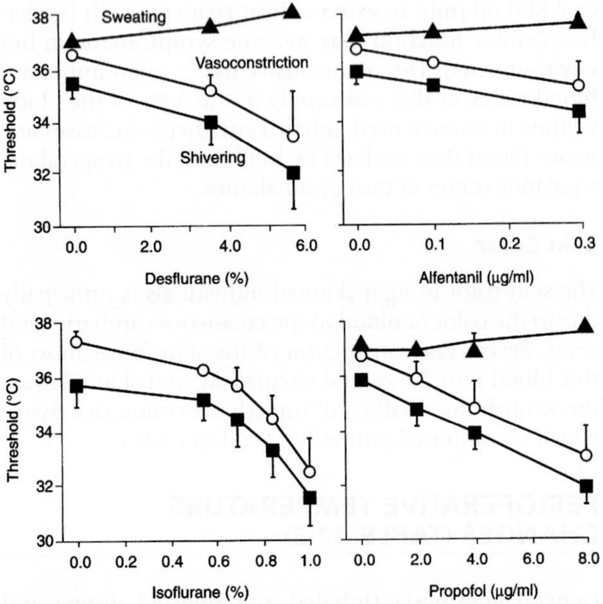

Figure 42-1. Changes in the thermoregulatory threshold for sweating, vasoconstriction, and shivering in the presence of increasing concentrations of inhaled or injected anesthetics. (From Sessler DI. Mild perioperative hypothermia. *N Engl J Med* 1997;336:1630–1637; with permission.)

thermoregulation in a dose-dependent manner and inhibit vasoconstriction and shivering about three times as much as they restrict sweating (Figure 42-1).

Sequence of Temperature Changes during Anesthesia

Tonic thermoregulatory vasoconstriction maintains a temperature gradient between the core and periphery of 2 to 4°C. Under general anesthesia, tonic vasoconstriction is attenuated, and heat contained in the core compartment will move to the periphery, thus allowing the core temperature to decrease towards the anesthetic-induced lowered threshold for vasoconstriction. This core to peripheral heat redistribution is responsible for the 1 to 5°C decrease in core temperature that occurs during the first hour of general anesthesia (Figure 42-2). After the first hour of general anesthesia, the core temperature usually decreases at a slower rate, reflecting continuing heat loss to the environment, which exceeds the metabolic production of heat. After 3 to 5 hours of anesthesia, the core temperature often stops decreasing. This thermal plateau may reflect a steady state in which heat loss equals heat production. Decreases in core temperature of a similar or greater magnitude to those experienced during general anesthesia may occur during spinal or epidural techniques. Combined general and regional

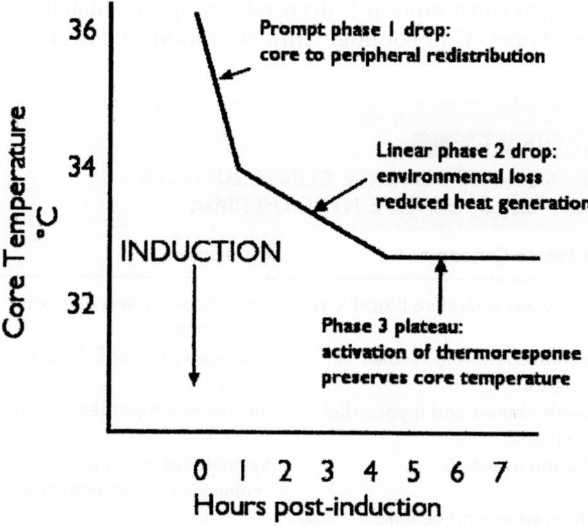

Figure 42-2. Graphic representation of the typical triphasic core temperature pattern that occurs after induction of anesthesia. Note that the phase 3 plateau may not occur, particularly during regional anesthesia or during combined regional and general anesthesia. Although core temperature is preserved during the phase 3 plateau, heat will continue to be lost to the environment from the peripheral compartment.

anesthetic techniques predispose the patient to a greater degree of heat loss than either technique used alone.

Adverse Consequences of Perioperative Hypothermia (Table 42-3)

Shivering occurs in approximately 40% of unwarmed patients who are recovering from general anesthesia and is associated with substantial sympathetic nervous system activation and discomfort from the sensation of cold.

BENEFICIAL EFFECTS OF HYPOTHERMIA

Oxygen consumption is decreased by approximately 5% to 7% per °C of cooling. Thus, even moderate decreases

TABLE 42-3.
IMMEDIATE ADVERSE CONSEQUENCES OF PERIOPERATIVE HYPOTHERMIA

Adverse Outcome	Mechanism
Increased operative blood loss	Coagulopathy and platelet dysfunction
Increased morbid cardiac events	Increased myocardial work load
Dysrhythmias and myocardial ischemia	Increased sympathetic activity
Wound infection	Sympathetic mediated cutaneous vasoconstriction
Delayed wound healing	
Delayed anesthetic emergence	Decreased drug metabolism and increased volatile agent solubility, decreased MAC
Delayed recovery room discharge	Post-anesthetic shivering, delayed recovery

in core temperature of 1 to 3°C below normal provide substantial protection against cerebral ischemia and arterial hypoxemia. Mild hypothermia (33 to 36°C) may be recommended during operations likely to be associated with cerebral ischemia, such as carotid endarterectomy, aneurysm clipping, and cardiac surgery.

MEASUREMENT OF BODY TEMPERATURE (TABLE 42-4)

PREVENTION OF PERIOPERATIVE HYPOTHERMIA (TABLE 42-5 AND FIG. 42-3)

TABLE 42-4.
MEASUREMENT OF BODY TEMPERATURE

Esophagus (about 24 cm beyond the corniculate cartilages or site of the loudest heart sounds heard through an esophageal stethoscope gives a reliable approximation of blood and cerebral temperature)
Nasopharyngeal (probe positioned behind the soft palate gives a less reliable measure of cerebral temperature than a correctly positioned esophageal probe; leakage of gases around the tracheal tube may influence the measurement)
Rectal (heat-producing bacteria in the gastrointestinal tract, cold blood returning from the lower limbs, and insulation of the probe by feces may influence readings)
Bladder (readings subject to a prolonged response time)
Tympanic membrane (rapidly responsive and accurate estimate of hypothalamic temperature; correlates with esophageal temperature; infrared thermometers allow nontraumatic measurement)
Pulmonary artery (best continuous estimate of body temperature)
Skin (reflects temperature of area being measured)

TABLE 42-5.

PREVENTION OF PERIOPERATIVE HYPOTHERMIA

Warm intravenous fluids
High ambient room temperature
Cover skin
Forced air warming (most effective method available)

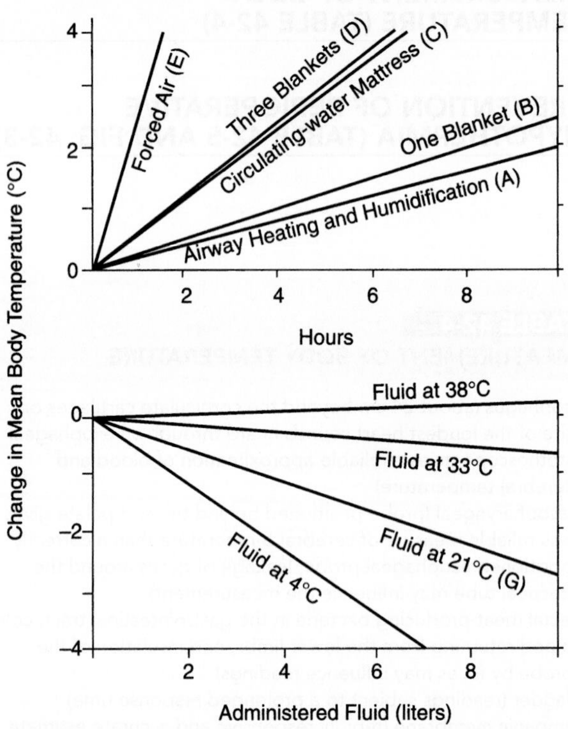

Figure 42-3. The effects of different warming techniques on mean body temperature plotted according to the elapsed hours of treatment (top) and changes in mean body temperature according to the volume of fluid administered (bottom). (From Sessler DI. Mild perioperative hypothermia. *N Engl J Med* 1997; 336:1630–1637; with permission.)

Autonomic Nervous System

43

The autonomic nervous system (ANS) controls the visceral functions of the body and is divided into the sympathetic, parasympathetic, and enteric nervous systems (Stoelting RK, Hillier SC. Autonomic nervous system. In: *Pharmacology and Physiology in Anesthetic Practice*. 4th ed. Philadelphia, Lippincott Williams & Wilkins, 2006: 694–704). The sympathetic and the parasympathetic nervous systems usually function as physiologic antagonists so that the activity of organs innervated by other divisions of the ANS represents a balance of the influence of each component (Table 43-1). Although the gastrointestinal tract is influenced by sympathetic and parasympathetic nervous system activity, it is the enteric nervous system, through the myenteric and submucous plexi, that regulates digestive activity even in the presence of spinal cord transection. An understanding of the anatomy and physiology of the ANS is useful for predicting the pharmacologic effects of drugs that act on either the sympathetic nervous system or the parasympathetic nervous system (Table 43-2).

ANATOMY OF THE SYMPATHETIC NERVOUS SYSTEM

Nerves

The nerves of the sympathetic nervous system arise from the thoracolumbar (T1 to L2) segments of the spinal cord (Fig. 43-1). Each nerve of the sympathetic nervous system consists of a preganglionic neuron and a postganglionic neuron (Fig. 43-2).

TABLE 43-1.

RESPONSES EVOKED BY AUTONOMIC NERVOUS SYSTEM STIMULATION

	Sympathetic Nervous System Stimulation	Parasympathetic Nervous System Stimulation
Heart		
Sinoatrial node	Increase heart rate	Decrease heart rate
Atrioventricular node	Increase conduction velocity	Decrease conduction velocity
His-Purkinje system	Increase automaticity,conduction velocity	Minimal effect
Ventricles	Increase contractility,conduction velocity	Minimal effects, slight decrease in contractility (?)
Bronchial smooth muscle	Relaxation	Contraction
Gastrointestinal tract		
Motility	Decrease	Increase
Secretion	Decrease	Increase
Sphincters	Contraction	Relaxation
Gallbladder	Relaxation	Contraction
Urinary bladder		
Smooth muscle	Relaxation	Contraction
Sphincter	Contraction	Relaxation
Uterus	Contraction	Variable
Ureter	Contraction	Relaxation

TABLE 43-1.
(Continued)

	Sympathetic Nervous System Stimulation	Parasympathetic Nervous System Stimulation
Eye		
Radial muscle	Mydriasis	
Sphincter muscle	Miosis	
Ciliary muscle	Relaxation for far vision	Contraction for near vision
Liver	Glycogenolysis Gluconeogenesis	Glycogen synthesis
Pancreatic β-cell secretion	Decrease	
Salivary gland secretion	Increase	Marked increase
Sweat glands	Increase*	Increase
Apocrine glands	Increase	
Arterioles		
Coronary	Constriction (α) Relaxation (β)	Relaxation (?)
Skin and mucosa	Constriction	Relaxation
Skeletal muscle	Constriction (α) Relaxation (β)	Relaxation
Pulmonary	Constriction	Relaxation

*Postganglionic sympathetic fibers to sweat glands are cholinergic.

TABLE 43-2.

MECHANISM OF ACTION OF DRUGS THAT ACT ON THE AUTONOMIC NERVOUS SYSTEM

Mechanism	Site	Drug
Inhibition of neurotransmitter synthesis	SNS	α-Methyldopa
False neurotransmitter	SNS	α-Methyldopa
Inhibition of uptake of neurotransmitter	SNS	Tricyclic antidepressants, cocaine, ketamine (?)
Displacement of neurotransmitter from storage sites	SNS	Amphetamine
	PNS	Carbachol
Prevention of neurotransmitter release	SNS	Bretylium
	PNS	Botulinum toxin
Mimic action of neurotransmitter at receptor	SNS	
	α-1	Phenylephrine, methoxamine
	α-2	Clonidine dexmedetomidine
	β-1	Dobutamine
	β-2	Terbutaline, albuterol

TABLE 43-2.
(Continued)

Mechanism	Site	Drug
Inhibition of action of neurotransmitter on postsynaptic receptor	SNS	
	α-1	
	α-2	Prazosin
	α-1 and α-2	Yohimbine
	β-1	Phentolamine
	β-1 and β-2	Metoprolol, esmolol
		Propranolol
	PNS	
	M1	Pirenzepine
	M1, M2	Atropine
	N1	Hexamethonium
	N2	d-Tubocurarine
Inhibition of metabolism of neurotransmitter	SNS	Monoamine oxidase inhibitors
	PNS	Neostigmine, pyridostigmine, edrophonium

PNS, parasympathetic nervous system; SNS, sympathetic nervous system.

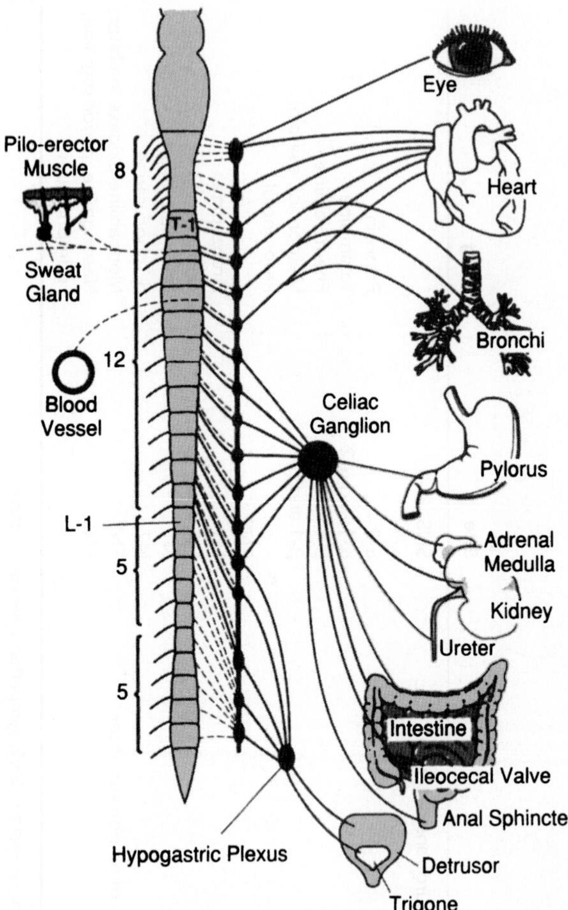

Figure 43-1. Anatomy of the sympathetic nervous system. Dashed lines represent postganglionic fibers in gray rami leading to spinal nerves for subsequent distribution to blood vessels and sweat glands. (From Guyton AC, Hall JE. *Textbook of Medical Physiology*, 10th ed. Philadelphia. Saunders, 2000; with permission.)

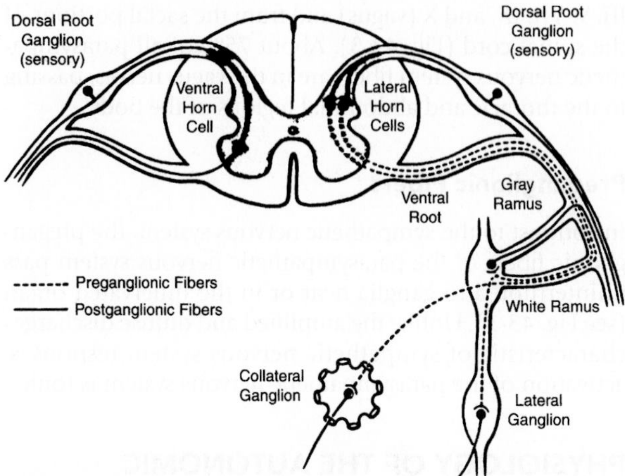

Figure 43-2. Anatomy of a sympathetic nervous system nerve. Preganglionic fibers pass through the white ramus to a paravertebral ganglia, where they may synapse, course up the sympathetic chain to synapse at another level, or exit the chain without synapsing to pass to an outlying collateral ganglion.

Preganglionic Neurons

The cells bodies of preganglionic neurons are located in the intermediolateral horn of the spinal cord. Fibers from these preganglionic cell bodies leave the spinal cord with anterior (ventral) nerve roots and pass via white rami into one of 22 pairs of ganglia composing the paravertebral sympathetic chain. The fibers of the sympathetic nervous system are not necessarily distributed to the same part of the body as the spinal nerve fibers from the same segments.

ANATOMY OF THE PARASYMPATHETIC NERVOUS SYSTEM

Nerves

The nerves of the parasympathetic nervous system leave the central nervous system (CNS) through cranial nerves

III, V, VII, IX, and X (vagus) and from the sacral portions of the spinal cord (Fig. 43-3). About 75% of all parasympathetic nervous system fibers are in the vagus nerves, passing to the thoracic and abdominal regions of the body.

Preganglionic Fibers

In contrast to the sympathetic nervous system, the preganglionic fibers of the parasympathetic nervous system pass uninterrupted to ganglia near or in the innervated organ (see Fig. 43-3). Unlike the amplified and diffuse discharges characteristic of sympathetic nervous system responses, activation of the parasympathetic nervous system is tonic.

PHYSIOLOGY OF THE AUTONOMIC NERVOUS SYSTEM

Postganglionic Fibers

The postganglionic fibers of the sympathetic nervous system secrete norepinephrine as the neurotransmitter and are classified as *adrenergic* (Fig. 43-4). The postganglionic fibers of the parasympathetic nervous system secrete acetylcholine as the neurotransmitter and are classified as *cholinergic* fibers (see Fig. 43-4).

Preganglionic Neurons

All preganglionic neurons of the sympathetic and parasympathetic nervous system release acetylcholine as the neurotransmitter and are thus classified as cholinergic fibers (acetylcholine release at preganglionic fibers activates both sympathetic and parasympathetic postganglionic neurons).

Norepinephrine as a Neurotransmitter

The synthesis of norepinephrine involves a series of enzyme-controlled steps that begin in the cytoplasm of

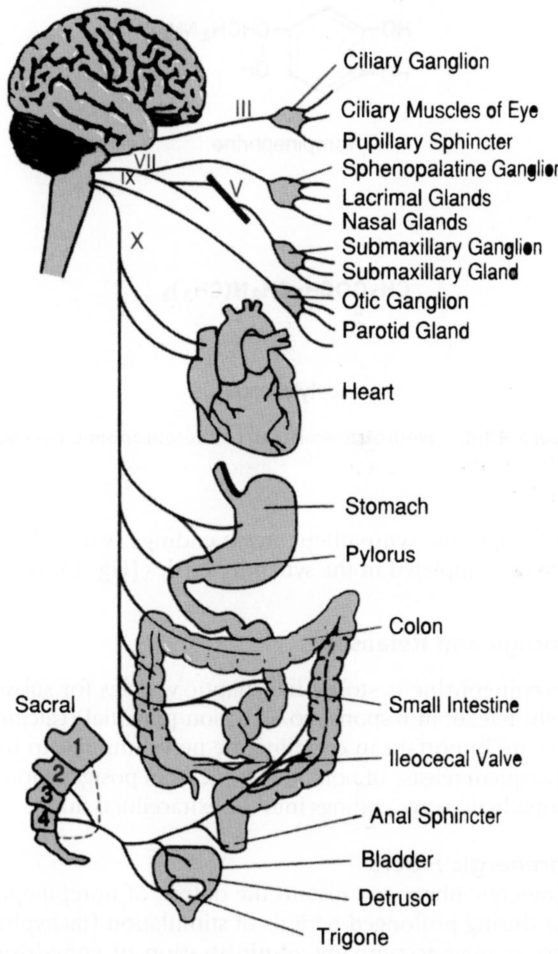

Figure 43-3. Anatomy of the parasympathetic nervous system. (From Guyton AC, Hall JE. *Textbook of Medical Physiology*, 10th ed. Philadelphia. Saunders, 2000; with permission.)

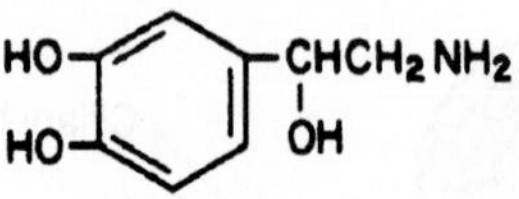

$$HO-C_6H_3(OH)-CH(OH)CH_2NH_2$$

Norepinephrine

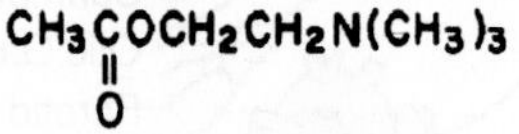

$$CH_3C(=O)OCH_2CH_2N(CH_3)_3$$

Acetylcholine

Figure 43-4. Neurotransmitters of the autonomic nervous system.

postganglionic sympathetic nerve endings (varicosities) and are completed in the synaptic vesicles (Fig. 43-5).

Storage and Release

Norepinephrine is stored in synaptic vesicles for subsequent release in response to an action potential (calcium ions are important in coupling the nerve impulse to the subsequent release of norepinephrine from postganglionic sympathetic nerve endings into the extracellular fluid).

Adrenergic Fibers

Adrenergic fibers can sustain the output of norepinephrine during prolonged periods of stimulation (tachyphylaxis as may accompany administration of ephedrine, and other indirect-acting sympathomimetics may reflect depletion of the limited pool of neurotransmitters).

Norepinephrine

The termination of action of norepinephrine is by (a) uptake (reuptake) back into postganglionic sympathetic

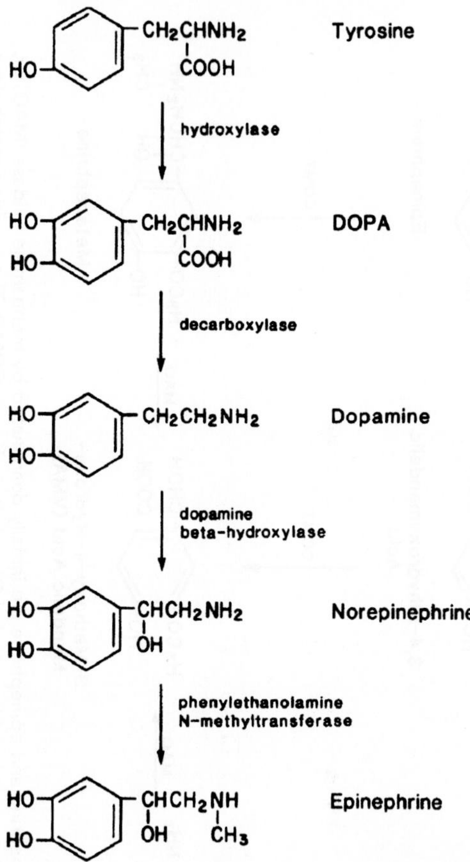

Figure 43-5. Steps in the enzymatic synthesis of endogenous catecholamines and neurotransmitters.

nerve endings (the most important mechanism for terminating the action of this neurotransmitter on receptors), (b) dilution by diffusion from receptors, and (c) metabolism by the enzymes monoamine oxidase (MAO) and catechol-O-methyltransferase (COMT) (Fig. 43-6).

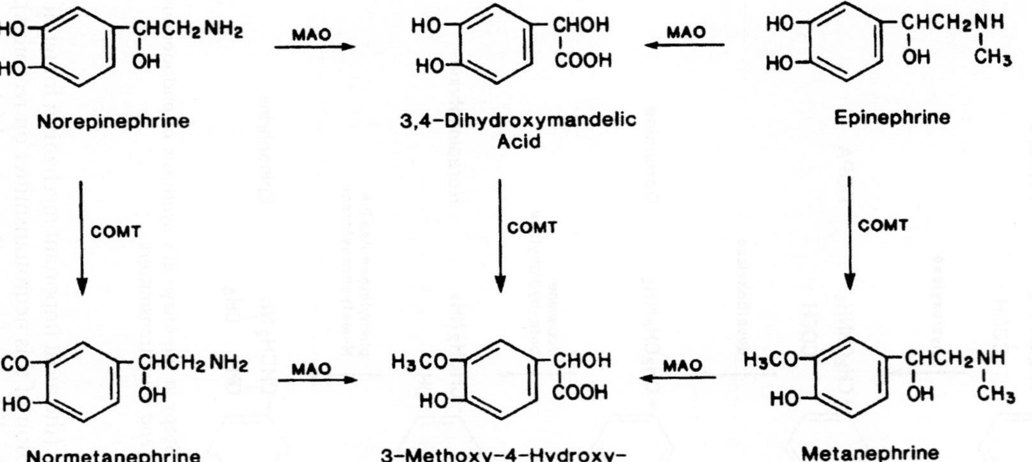

Figure 43-6. Norepinephrine and epinephrine are initially deaminated by monoamine oxidase (MAO) or, alternatively, they are first methylated by catechol-O-methyltransferase (COMT). The resulting metabolites are then further metabolized by the other enzyme (MAO or COMT) to form the principal end-metabolite, 3-methoxy-4-hydroxymandelic acid (vanillylmandelic acid, or VMA).

Acetylcholine as a Neurotransmitter

The synthesis of acetylcholine occurs in the cytoplasm of varicosities of the preganglionic and postganglionic parasympathetic nerve endings (choline acetyltransferase catalyzes the combination of choline with acetyl coenzyme A to form acetylcholine).

Storage and Release

Acetylcholine is stored in synaptic vesicles for release in response to an action potential (calcium ions bind to sites on axonal and vesicular membranes, resulting in the extrusion of the contents of the synaptic vesicles).

Metabolism

Acetylcholine has a brief effect at receptors (<1 ms) because of its rapid hydrolysis by acetylcholinesterase (true cholinesterase) to choline and acetate. Plasma cholinesterase (pseudocholinesterase) hydrolyzes acetylcholine too slowly to be physiologically important, and its absence in plasma cholinesterase produces no detectable clinical signs or symptoms until a drug such as succinylcholine or mivacurium is administered.

INTERACTIONS OF NEUROTRANSMITTERS WITH RECEPTORS (TABLE 43-3)

Norepinephrine Receptors

The pharmacologic effects of catecholamines led to the original concept of α- and β-adrenergic receptors. The subdivision of these receptors into α-1 (postsynaptic), α-2 (presynaptic), β-1 (cardiac), and β-2 (noncardiac) allows an understanding of drugs that act as either agonists or antagonists at these sites (see Table 43-2).

Dopamine Receptors

Dopamine receptors are also subdivided as dopamine1 (postsynaptic) and dopamine2 (presynaptic). The activation

TABLE 43-3.

CLASSIFICATION AND CHARACTERIZATION OF ADRENERGIC AND CHOLINERGIC RECEPTORS

Classification	Molecular Pharmacology	Signal Transduction	Effectors
Adrenergic Receptors			
α-1	α-1A1D	Gq11	Activates phospholipase C
	α-1B	Gq11	Activates phospholipase C
	α-1C	Gq11	Activates phospholipase C
α-2	α-2A	Gi and Go	Inhibits adenylate cyclase, calcium and potassium ion channels
	α-2B	Gi and Go	Inhibits adenylate cyclase, calcium and potassium ion channels
	α-2C	Gi and Go	Inhibits adenylate cyclase, calcium and potassium ion channels

TABLE 43-3.
(continued)

Classification	Molecular Pharmacology	Signal Transduction	Effectors
β-1	β-1	Gs	Stimulates adenylate cyclase and calcium ion channels
β-2	β-2	Gs	Stimulates adenylate cyclase and calcium ion channels
β-3	β-3	Gs	Stimulates adenylate cyclase and calcium ion channels
Cholinergic Receptors			
Nicotinic	Autonomic ganglia	Neuromuscular junction Central nervous system	Ion channels
Muscarinic	M_1	Gq	Phospholipase activation
	M_3	Gq	Phospholipase activation
	M_5	Gq	Phospholipase activation
	M_2	G1 and Go	Inhibits adenylate cyclase
	M_4	G1 and Go	Inhibits adenylate cyclase

of dopamine1 receptors is responsible for vasodilation of the splanchnic and renal circulations. Presynaptic α- and dopamine2 receptors function as a negative feedback loop so that their activation inhibits the subsequent release of neurotransmitter (Table 43-4).

Postsynaptic α-2 Receptors

In the CNS, the stimulation of postsynaptic α-2 receptors (clonidine, dexmedetomidine) results in enhanced potassium ion conductance and membrane hyperpolarization manifesting as decreased anesthetic requirements.

Signal Transduction

Signal transduction is the process by which the extracellular signal created by adrenergic receptor stimulation is transformed into an intracellular signal (α-1 and β-receptors are coupled to G proteins, and activated G proteins modulate either the synthesis or availability of intracellular cytoplasmic messengers and ultimately the activation of protein kinases and the phosphorylation of target proteins).

Catecholamines

Catecholamines encountering β-adrenergic receptors results in dramatic increases in intracellular cyclic adenosine monophosphate (cAMP).

Cyclic Adenosine Monophosphate

The resulting increased intracellular concentration of cAMP then initiates a series of intracellular events—cascading protein phosphorylation reactions and stimulation of the sodium-potassium pump—that result in the metabolic and pharmacologic effects considered typical of β-adrenergic or dopaminergic receptor stimulation by norepinephrine, epinephrine, dopamine, or agonist drugs.

α-Receptors

In contrast to β-receptors, α-1 receptors facilitate calcium ion movement into cells and stimulate the hydrolysis of

TABLE 43-4.
RESPONSES EVOKED BY SELECTIVE STIMULATION OF ADRENERGIC RECEPTORS

α-1 (postsynaptic) Receptors
- Vasoconstriction
- Mydriasis
- Relaxation of gastrointestinal tract
- Contraction of gastrointestinal sphincters
- Contraction of bladder sphincter

α-2 (presynaptic) Receptors
- Inhibition of norepinephrine release

α-2 (postsynaptic) receptors
- Platelet aggregation
- Hyperpolarization of cells in the central nervous system

β-1 (postsynaptic) receptors
- Increased conduction velocity
- Increased automaticity
- Increased contractility

β-2 (postsynaptic) receptors
- Vasodilation
- Bronchodilation
- Gastrointestinal relaxation
- Uterine relaxation
- Bladder relaxation
- Glycogenolysis
- Lipolysis

Dopamine1 (postsynaptic) receptors
- Vasodilation

Dopamine2 (presynaptic) receptors
- Inhibition of norepinephrine release

---

polyphosphoinositides. α-2 and dopamine2 receptors inhibit adenylate cyclase.

Adrenergic Receptor Concentrations

Concentrations of β-adrenergic receptors are not fixed but parallel concentrations of norepinephrine present in the synaptic cleft and plasma; desensitization reflects the rapid waning of responses to hormones and neurotransmitters despite a continuous exposure to adrenergic agonists, whereas down-regulation occurs only hours after exposure to agonists.

Rebound Tachycardia and Myocardial Ischemia

Changes in adrenergic receptor activity are consistent with rebound tachycardia and myocardial ischemia that may accompany the sudden discontinuation of chronic β-adrenergic receptor blockers.

Congestive Heart Failure

Chronic congestive heart failure (CHF) results in the depletion of catecholamines in the myocardium and compensatory increases in plasma concentrations of norepinephrine to maintain systemic vascular resistance and perfusion pressure. Accompanying decreases in the concentrations of β-1 receptors in the heart are responsible for the failure of β-agonists to effectively treat CHF.

Acetylcholine Receptors (See Table 43-3)

Nicotinic Receptors

Acetylcholine can affect nicotinic receptors at either the neuromuscular junction or autonomic ganglia or muscarinic receptors. Nicotinic receptors belong to the superfamily of ligand-gated ion channels, which includes glutamate and glycine receptors.

When acetylcholine occupies both α-subunits, the channel opens and ions flow. If only one site is occupied, the channel remains closed and no flow of ions or change in electrical potential occurs.

Muscarinic Receptors

In contrast to ligand-gated nicotinic receptors, muscarinic receptors belong to the superfamily of G protein–coupled receptors.

Signal Transduction

Odd numbered muscarinic receptors (M_1, M_3, and M_5) work predominantly through the hydrolysis of phosphoinositide and release of intracellular calcium, whereas even number receptors (M_2 and M_4) work primarily through Gi proteins to regulate adenylate cyclase.

Like other G-protein coupled receptors, the response of muscarinic receptors to changes in concentrations is slow.

RESIDUAL AUTONOMIC NERVOUS SYSTEM TONE

The sympathetic and parasympathetic nervous systems are continually active, and this basal rate of activity is referred to as sympathetic or parasympathetic tone. This basal response permits alterations in sympathetic or parasympathetic nervous system activity to either increase or decrease responses at innervated organs.

In addition to continual direct sympathetic nervous system stimulation, a portion of overall sympathetic tone reflects the basal secretion of norepinephrine and epinephrine by the adrenal medulla.

Determination of Autonomic Nervous System Function (Table 43-5)

Aging and Autonomic Nervous System Dysfunction

Common clinical manifestations of ANS dysfunction in elderly patients include orthostatic hypotension, postprandial hypotension, hypothermia, and heat stroke. Clinically, an attenuation of the physiologic responses to β-adrenergic stimulation occurs in the elderly (exogenous β-adrenergic agonists have less profound effects on heart rate).

Diabetic Autonomic Neuropathy

Diabetic autonomic neuropathy is present in 20% to 40% of insulin-dependent diabetic patients.

TABLE 43-5.
CLINICAL ASSESSMENT OF AUTONOMIC NERVOUS SYSTEM FUNCTION

Clinical Observation	Method of Measurement	Normal Value
Parasympathetic Nervous System		
Heart rate response to Valsalva	Patient blows into a mouthpiece maintaining a pressure of 40 mmHg for 15 seconds.	
	The Valsalva ratio is the ratio of the longest R-R interval on the electrocardiogram immediately after release to the shortest R-R interval during the maneuver.	Ratio >1.21
Heart rate response to standing	Heart rate is measured as patient changes from the supine to standing position (increase maximal around 15th beat after standing and slowing maximal around 30th beat).	
	The response to standing is expressed as the "30"15" ratio and is the ratio of the longest R-R interval (around 30th beat) to the shortest R-R interval (around 15th beat).	Ratio >1.04
Heart response to deep breathing	Patient takes six deep breaths in 1 minute.	
	The maximum and minimum heart rates during each cycle are measured and the mean of the differences (maximum heart rate – minimum heart rate) during three	Mean difference >15 bpm

TABLE 43-5.
(continued)

Clinical Observation	Method of Measurement	Normal Value
	successive breathing cycles is taken as the maximum – minimum heart rate.	
Sympathetic Nervous System		
Blood pressure response to standing	The patient changes from the supine to standing position and the standing systolic blood pressure is subtracted from the supine systolic blood pressure.	Difference <10 mmHg
Blood pressure response to sustained handgrip	The patient maintains a handgrip of 30% of maximum squeeze for up to 5 minutes. The blood pressure is measured every minute and the initial diastolic blood pressure is subtracted from the diastolic blood pressure just prior to release.	Difference >16 mmHg

Common manifestations of diabetic autonomic neuropathy include impotence, diarrhea, postural hypotension, sweating abnormalities, and gastroparesis.

When impotence or diarrhea are the sole manifestations of autonomic neuropathy, little impact on survival is present, whereas 5-year mortality rates may exceed 50% when postural hypotension or gastroparesis are present.

Chronic Sympathetic Nervous System Stimulation

Chronic stimulation of the sympathetic nervous system may increase morbidity and mortality. Interventions that attenuate stress responses during the entire perioperative period (continuous epidural infusions of local anesthetics, perioperative administration of β-adrenergic blocking drugs and α-2 agonists) may influence morbidity and mortality rates.

Acute Denervation

The acute denervation of sympathetic nervous system tone, as produced by a regional anesthetic or spinal cord transection, results in immediate maximal vasodilation of blood vessels (spinal shock).

Denervation Hypersensitivity

Denervation hypersensitivity is the increased responsiveness of the innervated organ to norepinephrine or epinephrine; this develops during the first week or so after an acute interruption of ANS innervation. It presumably reflects the proliferation of receptors (up-regulation) on postsynaptic membranes that occurs when norepinephrine or acetylcholine is no longer released at synapses.

ADRENAL MEDULLA

Epinephrine and norepinephrine released by the adrenal medulla function as hormones and not as neurotransmitters.

Synthesis

In the adrenal medulla, most of the formed norepinephrine is converted to the hormone epinephrine by the action of phenylethanolamine-N-methyltransferase. The activity of this enzyme is enhanced by cortisol; stress that releases glucocorticoids also results in the increased synthesis and release of epinephrine.

Release

The triggering event in the release of epinephrine and norepinephrine from the adrenal medulla is the liberation of acetylcholine by preganglionic cholinergic fibers.

Norepinephrine and Epinephrine Release

Norepinephrine and epinephrine released from the adrenal medulla evoke responses similar to the direct stimulation of the sympathetic nervous system. The difference, however, is that effects are greatly prolonged (10 to 30 seconds), compared with the brief duration of action on receptors that is produced by norepinephrine released as a neurotransmitter from postganglionic sympathetic nerve endings.

Circulating Epinephrine

The effects of circulating epinephrine differ from those of norepinephrine in that the cardiac and metabolic effects of epinephrine are greater, whereas a relaxation of blood vessels in skeletal muscles reflects a predominance of β- over α-effects at low concentrations of epinephrine.

Metabolic Rate

The metabolic rate of all cells can be influenced by hormones released from the adrenal medulla, even though these cells are not directly innervated by the sympathetic nervous system.

Pain

44

Pain is a complex phenomenon and includes both sensory-discriminative and motivational-affective components (Stoelting RK, Hillier SC. Pain. In: *Pharmacology and Physiology in Anesthetic Practice*. 4th ed. Philadelphia, Lippincott Williams & Wilkins, 2006:705–715). A failure to appreciate the complex factors that affect the experience of pain and reliance entirely upon physical examination findings and laboratory tests may lead to misunderstanding and the inadequate treatment of pain. The nociceptive system is highly complex and highly adaptable. Sensitivity of most of its components can be reset by a variety of physiologic and pathologic conditions. Innovative medications are available that target the causes of pain through actions on pain transduction, transmission, interpretation, and modulation in both the peripheral nervous system (PNS) and the central nervous system (CNS) (Table 44-1).

SOCIAL IMPACT

It is estimated that chronic pain may affect as many as 40% of the adult population. The costs to society related to chronic pain are immense.

NEUROBIOLOGY OF PAIN

Experience of Pain

The experience of pain involves a series of complex neurophysiologic processes that reflect four distinct components—transduction, transmission, modulation, and perception.

TABLE 44-1.
TREATMENT OF NEUROPATHIC PAIN WITH ADJUVANT DRUGS

Drug	Mechanism of Action
Carbamazepine	Sodium ion channel blockade
Gabapentin	Effects on calcium ion channels (?)
Lidocaine patch	Sodium ion channel blockade Mechanical protection of allodynic skin
Mexiletine	Sodium ion channel blockade
Phenytoin	Sodium ion channel blockade
Nortriptyline	Neurotransmitter reuptake inhibitor
Desipramine	Neurotransmitter reuptake inhibitor
Corticosteroids	Antiinflammatory effects Sodium ion channel blockade Decreased capillary permeability
Clonidine	α-Adrenergic blockade

Transduction

Transduction is the process by which a noxious stimulus is converted to an electrical impulse in sensory nerve endings.

Transmission

Transmission is the conduction of these electrical impulses to the CNS, with the major connections for these nerves being in the dorsal horn of the spinal cord and thalamus with projections to the cingulate, insular, and somatosensory cortexes.

Modulation

Modulation of pain is the process of altering pain transmission. It is likely that both inhibitory and excitatory mechanisms modulate pain (nociceptive) impulse transmission in the PNS and CNS.

Perception

Pain perception is thought to occur at the thalamus, with the cortex being important for discrimination of specific sensory experiences.

MODULATION OF NOCICEPTION

Peripheral Modulation

The peripheral modulation of nociceptive stimuli occurs either through the liberation or elimination of chemicals in the vicinity of the nociceptor.

Tissue Injury

Tissue injury activates nociceptors in the periphery by causing the release of neurotransmitters, such as substance P and glutamate, which directly activate nociceptors.

Other Mediators

Other mediators (bradykinin, histamine, prostaglandins, serotonin, potassium and hydrogen ions, and lactic acid) further sensitize and excite nociceptors and act as mediators of inflammation.

Spinal Modulation

Nociceptive Afferent Signals

The excitatory amino acid transmitters glutamate and aspartate and several neuropeptides (vasoactive intestinal peptide, calcitonin, neuropeptide Y) modulate transmission of nociceptive afferent signals in the spinal cord.

Substance P

Substance P is also an important neuromodulator that can enhance or aggravate pain.

Inhibitory Substances

Inhibitory substances involved in the regulation of afferent impulses in the dorsal horn include γ-aminobutyric acid (GABA), glycine, enkephalins, endorphins, norepinephrine, dopamine, and adenosine.

Supraspinal Modulation

Descending Inhibitory Tracts

Descending inhibitory tracts at the brain stem level originate from cell bodies located in the region of the periaqueductal gray matter.

Nerve Fibers

Nerve fibers identified as participants in inhibitory modulation include the opioid system and associated neurotransmitters (endorphins, enkephalins, other neuropeptides).

A-δ and C Fibers

Neurotransmitters released from these projections hyperpolarize A-delta and C fibers.

Monoamine Pathway

In addition to opioid descending inhibitory pathways, a monoamine pathway originates from locations in the periaqueductal gray matter.

Cognitive Modulation

The cognitive modulation of pain involves the patient's ability to relate a painful experience to another event (pain experience in a pleasant environment elicits a less intense response than pain experienced in a setting of depression). Another area of perception is attention, which presumes that only a fixed number of afferent impulses can reach cortical centers. If a patient in pain concentrates on separate and unrelated images, it is possible to decrease the effects of painful sensations (biofeedback or hypnosis).

Neuroplasticity

Neuroplasticity describes the dynamic modulation of neural impulses.

Peripheral Nerves

As peripheral nerve firing increases, other changes also occur in the excitability of spinal cord neurons, altering their response to afferent impulses.

Central Sensitization

Central sensitization to afferent impulses results from a functional change in spinal cord processing. The temporal summation of the number and duration of action potentials elicited per stimulus (wind-up phenomenon) results in a persistence of action potentials for up to 60 seconds after the discontinuance of the stimulus, and results in a change in spinal cord processing that can last for 1 to 3 hours.

Spinal Cord Synaptic Plasticity

Spinal cord synaptic plasticity involves the binding of glutamate to the NMDA receptors as well as binding of substance P and neurokinins.

PERIPHERAL NERVE PHYSIOLOGY

Nociceptors

Nociceptors (pain receptors) are free nerve ending receptors present in skin, muscles, joints, viscera, and vasculature.

Failure of Pain Receptors

The failure of pain receptors to adapt is protective because it allows the individual to remain aware of continued tissue damage. Specific types of nociceptors react to different types of stimuli.

Visceral Nociceptors

Visceral nociceptors, unlike cutaneous nociceptors, are not designed solely as pain receptors, because internal organs are infrequently exposed to potentially damaging events. Many damaging stimuli (cutting, burning, clamping) produce no pain when applied to visceral structures.

Transduction

Mechanical, thermal, or chemical energy is converted into an electrical action potential (transduction) capable of propagating (transmission) along the nerve fiber toward the spinal cord when the resting threshold of a nociceptor is exceeded.

Inflammatory Mediators

Inflammatory mediators (bradykinin, prostaglandins, serotonin, histamine, cytokines) are released in response to tissue injury.

Bradykinin

Bradykinin is viewed as the first mediator to cause activation of second messengers, resulting in increased sodium ion channel conductance and sensitization.

Prostaglandins

Prostaglandins enhance the activity of bradykinin and contribute to inflammatory responses.

A-δ Fibers and C Fibers

Exposure to inflammatory mediators causes A-δ fibers and C fibers to undergo peripheral sensitization so that their stimulus thresholds are decreased and their firing and intensity is increased and prolonged.

Acute Inflammation

In the majority of cases of acute inflammation, the process naturally resolves as tissues heal, peripheral sensitization diminishes, and nociceptors return to their original resting threshold.

Chronic Pain

Chronic pain occurs when the conditions associated with inflammation do not resolve. This results in persistent pain sensations from a normally painful stimuli (hyperalgesia) and the occurrence of pain sensations in response to normally nonpainful stimuli (allodynia).

Hyperalgesia

Hyperalgesia is a decrease in the pain threshold in an area of inflammation so that even trivial stimuli cause pain.

Transmission

Pain signals are transmitted from nociceptors along myelinated A-δ fibers (rapid conduction for early response) and unmyelinated C fibers (slow conduction for more delayed response). These afferent fibers enter the spinal cord through the dorsal nerve roots and terminate on cells in the dorsal horn.

Fast and Slow Pain (Figs. 44-1 and 44-2)

Fast Pain

Fast pain (Fig. 44-1) is a short, well-localized, stabbing sensation that is matched to the stimulus, such as a pinprick or surgical skin incision. This pain starts abruptly when the stimulus is applied and ends promptly when the stimulus is removed.

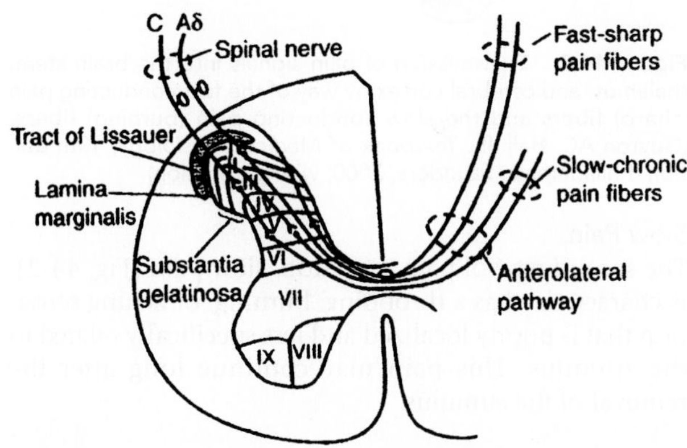

Figure 44-1. Transmission of both fast-sharp and slow-chronic pain signals into and through the cord on their way to the brain. (Guyton AC, Hall JE. *Textbook of Medical Physiology*, 10th edition. Philadelphia; Saunders, 2000; with permission).

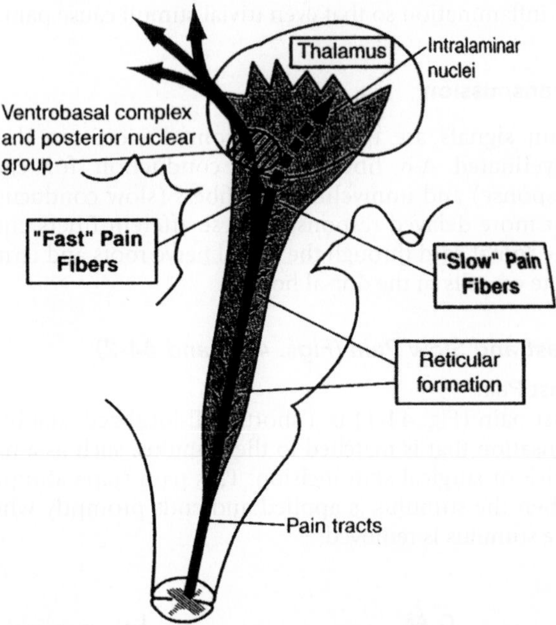

Figure 44-2. Transmission of pain signals into the brain stem, thalamus, and cerebral cortex by way of the fast conducting pain (sharp) fibers and the slow conducting pain (burning) fibers. (Guyton AC, Hall JE. *Textbook of Medical Physiology*, 10th edition. Philadelphia. Saunders, 2000; with permission).

Slow Pain

The second type of pain sensation, slow pain (Fig. 44-2), is characterized as a throbbing, burning, or aching sensation that is poorly localized and less specifically related to the stimulus. This pain may continue long after the removal of the stimulus.

Temperature versus Pain

The nerve fibers for temperature follow the same pathways as fibers for pain. Indeed, artificially applied pain in the form of a heat stimulus causes pain in almost all individuals when skin temperature exceeds 43°C (pain threshold).

Neuropathic Pain

Neuropathic pain of a peripheral origin is a distinct type of chronic pain that occurs in the complete absence of an inflammatory reaction. Direct damage to a peripheral nerve results in a continual ectopic spontaneous discharge of pain signals (neuropathic pain). This peripheral sensitization can contribute to secondary hyperalgesia and central sensitization.

CENTRAL NERVOUS SYSTEM PHYSIOLOGY

Pain transmission from peripheral nociceptors to the spinal cord and higher structures of the CNS is a dynamic process involving several pathways, numerous receptors, neurotransmitters, and secondary messengers. The dorsal horn functions as a relay center for nociceptive and other sensory activity. The degree of activation of ascending pain projection systems depends on multiple factors (Table 44-2).

Dorsal Horn and Ascending Nociceptive Pathway

The dorsal horn consists of six laminae (see Fig. 44-1).

TABLE 44-2.
FACTORS THAT INFLUENCE THE ACTIVATION OF ASCENDING PAIN SYSTEMS

Degree of activation of segmental and descending inhibitory neurons in the dorsal horn
Preexisting concentrations of excitatory neurotransmitters
Level of activation of inhibitory neurotransmitters
Intensity of noxious stimulus
Degree of sensitization of nociceptors in the periphery

Laminae

Laminae I and II are the sites of termination of afferent C-fibers and these two laminae are known as the *substantia gelatinosa*.

Lamina V is the site of second-order wide dynamic range (WDR) and nociceptive-specific (NS) neurons that receive input from nociceptive and nonnociceptive neurons. The NS neurons respond only to noxious stimuli in their peripheral environment, whereas WDR neurons respond to innocuous and noxious stimuli of many types.

Transmission and Modulation

The dorsal horn and its laminae serve as the receiving site for activity initiated on the arrival of action potentials from the periphery via primary afferent neurons. Two main classes of neurotransmitters are associated with primary afferent nociceptive transmission in the dorsal horn—excitatory amino acids, such as glutamate, and neurokinin peptides, such as substance P.

Thalamus and Cerebral Cortex

After leaving the dorsal horn and ascending via the spinothalamic and other pain pathways, nociceptive action potentials reach higher brain centers (reticular formation, midbrain, hypothalamus, cerebral cortex). Pain impulses travel from the thalamus to the somatosensory areas of the cerebral cortex.

Gate Control Theory

Both tactile and thermal afferent stimulation has inhibitory influences on pain perception. The basis of the gate control theory is that A-δ fiber stimulation activates interneurons in the dorsal horn that inhibit the activity of nociceptive transmission neurons. This inhibition is the basis of transcutaneous electrical nerve stimulation, as well as spinal cord and thalamic stimulation for pain control.

Gate cells screen action potentials by determining which ones are transmitted to the CNS for perception.

Glutamate

Glutamate is an excitatory amino acid that is released from presynaptic endings of the primary afferent neurons terminating in the dorsal horn. This release results in the activation of kainate, α-amino-3-hydroxy-5-methyl-4-isoxazoleproprionate (AMPA), and N-methyl-D-aspartate (NMDA) receptors. Much like peripheral modulators (bradykinin), glutamate acts as a central pain mediator at nearly all secondary afferent neurons involved in nociceptive processing.

NMDA Receptors

Glutamate is rapidly removed from the synaptic cleft and, thus, no activity occurs at NMDA receptors in normal nociceptive transmission processes. In the presence of persistent pain arising from abnormal conditions (peripheral sensitization, neuropathic pain, chronic pain), the frequency of pain signal transmission increases, resulting in increased amounts of glutamate available in synaptic clefts. The activation of NMDA receptors serves to activate secondary messengers and enzymatic processes and generates various substances (nitric oxide) that are believed to contribute to the enhanced neuronal sensitivity known as central sensitization.

Central Sensitization

Central sensitization is believed to be the origin of many chronic pain conditions. Central sensitization describes the increased excitability of secondary afferent neurons evoked by neurochemical changes resulting from activation of NMDA receptors. It is likely that many chronic pain conditions reflect a central sensitization that results from the chronic input from the PNS into the spinal cord and the subsequent activation of NMDA receptors.

Persistent Pain and Anatomical Changes

Persistent pain can lead to anatomical changes in both the PNS and CNS. Following nerve injury, a variety of neuronal plasticity changes occur, such as sprouting of dendrites on neurons projecting to the dorsal horn or ingrowth of sympathetic fibers into the dorsal root ganglia.

NMDA Receptors and Tolerance

NMDA receptors are important in facilitating central sensitization and development of opioid tolerance.

Stressors

Emotional or physical stress exacerbates central neuropathic pain but seldom accompanies peripheral neuropathic pain.

Defining Central Neuropathic Pain

The most common description of spontaneous pain of central neuropathic pain is burning or scalding.

Glial Cells

Glial cells have important neuromodulatory and neurotrophic effects, and they are critically important in providing immune function following injury, inflammation, or infection.

Preemptive Analgesia

Preemptive analgesia is based on the concept that blocking nociceptive afferent inputs or their effects on dorsal horn neurons before the start of tissue injury may delay or halt the process of central sensitization. Comprehensive preemptive strategies must start before the painful stimulus (surgical incision) and be maintained during the entire period of intense nociceptive stimulation (perioperative analgesia).

ENDOGENOUS PAIN SUPPRESSION PATHWAYS (FIG. 44-3 AND TABLE 44-3)

Descending Pain Pathways

Descending pain pathways are activated as a result of pain detection, discrimination, and perception at the

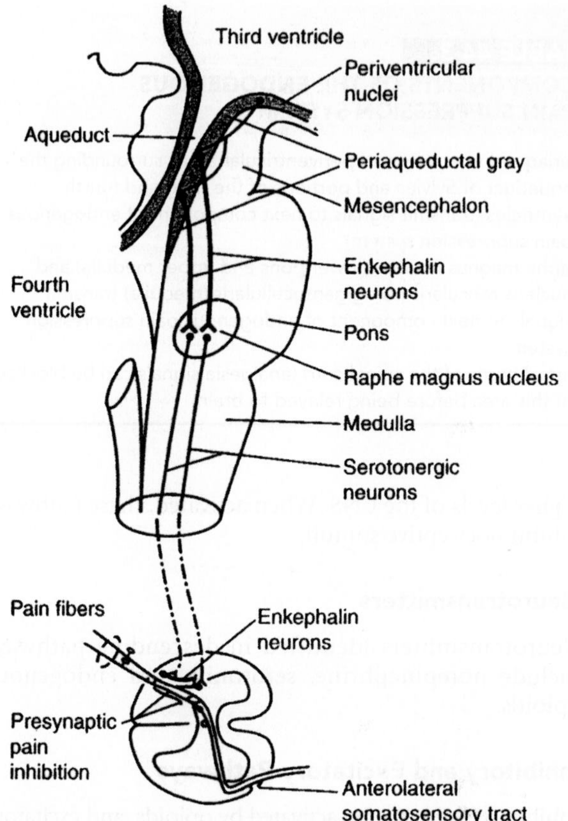

Figure 44-3. Analgesia system of the brain and spinal cord demonstrating inhibition of incoming pain signals at the cord level and the presence of enkephalin-secreting neurons that suppress pain signals in both the spinal cord and brain stem. (Guyton AC, Hall JE. *Textbook of Medical Physiology*, 10th edition. Philadelphia. Saunders, 2000; with permission).

TABLE 44-3.
COMPONENTS OF THE ENDOGENOUS PAIN SUPPRESSION SYSTEM

Periaqueductal gray and periventricular areas surrounding the aqueduct of Sylvius and portions of the third and fourth ventricles (transmit signals to next component of endogenous pain suppression system)
Raphe magnus nucleus (lower pons and upper medulla) and nucleus reticularis paragigantocellularis (medulla) transmit signals to next component of endogenous pain suppression system
Dorsal horns of the spinal cord (analgesia signals can be blocked at this area before being relayed to brain)

higher levels of the CNS. When activated, these pathways inhibit nociceptive stimuli.

Neurotransmitters

Neurotransmitters identified in descending pathways include norepinephrine, serotonin, and endogenous opioids.

Inhibitory and Excitatory Pathways

Inhibitory pathways are activated by opioids, and excitatory pathways are inhibited by opioids, thus providing the mechanism of analgesia induced by drugs such as morphine.

Tricyclic Antidepressants

Tricyclic antidepressants block the presynaptic reuptake of serotonin and norepinephrine and thus augment their postsynaptic actions in descending pain suppression pathways.

CLASSIFICATION OF PAIN (TABLE 44-4)

TABLE 44-4.
PHYSIOLOGIC PAIN CATEGORIES

	Example	Mechanism
Nociceptive	Arthritis Bone fracture Bone metastasis Cellulitis	Activation of nociceptors
Visceral	Pancreatic Peptic ulcer Myocardial infarction	Activation of nociceptors
Neuropathic	Posthepatic neuralgia Diabetic neuropathy Poststroke pain Trigeminal neuralgia	Ectopic discharges in the nervous system Spontaneous activity in nerves Neuroma formation
Complex regional pain syndrome	Persistent focal pain after trauma with or without evidence of sympathetic nervous system involvement	Sensitization of spinal neurons

Adapted from Galer B, Gammaitoni A, Alvarez NA. Pain. *Sci Am Med* 2002:11:XIV:1–27.

Acute and Chronic Pain

Acute Pain

Acute pain is generally associated with well-defined tissue damage and is of limited duration, after which nociceptors return to a normal resting stimulus threshold. Treatment approaches include common analgesic medications (opioids and nonopioids).

Chronic Pain

Chronic pain can be categorized as malignant or nonmalignant. Chronic pain may have both nociceptive and neuropathic elements.

Autonomic Nervous System

Patients with acute pain or chronic pain may exhibit autonomic nervous system signs and symptoms (tachycardia, increased blood pressure, diaphoresis, rapid breathing) when pain is present. Guarding is more common in patients with chronic pain who manifest allodynia.

Nociceptive and Neuropathic Pain

Organic pain may be subdivided into nociceptive or neuropathic pain. Nociceptive pain includes visceral and somatic pain and refers to pain due to the peripheral stimulation of nociceptors in visceral or somatic structures.

Nociceptive pain is usually responsive to opioid or nonopioid analgesics.

Neuropathic pain involves peripheral or central afferent neural pathways and commonly is described as burning or lancinating pain (often responds poorly to opioid analgesics).

Visceral Pain

Visceral pain typically radiates and may be referred to surface areas of the body far removed from the painful viscus but with the same dermatome origin as the diseased viscus.

Visceral pain, like deep somatic pain, initiates the reflex contraction of nearby skeletal muscles, which makes the abdominal wall rigid when inflammatory processes involve the peritoneum.

Visceral pain due to malignant invasion of a hollow or solid viscus is often described as diffuse, gnawing, or cramping if a hollow viscus is involved and as sharp or aching if a solid viscus is involved.

Somatic Pain

Somatic pain is described as sharp, stabbing, well-localized pain that typically arises from the skin, skeletal muscles, and peritoneum.

Pain from a surgical incision, the second stage of labor, or peritoneal irritation is somatic pain.

The presence of both visceral and somatic pain pathways can result in the localization of pain from viscera to dual surface areas of the body at the same time.

Sympathetic Nervous System Responses

Painful stimulation may evoke reflex increases in sympathetic nervous system efferent activity. It is possible that associated vasoconstriction leads to acidosis, tissue ischemia, and the release of chemicals that further activate pain receptors.

The resulting sustained, painful stimulation produces further increases in sympathetic nervous system activity, and the vicious cycle termed *reflex sympathetic dystrophy* (complex regional pain syndrome) may develop.

Sites Amenable to Surgical Section of Pain Pathways

Surgical section through the anterolateral quadrant of the spinal cord (cordotomy) at the thoracic level interrupts the anterolateral spinothalamic tract and relieves pain from the limb on the side opposite the cord transection.

Cordotomy may be unsuccessful, because some pain fibers do not cross to the opposite side of the spinal cord until they have reached the brain. Pain that is more intense than the original pain may develop several months after the cordotomy.

EMBRYOLOGIC ORIGIN AND LOCALIZATION OF PAIN

The position in the spinal cord to which visceral afferent fibers pass for each organ depends on the segment (dermatome) of the body from which the organ developed embryologically (Fig. 44-4).

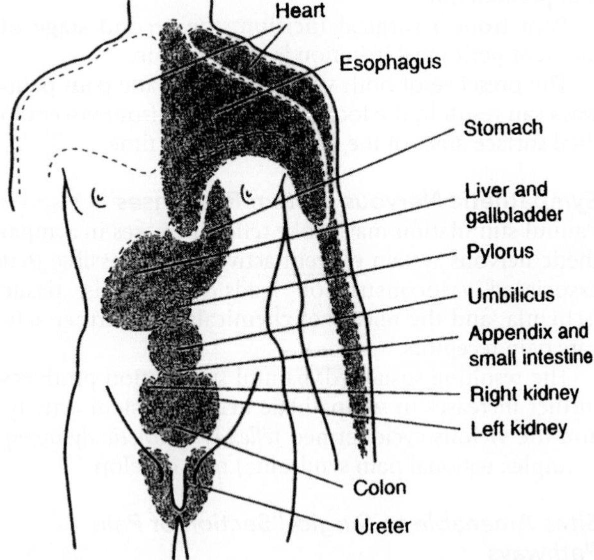

Figure 44-4. Surface area of referred pain from different visceral organs. (Guyton AC, Hall JE. *Textbook of Medical Physiology*, 10th edition. Philadelphia. Saunders, 2000; with permission).

Systemic Circulation

45

The systemic circulation supplies blood to all the tissues of the body except the lungs (Stoelting RK, Hillier SC. Systemic circulation. In: *Pharmacology and Physiology in Anesthetic Practice.* 4th ed. Philadelphia, Lippincott Williams & Wilkins, 2006:716–732).

ENDOTHELIAL FUNCTION

The endothelium promotes vasodilatation and confers anti-thrombotic and anti-adhesive properties to the vessel wall. The endothelium also regulates vascular permeability, smooth muscle proliferation, and has an important role in the regulation of glucose and lipid metabolism.

Endothelial Function and Regulation of Vascular Tone

Under physiologic conditions, local vascular pressure and flow are the primary stimuli for endothelial vasoactive substance release.

Nitric oxide and prostacyclin are powerful vasodilators released by endothelial cells and both also inhibit platelet aggregation and thrombosis. Continuous nitric oxide production maintains vascular tone in a normally low state.

COMPONENTS OF THE SYSTEMIC CIRCULATION (TABLE 45-1)

TABLE 45-1.
COMPONENTS OF THE SYSTEMIC CIRCULATION

Arteries (transmit blood under high pressure)
Arterioles (contract and dilate to control blood flow into capillaries)
Capillaries (sites for transfer of oxygen and nutrients and receipt of metabolic byproducts)
Venules (collect blood from capillaries for delivery to veins)
Veins (contract or expand to store blood, venous pump mechanism)

PHYSICAL CHARACTERISTICS OF THE SYSTEMIC CIRCULATION (FIGS. 45-1 AND 45-2) (TABLE 45-2)

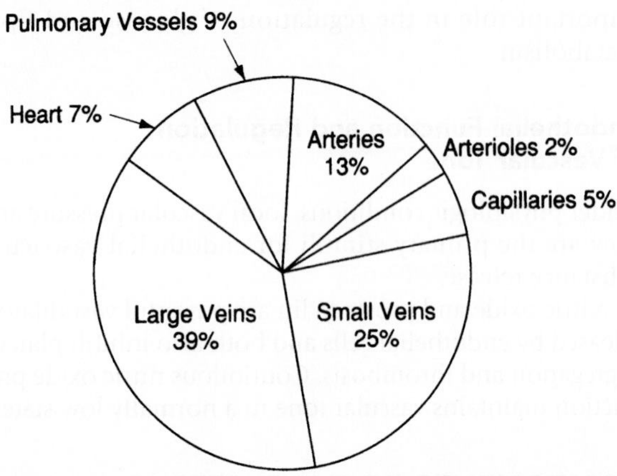

Figure 45-1. Distribution of blood volume in the systemic and pulmonary circulation. (From Guyton AC, Hall JE. *Textbook of Medical Physiology*, 10th ed. Philadelphia: Saunders, 2000; with permission.)

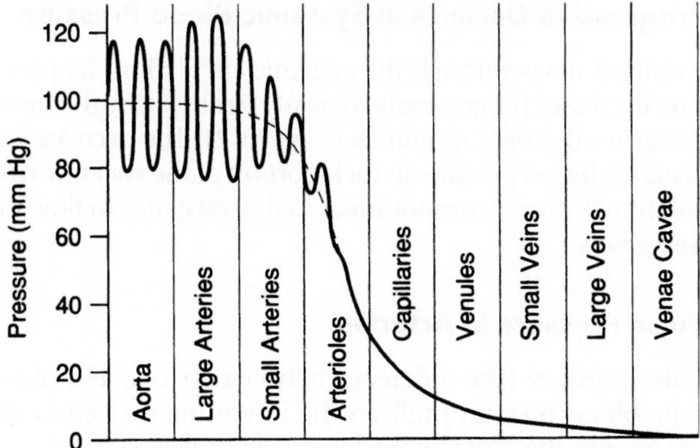

Figure 45-2. Systemic blood pressure decreases as blood travels from the aorta to large veins. (From Guyton AC, Hall JE. *Textbook of Medical Physiology*, 10th ed. Philadelphia: Saunders, 2000; with permission.)

TABLE 45-2.
NORMAL PRESSURES IN THE SYSTEMIC CIRCULATION

	Mean Value (mm Hg)	Range (mm Hg)
Systolic blood pressure*	120	90–140
Diastolic blood pressure*	80	70–90
Mean arterial pressure	92	77–97
Left ventricular end-diastolic pressure	6	0–12
Left atrium		
a wave	10	2–12
v wave	13	6–20
Right atrium		
a wave	6	2–10
c wave	5	2–10
v wave	3	0–8

*Measured in the radial artery.

Progressive Declines in Systemic Blood Pressure

As blood flows through the systemic circulation, its pressure decreases progressively to nearly 0 mm Hg by the time it reaches the right atrium (see Fig. 45-2). The decrease in systemic blood pressure in each portion of the systemic circulation is directly proportional to the resistance to flow in the vessels.

Pulse Pressure in Arteries

Pulse pressure (the difference between systolic and diastolic blood pressure) reflects the intermittent ejection of blood into the aorta by the heart (see Table 45-1).

Factors Altering Pulse Pressure (Table 45-3)

Enhancement of the pulse pressure often occurs as the pressure wave is transmitted peripherally; this augmentation of the peripheral pulse pressure must be recognized whenever systemic blood pressure measurements are made in peripheral arteries (Fig. 45-3).

Pulse pressure becomes progressively less as blood passes through small arteries and arterioles, until it becomes almost absent in capillaries.

Measurement of Blood Pressure by Auscultation

Measurement of blood pressure by auscultation uses the principle that blood flow in large arteries is laminar and not audible.

TABLE 45-3.
FACTORS ALTERING PULSE PRESSURE

Left ventricular stroke volume
Velocity of blood flow
Compliance of the arterial tree

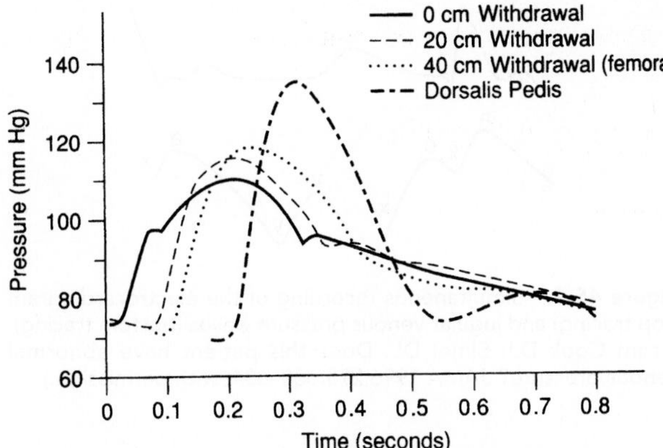

Figure 45-3. There is enhancement of the pulse pressure as the systemic blood pressure is transmitted peripherally. (From Guyton AC, Hall JE. *Textbook of Medical Physiology*, 10th ed. Philadelphia: Saunders, 2000; with permission.)

If blood flow is arrested by an inflated cuff, and the pressure in the cuff is released slowly, audible tapping sounds (Korotkoff sounds) can be heard when the pressure of the cuff decreases just below systolic blood pressure and blood starts flowing in the brachial artery. This method usually produces values within 10% of those determined by direct measurement from the arteries.

Right Atrial Pressure

Right atrial pressure is regulated by a balance between venous return and the ability of the right ventricle to eject blood.

Central Venous Pressure

Pressure in the right atrium is commonly designated the central venous pressure.

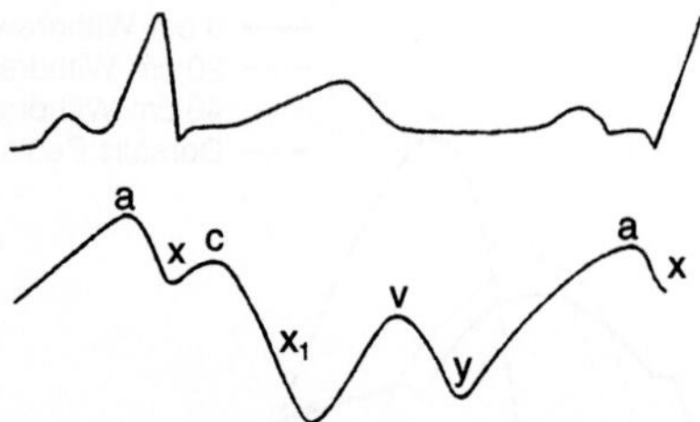

Figure 45-4. Simultaneous recording of the electrocardiogram (top tracing) and jugular venous pressure waves (bottom tracing). (From Cook DJ, Simel DL. Does this patient have abnormal venous pressure? *JAMA* 1996;275:630–634; with permission.)

Jugular Venous Pressure

The normal jugular venous pressure reflects phasic changes in the right atrium and consists of three positive waves and three negative troughs (Fig. 45-4). Abnormalities of these venous waveforms may be useful in the diagnosis of various cardiac conditions (Table 45-4).

Effect of Hydrostatic Pressure

Pressure in the veins below the heart is increased and that in veins above the heart is decreased by the effect of gravity (Fig. 45-5).

As a guideline, pressure changes 0.77 mm Hg for every centimeter the vessel is above or below the heart.

Venous Valves and the Pump Mechanism

Valves in veins are arranged so that the direction of blood flow can be toward the heart only. In a standing human, movement of the legs compresses skeletal muscles and veins so that blood is directed toward the heart.

Reference Level for Measuring Venous Pressure

Tricuspid Valve as Reference Point

Hydrostatic pressure does not alter venous or arterial pressures that are measured at the level of the tricuspid

TABLE 45-4.
ABNORMALITIES OF JUGULAR VENOUS PRESSURE WAVEFORMS

Waveform	Cardiac Abnormality
Absent a wave	Atrial fibrillation Sinus tachycardia
Flutter waves	Atrial flutter
Prominent a waves	First-degree atrioventricular heart block
Large a wave	Tricuspid stenosis Pulmonary hypertension Pulmonic stenosis Right atrial myxoma
Cannon a waves	Atrioventricular dissociation Ventricular tachycardia
Absent x wave descent	Tricuspid regurgitation
Large cv waves	Tricuspid regurgitation Constrictive pericarditis
Slow y wave descent	Tricuspid stenosis Right atrial myxoma
Rapid y wave descent	Tricuspid regurgitation Atrial septal defect Constrictive pericarditis
Absent y wave descent	Cardiac tamponade

Adapted from Cook DJ, Simel DL. Does this patient have abnormal central venous pressure? *JAMA* 1996; 275:630–634.

valve. (Reference point for pressure measurement is considered to be the level of the tricuspid valve.)

External reference points for the level of the tricuspid valve in a supine individual are about one-third the distance from the anterior chest and about one-fourth the distance above the lower end of the sternum.

A precise hydrostatic point to which pressures are referenced is essential for the accurate interpretation of venous pressure measurements (each centimeter below the hydrostatic point adds 0.77 mm Hg to the measured

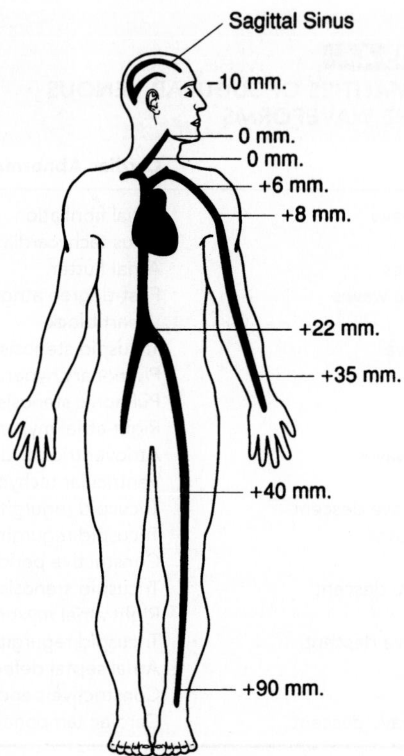

Figure 45-5. Effect of hydrostatic pressure on venous pressures throughout the body. (From Guyton AC, Hall JE. *Textbook of Medical Physiology*, 10th ed. Philadelphia: Saunders, 2000; with permission.)

pressure, whereas 0.77 mm Hg is subtracted for each centimeter above this point).

Conversion Factors

A venous pressure measurement in millimeters of mercury can be converted to centimeters of water by multiplying the pressure by 1.36, which adjusts for the density of mercury relative to water (10 mm Hg equals 13.6 cm H_2O). Conversely, dividing the central venous pressure measurement in centimeters of water by 13.6 converts this value to an equivalent pressure in millimeters of mercury.

PHYSICAL CHARACTERISTICS OF BLOOD

Hematocrit

The percentage of blood comprising erythrocytes is the hematocrit, which to a large extent determines the viscosity of blood (Fig. 45-6).

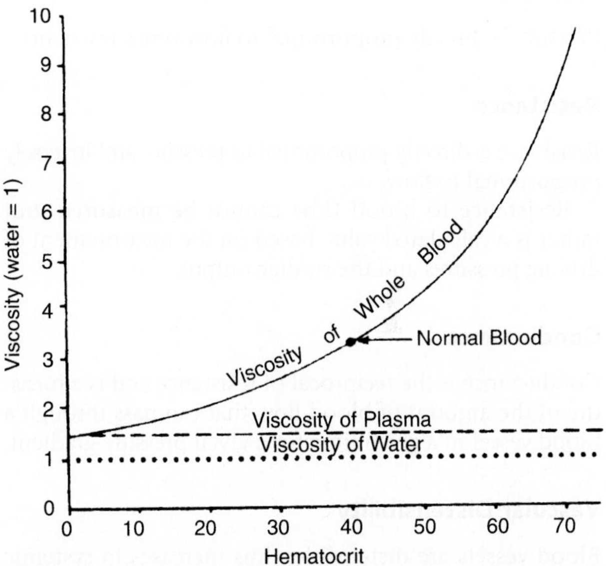

Figure 45-6. Hematocrit greatly influences the viscosity of blood. (From Guyton AC, Hall JE. *Textbook of Medical Physiology*, 10th ed. Philadelphia: Saunders, 2000; with permission.)

Plasma

Plasma is considered extracellular fluid; it is identical to interstitial fluid except for its greater concentrations of proteins (albumin, globulin, fibrinogen). The primary function of albumin is to create colloid osmotic pressure, which prevents fluid from leaving the capillaries.

DETERMINANTS OF TISSUE BLOOD FLOW

Tissue blood flow is directly proportional to the pressure difference between two points (not absolute pressure) and inversely proportional to resistance to flow through the vessel.

Pressure

Pressure is directly proportional to flow times resistance.

Resistance

Resistance is directly proportional to pressure and inversely proportional to flow.

Resistance to blood flow cannot be measured, but rather is a calculated value based on the measurement of driving pressures and the cardiac output.

Conductance

Conductance is the reciprocal of resistance and is a measure of the amount of blood flow that can pass through a blood vessel in a given time for a given pressure gradient.

Vascular Distensibility

Blood vessels are distensible, thus increases in systemic blood pressure cause the vascular diameter to increase, which in turn decreases resistance to blood flow. Decreases in intravascular pressure increase the resistance to blood flow.

Vascular Compliance

The volume of blood normally present in all veins is about 2,500 mL, whereas the arterial system contains only about 750 mL of blood when the mean arterial pressure is 100 mm Hg.

Blood Loss

The enhancement of sympathetic nervous system activity to the blood vessels, especially the veins, decreases the dimensions to the circulatory system, and the circulation continues to function almost normally even when as much as 25% of the total blood volume has been lost.

CONTROL OF TISSUE BLOOD FLOW (TABLES 45-5 AND 45-6)

Cerebral Blood Flow

A high cerebral blood flow limits the excessive accumulation of hydrogen ions and carbon dioxide in the brain.

Skeletal Muscle Blood Flow

Skeletal muscles represent 35% to 40% of body mass but receive only about 15% of the total cardiac output,

TABLE 45-5.
CONTROL OF TISSUE BLOOD FLOW

Local control (based on the need for delivery of oxygen or other nutrients)
Autoregulation (local mechanism in which a specific tissue is able to maintain a relatively constant blood flow over a wide range of mean arterial pressures)
Long-term control (change in vascularity of tissues with sustained increases in blood pressure, increased metabolism, inadequate oxygen delivery)
Autonomic nervous system control (norepinephrine influences resistance to redistribute tissue blood flow; prominent in the kidneys and skin and minimal in the cerebral circulation)

TABLE 45-6.
TISSUE BLOOD FLOW

	Approximate blood flow		
	(mL/minute)	(mL/100 g/minute)	Cardiac Output (% of total)
Brain	750	50	15
Liver	1,450	100	29
Portal vein	1,100		
Hepatic artery	350		
Kidneys	1,000	320	20
Heart	225	75	5
Skeletal muscles	750	4	15 (at rest)
Skin	400	3	8
Other tissues	425	2	8
Total	5,000		100

Adapted from Guyton AC, Hall JE. *Textbook of Medical Physiology*, 10th ed. Philadelphia: Saunders, 2000.

reflecting the low metabolic rate of inactive skeletal muscles.

Mean Arterial Blood Pressure

Mean arterial blood pressure is the most important determinant of tissue blood flow, because it is the average, tending to drive blood through the systemic circulation.

REGULATION OF SYSTEMIC BLOOD PRESSURE (TABLE 45-7)

Reciprocal changes in cardiac output and systemic vascular resistance maintains systemic blood pressure over a narrow range.

TABLE 45-7.
REGULATION OF SYSTEMIC BLOOD PRESSURE

Rapid-Acting Mechanisms (adapt to new levels of systemic blood pressure)
- Baroreceptor reflexes

Chemoreceptor Reflexes
- Atrial reflexes
- Central nervous system ischemic reflex (Cushing reflex)

Moderately Rapid-Acting Mechanisms
- Hormonal induced vasoconstriction
- Catecholamines
- Renin-angiotensin
- Antidiuretic hormone

Intrinsic
- Capillary fluid shift
- Stress-relaxation of blood vessels

Long-Term Mechanisms (delayed onset but do not adapt)
- Renal-body fluid system
- Renin-Angiotensin System
- Aldosterone (retain sodium and water)

REGULATION OF CARDIAC OUTPUT AND VENOUS RETURN

Determinants of Cardiac Output

Venous return is more important than myocardial contractility in determining cardiac output.

Decreased Cardiac Output

Any factor that interferes with venous return can lead to decreased cardiac output (hemorrhage, acute venodilation as produced by spinal anesthesia, positive pressure ventilation).

Increased Cardiac Output

Factors that increase cardiac output are associated with decreases in systemic vascular resistance (anemia, increased blood volume, exercise, arteriovenous shunts associated with hemodialysis)

Increased Myocardial Contractility

Sympathetic nervous system stimulation increases myocardial contractility and heart rate to increase cardiac output beyond that possible from venous return alone.

Maximal stimulation by the sympathetic nervous system can double cardiac output. A sympathetic nervous system–induced increase of cardiac output is only transient. Typically, inotropic interventions evoke responses through increases in myoplasmic calcium concentrations and less often by increasing the sensitivity of the contractile components to calcium. It is difficult to separate changes in myocardial contractility from changes in preload.

Regardless of the mechanisms for increased myocardial contractility, the effects of positive inotropic interventions are additive to the effects of increasing the preload.

Ventricular Function Curves

Ventricular function curves (Frank-Starling curves) depict the cardiac output at different atrial (ventricular end-diastolic) filling pressures (Fig. 45-7).

Pressure-Volume Loops

Pressure-volume loops describe the dynamic characteristics of cardiac function (Fig. 45-8).

Shock Syndromes

Shock syndromes are caused by inadequate tissue blood flow and oxygen delivery to cells, resulting in a generalized deterioration of organ function. The usual cause of inadequate tissue perfusion is inadequate cardiac output due to decreased venous return or myocardial depression. An important feature of persistent shock is the eventual progressive deterioration of the heart.

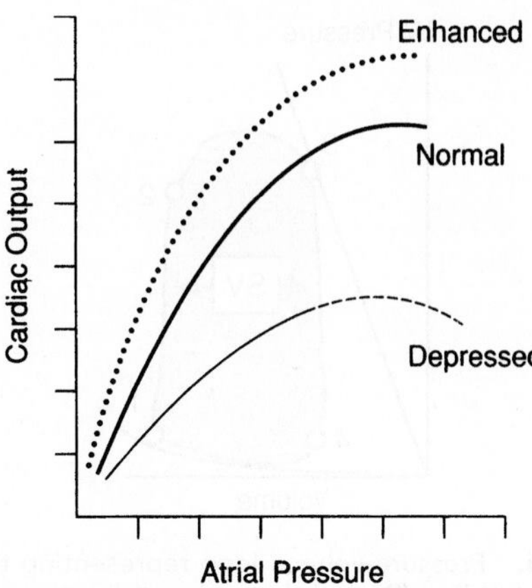

Figure 45-7. Ventricular function curves (Frank-Starling curves) depict the volume of forward ventricular ejection (cardiac output) at different atrial filling pressures and varying degrees of myocardial contractility.

Hemorrhagic Shock

Hemorrhage is the most common cause of shock due to decreased venous return.

Nonhemorrhagic Shock

Loss of plasma from the circulation in the absence of blood loss can result in shock similar to that produced by hemorrhage (intestinal obstruction, burns).

Hypovolemic Shock

Hypovolemic shock that results from plasma loss has the same clinical characteristics as hemorrhagic shock except that the selective loss of plasma greatly increases the viscosity of blood and exacerbates sluggishness of blood flow.

Neurogenic Shock

Neurogenic shock occurs in the absence of blood loss when vascular capacity increases so greatly that even a

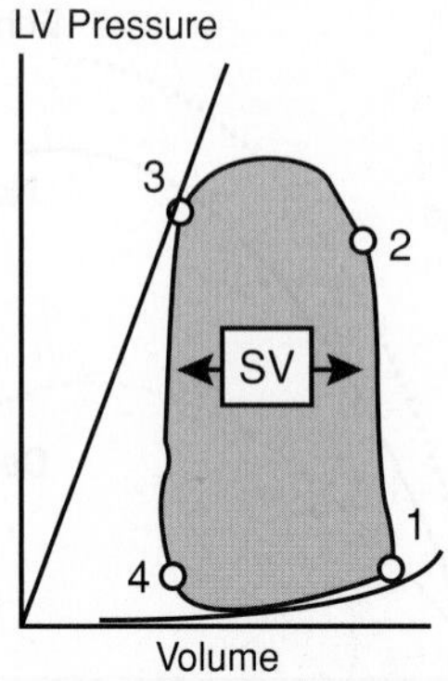

Figure 45-8. Pressure-volume loop representing the cardiac cycle. The end-diastolic and the end-systolic pressure-volume relationships represent the boundaries for the loops. The width of the pressure-volume loop represents the stroke volume (SV). Increases or decreases in myocardial contractility make the end-systolic pressure volume relationship steeper or shallower. The four segments of the loop (isovolumic contraction, ejection, isovolumic relaxation, ventricular filling) for the left ventricle are depicted in succession by mitral valve closure (1), aortic valve opening (2), aortic valve closure (3), mitral valve opening (4).

normal blood volume is not capable of maintaining venous return and cardiac output (acute spinal cord transection, spinal or epidural anesthesia).

Septic Shock

Septic shock is characterized by profound peripheral vasodilation, increased cardiac output secondary to decreased systemic vascular resistance, and the development of disseminated intravascular coagulation.

Causes of septic shock are most often release of endotoxins from ischemic portions of the gastrointestinal tract or bacteremia due to extension of urinary tract infections. The septic response is likely to reflect a systemic inflammatory response produced by exposure to bacterial cell products that ultimately lead to a progressively dysfunctional host response and multisystem organ failure.

Immunosuppressed and elderly patients are vulnerable to the development of sepsis and associated septic shock.

Measurement of Cardiac Output

Fick Method

Cardiac output is calculated as oxygen consumption divided by the arteriovenous difference for oxygen.

Indicator Dilution Method

A nondiffusible dye (indocyanine green) is injected into the right atrium (or central venous circulation), and the concentration of dye is subsequently measured continuously in the arterial circulation by a spectrophotometer.

Thermodilution Method

Thermodilution cardiac outputs are determined by measuring the change in blood temperature between two points (right atrium and pulmonary artery) after injection of a known volume of cold saline solution at the proximal right atrial port.

The change in blood temperature as measured at the distal pulmonary artery port is inversely proportional to pulmonary blood flow (the extent to which the cold saline solution is diluted by blood), which is equivalent to cardiac output.

The advantages of this technique, compared with the indicator dilution method, include the dissipation of cold in tissues so recirculation is not a problem, and safety of repeated and frequent measurements because saline is innocuous.

FETAL CIRCULATION (FIG. 45-9)

Placenta

In utero, the placenta acts as the fetal lung, and oxygenated blood (saturation about 80%) from the placenta passes through a single umbilical vein to the fetus.

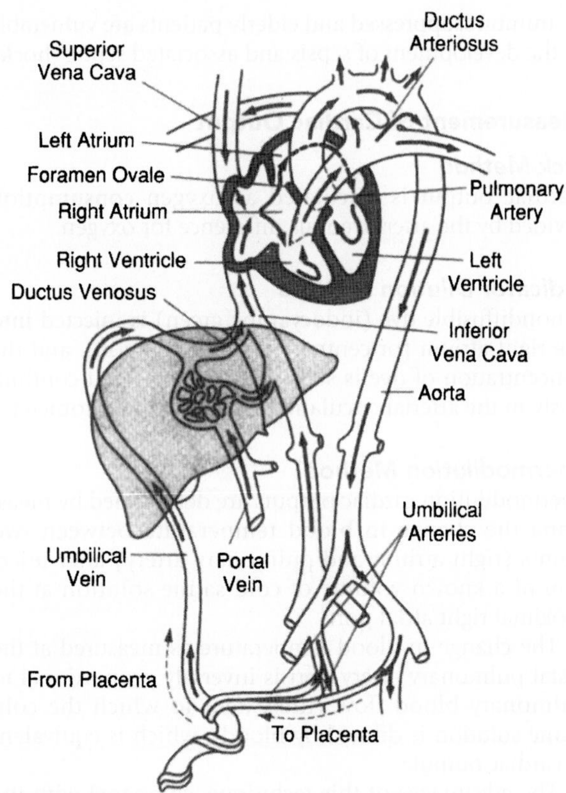

Figure 45-9. The placenta acts as the lungs for the fetus. Most of the oxygenated blood reaching the fetal heart via the umbilical vein and inferior vena cava is diverted through the foramen ovale and pumped out the aorta to the head. Deoxygenated blood returned via the superior vena cava is mostly pumped through the pulmonary artery and ductus arteriosus to the feet and umbilical arteries. (From Ganong WF. *Review of Medical Physiology*, 21st ed. New York, Lange Medical Books/McGraw Hill, 2003; with permission).

Fetal Hemoglobin

Fetal hemoglobin differs from adult hemoglobin in binding oxygen less avidly, thus maximizing oxygen transfer to tissues despite low hemoglobin saturations with oxygen.

Birth

The principal changes in the fetal circulation at birth are increased systemic vascular resistance and systemic blood pressure due to the cessation of blood flow through the placenta. In addition, pulmonary vascular resistance decreases dramatically upon expansion of the lungs, leading to a marked increase in pulmonary blood flow.

Foramen Ovale

These alterations in pulmonary and systemic vascular resistance change the pressure gradient across the foramen ovale, causing the flaplike valve that is present on the left atrial septum to occlude the opening.

Ductus Arteriosus

Flow through the ductus arteriosus decreases after birth due to constriction of the muscular wall of this vessel on exposure to higher concentrations of oxygen.

Microcirculation and Lymphatics

46

The circulation is designed to supply tissues with blood in amounts commensurate with their needs for oxygen and nutrients (Stoelting RK, Hillier SC. Microcirculation and lymphatics. In: *Pharmacology and Physiology in Anesthetic Practice.* 4th ed. Philadelphia, Lippincott Williams & Wilkins, 2006:733–738). Capillaries, whose walls consist of a single layer of endothelial cells, serve as the site for the rapid transfer of oxygen and nutrients to tissues and the receipt of metabolic byproducts. Fluid and proteins that have escaped from the circulation are returned to the venous circulation by the lymphatic system.

MICROCIRCULATION

The microcirculation is defined as the circulation of blood through the smallest vessels of the body—arterioles, capillaries, and venules.

Anatomy of the Microcirculation (Table 46-1 and Fig. 46-1)

Capillary Walls

The capillary walls are about 1 μm thick, consisting of a single layer of endothelial cells surrounded by a thin basement membrane on the outside (Fig. 46-2).

TABLE 46-1.
ANATOMY OF THE VARIOUS TYPES OF BLOOD VESSELS

Vessel	Lumen Diameter	Approximate Cross-Sectional Area (cm2)	Percentage of Blood Volume Contained
Aorta	2.5 cm	2.5	
Artery	0.4 cm	20	13
Arteriole	30 μm	40	1
Capillary	5 μm	2,500	6
Venule	20 μm	250	
Vein	0.5 cm	80	64*
Vena cava	3 cm	8	
Heart			7
Pulmonary circulation		18	9

*Blood volume contained in venules, veins, and vena cava.

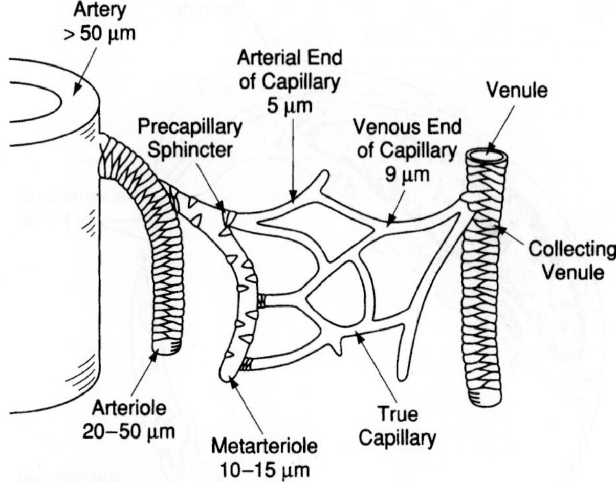

Figure 46-1. Anatomy of the microcirculation. (From Ganong WF. *Review of Medical Physiology*, 21st ed. New York. Lange Medical Books/McGraw-Hill, 2003; with permission.)

Cytoplasm

The cytoplasm of endothelial cells is attenuated to form gaps or pores that are 20 to 100 nm in diameter. These pores permit the passage of relatively large molecules.

Brain Circulation

In the brain, the capillaries resemble those in skeletal muscles, except the interdigitated junctions between endothelial cells are tighter (forming the blood-brain barrier), permitting the passage of only small molecules.

Gas Exchange

Oxygen and carbon dioxide are both lipid soluble and readily pass through endothelial cells.

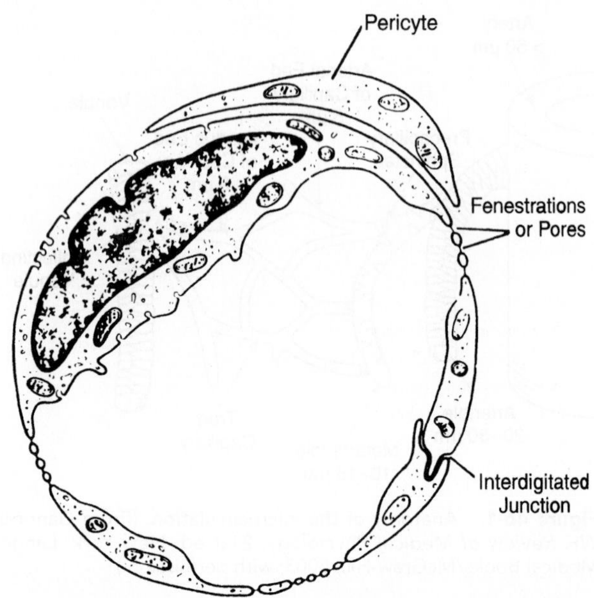

Figure 46-2. Capillaries include interdigitated junctions and pores to facilitate passage of lipid-insoluble ions and molecules. (From Ganong WF. *Review of Medical Physiology*, 21st ed. New York. Lange Medical Books/McGraw-Hill, 2003; with permission.)

Pressure

The thin walls of capillaries are able to withstand high intraluminal pressures because their small diameter prevents excessive wall tension (Laplace's law).

Blood Flow in Capillaries

The blood flow in capillaries is approximately 1 mm/s and is intermittent rather than continuous.

This intermittent blood flow reflects the contraction and relaxation of metarterioles and precapillary sphincters in alternating cycles of 6 to 12 times per minute (vasomotion).

A low P_{O_2} allows more blood to flow through capillaries to supply tissues (a form of autoregulation).

Vasoactive Role of the Capillary Endothelium

The endothelium is not inert but is an important source of substances that cause the contraction or relaxation of vascular smooth muscle (prostacyclin, nitric oxide, endothelin).

Fluid Movement across Capillary Membranes

Solvent and Solute Movement

Solvent and solute movement across capillary endothelial cells occurs by filtration, diffusion (most important), and pinocytosis.

Filtration is the net outward movement of fluid at the arterial end of capillaries.

Diffusion of fluid occurs in both directions across capillary membranes.

Filtration

The four pressures that determine whether fluid will move outward across capillary membranes (filtration) or inward across capillary membranes (reabsorption) are (a) capillary pressure, (b) interstitial fluid pressure, (c) plasma colloid osmotic pressure, and (d) interstitial fluid colloid osmotic pressure (Tables 46-2, 46-3, and 46-4).

Capillary Pressure

Capillary pressure tends to move fluid outward across the arterial ends of capillary membranes.

Interstitial Fluid Pressure

Interstitial fluid pressure tends to move fluid outward across capillary membranes.

Plasma Colloid Osmotic Pressure

Plasma colloid osmotic pressure is due principally to plasma proteins (albumin) and tends cause movement of fluid inward through capillary membranes.

TABLE 46-2.
FILTRATION OF FLUID AT THE ARTERIAL ENDS OF CAPILLARIES

Pressure Favoring Outward Movement	
Capillary pressure	25 mm Hg
Interstitial fluid pressure	−6.3 mm Hg
Interstitial fluid colloid osmotic pressure	5 mm Hg
Total	36.3 mm Hg
Pressure Favoring Inward Movement	
Plasma colloid osmotic pressure	28 mm Hg
Net filtration pressure	8.3 mm Hg

Interstitial Fluid Colloid Osmotic Pressure

Proteins present in the interstitial fluid are principally responsible for the interstitial fluid colloid osmotic pressure of about 5 mm Hg, which tends to cause movement of fluid outward across capillary membranes. Interstitial fluid protein content also remains low because proteins cannot readily diffuse across capillary mem-

TABLE 46-3.
REABSORPTION OF FLUID AT THE VENOUS ENDS OF CAPILLARIES

Pressure Favoring Outward Movement	
Capillary pressure	10 mm Hg
Interstitial fluid pressure	−6.3 mm Hg
Interstitial fluid colloid osmotic pressure	5 mm Hg
Total	21.3 mm Hg
Pressure Favoring Inward Movement	
Plasma colloid osmotic pressure	28 mm Hg
Net reabsorption pressure	6.7 mm Hg

TABLE 46-4.
MEAN VALUES OF PRESSURES ACTING ACROSS CAPILLARY MEMBRANES

Pressure Favoring Outward Movement	
Capillary pressure	17 mm Hg
Interstitial fluid pressure	−6.3 mm Hg
Interstitial fluid colloid osmotic pressure	5 mm Hg
Total	28.3 mm Hg
Pressure Favoring Inward Movement	
Plasma colloid osmotic pressure	28 mm Hg
Net overall filtration pressure	0.3 mm Hg

branes, and any that crosses are likely to be removed by lymph vessels.

Diffusion

Diffusion is the most important mechanism for the transfer of nutrients between the plasma and the interstitial fluid.

Lipid-Soluble Molecules

Oxygen, carbon dioxide, and anesthetic gases are examples of lipid-soluble molecules that can diffuse directly through capillary membranes independently of pores. The diffusion rate of lipid-soluble molecules across capillary membranes in either direction is proportional to the concentration difference between the two sides of the membrane. For this reason, large amounts of oxygen move from capillaries toward tissues, whereas carbon dioxide moves in the opposite direction.

Pinocytosis

Pinocytosis is the process by which capillary endothelial cells ingest small amounts of plasma or interstitial fluid, followed by migration to the opposite surface, where the fluid is released.

LYMPHATICS

Lymph vessels

Lymph vessels represent an alternate route by which excess fluids can flow from interstitial fluid spaces into the blood. The most important function of the lymphatic system is the return of protein into the circulation and maintenance of a low protein concentration in the interstitial fluid. Only cartilage, bone, epithelium, and tissues of the central nervous system are devoid of lymphatic vessels.

Anatomy

Thoracic and Right Lymphatic Duct

The terminal lymph vessels are the thoracic duct and the right lymphatic duct (Fig. 46-3). Avoidance of possible damage to the thoracic duct is often the reason to select

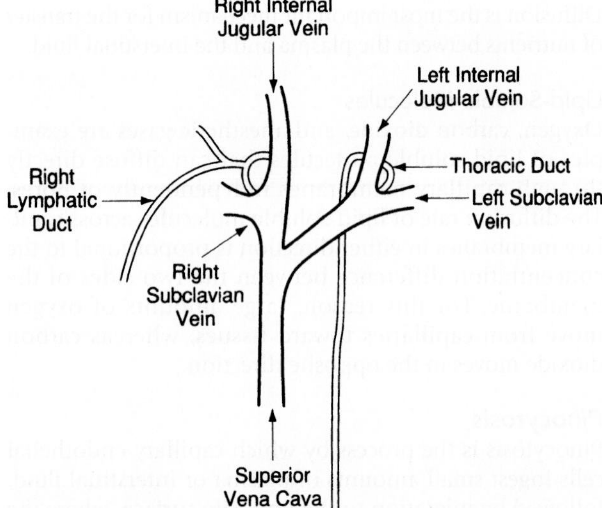

Figure 46-3. Depiction of the thoracic duct and right lymphatic duct as they enter the venous system.

the right side of the neck as the site for percutaneous placement of a venous catheter into the right internal jugular vein.

Valves

Lymph vessels contain flaplike valves between endothelial cells that open toward the interior, allowing the unimpeded entrance of interstitial fluid and proteins and the prevention of backflow.

Formation

Lymph is interstitial fluid that flows into lymphatic vessels. The lymphatic system is also one of the major channels for absorption of nutrients, especially fat, from the gastrointestinal tract.

Bacteria that enter lymph vessels are removed and destroyed by lymph nodes

Flow of Lymph

The flow of lymph through the thoracic duct is about 100 mL/hour. Skeletal muscle contraction and passive movements of the extremities facilitate the flow of lymph.

Edema

Edema is the presence of excess interstitial fluid in peripheral tissues. This results in positive pressure in interstitial fluid spaces and exceeds the ability of lymph vessels to transport the excess fluid.

Transudate and Exudate

Edema may also be accompanied by the presence of fluid in potential spaces such as the pleural cavity, pericardial space, peritoneal cavity, and synovial spaces. Fluid that collects in these spaces is called transudate if it is sterile and exudate if it contains bacteria.

Ascites

Excessive fluid in the peritoneal space—one of the spaces most prone to develop edema fluid—is called ascites. The peritoneal cavity is susceptible to the development of edema fluid because any increased pressure in the liver, as due to cirrhosis or cardiac failure, causes transudation of protein-containing fluids from the surface of the liver into the peritoneal cavity.

Causes of Edema

Causes of increased interstitial fluid volume that manifests as edema include (a) increased capillary pressure, (b) decreased plasma protein concentrations, (c) obstruction to lymph vessels, and (d) increased permeability of capillaries. Renal dysfunction leading to excessive retention of fluid is also a cause of edema.

Increased Capillary Pressure

Increased capillary pressure, as accompanies impaired venous return due to cardiac failure, results in the filtration of fluid from capillaries that exceeds reabsorption.

Decreased Plasma Protein Concentrations

Decreased plasma protein concentrations reduce the colloid osmotic pressure so that capillary pressure predominates and excess fluid leaves the circulation.

Obstruction of Lymph Vessels

The obstruction of lymph vessels results in an accumulation of protein in interstitial fluid. Edema due to this cause typically regresses over 2 to 3 months as new lymph vessels develop.

Pulmonary Circulation

47

The pulmonary circulation is a low-pressure, low-resistance system in series with the systemic circulation (Stoelting RK, Hillier SC. Pulmonary circulation. In: *Pharmacology and Physiology in Anesthetic Practice*. 4th ed. Philadelphia, Lippincott Williams & Wilkins, 2006:739–746). Blood passes through pulmonary capillaries in about 1 s, during which time it is oxygenated and excess carbon dioxide is removed.

ANATOMY

Ventricles

Anatomically, the right ventricle is wrapped halfway around the left ventricle; the semilunar shape of the right ventricle allows it to pump with a minimal shortening of its muscle fibers.

Pulmonary Artery

The pulmonary artery extends only about 4 cm beyond the apex of the right ventricle before division into the right and left main pulmonary arteries. The large diameter and distensibility of the pulmonary arteries allows the pulmonary circulation to easily accommodate the stroke volume of the right ventricle.

Pulmonary Capillaries

The pulmonary capillaries supply the estimated 300 million alveoli, providing a gas-exchange surface of 70 m^2.

Vasomotor Tone

Despite the presence of autonomic nervous system innervation, the resting vasomotor tone is minimal, and the larger pulmonary vessels are almost maximally dilated in the normal resting state.

Pressure Gradients

If alveolar pressure exceeds intravascular pressure, as occurs during positive-pressure ventilation of the lungs, pulmonary capillaries collapse and blood flow ceases.

Bronchial Circulation

After bronchial arterial blood has passed through supporting tissues, the majority of it empties into pulmonary veins and enters the left atrium rather than passing back to the right atrium. The entrance of deoxygenated blood into the left atrium dilutes oxygenated blood and accounts for an anatomic shunt that is equivalent to ~1% to 2% of the cardiac output.

Pulmonary Lymph Vessels

Pulmonary lymphatic flow facilitates the removal of edema fluid from alveolar spaces.

INTRAVASCULAR PRESSURES

Pressures in the pulmonary circulation are about one-fifth those present in the systemic circulation (Fig. 47-1).

Pulmonary Pressure

The normal pressure in the pulmonary artery is about 22/8 mm Hg, with a mean pulmonary artery pressure of

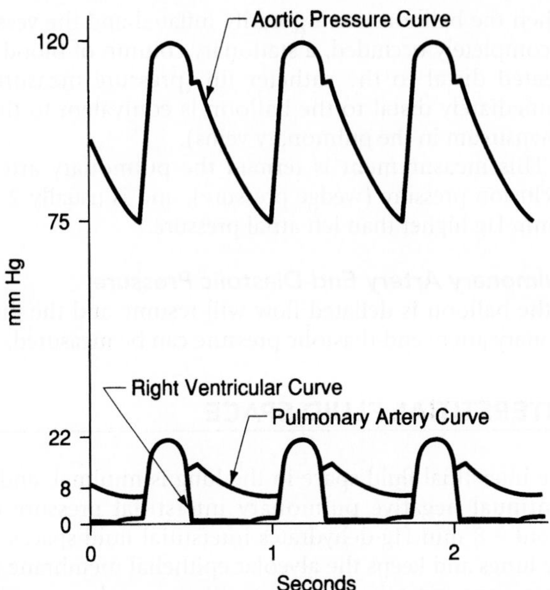

Figure 47-1. Comparison of intravascular pressures in the systemic and pulmonary circulations. (From Guyton AC, Hall JE. *Textbook of Medical Physiology*, 10th ed. Philadelphia: Saunders, 2000; with permission.)

13 mm Hg. The mean pulmonary capillary pressure is about 10 mm Hg, and the mean pressure in the pulmonary veins is about 4 mm Hg, so that the pressure gradient across the pulmonary circulation is only 9 mm Hg.

Overall, the resistance to blood flow in the pulmonary circulation is about one-tenth the resistance in the systemic circulation.

Measurement of Left Atrial Pressure

Pulmonary Artery Occlusion Pressure

The left atrial pressure can be estimated by inserting a balloon-tipped catheter into a small pulmonary artery.

When the balloon is temporarily inflated and the vessel is completely occluded, a stationary column of blood is created distal to the catheter tip (pressure measured immediately distal to the balloon is equivalent to that downstream in the pulmonary veins).

This measurement is termed the pulmonary artery occlusion pressure (wedge pressure), and is usually 2 to 3 mm Hg higher than left atrial pressure.

Pulmonary Artery End-Diastolic Pressure

If the balloon is deflated flow will resume and the pulmonary artery end-diastolic pressure can be measured.

INTERSTITIAL FLUID SPACE

The interstitial fluid space in the lung is minimal, and a continual negative pulmonary interstitial pressure of about −8 mm Hg dehydrates interstitial fluid spaces of the lungs and keeps the alveolar epithelial membrane in close approximation to the capillary membranes. The diffusion distance between gas in the alveoli and the capillary blood is minimal, averaging about 0.4 μm.

Another consequence of negative pressure in pulmonary interstitial spaces is that it pulls fluid from alveoli through alveolar membranes and into interstitial fluid spaces, keeping the alveoli dry.

PULMONARY BLOOD VOLUME

Blood volume in the lungs is about 450 mL. Of this amount, about 70 mL is in capillaries, and the remainder is divided equally between pulmonary arteries and veins.

Postural Changes

Pulmonary blood volume can increase up to 40% when an individual changes from the standing to the supine position (responsible for the decrease in vital capacity in the supine position and the occurrence of orthopnea in the presence of left ventricular failure).

PULMONARY BLOOD FLOW AND DISTRIBUTION

Optimal oxygenation depends on matching ventilation to pulmonary blood flow.

Shunt

Shunt occurs in lung areas that are partially but inadequately perfused, whereas *dead space ventilation* occurs in lung areas that are ventilated but inadequately perfused (Fig. 47-2).

Pao_2

Decreases in Pao_2 cause increases in pulmonary artery and right ventricular pressures.

Endothelial Regulation of Pulmonary Blood Flow

Nitric Oxide

Nitric Oxide (NO) is synthesized in endothelial cells by nitric oxide synthase (NOS). NO diffuses from its site

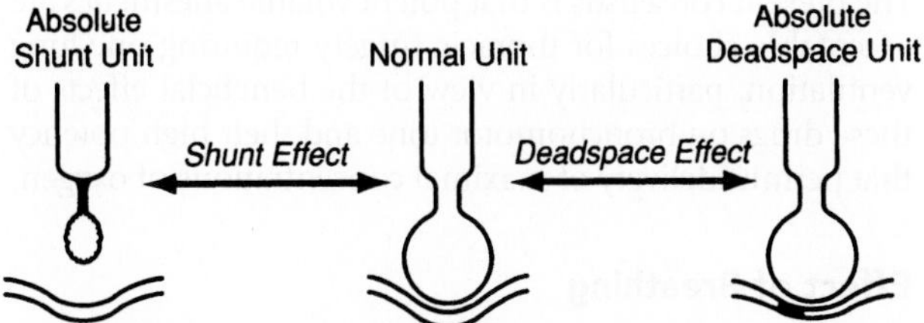

Figure 47-2. Gas exchange is maximally effective in normal lung units with optimal ventilation to perfusion (V/Q) relationships. The continuum of (V/Q) relationships is depicted by the ratios between normal and absolute shunt or dead space units.

of production, usually endothelial cells, into adjacent pulmonary vascular smooth muscle cells. NO induces vasorelaxation by stimulating the production of cyclic guanosine monophosphate (cGMP) by the enzyme guanylate cyclase.

Endothelin

Endothelin is a potent endogenous peptide vasoconstrictor that also promotes smooth muscle proliferation.

Prostacyclin

Prostacyclin is a potent vasodilatory prostaglandin released by the pulmonary endothelium. Prostacyclin is also an extremely potent inhibitor of platelet aggregation and vascular smooth muscle proliferation.

Hypoxic Pulmonary Vasoconstriction

Alveolar hypoxia

Alveolar hypoxia ($Pa{O_2}$ <70 mm Hg) evokes vasoconstriction in the pulmonary arterioles supplying the affected alveoli; the net effect is to divert blood flow away from poorly ventilated alveoli. As a result, the shunt effect is minimized, and the resulting $Pa{O_2}$ is maximized.

One-Lung Ventilation

The present consensus is that potent volatile anesthetics are acceptable choices for thoracic surgery requiring one-lung ventilation, particularly in view of the beneficial effects of these drugs on bronchomotor tone and their high potency that permits delivery of maximal concentrations of oxygen.

Effect of Breathing

Spontaneous Respiration

During spontaneous respiration, venous return to the heart is increased due to the contraction of the diaphragm and abdominal muscles, which decreases intrathoracic pressure.

Positive Pressure Ventilation

In contrast to spontaneous breathing, positive pressure ventilation increases intrathoracic pressure and thus impedes venous return to the heart and decreases right ventricular stroke volume.

Hydrostatic Pressure Gradients

Blood flow to the lungs in the upright position is to a certain extent gravity dependent. Traditionally, the lung is divided into three blood flow zones, reflecting the impact of alveolar pressure, pulmonary artery pressure, and pulmonary venous pressure on the caliber of pulmonary blood vessels (Fig. 47-3).

Topographic Distribution of Pulmonary Blood Flow

The "zone" model of the lung predicts that greater blood flow will occur in those areas of the lung that are below the level of the heart and less flow will occur in areas above the level of the heart. The prediction that

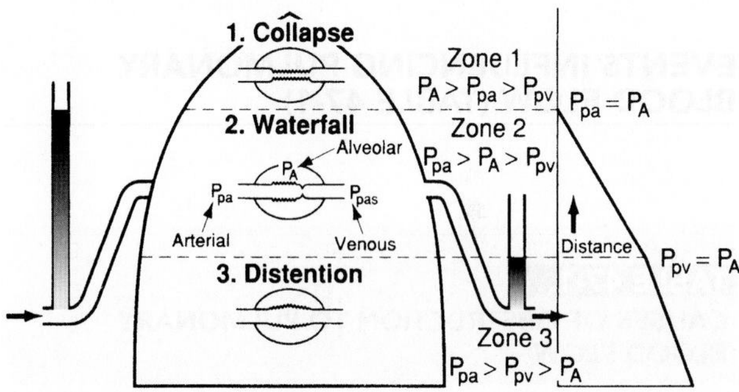

Figure 47-3. The lung is divided into three pulmonary blood flow zones reflecting the impact of alveolar pressure (PA), pulmonary artery pressure (Ppa), and pulmonary venous pressure (Ppv) on the caliber of pulmonary blood vessels. (From West JB, Dollery CT, Naimark A. Distribution of blood flow in isolated lung: relation to vascular and alveolar pressures. *J Appl Physiol* 1964;19:713–718; with permission.)

pulmonary blood flow is uniform in isogravitational planes is incorrect, because other factors predominate over gravitational effects on pulmonary blood flow.

PULMONARY EDEMA

Pulmonary edema is present when excessive quantities of fluid are present, either in pulmonary interstitial spaces or in alveoli.

Causes

The most common cause of acute pulmonary edema is greatly increased pulmonary capillary pressure resulting from left ventricular failure and pooling of blood in the lungs.

Pulmonary edema can also result from the local capillary damage that occurs with inhalation of acidic gastric fluid or irritant gases, such as smoke; this illustrates the difference between *permeability* pulmonary edema in contrast to *hydrostatic* pulmonary edema.

EVENTS INFLUENCING PULMONARY BLOOD FLOW (TABLE 47-1)

TABLE 47-1.
CAUSES OF OBSTRUCTION TO PULMONARY BLOOD FLOW

Pulmonary embolism (tachypnea and dyspnea, vasospasm)
Atelectasis
Pulmonary emphysema (pulmonary hypertension)
Anthracosis (pulmonary hypertension with exercise)

Heart

48

CARDIAC PHYSIOLOGY

The heart can be characterized as a pulsatile four-chamber pump composed of two atria (primer pumps to the ventricles) and two ventricles (power pumps) (Stoelting RK, Hillier SC. Heart. In: *Pharmacology and Physiology in Anesthetic Practice*. 4th ed. Philadelphia, Lippincott Williams & Wilkins, 2006:747–758). *Systole* means "contraction" and is the time interval between closure of the tricuspid and mitral valves and closure of the pulmonary and aortic valves. *Diastole* is a period of relaxation corresponding to the interval between the closure of the pulmonary and aortic valves and the closure of the tricuspid and mitral valves.

Cardiac Muscle

Syncytium Cells

Cardiac muscle is a *syncytium,* in which the cells are so tightly bound together that when one of these cells becomes excited, the action potential spreads to all of them.

Atrioventricular Bundle

The cardiac action potential is conducted from the atrial syncytium to the ventricular syncytium by a specialized conduction pathway known as the atrioventricular bundle.

Cardiac Action Potential

The normal cardiac action potential results from time-dependent changes in the permeability of cardiac muscle

TABLE 48-1.
ION MOVEMENT DURING PHASES OF THE CARDIAC ACTION POTENTIAL

Phase	Ion	Movement Across Cell Membranes
0	Sodium	In
1	Potassium	Out
	Chloride	In
2	Calcium	In
	Potassium	Out
3	Potassium	Out
4	Sodium	In

cell membranes to sodium, potassium, calcium, and chloride ions during phases 0 to 4 of the action potential (Table 48-1) (Fig. 48-1).

Depolarization

In nonpacemaker contractile atrial and ventricular cardiac cells, phase 4 is constant during diastole, and these cells remain at rest until activated by a propagated cardiac impulse or an external stimulus. In contrast, pacemaker cardiac cells exhibit spontaneous phase 4 depolarization until the threshold potential is reached (about −70 mV), resulting in self-excitation and the propagation of a cardiac action potential.

The rate of depolarization during phase 0 is referred to as V_{max} (reflection of myocardial contractility).

Frequency of Discharge

The frequency of discharge of cardiac pacemaker cells is determined by the rate of phase 4 depolarization, the threshold potential, and the resting transmembrane potential (Fig. 48-2).

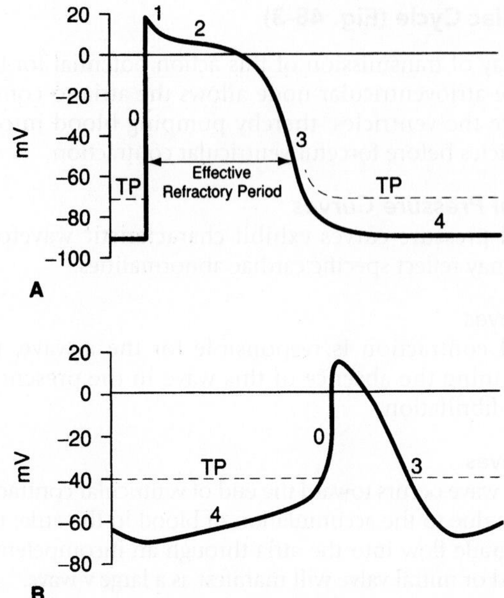

Figure 48-1. Cardiac action potential recorded from a ventricular contractile cell **(A)** or an atrial pacemaker cell **(B)**. (TP, threshold potential.)

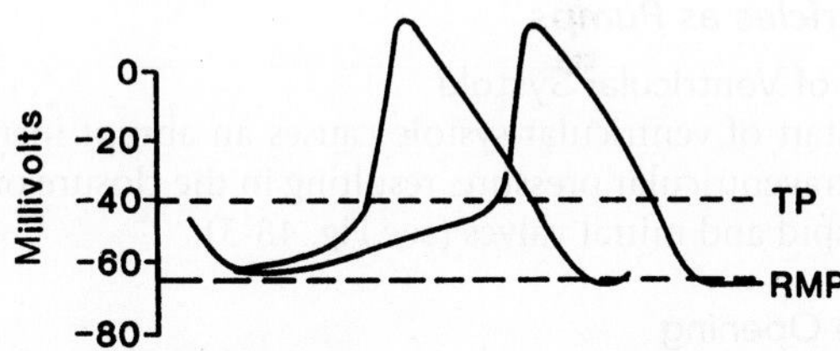

Figure 48-2. The rate of pacemaker discharge is dependent on the slope of spontaneous phase 4 depolarization, negativity of the threshold potential (TP), and negativity of the resting transmembrane potential (RMP).

Cardiac Cycle (Fig. 48-3)

A delay of transmission of this action potential for 0.1 s in the atrioventricular node allows the atria to contract before the ventricles, thereby pumping blood into the ventricles before forceful ventricular contraction.

Atrial Pressure Curves

Atrial pressure curves exhibit characteristic waveforms that may reflect specific cardiac abnormalities.

A Waves

Atrial contraction is responsible for the a wave, thus explaining the absence of this wave in the presence of atrial fibrillation.

V Waves

The v wave occurs toward the end of ventricular contraction and is due to the accumulation of blood in the atria; thus, retrograde flow into the atria through an incompetent tricuspid or mitral valve will manifest as a large v wave.

Atria as Pumps

At the conclusion of ventricular systole, and when ventricular pressures decrease rapidly, the higher pressures in the atria force the valves open and allow blood to flow rapidly into the ventricles.

Ventricles as Pumps

Start of Ventricular Systole

The start of ventricular systole causes an abrupt increase in intraventricular pressure, resulting in the closure of the tricuspid and mitral valves (see Fig. 48-3).

Valve Opening

An additional 0.02 to 0.03 s is required for each ventricle to develop sufficient pressure to open the pulmonary and aortic valves, which are kept closed by the back pressure of blood in the pulmonary artery and aorta (isovolemic contraction).

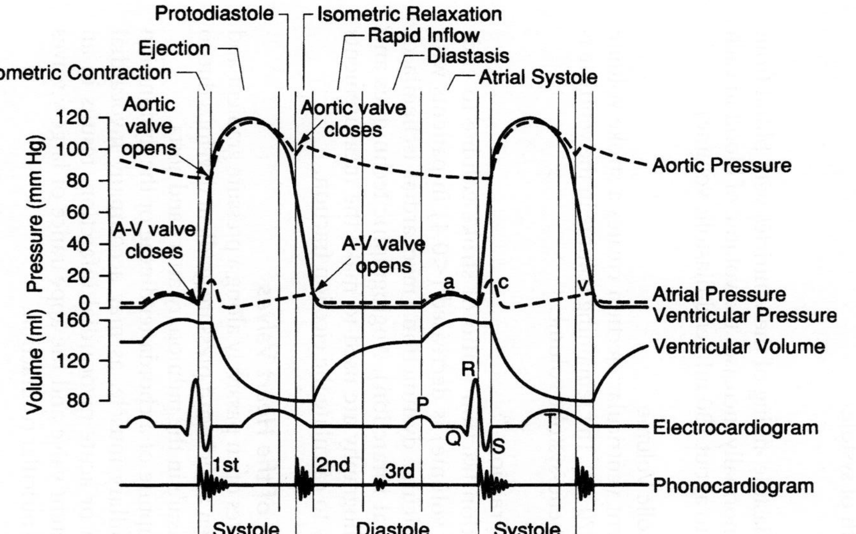

Figure 48-3. Events of the cardiac cycle, including changes in intravascular pressures, ventricular volume, electrocardiogram, and phonocardiogram. (A-V, atrioventricular.) (From Guyton AC, Hall JE. *Textbook of Medical Physiology*, 10th ed. Philadelphia: Saunders, 2000; with permission.)

Ventricular Ejection

When intraventricular pressures are sufficient, the pulmonary and aortic valves open, and about 60% of the total ventricular ejection of blood occurs during the first one-fourth of systole.

Diastole

During diastole, filling of the ventricles with blood from the atria normally increases the volume of blood in each ventricle to about 130 mL (end-diastolic volume).

End-Systolic Volume

Subsequent ventricular ejection creates a stroke volume of about 70 mL. The remaining volume in the ventricle is called the end-systolic volume.

Ejection Fraction

The ejection fraction (ratio of stroke volume to end-diastolic volume) is decreased (<0.4) in patients with left ventricular dysfunction (myocardial ischemia or myocardial infarction). Angiographic techniques and echocardiography are used to make the measurements necessary to calculate the ejection fraction.

Function of the Heart Valves

Heart valves open passively along a pressure gradient and close when a backward pressure gradient develops due to high pressure in the pulmonary artery and aorta.

The rupture of a chorda tendineae or the dysfunction of a papillary muscle, as may accompany myocardial ischemia or acute myocardial infarction, results in an incompetent valve and the appearance of large v waves during ventricular contraction.

Work of the Heart

The heart accounts for 12% of total body heat production, although it represents only 0.5% of the body weight. The energy required for the work of the heart is derived mainly from the metabolism of fatty acids.

Intrinsic Autoregulation of Cardiac Function

The intrinsic ability of the heart to adapt to changing venous return (preload) reflects the increased stretch of cardiac muscle produced by an increased filling of the ventricles from the atria (Frank-Starling law of the heart).

Neural Control of the Heart

Innervation

The atria are abundantly innervated by the sympathetic and parasympathetic nervous systems, but the ventricles are supplied principally by the sympathetic nervous system.

Sympathetic Nervous System Stimulation

Maximal sympathetic nervous system stimulation can increase cardiac output by about 100% above normal.

CORONARY BLOOD FLOW

Systolic Interruption of Flow

Unique features of coronary blood flow include the interruption of blood flow during systole, due to mechanical compression of vessels by myocardial contraction and the absence of anastomoses between the left and right coronary arteries.

Maximal Oxygen Extraction

Another characteristic of the coronary circulation is the maximal oxygen extraction (about 70%) that occurs, resulting in a coronary venous oxygen saturation of about 30%.

Anatomy of the Coronary Circulation (Fig. 48-4)

Coronary Arteries

Coronary arteries lie predominantly on the epicardial surface of the heart and serve principally as conductance vessels that offer little resistance to coronary blood flow.

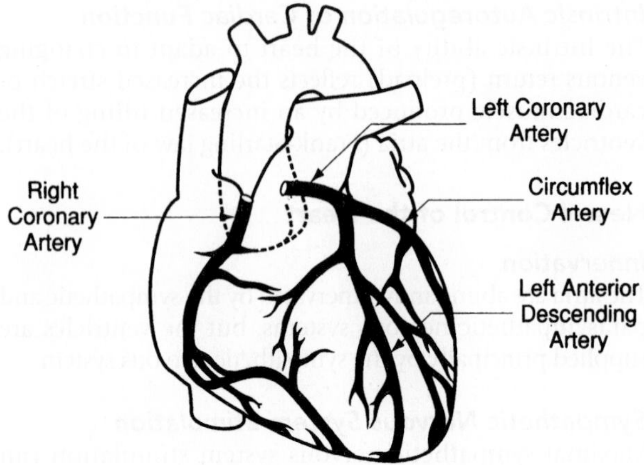

Figure 48-4. Anatomy of the coronary circulation.

Coronary Arterioles

The second type of vessels are small coronary arterioles that ramify throughout the cardiac muscle. These arterioles impose a highly variable resistance and regulate the distribution of blood flow in the myocardium.

Atherosclerosis

Atherosclerosis characterized as coronary artery disease involves the epicardial coronary arteries and not the coronary arterioles.

Coronary Blood Flow

It is estimated that at least 75% of total coronary blood flow occurs during diastole.

Systolic Blood Flow

During systole, blood flow through the subendocardial arteries of the left ventricle decreases to almost zero, which is consistent with the observation that the subendocardial region of the left ventricle is the most common site for myocardial infarction.

Tachycardia

Tachycardia, with an associated decrease in the time for coronary blood flow to occur during diastole, further jeopardizes the adequacy of myocardial oxygen delivery, particularly if coronary arteries are narrowed by atherosclerosis.

Determinants of Coronary Blood Flow (Table 48-2)

Myocardial Oxygen Consumption

Sympathetic nervous system stimulation, with associated increases in heart rate, systemic blood pressure, and myocardial contractility, results in increased myocardial oxygen consumption.

Increases in heart rate that shorten diastolic time for coronary blood flow are likely to increase myocardial oxygen consumption more than increases in systemic blood pressure, which are likely to offset increased oxygen demands by enhanced pressure-dependent coronary blood flow.

Increasing venous return (volume work) is the least costly means of increasing cardiac output in terms of myocardial oxygen consumption.

Nervous System Innervation

Coronary arteries contain α-, β-, and histamine receptors.

Coronary Artery Steal

Coronary artery steal is an absolute decrease in collateral-dependent myocardial perfusion at the expense of an

TABLE 48-2.
DETERMINANTS OF CORONARY BLOOD FLOW

Local metabolic needs (especially for oxygen)
Local vasodilator substance (adenosine)
Arterial blood pressure (particularly important in maintaining coronary blood flow through atherosclerotic arteries)

increase in blood flow to a normally perfused area of myocardium, as may follow the drug-induced vasodilation of coronary arterioles.

DYNAMICS OF HEART SOUNDS

First and Second Heart Sounds

The closure of the mitral and tricuspid valves produces the first heart sound, whereas the second heart sound is due to the closure of the aortic and pulmonary valves (Fig. 48-5).

Fourth Heart Sound

The fourth heart sound is caused by a rapid inflow of blood into the ventricles due to atrial contraction.

Abnormal Heart Sounds (Table 48-3)

CONDUCTION OF CARDIAC IMPULSES (FIG. 48-6)

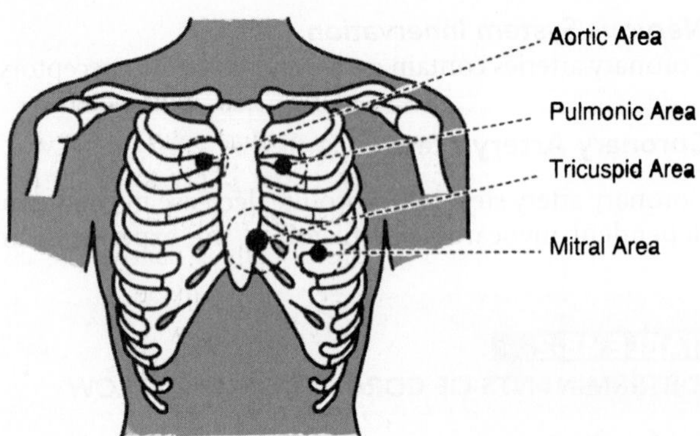

Figure 48-5. Optimal sites for auscultation of heart sounds due to opening or closure of specific cardiac valves. (From Guyton AC, Hall JE. *Textbook of Medical Physiology*, 10th ed. Philadelphia: Saunders, 2000; with permission.)

TABLE 48-3.
HEART MURMURS

	Timing of Murmur*
Aortic stenosis	Systole
Aortic regurgitation	Diastole
Mitral stenosis	Diastole
Mitral regurgitation	Systole
Patent ductus arteriosus	Continuous
Atrial septal defect	Systole
Ventricular septal defect	Systole

*Pulmonary and tricuspid stenosis or regurgitation produces murmurs during the cardiac cycle corresponding to the similar aortic or mitral valve abnormality.

Sinoatrial Node

The sinoatrial node is a specialized cardiac muscle that is continuous with atrial fibers, so that a cardiac action potential that begins in the sinoatrial node spreads immediately into the atria.

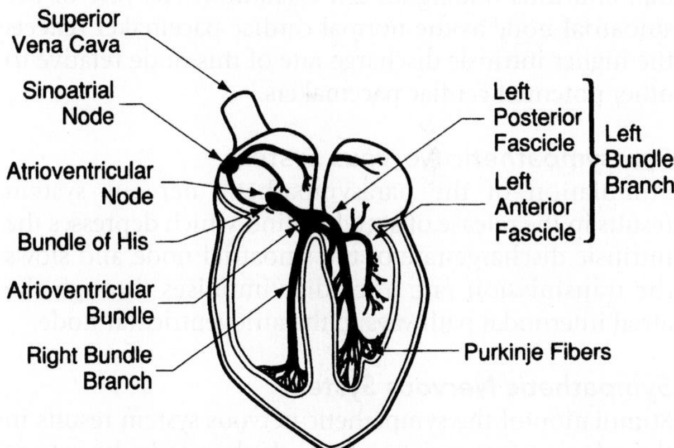

Figure 48-6. Anatomy of the conduction system for transmission of cardiac impulses.

Internodal Pathways

Internodal pathways conduct cardiac impulses from the sinoatrial to the atrioventricular node more rapidly than in the general mass of atrial muscle.

Atrioventricular Node

A delay of transmission of cardiac impulses occurs in the atrioventricular node that allows the atria to empty blood into the ventricles before ventricular systole is initiated.

Purkinje Fibers

Purkinje fibers that pass from the atrioventricular node through the atrioventricular bundle and into the ventricles are large fibers that transmit cardiac impulses so rapidly that both ventricles contract at almost exactly the same time.

Cardiac Pacemakers

A cardiac pacemaker cell is one that undergoes spontaneous phase 4 depolarization to reach threshold potential, and thus undergoes self-excitation. The role of the sinoatrial node as the normal cardiac pacemaker reflects the higher intrinsic discharge rate of this node relative to other potential cardiac pacemakers.

Parasympathetic Nervous System

Stimulation of the parasympathetic nervous system results in the release of acetylcholine, which depresses the intrinsic discharge rate of the sinoatrial node and slows the transmission rate of cardiac impulses through the atrial internodal pathways to the atrioventricular node.

Sympathetic Nervous System

Stimulation of the sympathetic nervous system results in the release of norepinephrine, which speeds the rate of spontaneous phase 4 depolarization and thus increases the intrinsic rate of discharge of the sinoatrial node.

CIRCULATORY EFFECTS OF HEART DISEASE

Valvular Heart Disease

Valvular heart disease produces circulatory effects related to volume overload (regurgitant lesions) or pressure overload (stenotic lesions) of the atria or ventricles.

Congenital Heart Disease

Congenital heart disease produces circulatory effects predominantly due to the presence of a left-to-right or right-to-left intracardiac shunt.

Left-to-Right Intracardiac Shunt

Pulmonary blood flow is greatly increased in the presence of a left-to-right intracardiac shunt, necessitating an increased cardiac output that often leads to cardiac failure.

Right-to-Left Intracardiac Shunt

Right-to-left intracardiac shunts are characterized by decreased pulmonary blood flow, direct return of venous blood to the systemic circulation, and chronic arterial hypoxemia.

Aortic Valve Disease

Aortic stenosis or aortic regurgitation results in a decrease in forward left ventricular stroke volume. Compensatory responses to offset this decreased cardiac output include left ventricular hypertrophy (four to five times normal size) and an increased circulating blood volume that facilitates venous return.

Myocardial Ischemia

Myocardial ischemia is often present, reflecting inadequate coronary blood flow due to higher intraventricular pressures (aortic stenosis) or low diastolic pressures (aortic regurgitation).

Mitral Valve Disease

Mitral stenosis or mitral regurgitation results in an accumulation of blood in the left atrium and accompanying increases in left atrial pressure.

Pulmonary Edema

Pulmonary edema is likely when left atrial pressure exceeds 30 mm Hg.

Atrial Fibrillation

Increased left atrial pressure predisposes to atrial fibrillation, because the associated enlargement of the left atrium increases the distance cardiac impulses must travel, thus increasing the likelihood of reentry.

Patent Ductus Arteriosus

Patent ductus arteriosus results in the backward flow of blood from the aorta into the pulmonary artery. Increased pulmonary blood flow results in increased pulmonary artery pressures and right ventricular hypertrophy.

Atrial Septal Defect

Increased pulmonary blood flow due to an atrial septal defect via a patent foramen ovale or a defect in the atrial septum eventually results in pulmonary hypertension, right ventricular hypertrophy, and right ventricular failure.

Ventricular Septal Defect

Ventricular septal defect produces a left-to-right intracardiac shunt leading to right ventricular hypertrophy and, ultimately, pulmonary hypertension.

Tetralogy of Fallot

Tetralogy of Fallot is the classic cause of right-to-left intracardiac shunt.

Abnormalities associated with tetralogy of Fallot include an aorta that overrides the interventricular septum, pulmonary artery narrowing, a ventricular septal defect, and right ventricular hypertrophy.

The major physiologic derangement caused by tetralogy of Fallot is shunting of as much as 75% of returning venous blood through the ventricular septal defect directly to the aorta, resulting in decreased pulmonary blood flow and profound arterial hypoxemia, even at birth.

MYOCARDIAL INFARCTION (TABLE 48-4)

Etiology

Humans with coronary artery disease have few collateral communications between the large epicardial coronary arteries. Consequently, acute occlusion of an epicardial coronary artery leads rapidly to transmural infarction.

Cardiac Cell Death

The magnitude of cardiac cell death after a myocardial infarction is determined by the product of the degree of ischemia and metabolism of the heart muscle. This emphasizes the need to avoid sympathetic nervous system stimulation after an acute myocardial infarction.

ANGINA PECTORIS

Angina pectoris occurs when myocardial oxygen requirements exceed delivery, as may occur during exercise or an

TABLE 48-4.
MAJOR CAUSES OF MORTALITY AFTER A MYOCARDIAL INFARCTION

Decreased cardiac output
Pulmonary edema
Ventricular fibrillation
Rupture of the infarcted area

event associated with stimulation of the sympathetic nervous system. Distribution of pain into the arms and neck reflects the embryonic origin of the heart and arms in the neck.

CARDIAC FAILURE

Cardiac failure manifests as decreased cardiac output or pulmonary edema, with selective left ventricular failure occurring 30 times more often than selective right ventricular failure.

Dyspnea

Dyspnea reflects increased left atrial pressure and an accumulation of fluid in the lungs, whereas selective increases in right atrial pressure manifest as hepatomegaly, ascites, and peripheral edema.

Decreased Cardiac Output

Chronic decreases in cardiac output result in the renal-induced retention of fluid in an effort to improve venous return to the heart.

Diastolic Heart Failure

Diastolic dysfunction is an important cause of heart failure, particularly in the elderly population. More than 40% of patients with symptomatic congestive cardiac failure have normal systolic function that is accompanied by diminished diastolic function.

Perioperative diastolic dysfunction may reduce the patient's ability to tolerate perioperative changes in blood volume, heart rate and rhythm, and positive pressure ventilation.

The Electrocardiogram and Analysis of Cardiac Dysrhythmias

49

ELECTROCARDIOGRAM

Because body fluids are good conductors, it is possible to record the sum of the action potentials of myocardial fibers on the surface of the body through the electrocardiogram (ECG) (Table 49-1) (Stoelting RK, Hillier SC. The electrocardiogram and analysis of cardiac dysrhythmias. In: *Pharmacology and Physiology in Anesthetic Practice.* 4th ed. Philadelphia, Lippincott Williams & Wilkins, 2006:759–768). The normal ECG consists of a P-wave (atrial depolarization), a QRS complex (ventricular depolarization), and a T-wave (ventricular repolarization) (Fig. 49-1).

Recording the Electrocardiogram

Grid Paper

Paper used for recording the ECG is designed such that each horizontal line corresponds to 0.1 mV and each vertical line corresponds to 0.04 s, assuming proper calibration and paper speed of the recording device (see Fig. 49-1).

Duration of Events

The duration of events during the conduction of the cardiac impulse can be calculated from a recording of the ECG (Table 49-1).

TABLE 49-1.

INTERVALS AND CORRESPONDING EVENTS ON THE ELECTROCARDIOGRAM

	Average	Range	Events in Heart
P-R interval* (s)	0.18	0.12–0.20	Atrial depolarization and conduction through the atrioventricular node
QRS duration (s)	0.08	0.05–0.10	Ventricular depolarization
Q-T interval* (s)	0.40	0.26–0.45	Ventricular depolarization and repolarization
S-T segment (s)	0.32		

*Dependent on heart rate.

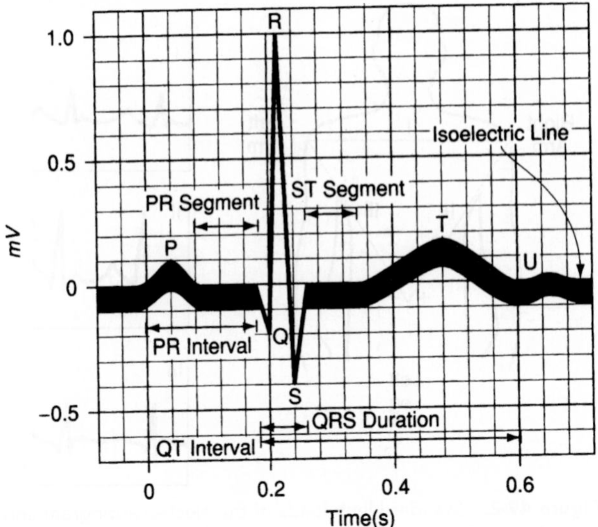

Figure 49-1. The normal waves and intervals on the electrocardiogram.

P-R Interval

The interval between the beginning of atrial contraction and the beginning of ventricular contraction is the P-R interval. The P-R interval depends on heart rate, averaging 0.18 s at a rate of 70 beats/minute and 0.14 s at a rate of 130 beats/minute.

QRS Complex and Q-T Interval

The QRS complex reflects ventricular depolarization, whereas the Q-T interval represents the time necessary for complete depolarization and repolarization of the ventricle. Like the P-R interval, the Q-T interval depends on heart rate.

Electrocardiogram Leads (Fig. 49-2)

Chest Leads (Table 49-2)

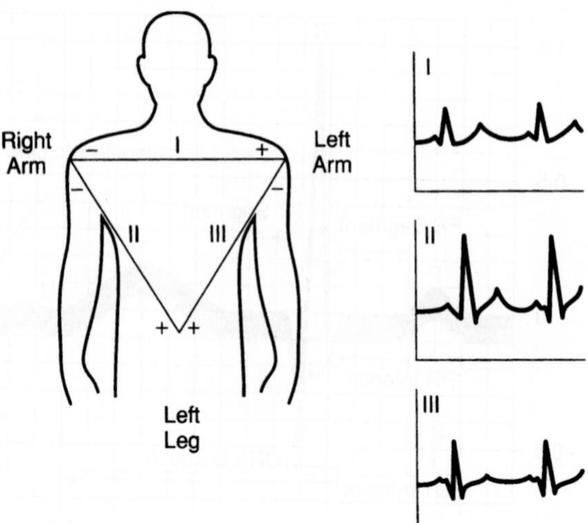

Figure 49-2. Standard limb leads of the electrocardiogram and typical recordings.

Auqmented Limb Leads

Augmented limb leads are similar to the standard limb leads except that the recording from the right-arm lead (aVR) is inverted. When the positive terminal is on the right arm, the lead is aVR; when on the left arm, the lead is aVL; and when on the left leg, the lead is aVF.

TABLE 49-2.
PLACEMENT OF PRECORDIAL LEADS

V1	Fourth intercostal space at the right sternal border
V2	Fourth intercostal space at the left sternal border
V3	Equidistant between V2 and V4
V4	Fifth intercostal space in the left midclavicular line
V5	Fifth intercostal space in the left anterior axillary line
V6	Fifth intercostal space in the left midaxillary line

Interpretation of the Electrocardiogram

Abnormalities

Abnormalities of the heart can be detected by analyzing the contours of the different waves in the various ECG leads. When one ventricle of the heart hypertrophies, the axis of the heart shifts toward the enlarged ventricle. The predominant direction of the vector through the heart during depolarization and repolarization of the ventricles is from the base to the apex.

Abnormalities of the QRS Complex

Hypertrophy of Ventricles

Hypertrophy of the ventricles prolongs the duration of the QRS complex (>0.1 s), reflecting the longer pathway the ventricular depolarization wave must travel.

Blockade of Purkinje Fibers

A blockade of the Purkinje fibers necessary for the conduction of the cardiac impulse greatly slows conduction and prolongs the duration of the QRS complex.

Ventricular Hypertrophy

The most frequent cause of high-voltage QRS complexes (>4 mV) is ventricular hypertrophy.

Decreased Voltage in the Standard Limb Leads (Table 49-3)

Current of Injury

A current of injury is due to the inability of damaged areas of the heart to undergo repolarization during diastole.

Myocardial Ischemia

Specific leads of the ECG are more likely than others to reflect myocardial ischemia that develops in those areas of the myocardium supplied by an individual coronary artery (Table 49-4).

TABLE 49-3.
CAUSES OF DECREASED VOLTAGE ON THE ELECTROCARDIOGRAM RECORDED FROM STANDARD LIMB LEADS

Multiple small myocardial infarctions
Rotation of the apex of the heart toward the anterior chest wall
Abnormal conditions around the heart
- Pericardial fluid
- Pulmonary emphysema

S-T Segment

An estimated 80% to 90% of S-T segment information contained in the conventional 12-lead ECG is present on lead V5.

Cardiac Dysrhythmias

Lead II has special value in the diagnosis of inferior wall myocardial ischemia and the origin of cardiac dysrhythmias.

Myocardial Infarction

Infarction of the cardiac muscle results in a deep Q-wave in the ECG leads recording from the infarcted area. The Q-wave occurs because no electrical activity is present in the infarcted area.

Anterior Wall Myocardial Infarction

In the presence of an old anterior wall myocardial infarction, a Q-wave develops in lead I because of loss of muscle mass in the anterior wall of the left ventricle.

Posterior Wall Myocardial Infarction

In posterior wall myocardial infarction, a Q-wave develops in lead III because of the loss of cardiac muscle in the posterior apical part of the ventricles.

TABLE 49-4.

RELATIONSHIP OF THE ELECTROCARDIOGRAM LEAD REFLECTING MYOCARDIAL ISCHEMIA TO THE AREAS OF MYOCARDIUM INVOLVED

Electrocardiogram Lead	Coronary Artery Responsible for Ischemia	Area of Myocardium Supplied by Coronary Artery
II, III, aVF	Right coronary artery	Right atrium Interatrial septum Right ventricle Sinoatrial node Atrioventricular node Inferior wall of left ventricle
V3–V6	Left anterior descending coronary artery	Anterior and lateral wall of left ventricle
I, aVL	Circumflex coronary artery	Lateral wall of left ventricle Sinoatrial node Atrioventricular node

Abnormalities of the T-Wave

The T-wave becomes abnormal when the normal sequence of repolarization does not occur.

Myocardial ischemia is the most common cause of prolonged depolarization of cardiac muscle. Myocardial ischemia also leads to elevation of the S-T segment on the ECG. To be clinically significant, the S-T elevation should be at least 1 mm above the baseline.

CARDIAC DYSRHYTHMIAS (TABLE 49-5)

Mechanisms (Table 49-6)

Perioperative Cardiac Dysrhythmias

Perioperative cardiac dysrhythmias are most likely to occur in patients with preexisting heart disease (coronary artery disease, valvular heart disease, cardiomyopathies) in the presence of a transient physiologic imbalance (ischemia, catecholamines, electrolyte abnormalities, laryngoscopy, and tracheal intubation).

TABLE 49-5.
DIAGNOSIS OF CARDIAC DYSRHYTHMIAS FROM THE ELECTROCARDIOGRAM

Are P-waves present, and what is their relationship to the QRS complexes?
Are the amplitudes, durations, and contours of the P-waves, P-R intervals, QRS complexes, and Q-T intervals normal?
During tachycardia, is the R-P long and P-R interval short (or vice versa)?
What are the atrial and ventricular discharge rates (same or different)?
Are the P-P and R-R intervals regular or irregular?

Adapted from Atlee JL. Perioperative cardiac dysrhythmias: diagnosis and management. *Anesthesiology* 1997; 86:1397–1424.

TABLE 49-6.
MECHANISMS OF CARDIAC DYSRHYTHMIAS

Altered automaticity of pacemaker cardiac cells
Ectopic pacemaker (premature contraction, focal area of myocardial ischemia)
Altered excitability of myocardial cells
Altered conduction of cardiac impulses through specialized conduction systems of the heart
- Heart block (atrioventricular bundle or one of the bundle branches)
- Excessive parasympathetic nervous system stimulation
- Drug-induced (digitalis, β-adrenergic antagonists)
- Myocardial infarction
- Age-related degeneration

Reentry
- Preexcitation syndromes

Anesthesia
- Nodal rhythm and increased ventricular automaticity
- Altered sinoatrial node automaticity and prolonged His-Purkinje conductions times

Autonomic nervous system imbalance (drugs, surgical stimulation)

Manifestations of these alterations may be the appearance of an ectopic cardiac pacemaker, development of heart block, or appearance of a reentry circuit.

Type of Cardiac Dysrhythmias

Sinus Tachycardia

Sinus tachycardia (heart rate >100 beats/minute) is often due to sympathetic nervous system stimulation, as may occur during a noxious stimulus in the presence of low concentrations of anesthetic drugs.

Body Temperature

Increased body temperature increases the heart rate by approximately 18 beats/minute for every degree Celsius increase.

Carotid Sinus–Mediated Reflex Stimulation

Carotid sinus–mediated reflex stimulation of the heart rate accompanies decreases in systemic blood pressure as produced by vasodilator drugs or acute hemorrhage.

Sinus Bradycardia

Sinus bradycardia (heart rate <60 beats/minute) accompanies parasympathetic nervous system stimulation of the heart. Bradycardia that occurs in physically conditioned athletes reflects the ability of their hearts to eject a greater stroke volume with each contraction, compared with the less conditioned heart.

Sinus Dysrhythmias

Sinus dysrhythmias are present during normal breathing with the heart rate (R-R intervals) varying approximately 5% during various phases of the resting breathing cycle; this most likely reflects baroreceptor reflex activity and changes in the negative intrapleural pressures that elicit a waxing and waning Bainbridge reflex. The absence of phasic changes suggests autonomic nervous system dysfunction, as may accompany diabetes mellitus.

Atrioventricular Heart Block

First-Degree Atrioventricular Heart Block

First-degree atrioventricular heart block is considered to be present when the P-R interval is >0.2 s at a normal heart rate.

Second-Degree Atrioventricular Heart Block

Second-degree atrioventricular heart block is classified as Wenckebach phenomenon (type I) or Mobitz (type II) heart block. Wenckebach phenomenon is characterized by a progressive prolongation of the P-R interval until conduction of the cardiac impulse is completely interrupted and a P-wave is recorded without a subsequent QRS complex. Mobitz heart block is the occurrence of a nonconducted atrial impulse without a prior change in the P-R interval.

Third-Degree Atrioventricular Heart Block

Third-degree atrioventricular heart block occurs during a complete block of the transmission of cardiac impulses from the atria to the ventricles. The P-waves are dissociated from the QRS complexes, and the heart rate depends on the intrinsic discharge rate of the ectopic pacemaker beyond the site of conduction block. If the ectopic pacemaker is near the atrioventricular node, the QRS complexes appear normal, and the heart rate is typically 40 to 60 beats/minute. When the site of the block is infranodal, the escape ventricular pacemaker often has a discharge rate of <40 beats/minute, and the QRS complexes are wide, resembling a bundle branch block. Occasionally, the interval of ventricular standstill at the onset of third-degree heart block is so long that death occurs. Temporary cardiac pacing may be provided through an intravenous infusion of isoproterenol (a chemical cardiac pacemaker) or a transvenous artificial cardiac pacemaker.

Premature Atrial Contractions

Premature atrial contractions are recognized by an abnormal P-wave and a shortened P-R interval. Premature atrial contractions are usually benign and often occur in individuals without heart disease.

Premature Nodal Contractions

Premature nodal contractions are characterized by the absence of P-waves preceding the QRS complexes.

Premature Ventricular Contractions

Premature ventricular contractions result from an ectopic pacemaker in the ventricles.

The QRS complex of the ECG is typically prolonged, because the cardiac impulse is conducted mainly through the slowly conducting muscle of the ventricle rather than the Purkinje fibers.

A compensatory pause after a premature ventricular contraction occurs because the first impulse from the sinoatrial node reaches the ventricle during its refractory period. When a premature ventricular contraction occurs, the ventricle may not have filled adequately with blood, and the stroke volume resulting from this contraction fails to produce a detectable pulse.

Premature ventricular contractions often reflect significant cardiac disease (myocardial ischemia).

Atrial Paroxysmal Tachycardia

Atrial paroxysmal tachycardia is caused by the rapid rhythmic discharge of impulses from an ectopic atrial pacemaker. The rhythm on the ECG is perfectly regular, and the P-waves are abnormal, often inverted, indicating a site of origin other than the sinoatrial node.

Typically, the onset of atrial paroxysmal tachycardia is abrupt (a single beat) and may end just as suddenly with the pacemaker shifting back to the sinoatrial node.

Atrial paroxysmal tachycardia can be terminated by producing parasympathetic nervous system stimulation at the heart with drugs (adenosine) or by unilateral external pressure applied to the carotid sinus.

Nodal Paroxysmal Tachycardia

Nodal paroxysmal tachycardia resembles atrial paroxysmal tachycardia, except P-waves are not identifiable on the ECG.

Ventricular Tachycardia

Ventricular tachycardia on the ECG resembles a series of ventricular premature contractions that occur at a rapid and regular rate. Stroke volume is often severely depressed during ventricular tachycardia, because the ventricles have insufficient time for cardiac filling.

Sustained ventricular tachycardia may necessitate termination using electrical cardioversion.

This cardiac dysrhythmia predisposes to ventricular fibrillation.

Atrial Flutter

Atrial flutter on the ECG is characterized by the 2:1, 3:1, or 4:1 conduction of atrial impulses to the ventricle. P-waves have a characteristic saw-toothed appearance, especially in leads II, III, aVF, and V1.

Atrial Fibrillation

Atrial fibrillation is characterized by normal QRS complexes occurring at a rapid and irregular rate in the absence of identifiable P-waves. Stroke volume is decreased during atrial fibrillation, because the ventricles do not have sufficient time to fill optimally between cardiac cycles.

A pulse deficit (heart rate by palpation is less than that calculated from the ECG) reflects the inability of each ventricular contraction to eject a sufficient stroke volume to produce a detectable peripheral pulse.

A risk of thromboembolism exists in patients with atrial fibrillation who are not treated with anticoagulants.

Ventricular Fibrillation

Ventricular fibrillation on the ECG is characterized by an irregular wavy line with voltages that range from 0.25 to 0.5 mV. A total incoordination of contractions occurs, with cessation of any effective pumping activity and disappearance of detectable systemic blood pressure.

The only effective treatment of ventricular fibrillation is the delivery of direct electric current through the ventricles (defibrillation), which simultaneously depolarizes all ventricular muscle. This depolarization allows the reestablishment of a cardiac pacemaker at a site other than the irritable focus that was responsible for ventricular fibrillation.

The Lungs

50

ANATOMY

Thoracic Cage

The thoracic cage is composed of 12 thoracic vertebral bodies, the ribs, and the sternum (Stoelting RK, Hillier SC. The lungs. In: *Pharmacology and Physiology in Anesthetic Practice*. 4th ed. Philadelphia, Lippincott Williams & Wilkins, 2006:769–780). The suprasternal notch (upper border of the manubrium between the sternoclavicular joints) is in the same horizontal plane as the midportion of the second thoracic vertebra.

Tracheal Tube Placement

The second thoracic vertebra is a useful radiologic landmark because it corresponds to the midportion of the trachea, which is a desirable location for the distal tip of a tracheal tube.

External palpation of tracheal tube cuff inflation in the suprasternal notch is an indirect method for confirming that the distal end of a tracheal tube is properly positioned above the carina.

Trachea

The adult trachea is a fibromuscular tube, approximately 10 to 12 cm in length. It begins at the level of the sixth cervical vertebra and extends downward until it bifurcates at the carina, opposite the fifth thoracic vertebra.

Bronchus

The bifurcation of the trachea at the carina gives rise to the right and left main stem bronchus. The right main stem bronchus extends approximately 2.5 cm before its initial division into the bronchus to the right upper and middle lobes with a continuation as the right lower lobe bronchus. The left main stem bronchus extends approximately 5 cm before its initial division.

The short length of the right main stem bronchus increases the technical difficulty in placing a right endobronchial tube (double-lumen tube) without obstructing the orifice to the right upper lobe.

An anomalous right upper lobe bronchus from the trachea (above the carina) is present in approximately 1 in 250 individuals.

Regulation of Airway Caliber

In health, airway caliber is determined actively by the state of contraction of airway smooth muscle and passively by the state of inflation of the lung.

Increased Lung Volume

Increases in lung volume are accompanied by increases in airway diameter because the airways are tethered by the surrounding lung parenchyma. As lung volumes decrease below functional residual capacity (FRC), significant increases in airway resistance occur.

Parasympathetic Stimulation

The pharmacologic blockade of parasympathetic pathways or surgical transection of the vagus nerves causes bronchodilation, demonstrating that airway smooth muscle is tonically contracted by the parasympathetic nerves.

Innervation of Bronchioles

Airway muscle tone is also influenced by nonadrenergic, noncholinergic innervation of the bronchioles. Histamine stimulates H_1 receptors (bronchoconstriction) and H_2 receptors (bronchodilation), but the predominant effect is bronchoconstriction.

TABLE 50-1.
INNERVATION OF THE LARYNX

Sensory Innervation
- Glossopharyngeal nerve (posterior tongue, pharynx)
- Superior laryngeal nerve (epiglottis, larynx to level of false vocal cords)
- Recurrent laryngeal nerve (vocal cords, upper trachea)

Motor Innervation
- Recurrent laryngeal nerve
- Superior laryngeal nerve (cricothyroid muscles)

Innervation of the Larynx (Table 50-1)

Cough Reflex

The administration of general anesthesia, local anesthesia to the airway, opioids, and benzodiazepines, all cause cough reflex suppression. Thus, the clearance of secretions and foreign material from the airway is likely to be impaired during the perioperative period.

Increasing age is associated with depression of the cough reflex.

Sneeze Reflex

The sneeze reflex is similar to the cough reflex except that it facilitates the clearance of secretions from the nasal passageways, rather than passageways below the nose.

MECHANICS OF BREATHING

Diaphragm

The diaphragm is the principal muscle of breathing, accounting for approximately 75% of the air that enters the lungs during spontaneous inspiration. It causes gas flow into the chest by decreasing intrathoracic pressure to less than atmospheric pressure.

Innervation

Motor innervation of the diaphragm is via the phrenic nerves.

Intercostal Muscle

During quiet breathing, the contribution of intercostal muscle contraction to inspiration is small.

Oxygen Cost

The oxygen cost of breathing is usually <5% of minute oxygen consumption. When the rate of breathing increases, or airways are narrowed, a large proportion of work is spent in overcoming the resistance to gas flow.

Exhalation

In contrast to inspiration, normal exhalation is a passive event, utilizing the elastic recoil of the lungs, chest wall, and abdominal structures. An important additional deflating force is the surface tension of the fluid lining the alveoli. Abdominal muscles are the important muscles of exhalation during exertion.

Paralysis of Abdominal Muscles

The paralysis of the abdominal muscles produced by regional anesthesia does not influence resting alveolar ventilation, but the patient's ability to cough and clear secretions may be compromised.

Alveolar Volume and Distribution of Ventilation

Alveolar volume is not uniform throughout the lungs because of differences in the distending pressures to which alveoli are subjected (alveoli in lung apices are more expanded than those at the lung bases).

Nitrogen Washout Test

The distribution of ventilation in the lungs and the volume at which airways in lung bases begin to close can be assessed by the single breath nitrogen washout test (Fig. 50-1).

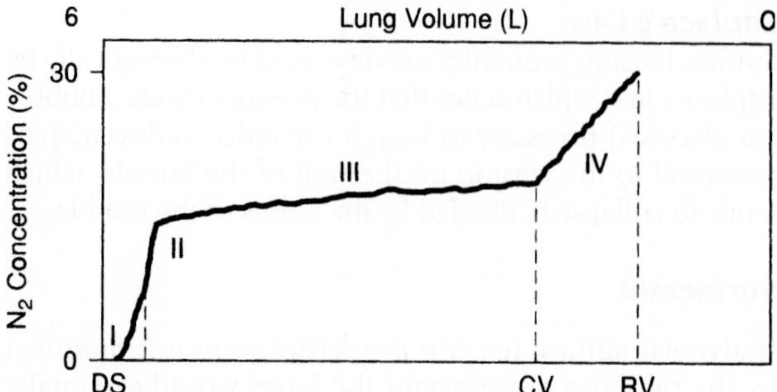

Figure 50-1. Single-breath nitrogen washout curve reflecting dead space volume (phase I), exhalation of alveolar gas (phases II and III), and airway closure in the lung bases (phase IV). (CV, closing volume; DS, dead space; RV, residual volume.)

Pneumothorax

When air enters the pleural space via a rupture in the lung or a hole in the chest wall, the lung on the affected side collapses because of its elastic recoil. The intrapleural pressure on the affected side is now atmospheric, thus shifting the mediastinum towards the normal side, which has a subatmospheric pressure (may cause a kinking of major vessels).

Tension pneumothorax occurs when air is allowed to enter during inspiration but cannot exit during exhalation. As with an open pneumothorax, a shift of the mediastinum occurs toward the intact lung, with a kinking of the great vessels and the development of arterial hypoxemia. Lifesaving treatment is decompression of the pneumothorax by insertion of a chest tube and removing the air.

SURFACE TENSION AND PULMONARY SURFACTANT

Surface Tension

Surface tension results from the attraction between the molecules of the fluid film that lines the alveoli (tends to reduce alveolar diameter).

Laplace's Law

Surface tension properties are described mathematically by Laplace's law, which states that the pressure inside a bubble (or alveolus) necessary to keep it expanded is directly proportional to the tension on the wall of the bubble, which tends to collapse it, divided by the radius of the bubble.

Surfactant

If alveolar surface tension properties were not modified by the presence of surfactant the lungs would eventually become collapsed, stiff, and fluid filled.

Surfactant is a lipoprotein secreted by type II alveolar cells (pneumocytes) lining the alveoli.

Development

Surfactant is first produced between 28 and 32 weeks. When the premature delivery of an infant is anticipated, the formation of pulmonary surfactant may be hastened by the administration of corticosteroids to the parturient.

Composition and Action

The phospholipid component of pulmonary surfactant, dipalmitoyl phosphatidylcholine (DPPC), decreases the surface tension of fluids lining the alveoli. Alveoli with small diameters have a lower surface tension because DPPC molecules densely populate the lining fluid. As an alveolus increases in size, the pulmonary surfactant becomes diluted at the surface of the alveolar lining fluid, thus diminishing its surface tension reducing effect.

Alveolar Size

Pulmonary surfactant helps to stabilize the sizes of alveoli, reducing surface tension in larger alveoli to a lesser extent than in smaller alveoli. The net effect is the maintenance of consistent alveolar diameter and stability.

Respiratory Distress Syndrome

The absence or inadequate amounts of pulmonary surfactant is characteristic of respiratory distress syndrome of the neonate.

Changes in Alveolar Size

When the surface area of the surfactant film is kept small, a rearrangement of molecules occurs, causing surface tension to increase with time. Therefore, peripheral alveoli tend to collapse during prolonged periods of shallow breathing. A single large breath, vital capacity maneuver, or sigh, re-expands these alveoli, increasing their surface area, thus restoring normal surface tension.

COMPLIANCE

Compliance is expressed as the increase in the gas volume of the lungs for each unit increase of alveolar pressure.

LUNG VOLUMES AND CAPACITIES

A lung capacity is the sum of two or more lung volumes (Table 50-2 and Fig. 50-2).

TABLE 50-2.
LUNG VOLUMES AND CAPACITIES

	Abbreviation	Normal Adult Value
Tidal volume	VT	500 (6–8 mL/kg)
Inspiratory reserve volume	IRV	3,000 mL
Expiratory reserve volume	ERV	1,200 mL
Residual volume	RV	1,200 mL
Inspiratory capacity	IC	3,500 mL
Functional residual capacity	FRC	2,400 mL
Vital capacity	VC	4,500 mL (60–70 mL/kg)
Forced exhaled volume in 1 second	FEV_1	80%
Total lung capacity	TLC	5,900 mL

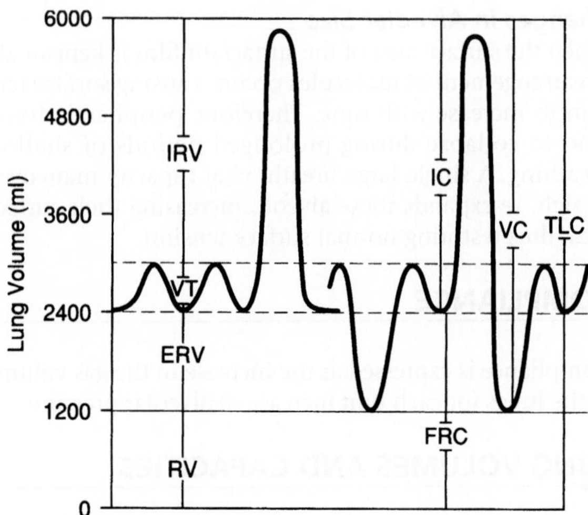

Figure 50-2. Schematic diagram of breathing excursions at rest and during maximal inhalation and/or exhalation (see Table 50-1 for definition of abbreviations). Lung capacities are the sum of two or more lung volumes.

Gender

Lung volumes and capacities are approximately 25% less in females than in males.

Position

Lung volumes and capacities also change with body position, most of them decreasing when the patient is supine and increasing when the patient is standing.

Airway Obstruction

In diseases associated with airway obstruction (asthma, bronchitis, emphysema) it is usually much more difficult to exhale than to inhale; this is associated with gas trapping, which leads to an increased residual volume and total lung capacity.

Functional Residual Capacity

Functional residual capacity (FRC) is the volume remaining in the lungs at the end of a normal quiet expiration.

Normal Function

The FRC buffers alveolar gas tensions against abrupt alterations in $Pa{O_2}$ and $Pa{CO_2}$ during the respiratory cycle. In the presence of a decreased FRC, transient interruptions in breathing, as during direct laryngoscopy, may result in rapid changes in $Pa{O_2}$.

Breathing 100% oxygen offsets the effect of apnea on $Pa{O_2}$, especially when the FRC is decreased, as in the parturient.

Effects of Anesthesia

After the induction of anesthesia and placement of a tracheal tube, a decrease in the FRC occurs of approximately 450 mL, regardless of whether neuromuscular blockade is present.

Reductions in FRC alter the distribution of ventilation so that regional ventilation will be diverted towards the nondependent portions of the lung. Because perfusion remains distributed in a gravity-dependent manner toward the dependent regions, ventilation/perfusion mismatching will occur. These factors, combined with alveolar collapse in dependent regions, are responsible for the right-to-left shunt—equivalent to approximately 10% of the cardiac output—that typically accompanies general anesthesia.

Positive end-expiratory pressure decreases this shunt by reinflating previously collapsed areas of the lung.

Vital Capacity (Table 50-3)

Forced exhaled vital capacity is the volume of gas that can be rapidly and maximally exhaled starting from total lung capacity.

It is customary to measure the volume of exhaled gases after 1 second (FEV_1) and 3 seconds (FEV_3). In normal

TABLE 50-3.
FACTORS INFLUENCING VITAL CAPACITY (VC)

Body build (tall thin person has larger VC than obese person)
Respiratory muscle conditioning (VC larger in athletes)
Fibrotic changes in lungs associated with asthma (decreased VC)
Pulmonary edema (decreased VC)

individuals, the FEV_1 is >80% of the VC (Fig. 50-3). In the presence of obstructive airway disease, this value is <50%.

Midexpiratory Flow Rate

Measurement of the mean airflow rate over the middle half of the forced VC is the forced midexpiratory flow rate

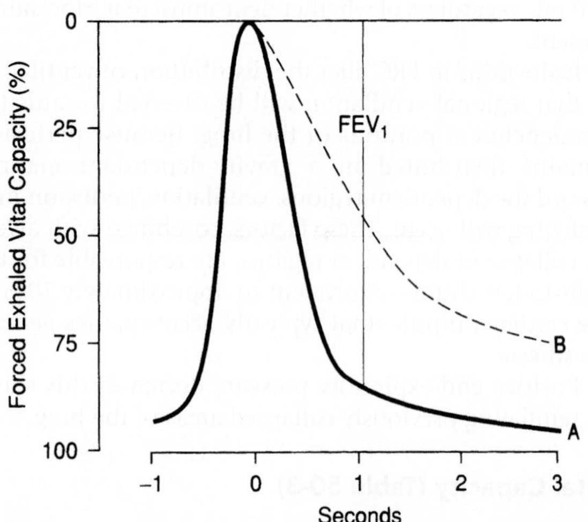

Figure 50-3. Schematic diagram of forced exhaled volume in normal individuals **(A)** and in individuals with obstructive airway disease **(B)**. A normal individual can exhale approximately 80% of the vital capacity in 1 s (FEV_1), compared with approximately 50% in 1 s in individuals with obstructive airway disease.

(MEFR 25%–75%). Reduction in this flow rate is a sensitive index of airway obstruction.

MINUTE VENTILATION

The minute ventilation represents the total amount of gas moved into the lungs each minute (tidal volume times breathing frequency). The average minute ventilation is approximately 6 liters.

Alveolar Ventilation

Alveolar ventilation is the volume of gas each minute that enters those areas of the lungs capable of participating in gas exchange with pulmonary capillary blood.

Alveolar ventilation is less than minute ventilation because a portion of the inhaled gases resides in those portions of the airway (dead space estimated to be 150 mL) that do not participate in gas exchange with pulmonary capillary blood. The $Paco_2$, and to a lesser extent the Pao_2, are determined by alveolar ventilation.

Dead Space

Anatomic Versus Physiologic Dead Space

Anatomic dead space includes those areas of the respiratory tract (nasal passageways, pharynx, trachea, and bronchi) that do not normally participate in gas exchange with pulmonary capillary blood. Physiologic dead space is the gas volume of alveoli that are not functional or only partially functional because of absent or poor blood flow through corresponding pulmonary capillaries (wasted ventilation).

Gas Exchange

Gas being exhaled from dead space (2 mL/kg or approximately 150 mL in an adult) contains no nitrogen (see Fig. 50-1). During exhalation, gas in dead space is exhaled before gas coming from the alveoli.

Anesthetic Breathing Systems

Anesthetic breathing systems are designed to preferentially conserve dead space gas (oxygen and anesthetic are not removed, and the gas is devoid of carbon dioxide) and to eliminate alveolar gas (oxygen and anesthetic are depleted, and carbon dioxide is added).

Conceptually, rebreathing dead space gas is similar to delivering fresh gases from the anesthesia machine.

CONTROL OF VENTILATION

Many of the drugs used in the perioperative period to provide anesthesia, amnesia, and analgesia have profound effects upon the control of ventilation (respiratory depression).

Chemoreceptors

The fine control of ventilation is provided by the respiratory center under the influence of chemical stimuli from chemoreceptors.

$Pa{CO_2}$

The major factor in the regulation of alveolar ventilation is the $Pa{CO_2}$ rather than the $Pa{O_2}$. A 50% increase in $Pa{CO_2}$ evokes a tenfold increase in alveolar ventilation, and a $Pa{O_2}$ of 40 mm Hg evokes a 1.5-fold increase in alveolar ventilation.

Medullary Vasomotor Center

The stimulation of the medullary vasomotor center is associated with a spillover of impulses to the nearby respiratory center (decreases in systemic blood pressure, which evoke increases in sympathetic nervous system activity from the vasomotor center; also evoke increases in alveolar ventilation due to the increased activity of the respiratory center).

Respiratory Center (Fig. 50-4)

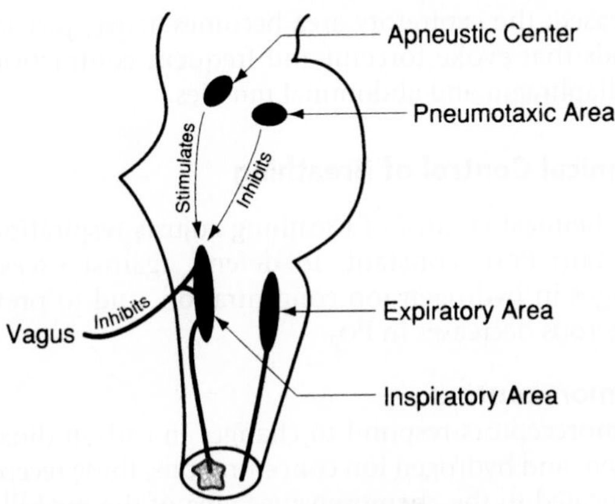

Figure 50-4. The respiratory center is located bilaterally in the reticular substance of the medulla oblongata and pons. (Redrawn from Guyton AC, Hall JE. *Textbook of Medical Physiology*, 10th ed. Philadelphia: Saunders, 2000; with permission.)

Inspiratory Area

Rhythmic inspiratory cycles are generated in the inspiratory area, located bilaterally in the dorsal portion of the medulla.

Pneumotaxic Area

Signals from the pneumotaxic area are transmitted to the inspiratory area and trigger the termination of inspiration, thus limiting lung inflation.

Apneustic Center

When apneustic center activity is unmasked because of damage to the pneumotaxic area, the pattern of breathing is maximal lung inflation with occasional brief expiratory gasps (apneuses).

Expiratory Area

At rest, exhalation results from a passive recoil of the elastic structure of the lungs and surrounding chest wall and requires no motor activity. When alveolar ventilation is increased, the expiratory area becomes active, providing signals that evoke forceful and frequent contraction of the diaphragm and abdominal muscles.

Chemical Control of Breathing

The chemical control of breathing adjusts respiration to maintain PCO_2 constant, to defend against excessive changes in hydrogen ion concentration, and to prevent dangerous decreases in PO_2.

Chemoreceptors

Chemoreceptors respond to changes in carbon dioxide, oxygen, and hydrogen ion concentrations; these receptors are located in the chemosensitive area of the medulla or in peripheral chemoreceptors.

Chemosensitive Area

The chemosensitive area (also known as medullary chemoreceptors) is located a few microns below the surface of the medulla (Fig. 50-5).

Hydrogen

Hydrogen ions are the most important stimulus of the chemosensitive area, but these ions do not easily cross the blood-brain barrier to enter the cerebrospinal fluid.

Carbon Dioxide

Carbon dioxide stimulates the chemosensitive area through its reaction with water in the cerebrospinal fluid to form carbonic acid and subsequent dissociation to hydrogen ions. It is estimated that 70% to 80% of the ventilatory response to carbon dioxide reflects an activation of the chemosensitive area.

The effect of increased $PaCO_2$ on alveolar ventilation peaks within 1 minute. After several hours, however, the stimulant effect wanes, reflecting the active transport (ion pump) of bicarbonate ions into the cerebrospinal fluid from the blood to return the cerebrospinal fluid pH to a normal value of 7.32.

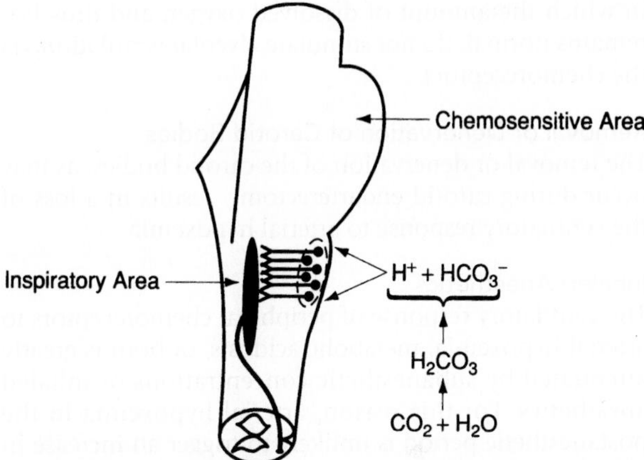

Figure 50-5. The chemosensitive area, located a few microns below the ventral surface of the medulla, transmits stimulatory impulses to the inspiratory area. This chemosensitive area is highly responsive to hydrogen ions (H+) in the cerebrospinal fluid that result from hydration of carbon dioxide. (From Guyton AC, Hall JE. *Textbook of Medical Physiology*, 10th ed. Philadelphia: Saunders, 2000; with permission.)

Peripheral Chemoreceptors

Carotid and Aortic Bodies

The carotid and aortic bodies are chemoreceptors located outside the central nervous system that are responsive to changes in PO_2, PCO_2, and the concentration of hydrogen ions. The hypoxic ventilatory response is potent and is predominantly mediated via the carotid body chemoreceptors.

Blood Flow

Blood flow through the peripheral chemoreceptors is the highest of any tissue in the body (metabolic needs of chemoreceptor tissues can be met almost entirely by dissolved oxygen). It is the PaO_2 and not the arterial hemoglobin saturation with oxygen (SaO_2) that determines the stimulation level of the peripheral chemoreceptors. This is the reason that anemia or carbon monoxide poisoning, in which the amount of dissolved oxygen and thus PO_2 remains normal, do not stimulate alveolar ventilation via the chemoreceptors.

Removal or Denervation of Carotid Bodies

The removal or denervation of the carotid bodies, as may occur during carotid endarterectomy, results in a loss of the ventilatory response to arterial hypoxemia.

Inhaled Anesthetics

The ventilatory response of peripheral chemoreceptors to arterial hypoxemia, metabolic acidosis, or both is greatly attenuated by subanesthetic concentrations of inhaled anesthetics. For this reason, arterial hypoxemia in the postanesthetic period is unlikely to trigger an increase in alveolar ventilation.

EFFECTS OF SLEEP ON BREATHING

Decreases in the level of environmental stimulation during sleep are associated with modest increases in $PaCO_2$, and the ventilatory response to carbon dioxide is decreased.

Persons with depressed ventilatory responses to hypercapnia and hypoxia while awake breathe even less during sleep, compared with those who show normal awake responses.

APNEIC PERIODS DURING SLEEP

Sleep apneas are classified as central (cessation of respiratory efforts) or obstructive (despite respiratory efforts, air flow ceases because of total upper airway obstruction).

Sleep Apnea

Sleep apnea is defined as the cessation of airflow at the mouth and nostril for >10 seconds, occurring more than 15 times per hour.

Snoring

Snoring is a manifestation of partial obstruction of the upper airway at sites including the pharynx and oropharynx.

Polycythemia and Pulmonary Hypertension

Recurrent episodes of arterial hypoxemia and hypercarbia may lead to polycythemia and pulmonary hypertension.

PERIODIC BREATHING

Periodic or Cheyne-Stokes breathing is characterized by a waxing and waning pattern of ventilation (apneic periods that last for up to 20 seconds followed by periods of hyperventilation). Cheyne-Stokes breathing is seen most often in patients with brain injury, congestive cardiac failure, and uremia.

NONVENTILATORY FUNCTIONS OF THE LUNGS

The nonventilatory functions of the lungs include a number of metabolic functions (synthesis, release, and removal of biologically active substances). The majority of exogenous substances removed by passage through the pulmonary circulation are not metabolized but instead are bound to components of lung tissue.

Pulmonary Gas Exchange and Blood Transport of Gases

51

PULMONARY GAS EXCHANGE

The primary function of the lungs is to provide for the optimal exchange of oxygen and carbon dioxide between the ambient environment and pulmonary capillaries (Stoelting RK, Hillier SC. Pulmonary gas exchange and blood transport of gases. In: *Pharmacology and Physiology in Anesthetic Practice*. 4th ed. Philadelphia, Lippincott Williams & Wilkins, 2006:781–791). Alveolar–capillary gas exchange is greatly dependent on the matching of regional alveolar ventilation with pulmonary capillary perfusion (V/Q).

Partial Pressure

The partial pressure (P) that a gas exerts is due to the constant impact of molecules in motion against a surface. In a mixture of gases, the partial pressure that each gas contributes to the total pressure is directly proportional to its relative concentration (Table 51-1).

Equilibrium is present when the number of molecules leaving the gas phase equals the number returning to the gas phase. At equilibrium, the partial pressure of the gas dissolved in the liquid phase is equal to the partial pressure of the gas in the gas phase and no net movement of gas occurs across the interface.

TABLE 51-1.
PARTIAL PRESSURES OF RESPIRATORY GASES AT SEA LEVEL (760 mm Hg)

Respiratory Gas	Inhaled Air (mm Hg)	Alveolar Gases (mm Hg)	Exhaled Gases (mm Hg)
Oxygen	159	104	120
Carbon dioxide	0.3	40	27
Nitrogen	597	569	566
Water	3.7	47	47

Vapor Pressure of Water

The pressure that water molecules exert to escape to the surface is the vapor pressure of water (47 mm Hg at 37°C).

Composition of Alveolar Gases

The composition of alveolar gases is different from the composition of inhaled (atmospheric) gases because (a) oxygen is constantly being absorbed from the alveoli, (b) carbon dioxide is constantly being added to the alveoli, and (c) dry inhaled gases are humidified by the addition of water vapor (see Table 51-1). Because the total partial pressure of gases in the alveoli remains unchanged, the addition of water vapor and carbon dioxide and removal of oxygen from the inhaled gases alters the delivered PO_2 from 159 mm Hg to 104 mm Hg and the PN_2 from 597 mm Hg to 569 mm Hg.

Partial Pressure of Oxygen

Alveolar partial pressure of oxygen (PAO_2) is determined by the rate of delivery of new oxygen by alveolar ventilation and the rate of absorption (250 mL/min) of oxygen into pulmonary capillary blood.

Inspired Partial Pressure of Oxygen

The inspired partial pressure of oxygen (PIO_2) is diluted by the vapor pressure of water (47 mm Hg) and the diffusion of carbon dioxide into the alveolus ($PACO_2$ 40 mm Hg). The impact of this dilution on the PAO_2 is magnified when the PIO_2 is decreased by a low PB (high altitude).

Supplemental Oxygen

Breathing supplemental oxygen offsets the dilutional effect of carbon dioxide and water vapor as well as the effect of altitude on PIO_2.

Partial Pressure of Carbon Dioxide

The alveolar partial pressure of carbon dioxide ($PACO_2$) is determined by the rate of carbon dioxide delivery to the alveoli from pulmonary capillary blood and the rate of removal of this carbon dioxide from the alveoli by alveolar ventilation.

The normal rate of delivery of carbon dioxide to alveoli by blood is 200 mL/minute. In the presence of a constant delivery of carbon dioxide to alveoli, the $PACO_2$ is directly proportional to alveolar ventilation.

Alveolar Gas Equation

The alveolar gas equation may be used clinically to calculate the gradient (or difference) between alveolar and arterial PO_2 (normally ~5 mm Hg). The alveolar to arterial oxygen gradient will increase as V/Q matching deteriorates.

Composition of Exhaled Gases

The composition of exhaled gases is determined by the proportion that is alveolar gas and the proportion that is dead space gas.

Dead Space Gas

The first portion of exhaled gas is from the large conducting airways (no gas exchange occurs) and is designated dead space gas (composition resembles inhaled gas).

End-Tidal Sampling

An analysis of the last portion of exhaled alveolar gas (end-tidal sample) is commonly used in the operating room to determine the composition of alveolar gas, including anesthetic concentrations. Minimum alveolar concentration (MAC) uses the alveolar concentration of the inhaled anesthetic as an index of anesthetic depth and to compare equal potent concentrations of inhaled anesthetics.

Gas Diffusion from Alveoli to Blood

Rate of Diffusion

The rate of gas diffusion across the alveolar–capillary membrane is determined by the solubility of the gas in the constituents of the membrane and the partial pressure difference across the membrane.

Gas Exchange

Carbon dioxide diffuses across the membrane approximately 20 times as rapidly as oxygen, and oxygen diffuses about twice as rapidly as nitrogen.

VENTILATION TO PERFUSION RATIO

The matching of ventilation to perfusion within the lung is crucial to the efficiency of gas exchange. In the presence of optimal V/Q matching, the $Pa{O_2}$ is approximately 104 mm Hg and the $Pa{CO_2}$ is 40 mm Hg.

A V/Q ratio of 0 is present when there is no ventilation to an alveolus that continues to be perfused by pulmonary capillary blood (shunt). A V/Q ratio equal to infinity means that there is ventilation but no pulmonary capillary blood flow to the alveolus (wasted ventilation).

Nitric Oxide

Low dose inhaled nitric oxide (NO) (< 2 ppm) is occasionally used to improve oxygenation in patients with acute respiratory distress syndrome (ARDS), a disease characterized by severe V/Q mismatch that causes refractory hypoxemia.

Physiologic Shunt

Physiologic shunt designates the 2% to 5% of the cardiac output that normally bypasses the lungs by flowing through bronchial veins into pulmonary veins or through thebesian and anterior cardiac veins into the left side of the heart (Table 51-2).

Physiologic Dead Space

Conducting airways that do not participate in gas exchange (anatomic dead space) and nonperfused alveoli that are ventilated but do not participate in gas exchange are designated as physiologic dead space. In health, the physiologic dead space is accounted for almost entirely by the anatomic dead space.

Tidal Volume

The ratio of physiologic dead space to tidal volume is calculated by measuring the tidal volume, the $PaCO_2$, and $PETCO_2$ (Table 51-3).

Increased Dead Space

In contrast to shunting, increased dead space tends to impair carbon dioxide elimination rather than oxygenation.

TABLE 51-2.
CALCULATION OF PHYSIOLOGIC SHUNT FRACTION

$$QS/QT = \frac{CcO_2 - CaO_2}{CcO_2 - CvO_2}$$

Q_S = amount of pulmonary blood flow not exposed to ventilated alveoli.
Q_T = total pulmonary blood flow.
CcO_2 = O_2 content of pulmonary capillary blood, mL/dL.
CaO_2 = O_2 content of arterial blood, mL/dL.
CvO_2 = O_2 content of mixed venous blood, mL/dL.

TABLE 51-3.
CALCULATION OF THE PHYSIOLOGIC DEAD SPACE TO TIDAL VOLUME RATIO

$$V_D/V_T = \frac{PaCO_2 - PETCO_2}{PaCO_2}$$

V_D/V_T = ratio of physiologic dead space to VT.
$PaCO_2$ = arterial partial pressure of CO_2, mm Hg.
$PETCO_2$ = mixed exhaled partial pressure of CO_2, mm Hg.

Anesthesia

During anesthesia, breathing systems may add additional dead space (apparatus dead space). Although it is important to avoid excessive apparatus dead space in all patients, infants are particularly vulnerable to respiratory compromise, because their tidal volumes are relatively small compared to breathing circuit volumes.

BLOOD TRANSPORT OF OXYGEN AND CARBON DIOXIDE

Oxygen Uptake into the Blood (Fig. 51-1)

Mixed venous blood is exposed to a PAO_2 of approximately 104 mm Hg, causing a rapid diffusion of oxygen down a ~60 mm Hg partial pressure gradient into pulmonary capillary blood. Blood leaving the pulmonary capillaries has a PO_2 of approximately 104 mm Hg, whereas the arterial blood, which is diluted by contributions from bronchial blood flow, has a PaO_2 of approximately 95 mm Hg (Fig. 51-2).

Diffusion of Oxygen from the Capillaries (Fig. 51-3)

Interstitial fluid PO_2 averages approximately 40 mm Hg, providing a large initial partial pressure gradient for the diffusion of oxygen from tissue capillaries having a PaO_2 near 95 mm Hg.

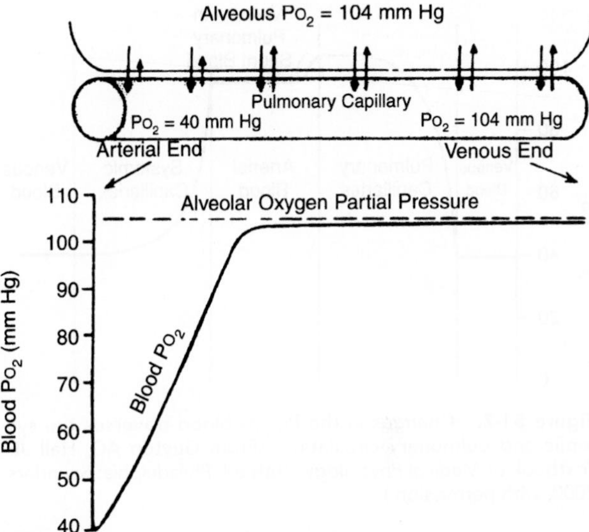

Figure 51-1. Schematic depiction of the uptake of oxygen by pulmonary capillary blood. (From Guyton AC, Hall JE. *Textbook of Medical Physiology*, 9th ed. Philadelphia: Saunders, 1996; with permission.)

Diffusion of Carbon Dioxide from Cells (Fig. 51-4)

The continuous formation of carbon dioxide in cells maintains a partial pressure gradient (1 to 6 mm Hg) for its diffusion into capillary blood.

Blood Transport of Oxygen

Approximately 97% of oxygen transported from alveoli to tissues is carried to tissues in chemical combination with hemoglobin, whereas approximately 3% of oxygen is transported in the dissolved state in plasma.

Oxygen Content of Hemoglobin

Each gram of hemoglobin can combine with approximately 1.34 mL of oxygen.

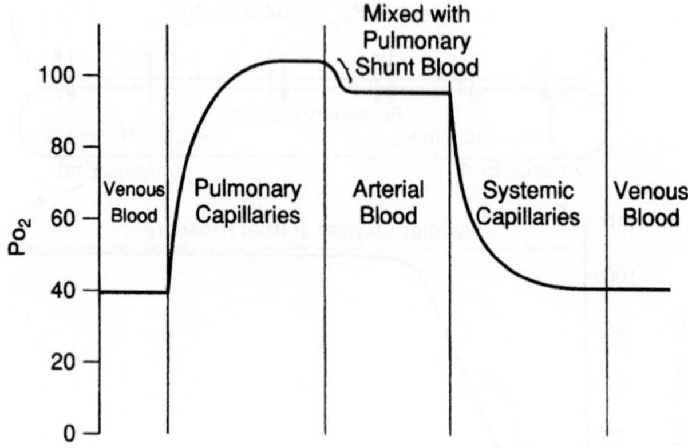

Figure 51-2. Changes in the P_{O_2} as blood traverses the systemic and pulmonary circulation. (From Guyton AC, Hall JE. *Textbook of Medical Physiology*, 10th ed. Philadelphia: Saunders, 2000; with permission.)

In the presence of a normal hemoglobin concentration of 15 g/dL, blood will carry approximately 20 mL of oxygen when the hemoglobin is 100% saturated. Approximately 5 mL of this 20 mL passes to tissues, thus decreasing the hemoglobin saturation with oxygen to approximately 75%, corresponding to a P_{VO_2} of approximately 40 mm Hg.

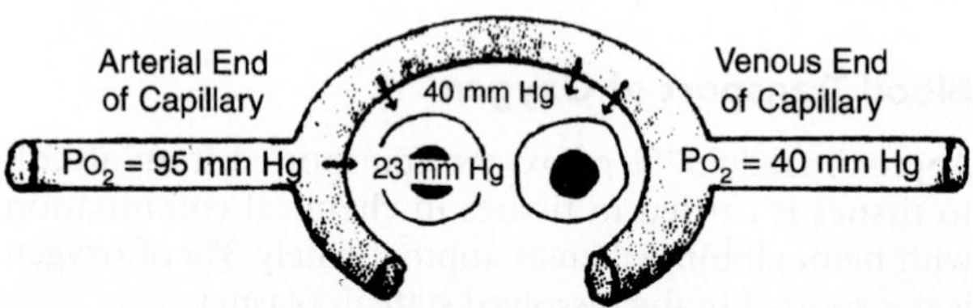

Figure 51-3. Schematic depiction of the diffusion of oxygen from tissue capillaries into the interstitial fluid. (From Guyton AC, Hall JE. *Textbook of Medical Physiology*, 10th ed. Philadelphia: Saunders, 2000; with permission.)

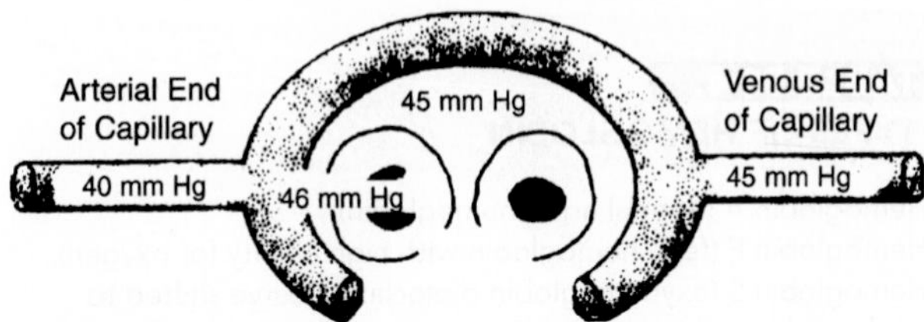

Figure 51-4. Schematic depiction of uptake of carbon dioxide by capillary blood. (From Guyton AC, Hall JE. *Textbook of Medical Physiology*, 10th ed. Philadelphia: Saunders, 2000; with permission.)

Oxygen Content of Plasma

The amount of oxygen dissolved in plasma is a linear function of the Po_2 (0.003 mL/mm Hg corresponding to 0.3 mL/100 dL when the Po_2 is 100 mm Hg). Under resting conditions, approximately 5 mL of oxygen is released to the tissues for every 100 dL of blood, resulting in a total delivery of oxygen to tissues of 250 mL/min when the cardiac output is 5 L/min.

Preoxygenation

Preoxygenation of the patient's lungs prior to the induction of anesthesia and tracheal intubation is intended to increase oxygen reserves in the lungs and thus delay the onset of arterial hypoxemia during apnea. Maximum alveolar preoxygenation in an adult during tidal volume breathing (100% oxygen via a face mask using a circle absorption system) requires at least 2.5 minutes.

Hemoglobin

The four heme molecules, each with a central iron atom, combine with globin, a globular protein synthesized in the ribosomes of the endoplasmic reticulum to form hemoglobin (Table 51-4).

Oxyhemoglobin Dissociation Curve (fig. 51-5)

Shift of the Oxyhemoglobin Dissociation Curve (Table 51-5)

TABLE 51-4.
TYPES OF HEMOGLOBIN

Hemoglobin A (normal adult hemoglobin)
Hemoglobin F (fetal hemoglobin with high affinity for oxygen)
Hemoglobin S (oxyhemoglobin dissociation curve shifted to right, sickle cells)
Myoglobin (present in skeletal muscles)
Neuroglobin (present in brain)

Partial Pressure of Oxygen at 50% Saturation

A shift of the oxyhemoglobin dissociation curve to the right is reflected by an increase in the P_{50} to >26 mm Hg,

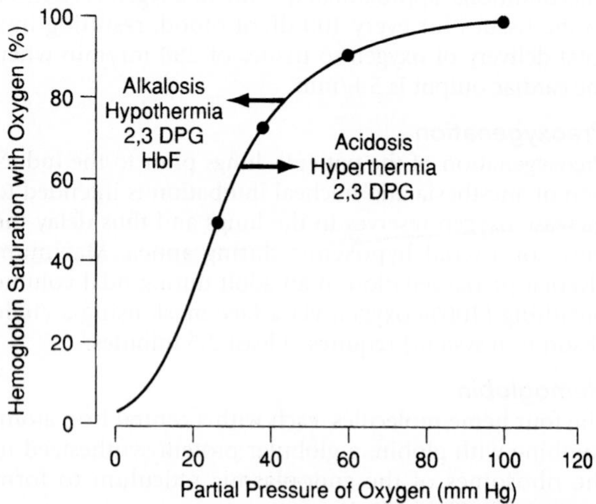

Figure 51-5. Oxyhemoglobin dissociation curve for hemoglobin A at pH level of 7.4 and 37° C. Changes in pH level, body temperature, concentration of 2,3-diphosphoglycerate (2,3-DPG), and the presence of different types of hemoglobin (HbF) shift the oxyhemoglobin dissociation curve to the left or right of its normal position.

TABLE 51-5.
FACTORS INFLUENCING THE POSITION OF THE OXYHEMOGLOBIN DISSOCIATION CURVE

Hydrogen ion concentration of the blood
Body temperature
Concentration of 2,3-diphosphoglycerate
Type of hemoglobin

whereas the P_{50} is <26 mm Hg when the oxyhemoglobin dissociation curve is shifted to the left.

A shift of the oxyhemoglobin dissociation curve to the left means that the Po_2 must decrease further before oxygen is released from hemoglobin to tissues.

Bohr Effect
The Bohr effect is the shift in the position of the oxyhemoglobin dissociation curve caused by carbon dioxide entering or leaving the blood.

2,3-Diphosphoglycerate
The effect of 2,3-DPG is to decrease the affinity of hemoglobin for oxygen (shifts the oxyhemoglobin dissociation curve to the right), thus causing oxygen to be released to tissues at a higher Pao_2 than in the absence of this substance.

Carbon Monoxide

Carbon monoxide competes with oxygen for binding at the same location on the hemoglobin molecule (a carbon monoxide partial pressure of 0.7 mm Hg can bind nearly all the hemoglobin sites normally occupied by oxygen).

Chemoreceptor Response
The Pao_2 remains normal despite the absence of oxyhemoglobin, reflecting the fact that dissolved oxygen determines the Po_2. Chemoreceptors that would otherwise

increase alveolar ventilation in response to hypoxemia are not stimulated because the $Pa{O_2}$ remains normal.

Treatment

The primary treatment of carbon monoxide poisoning is the administration of oxygen, to elevate the $Pa{O_2}$ and thus displace carbon monoxide from hemoglobin.

Anesthetics

Carbon monoxide formation may result from degradation of volatile anesthetics (desflurane>enflurane> isoflurane) by the strong base in desiccated carbon dioxide absorbents.

Carboxyhemoglobin

Carboxyhemoglobin does not influence the readings obtained by pulse oximetry.

Cyanosis

More than 5 g of reduced hemoglobin causes cyanosis, regardless of the overall concentration of oxyhemoglobin. Therefore, patients with polycythemia may appear cyanotic despite adequate arterial concentrations of oxygen, whereas the anemic patient may lack sufficient hemoglobin to produce enough reduced hemoglobin to cause cyanosis even in the presence of profound tissue hypoxia.

Blood Transport of Carbon Dioxide

Carbon dioxide formed as a result of metabolic processes in cells readily diffuses across cell membranes into capillary blood. Despite a small partial pressure difference between tissues and blood (1 to 6 mm Hg), the high solubility of carbon dioxide (20 times more soluble than oxygen) permits rapid transfer.

$Pv{CO_2}$ versus $Pa{CO_2}$

The $Pv{CO_2}$ is ~5 mm Hg greater than the $Pa{CO_2}$, reflecting the addition of carbon dioxide from the tissues;

this influx of carbon dioxide lowers the venous blood pH to 7.36, compared with an artereal pH of 7.4 in tissues).

Haldane Effect

The Haldane effect is the displacement of carbon dioxide from hemoglobin by oxygen that occurs at the lungs.

Body Stores of Carbon Dioxide

In contrast to total body oxygen stores of approximately 1.5 liters, an estimated 120 liters of carbon dioxide are dissolved in the body.

Apneic Oxygenation

In the presence of apnea but with the provision of oxygen (apneic oxygenation), the $Pa{CO_2}$ increases 5 to 10 mm Hg during the first minute of apnea (equilibration with venous blood) and then increases approximately 3 mm Hg/min, reflecting the metabolic production of carbon dioxide.

Respiratory Quotient

The respiratory quotient is the ratio of carbon dioxide output to oxygen uptake.

CHANGES ASSOCIATED WITH HIGH ALTITUDE (TABLE 51-6 and FIG. 51-6)

Inhaled Anesthetics

The pharmacologic effect of inhaled anesthetics is decreased as PB is reduced (60% inhaled nitrous oxide produces a partial pressure of 456 mm Hg at sea level compared with 314 mm Hg at 3,300 m). The inhaled concentration of nitrous oxide at 3,300 m elevation would have to be 87% to produce the same partial pressure produced by breathing 60% nitrous oxide at sea level.

Acclimatization to Altitude (Table 51-7)

TABLE 51-6.
EFFECTS OF ALTITUDE ON RESPIRATORY GASES WHILE BREATHING AIR

Altitude (m/ft)	PB (mmHg)	PIO_2 (mmHg)	PAO_2 (mmHg)	$PACO_2$ (mmHg)	SaO_2 (%)
Sea level	760	159	104	40	97
3,300/10,000	523	110 (436)*	67	36	90
6,600/20,000	349	73	40	24	70
9,900/30,000	226	47	21	24	20

*Breathing 100% oxygen.

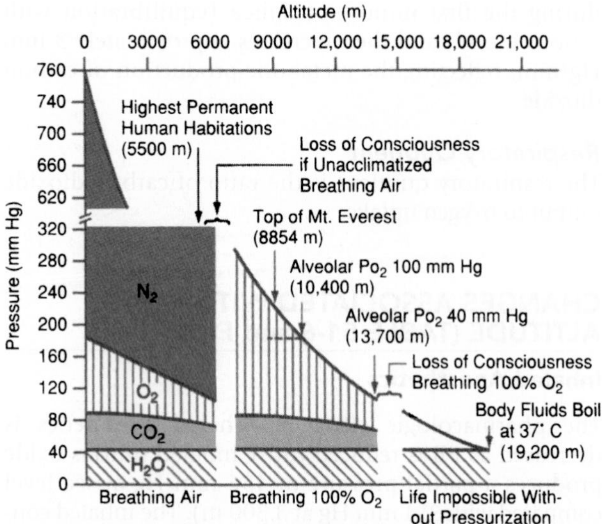

Figure 51-6. Composition of alveolar air breathing air (0 to 6,100 m) and 100% oxygen (6,100 to 13,700 m). (From Ganong WF. *Review of Medical Physiology*, 21st ed. New York, Lang Medical Books/McGraw Hill, 2003; with permission.)

TABLE 51-7.
COMPENSATORY RESPONSES EVOKED BY ASCENT TO ALTITUDE

Increased alveolar ventilation
Increased hemoglobin production
Increased 2,3-disphosphoglycerate concentrations
Increased diffusing capacity of the lungs
Increased vascularity of the tissues
Increased cellular use of oxygen

Acute Mountain Sickness

Acute mountain sickness is a syndrome of headache, insomnia, dyspnea, anorexia, and fatigue that has been described on rapid ascent to even intermediate altitude (2,000 m). High-altitude pulmonary edema and cerebral edema are serious forms of acute mountain sickness.

Chronic Mountain Sickness

An occasional sea level native who remains for prolonged periods at high altitude may develop chronic mountain sickness characterized by polycythemia, pulmonary hypertension, and right ventricular failure. Recovery is usually prompt when these individuals return to sea level, provided that pulmonary vascular remodeling has not caused an irreversible increase in pulmonary vascular resistance.

CHANGES ASSOCIATED WITH EXCESSIVE BAROMETRIC PRESSURE

The PB increases the equivalent of 1 atm for every 10 m below the surface of sea water (10.4 m for fresh water).

Nitrogen Narcosis

The increased PB below the surface of the water compresses gases in the lungs to smaller volumes, thus producing nitrogen narcosis.

Decompression Sickness

Decompression sickness (caisson disease) occurs when sudden decreases in the PB allow nitrogen bubbles to develop in body tissues and fluids

Hyperbaric Oxygen Therapy (Tables 51-8 and 51-9)

TABLE 51-8.
INDICATIONS FOR HYPERBARIC OXYGEN THERAPY

Decompression sickness
Air embolism
Carbon monoxide poisoning
Clostridial gangrene
Refractory osteomyelitis
Radiation necrosis
Profound anemia

TABLE 51-9.
COMPLICATIONS OF HYPERBARIC OXYGEN THERAPY

Tympanic membrane rupture
Nasal sinus trauma
Pneumothorax
Air embolism
Central nervous system toxicity
Oxygen toxicity

Acid–Base Balance

52

Hydrogen ion concentrations in the various compartments are precisely regulated (arterial pH 7.35 to 7.45) in the face of enormous variations in local production and clearance (Stoelting RK, Hillier SC. Acid-base balance. In: *Pharmacology and Physiology in Anesthetic Practice*. 4th ed. Philadelphia, Lippincott Williams & Wilkins, 2006: 792–800). The pH is equivalent to the negative logarithm of the hydrogen ion concentration expressed in nmol/L (a pH of 7.4 is equivalent to a hydrogen ion concentration of 40 nmol/L). The expression of the hydrogen ion concentration as pH masks large variations in hydrogen ion concentration despite small changes in pH (Table 52-1). For example, a pH range of 7.0 to 7.7 is associated with a five-fold change (100 nmol/L to 20 nmol/L) in hydrogen ion concentration (Table 52-1). The pH of venous blood and interstitial fluid is lower than that of arterial blood, approximately 7.35.

MECHANISMS FOR REGULATION OF HYDROGEN ION CONCENTRATION

Buffer Systems (Fig. 52-1)

Body fluids contain acid–base buffer systems that immediately combine with acid or alkali to prevent excessive changes in the hydrogen ion concentration.

Bicarbonate Buffering System

The bicarbonate buffering system consists of carbonic acid and sodium bicarbonate. The addition of a strong acid, such as hydrochloric acid, to the bicarbonate buffering

TABLE 52-1.
RELATION OF HYDROGEN ION CONCENTRATION TO pH

Hydrogen ions (nmol/L)	pH
100	7.00
80	7.10
63	7.20
50	7.30
42	7.38
40	7.40
38	7.42
32	7.50
25	7.60
20	7.70

system results in the conversion of the strong acid to weak carbonic acid (Fig. 52-2).

The bicarbonate buffer system accounts for >50% of the total buffering capacity of blood.

Hemoglobin Buffering System

Hemoglobin is a particularly effective buffer because it is localized in quantity in erythrocytes, it has a pK level of 6.8, which is close to the physiologic pH, and it has a buffering capacity that varies with oxygenation.

$$HHb \rightleftharpoons H^+ + Hb^-$$

$$HProt \rightleftharpoons H^+ + Prot^-$$

$$H_2PO_4^- \rightleftharpoons H^+ + HPO_4^{2-}$$

$$H_2CO_3 \rightleftharpoons H^+ + HCO_3^-$$

Figure 52-1. Buffering systems present in the body.

$$CO_2 + H_2O \rightleftharpoons H_2CO_3 \rightleftharpoons HCO_3^- + H^+$$

Figure 52-2. Hydration of carbon dioxide results in carbonic acid, which can subsequently dissociate into bicarbonate and hydrogen ions.

Protein Buffering System

Although the relatively low concentration of plasma proteins limits their role as extracellular buffers, hypoproteinemia will further reduce buffering capacity, especially in the critically ill patient.

Phosphate Buffering System

The phosphate buffering system is especially important in renal tubules, where phosphate is concentrated.

Intracellular pH Regulation

Although blood pH is commonly measured clinically, it is the intracellular pH that is of functional importance (Table 52-2).

TABLE 52-2.
INTRACELLULAR FUNCTIONS AFFECTED BY LOCAL pH

Cellular metabolism
Cytoskeletal structure
Muscle contractility
Cell–cell coupling
Membrane conductance
Intracellular messengers
Cell activation, growth, and proliferation
Cell volume regulation
Intracellular membrane flow

Ventilatory Responses

The ventilatory responses for regulation of pH manifest as alterations in the activity of the respiratory center within 1 to 5 minutes of the change in hydrogen ion concentration. As a result, alveolar ventilation increases or decreases to produce appropriate changes in the concentration of carbon dioxide. Doubling alveolar ventilation eliminates sufficient carbon dioxide to increase the pH to approximately 7.6. Conversely, decreasing alveolar ventilation to one-fourth of normal results in the retention of carbon dioxide sufficient to decrease the pH to approximately 7.0.

Degree of Ventilatory Response

Ventilatory responses cannot return the pH to 7.4 when a metabolic abnormality is responsible for the acid–base disturbance; this reflects the fact that the intensity of the stimulus responsible for increases or decreases in alveolar ventilation will begin to diminish as the pH returns toward 7.4. Most patients will not hyperventilate to below 20 mm Hg.

Renal Responses

Bicarbonate Conservation

Almost all filtered bicarbonate must be reabsorbed from the glomerular filtrate to maintain the normal plasma bicarbonate concentration (25 mEq/L) and plasma pH. Most bicarbonate reabsorption occurs in the proximal convoluted tubule (facilitated by carbonic anhydrase).

Carbonic anhydrase facilitates the dissociation of carbonic acid into water and carbon dioxide, which both enter the tubular cell. Carbon dioxide and water generate bicarbonate, which enters the peritubular circulation accompanied by sodium.

Renal Tubular Secretion of Hydrogen Ions

Hydrogen ions are actively secreted into renal tubules by epithelial cells lining proximal renal tubules, distal renal

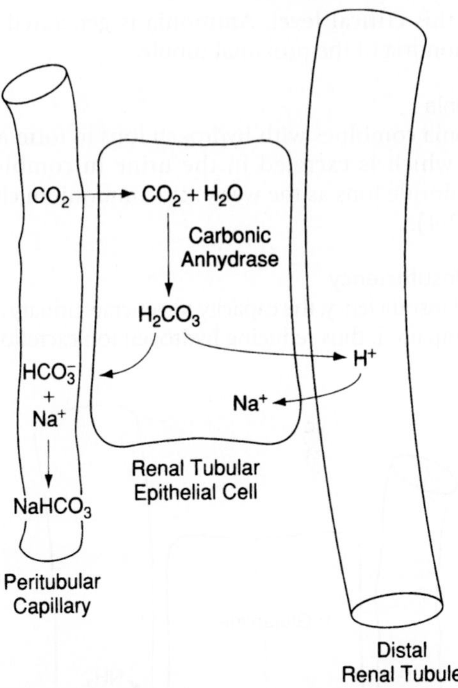

Figure 52-3. Schematic depiction of the renal tubular secretion of hydrogen ions, which are formed from the dissociation of carbonic acid in renal tubular epithelial cells.

tubules, and collecting ducts (Fig. 52-3). At the same time, sodium ions are reabsorbed in exchange for the secreted hydrogen ions and combine with bicarbonate ions in the peritubular capillaries. This process is facilitated by aldosterone.

Urinary pH Levels

Active hydrogen ion transport is inhibited when the urinary pH drops below 4.0. Thus, hydrogen ions must combine with ammonia and phosphate buffers in the renal tubular lumen to prevent the pH from decreasing below this critical level. Ammonia is generated in the mitochondria of the proximal tubule.

Ammonia

Ammonia combines with hydrogen ions to form ammonium, which is excreted in the urine in combination with chloride ions as the weak acid ammonium chloride (Fig. 52-4).

Renal Insufficiency

In renal insufficiency, the capacity to generate urinary ammonia is impaired, thus reducing hydrogen ion excretion.

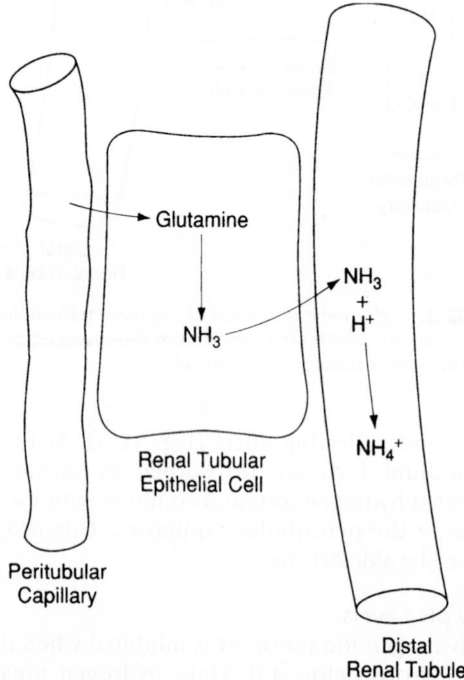

Figure 52-4. Ammonia formed in renal tubular epithelial cells combines with hydrogen ions in the renal tubules to form ammonium.

Regulation of Chloride

Extracellular fluid is electroneutral, so that the sum of the positive charges of all cations must equal the sum of negative charges of all anions. The chloride anion follows changes in the concentration of bicarbonate ions; as the most abundant extracellular anion, the physiologic manipulation of chloride is an important element of pH control.

Degree of Renal Compensation

Renal responses for the regulation of acid–base balance are slow to act (hours) but continue until the pH returns to almost 7.4. Thus, unlike ventilatory responses, which are rapid but incomplete, the value of renal regulation of hydrogen ion concentrations is not its rapidity but instead its ability to nearly completely neutralize any excess acid or alkali that enters the body fluids.

ACID–BASE DISTURBANCES (TABLE 52-3)

Respiratory Acidosis

Any event (drug or disease) that decreases alveolar ventilation results in an increased concentration of dissolved carbon dioxide in the plasma (increased $Paco_2$). By convention, carbonic acid resulting from dissolved carbon dioxide is considered a respiratory acid, and respiratory acidosis is present when the pH is <7.35.

Respiratory Alkalosis

Respiratory alkalosis is present when increased alveolar ventilation (low Pao_2, iatrogenic hyperventilation during anesthesia) removes sufficient carbon dioxide from the body to decrease the hydrogen ion concentration to the extent that the pH becomes >7.45.

Renal Compensation

The kidneys compensate over time for the loss of carbon dioxide by excreting bicarbonate ions in association with

TABLE 52-3.
CLASSIFICATION OF ACID–BASE DISTURBANCES

	pH	Pa_{CO_2}	Bicarbonate
Respiratory acidosis			
Acute	−−	+++	+
Chronic	NC	+++	++
Respiratory alkalosis			
Acute	++	−−−	−
Chronic	NC	−−−	−−
Metabolic acidosis			
Acute	−−−	−	−−−
Chronic	−	−−−	−−−
Metabolic alkalosis			
Acute	+++	+	+++
Chronic	++	++	+++

+, increase; −, decrease; NC, no change from normal.

sodium and potassium ions. This renal compensation is evident in individuals residing at altitude who have a nearly normal pH despite a low Pa_{CO_2}.

Metabolic Acidosis

Any acid formed in the body other than carbon dioxide is considered a metabolic acid, and its accumulation results in metabolic acidosis.

Lactic Acidosis

Severe reductions in hepatic blood flow, which occur during shock, will decrease hepatic lactate clearance. Lactic acid is a strong acid, and therefore dissociates almost completely under physiologic conditions into the lactate anion and a proton. A serum lactate >1.5 mmol/L upon admission is an independent predictor of mortality in critically ill patients.

Cardiac Effects

Metabolic acidosis impairs myocardial contractility and the responses to endogenous or exogenous catecholamines.

Hemodynamic deterioration is usually minimal when the pH remains >7.2 due to compensatory increases in sympathetic nervous system activity.

Respiratory Acidosis

Respiratory acidosis may produce more rapid and profound myocardial dysfunction than does metabolic acidosis, reflecting the ability of carbon dioxide to freely diffuse across cell membranes and exacerbate intracellular acidosis.

Treatment

The use of sodium bicarbonate to treat metabolic acidosis is questionable. Sodium bicarbonate administration increases the carbon dioxide load to the lungs, leading to further increases in arterial and intracellular P_{CO_2} if alveolar ventilation is not concomitantly increased.

Renal Failure

Renal failure prevents excretion of acids formed by normal metabolic processes, and metabolic acidosis occurs.

Dilutional Acidosis

Dilutional acidosis occurs when the plasma pH is decreased by extracellular volume expansion with solutions such as normal saline. Clinically, a hyperchloremic metabolic acidosis may accompany the large-volume infusion of isotonic saline. The measurement of the plasma lactic acid concentration and calculation of the anion gap from sodium, chloride, and bicarbonate permits a differentiation of dilutional acidosis from acidosis due to tissue hypoperfusion.

Metabolic Alkalosis

The causes of metabolic alkalosis include vomiting with excess loss of hydrochloric acid, nasogastric suction, chronic administration of thiazide diuretics, and excess secretion of aldosterone.

Compensation of Acid–Base Disturbances

Respiratory Acidosis

Respiratory acidosis is compensated for within 6 to 12 hours by the increased renal secretion of hydrogen ions, with a resulting increase in the plasma bicarbonate concentration. After a few days, the pH will be normal, despite the persistence of an increased $PaCO_2$. The sudden correction of chronic respiratory acidosis, through iatrogenic hyperventilation, may result in acute metabolic alkalosis, because increased plasma concentrations of bicarbonate cannot be promptly eliminated by the kidneys.

Respiratory Alkalosis

Respiratory alkalosis is compensated for by a decreased reabsorption of bicarbonate ions from the renal tubules. As a result, more bicarbonate ions are excreted in the urine, which decreases the plasma concentration of bicarbonate and returns the pH toward normal despite the persistence of a decreased $PaCO_2$.

Metabolic Acidosis

Metabolic acidosis stimulates alveolar ventilation, which causes the rapid removal of carbon dioxide from the body and decreases the hydrogen ion concentration toward normal. The compensation for metabolic acidosis is only partial as pH remains somewhat below normal.

Metabolic Alkalosis

Metabolic alkalosis diminishes alveolar ventilation, which in turn causes an accumulation of carbon dioxide and a subsequent increase in hydrogen ion concentration (compensation is only partial). The presence of paradoxical aciduria indicates electrolyte depletion.

The Anion Gap (Table 52-4)

For electroneutrality to occur, the concentration of the combined unmeasured anions must exceed that of the unmeasured cations by the same amount (Fig. 52-5).

TABLE 52-4.
MEASURED IONS COMMONLY USED IN ANION GAP CALCULATION

Electrolyte	Cations Value (mEq/L)	Electrolyte	Anions Value (mEq/L)
Sodium	140	Chloride	104
		Bicarbonate	24
Calcium	5	Phosphate	2
Magnesium	1.5	Sulphate	1
Potassium	4.5	Organic Acids	5
		Proteins	15
Total Cations	151	Total Anions	151

The term *anion gap* refers solely to the difference in concentration between the traditionally measured anions and cations (Fig. 52-6).

Metabolic acidosis is most often associated with an increase in the anion gap.

Effects of Temperature on Acid–Base Status

As blood is cooled, CO_2 becomes more soluble (partial pressure will decrease as the temperature falls). If the blood temperature is decreased by 10°C to 27°C, the pH will increase to 7.6.

Blood-gas Measurement

Two alternate blood-gas management strategies, α-stat and pH-stat, are utilized to interpret arterial blood gases

TOTAL CATION CHARGE = TOTAL ANION CHARGE

$$Na^+ + \text{unmeasured cations} = (HCO_3^- + Cl^-) + \text{unmeasured anions}$$

Figure 52-5. Calculation of electrochemical neutrality.

$$\text{Anion Gap} = Na^+ - (HCO_3^- + Cl^-)$$

Figure 52-6. Calculation of the anion gap.

during hypothermia in the operating room (Table 52-5). pH stat management seeks to return the pH and P_{CO_2} of hypothermic blood to normal. Alpha-stat management seeks to replicate the alkalinization of blood that occurs during cooling.

GASTRIC INTRAMUCOSAL pH

Acid–base changes in the gut may precede systemic changes in early shock.

TABLE 52-5.
COMPARISON OF pH STAT AND α-STAT BLOOD GAS MANAGEMENT STRATEGIES

	pH stat	α-Stat
CO_2 added to oxygenator	Yes	No
Enzyme function	Decreased	Near normal
Cerebral blood flow	Increased	Normal
Blood gas temperature correction required	Yes	No
Hb-O_2 dissociation curve	Less marked left shift	Marked left shift

Endocrine System

53

Endocrine glands secrete hormones into the blood for delivery to distant sites where a response is evoked (Stoelting RK, Hillier SC. Endocrine system. In: *Pharmacology and Physiology in Anesthetic Practice*. 4th ed. Philadelphia, Lippincott Williams & Wilkins, 2006:801–814). Unrecognized endocrine dysfunction is unlikely if it can be established that (a) body weight is unchanged, (b) heart rate and systemic blood pressure are normal, (c) glycosuria is absent, (d) sexual function is normal, and (e) no history of recent endocrine system–related medication is present.

MECHANISM OF HORMONE ACTION

The combination of the hormone and receptor activates adenylate cyclase, leading to the conversion of adenosine triphosphate (ATP) to cyclic adenosine monophosphate (cAMP). The resulting increased intracellular concentration of cAMP is responsible for initiating cellular responses attributed to the effects of hormones. An alternative mechanism of action for hormones is illustrated by corticosteroids that stimulate genes in cells to form specific intracellular proteins. These proteins then function as enzymes or carrier proteins, which, in turn, activate other functions of cells.

PITUITARY GLAND

The pituitary gland lies in the sella turcica at the base of the brain and is connected to the hypothalamus by the pituitary stalk. Physiologically, the gland is outside the blood-brain barrier and is divided into the anterior pituitary (adenohypophysis) and posterior pituitary (neurohypophysis) (Table 53-1). Hormones designated as hypothalamic-releasing hormones and hypothalamic-inhibitory hormones originating in the hypothalamus control secretions from the anterior pituitary (Table 53-2).

Anterior Pituitary (See Table 53-1)

Human Growth Hormone

Human growth hormone (HGH) stimulates the growth of all tissues in the body and evokes intense metabolic effects. The secretion of HGH is regulated by releasing inhibitory (somatostatin) hormones secreted by the hypothalamus, as well as by physiologic and pharmacologic events (Table 53-3).

Prolactin

Prolactin is responsible for the growth and development of the breast in preparation for breast-feeding (Table 53-4).

Gonadotropins

Luteinizing hormone (LH) and follicle-stimulating hormone (FSH) are gonadotropins responsible for pubertal maturation and the secretion of steroid sex hormones by the gonads of either sex.

Adrenocorticotropic Hormone (ACTH)

Adrenocorticotropic hormone (ACTH) is principally responsible for regulating the secretions of the adrenal cortex, especially cortisol. In addition, ACTH stimulates the formation of cholesterol in the adrenal cortex. Cholesterol is the initial building block for the synthesis of corticosteroids. The secretion of ACTH responds most dramatically to stress and is under the control of corticotropin-releasing hormone from the hypothalamus, as well as a negative-feedback mechanism that depends on the circulating plasma concentration of cortisol (Table 53-5). In the absence of ACTH, the adrenal cortex undergoes atrophy,

TABLE 53-1.
PITUITARY HORMONES

Hormone	Cell Type	Principal Action
Anterior pituitary		
Human growth hormone (HGH, somatotrophin)	Somatotropes	Accelerates body growth
Prolactin	Mammotrophs	Stimulates secretion of milk and maternal behavior, inhibits ovulation
Luteinizing hormone (LH)	Gonadotrophs	Stimulates ovulation in females and testosterone secretion in males
Follicle-stimulating hormone (FSH)	Gonadotrophs	Stimulates ovarian follicle growth in females and spermatogenesis in males
Adrenocorticotropic hormone (ACTH)	Corticotropes	Stimulates adrenal cortex secretion and growth
Thyroid-stimulating hormone (TSH)	Thyrotropes	Stimulates thyroid secretion and growth
β-Lipotropin	Corticotropes	Precursor of endorphins
Posterior pituitary		
Arginine vasopressin	Supraoptic nuclei	Promotes water retention and regulates plasma osmolarity
Oxytocin	Paraventricular	Causes ejection of milk and nuclei uterine contraction

TABLE 53-2.
HYPOTHALAMIC HORMONES

Hormone	Target Anterior Pituitary Hormone
Human growth hormone–releasing hormone	HGH
Human growth hormone–inhibiting hormone (somatostatin)	HGH, prolactin, TSH
Prolactin-releasing factor	Prolactin
Prolactin-inhibiting factor	Prolactin
Luteinizing hormone–releasing hormone	LH, FSH
Corticotropin-releasing hormone	ACTH, β-lipotropins, endorphins
Thyrotropin-releasing hormone	TSH

ACTH, adrenocorticotrophics hormone; FSH, follicle-stimulating hormone; HGH, human growth hormone; LH, luteinizing hormone; TSH, thyroid-stimulating hormone.

TABLE 53-3.
REGULATION OF HUMAN GROWTH HORMONE (HGH) SECRETION

Stimulation	Inhibition
HGH-releasing hormone	HGH-inhibiting hormone
Stress	HGH
Physiologic sleep	Pregnancy
Hypoglycemia	Hyperglycemia
Free fatty acid decrease	Free fatty acid increase
Amino acid increase	Cortisol
Fasting	Obesity
Estrogens	
Dopamine	
α-Adrenergic agonists	

TABLE 53-4.
REGULATION OF PROLACTIN SECRETION

Stimulation	Inhibition
Prolactin-releasing factor	Prolactin-inhibiting factor
Pregnancy	Prolactin
Suckling	Dopamine
Stress	L-dopa
Physiologic sleep	
Metoclopramide	
Cimetidine	
Opioids	
α-Methyldopa	

but the zona glomerulosa, which secretes aldosterone, is least affected (hypophysectomy has minimal effects on electrolyte balance). The chronic administration of corticosteroids leads to functional atrophy of the hypothalamic-pituitary axis; thus it is conceivable that stressful events during the perioperative period might evoke life-threatening hypotension. For this reason, it is a common

TABLE 53-5.
REGULATION OF ADRENOCORTICOTROPIC HORMONE (ACTH) SECRETION

Stimulation	Inhibition
Corticotropin-releasing hormone	ACTH
Cortisol decrease	Cortisol increase
Stress	Opioids
Sleep-wake transition	Etomidate
Hypoglycemia	Suppression of the hypothalamic-pituitary axis
Trauma	
α-Adrenergic agonists	
β-Adrenergic antagonists	

practice to administer supplemental exogenous corticosteroids to patients considered at risk, based on the suppression of the hypothalamic-pituitary axis. No evidence supports, however, that supplemental corticosteroids in excess of normal daily physiologic secretion are necessary or beneficial in the intraoperative and postoperative period.

Thyroid-Stimulating Hormone

Thyroid-stimulating hormone (TSH) causes proteolysis of thyroglobulin in the follicles of thyroid cells, with the resultant release of thyroid hormones into the circulation.

Posterior Pituitary

Arginine Vasopressin

Arginine vasopressin (AVP) (previously designated antidiuretic hormone, ADH) is responsible for conserving body water and regulating the osmolarity of body fluids (Table 53-6). Painful stimulation and hemorrhage, as associated with surgery, are potent events for evoking the release of AVP. Hydration and the establishment of an

TABLE 53-6.
REGULATION OF ARGININE VASOPRESSIN SECRETION

Stimulation	Inhibition
Increased plasma osmolarity	Decreased plasma osmolarity
Hypovolemia	Ethanol
Pain	α-Adrenergic agonists
Hypotension	Cortisol
Hyperthermia	Hypothermia
Stress	
Nausea and vomiting	
Opioids (?)	

adequate blood volume before the induction of anesthesia serve to maintain urine output, presumably by blunting the release of AVP associated with painful stimulation or fluid deprivation before surgery. The administration of morphine, and presumably other opioids, in the absence of painful stimulation does not evoke the release of AVP. Ethanol inhibits the secretion of AVP. Decreased urine output and fluid retention previously attributed to the release of AVP during positive pressure ventilation of the lungs are more likely due to changes in cardiac filling pressures that impair the release of atrial natriuretic hormone. Diabetes insipidus results when the destruction of neurons occurs in or near the supraoptic and paraventricular nuclei of the hypothalamus. It will not occur when the posterior pituitary alone is damaged, because the transected fibers of the pituitary stalk can still continue to secrete AVP. Diabetes insipidus, which develops in association with pituitary surgery, typically is due to trauma to the posterior pituitary and is usually transient.

Oxytocin

The primary role of oxytocin is to eject milk from the lactating mammary gland. Large amounts of oxytocin cause the sustained uterine contraction necessary for postpartum hemostasis.

THYROID GLAND

The principal hormonal secretions of the thyroid gland are thyroxine (T4) and triiodothyronine (T3). T3 is the most biologically active form of thyroid hormone (five times more active than T4) and is produced directly from tyrosine metabolism or from the conversion of T4 in peripheral tissues. In addition to thyroid hormones, the thyroid gland secretes calcitonin, which is important for calcium ion use. The most obvious effect of thyroid hormones is to increase minute oxygen consumption in nearly all tissues, with the brain being an important exception. The failure of thyroid hormones to greatly alter the minute oxygen consumption of the brain is consistent with the minimal changes in anesthetic requirements (MAC) that accompany hyperthyroidism or hypothyroidism. Cardiovascular changes are often the earliest clinical manifestations of abnormal thyroid hormone levels.

Mechanism of Action

It is generally believed that thyroid hormones exert most, if not all, of their effects through the control of protein synthesis. This most likely reflects the ability of thyroid hormones to activate the DNA transcription process in the cell nucleus, with the resulting formation of new cell proteins, including enzymes. Sympathomimetic effects that accompany thyroid hormone stimulation most likely reflect an increased number and sensitivity of β-adrenergic receptors in response to the release of T4 and T3.

Calcitonin

Calcitonin is a polypeptide hormone secreted by the thyroid gland; it causes a decrease in the plasma concentration of calcium ions.

PARATHYROID GLANDS

Parathyroid hormone is responsible for regulating the plasma concentration of calcium ions. Small decreases in the plasma concentration of calcium ions are potent stimulants for the release of parathyroid hormone. The most prominent effect of parathyroid hormone is to promote the mobilization of calcium from bones, reflecting the stimulation of osteoclastic activity. At the kidneys, parathyroid hormone increases the renal tubular reabsorption of calcium ions and inhibits the renal reabsorption of phosphate.

ADRENAL CORTEX

The two major classes of corticosteroids are mineralocorticoids and glucocorticoids (Table 53-7). Mineralocorticoids influence the plasma concentrations of sodium and potassium ions, whereas glucocorticoids influence carbohydrate, fat, and protein metabolism as well as exhibiting antiinflammatory effects. Anatomically, the adrenal cortex is divided into three zones designated the (a) zona glomerulosa that secretes mineralocorticoids, (b) zona fasciculata that secretes glucocorticoids, and (c) zona reticularis that secretes androgens and estrogens.

Mineralocorticoids

Aldosterone accounts for approximately 95% of the mineralocorticoid activity produced by corticosteroids.

Physiologic Effects

The principal functions of aldosterone are to sustain extracellular fluid volume by conserving sodium and to maintain a normal plasma concentration of potassium (aldosterone causes the absorption of sodium ions and simultaneous secretion of potassium ions). Water follows sodium, so that extracellular fluid volume tends to change in proportion to the rate of aldosterone secretion. When the plasma concentration of potassium is decreased approximately 50% due to the excess secretion of aldosterone, skeletal muscle weakness or even paralysis occurs, reflecting hyperpolarization of nerve and muscle membranes, which prevents transmission of action potentials.

Mechanism of Action

Aldosterone diffuses to the interior of renal tubular epithelial cells, where it induces DNA to form messenger RNA (mRNA) necessary for the transport of sodium and potassium ions.

TABLE 53-7.

PHYSIOLOGIC EFFECTS OF ENDOGENOUS CORTICOSTEROIDS (mg)

	Daily Secretion	Sodium Retention*	Glucocorticoid Effect*	Antiinflammatory Effect*
Aldosterone	0.125	3,000	0.3	Insignificant
Desoxycorticosterone	—	100	0	0
Cortisol	20	1	1	1
Corticosterone	Minimal	15	0.35	0.3
Cortisone	Minimal	0.8	0.8	0.8

*Relative to cortisol.

Regulation of Secretion

The most important stimulus for aldosterone secretion is an increase in the plasma potassium concentration. The renin-angiotensin system is also an important determinant of aldosterone secretion. Mineralocorticoid secretion is not under the primary control of ACTH. For this reason, hypoaldosteronism does not accompany a loss of ACTH secretion from the anterior pituitary.

Glucocorticoids

Cortisol

At least 95% of the glucocorticoid activity results from the secretion of cortisol.

Physiologic Effects (Table 53-8)

Developmental Changes

Plasma concentrations of cortisol increase progressively during the last trimester of pregnancy to reach a peak plasma concentration at term, thus permitting the maturation of a number of systems that are critical for survival with the onset of extrauterine life (surfactant, enzymes).

Gluconeogenesis

Cortisol stimulates gluconeogenesis by the liver as much as tenfold, reflecting principally a mobilization of amino

TABLE 53-8.
PHYSIOLOGIC EFFECTS OF CORTISOL

Increased gluconeogenesis
Protein catabolism
Fatty acid mobilization
Antiinflammatory effects
Increased number or responsiveness of β-adrenergic receptors (maintains systemic blood pressure)
Maintains normal responsiveness of arterioles to catecholamines
Inhibits bone formation

acids from extrahepatic sites and their transfer to the liver for conversion to glucose (results in hyperglycemia).

Protein Catabolism

Cortisol decreases protein stores in nearly all cells except hepatocytes, reflecting the mobilization of amino acids for gluconeogenesis (produces skeletal muscle weakness).

Fatty Acid Mobilization

Cortisol promotes the mobilization of fatty acids from adipose tissue and enhances the oxidation of fatty acids in cells. Despite these effects, excess amounts of cortisol cause the deposition of fat in the neck and chest regions, giving rise to a "buffalo-like" torso, because the deposition of fat at these sites occurs at a rate that exceeds its mobilization.

Antiinflammatory Effects

Cortisol in large amounts has antiinflammatory effects, reflecting its ability to stabilize lysosomal membranes and to decrease the migration of leukocytes into the inflamed area; this characteristic of cortisol secretion is important in attenuating inflammation associated with disease states such as rheumatoid arthritis and acute glomerulonephritis. The level of immunity against bacterial or viral infection is decreased, and fulminating infection can occur. Conversely, this ability of cortisol to suppress immunity is useful in decreasing the likelihood of immunologic rejection of transplanted tissues. The beneficial effect of cortisol in the treatment of allergic reactions reflects the prevention of inflammatory responses that are responsible for many of the life-threatening effects of an allergic reaction, such as laryngeal edema.

Mechanism of Action

Cortisol stimulates DNA-dependent synthesis of mRNA in the nuclei of responsive cells, leading to the synthesis of appropriate enzymes.

Regulation of Secretion

The most important stimulus for the secretion of cortisol (13 to 20 mg daily) is the release of ACTH from the anterior pituitary (see Table 53-5). The secretion of ACTH in the anterior pituitary is determined by two hypothalamic neurohormones (diurnal release of corticotropin-releasing hormone and AVP) that act synergistically. Circulating cortisol also exerts a direct negative-feedback effect on the hypothalamus and anterior pituitary to decrease the release of corticotropin-releasing hormone and ACTH from these respective sites. Stress, as associated with the intraoperative period, can override the normal negative-feedback control mechanisms, and plasma concentrations of cortisol are increased. Cortisol is secreted and released by the adrenal cortex at a basal rate of approximately 20 mg daily. In response to maximal stressful stimuli (sepsis, burns), the output of cortisol is increased to approximately 150 mg daily. Therefore, this amount should be sufficient replacement when provided to patients who lack adrenal function and who are acutely ill or undergoing major surgery.

Effect of Anesthesia and Surgery

Plasma cortisol concentrations typically increase (two- to tenfold) following the induction of anesthesia, during surgery, and in the postoperative period. Plasma cortisol concentrations typically return to normal levels within 24 hours postoperatively, but may remain elevated for as long as 72 hours depending on the severity of the surgical trauma. Plasma cortisol concentrations in the perioperative period reflect a response designed to provide protection during and after surgery. Supportive animal evidence is the observation that adrenalectomized animals receiving subphysiologic doses of cortisol experienced hemodynamic instability and increased mortality following surgery. Suppression of the hypothalamic-pituitary axis, as produced by the chronic administration of corticosteroids, also prevents the release of cortisol in response to stressful stimuli.

REPRODUCTIVE GLANDS

Testes

The testes secrete male sex hormones, which are collectively designated androgens. At most sites of action, testosterone is not the active form of the hormone being converted in target tissues to the more active dihydrotestosterone by a reductase enzyme.

Ovaries

The two ovarian hormones, estrogen and progesterone, are secreted in response to LH and FSH, which are released from the anterior pituitary in response to hypothalamic-releasing hormones.

Estrogens

Estrogens are responsible for the development of female sexual characteristics.

Progesterone

Progesterone is necessary for the preparation of the uterus for pregnancy and the breasts for lactation.

Menstruation

The overall duration of a normal menstrual cycle is 21 to 35 days and consists of three phases designated as follicular, ovulatory, and luteal. The increase in body temperature (approximately 0.5°C) that accompanies ovulation most likely reflects a thermogenic effect of progesterone.

Pregnancy

During pregnancy, the placenta forms large amounts of estrogens, progesterone, chorionic gonadotropin, and chorionic somatomammotropin. Chorionic gonadotropin prevents the usual involution of the corpus luteum, which would lead to the onset of menstrual bleeding.

This placental hormone is the first key hormone of pregnancy and can be detected in the maternal plasma within 9 days after conception, thus providing the basis for pregnancy tests. Increased plasma concentrations of progesterone are presumed to be the stimulus for the increased alveolar ventilation that accompanies pregnancy. The parturient with asthma may experience unpredictable changes in airway reactivity.

Menopause

The ovaries gradually become unresponsive to the stimulatory effects of LH and FSH, resulting in the disappearance of sexual cycles between the ages of 45 and 55 years. Sensations of warmth spreading from the trunk to the face (hot flashes) coincide with surges of LH secretion and are prevented by the exogenous administration of estrogens.

PANCREAS

The pancreas secretes digestive substances into the duodenum as well as four hormones (insulin, glucagon, somatostatin, pancreatin peptide) that are produced by the islets of Langerhans and released into the systemic circulation.

Insulin

Insulin is an anabolic hormone promoting the storage of glucose, fatty acids, and amino acids. The amount of insulin secreted daily is equivalent to approximately 40 units. In the systemic circulation, insulin has an elimination half-time of approximately 5 minutes, with >80% degraded in the liver and kidneys. Insulin binds to receptor proteins in cell membranes, leading to the activation of the glucose transport system. Activation of sodium-potassium ATPase in cell membranes by insulin results in movement of potassium ions into cells and a decrease in the plasma concentration of potassium.

TABLE 53-9.
REGULATION OF INSULIN SECRETION

Stimulation	Inhibition
Hyperglycemia	Hypoglycemia
β-Adrenergic agonists	β-Adrenergic antagonists
Acetylcholine	α-Adrenergic agonists
Glucagon	Somatostatin
	Diazoxide
	Thiazide diuretics
	Volatile anesthetics
	Insulin

Regulation of Secretion

The principal control of insulin secretion is via a negative-feedback effect of the blood glucose concentration of the pancreas (Table 53-9). Virtually no insulin is secreted by the pancreas when the blood glucose concentrations are <50 mg/dL, and maximum stimulation for the release of insulin occurs when blood glucose concentrations are >300 mg/dL. The pancreas is richly innervated by the autonomic nervous system, with insulin release occurring in response to β-adrenergic stimulation or release of acetylcholine. Conversely, α-adrenergic stimulation or β-adrenergic blockade results in the inhibition of insulin release. Oral glucose is more effective than glucose administered intravenously in evoking the release of insulin, suggesting the presence of an anticipatory signal from the gastrointestinal tract to the pancreas. Consistent with this is the more likely occurrence of glycosuria after intravenous rather than oral glucose administration.

Physiologic Effects

Insulin promotes the use of carbohydrates for energy while depressing the use of fats and amino acids. Insulin facilitates the storage of fat in adipose cells by inhibiting lipase enzyme, which normally causes the hydrolysis of triglycerides in fat cells. Brain cells are unique in that the permeability of their membranes to glucose does not depend on the presence of insulin. Lack of insulin causes the use of mainly fat, to the exclusion of glucose except by brain cells.

Diabetes Mellitus

Diabetes mellitus is a metabolic disease characterized by hyperglycemia that results from defects in insulin secretion and/or action of insulin. The presence of chronic hyperglycemia is associated with long-term damage and dysfunction of the kidneys, eyes, autonomic nervous system, heart, blood vessels, and microcirculation. The vast majority of cases of diabetes are either type 1 (insulin-dependent) or type 2 (non–insulin dependent) in an approximate ratio of 1 to 9 (Table 53-10). Even in the absence of overt diabetes, patients with latent disease release less insulin in response to glucose stimulation. The insulin-deficient liver is likely to use fatty acids to produce ketones, which can serve as an energy source for skeletal muscles and cardiac muscle. The production of ketones can lead to ketoacidosis, whereas urinary excretion of these anions contributes to the depletion of electrolytes, especially potassium. Low plasma concentrations

TABLE 53-10.
ETIOLOGIC CLASSIFICATION OF DIABETES MELLITUS

Type 1 diabetes mellitus (absolute insulin deficiency owing to pancreatic β-cell destruction)
Type 2 diabetes mellitus (insulin resistance vs. insulin deficiency)
Endocrinopathies (acromegaly, Cushing syndrome)
Drug-induced (glucocorticoids, thiazides)
Gestational diabetes mellitus
Genetic defects in pancreatic β-cell function
Genetic defects in insulin action (resistance)

insulin, although inadequate to prevent hyperglycemia, may be quite effective in blocking lipolysis. This differential effect of insulin explains the frequent observation in patients with diabetes mellitus that hyperglycemia can exist without the presence of ketone bodies. Ketosis can be reliably prevented by continuously providing all diabetic patients with glucose and insulin.

Glucagon

Glucagon is a catabolic hormone acting to mobilize glucose, fatty acids, and amino acids into the systemic circulation (Table 53-11). Glucagon is able to abruptly increase the blood glucose concentration by stimulating glycogenolysis in the liver.

TABLE 53-11.
REGULATION OF GLUCAGON SECRETION

Stimulation	Inhibition
Hypoglycemia	Hyperglycemia
Stress	Somatostatin
Sepsis	Insulin
Trauma	Free fatty acids
β-Adrenergic agonists	α-Adrenergic agonists
Acetylcholine	
Cortisol	

Kidneys

54

The principal function of the kidneys is to stabilize the composition of the extracellular fluid, as reflected by electrolyte and hydrogen ion concentrations (Stoelting RK, Hillier SC. Kidneys. In: *Pharmacology and Physiology in Anesthetic Practice*. 4th ed. Philadelphia, Lippincott Williams & Wilkins, 2006:815–828). The end-products of protein metabolism, such as urea, are excreted, whereas essential body nutrients, including amino acids and glucose, are retained. The kidneys also secrete hormones for the regulation of systemic blood pressure (angiotensin II, prostaglandins, kinins) and the production of erythrocytes (erythropoietin). The kidneys receive an estimated 20% of the cardiac output.

NEPHRON

The functional unit of the kidney is the nephron, which is composed of capillaries known as the *glomerulus* and a long tubule in which the fluid filtered through the glomerular capillaries is converted to urine on its way to the renal pelvis (Fig. 54-1).

Glomerulus

The glomerulus is formed only in the renal cortex by a tuft of capillaries that invaginate into the dilated blind end of the renal tubule known as Bowman's capsule. It is the pressure in glomerular capillaries that causes water and low molecular weight substances to filter into Bowman's capsule, which is in direct continuity with the proximal renal tubule.

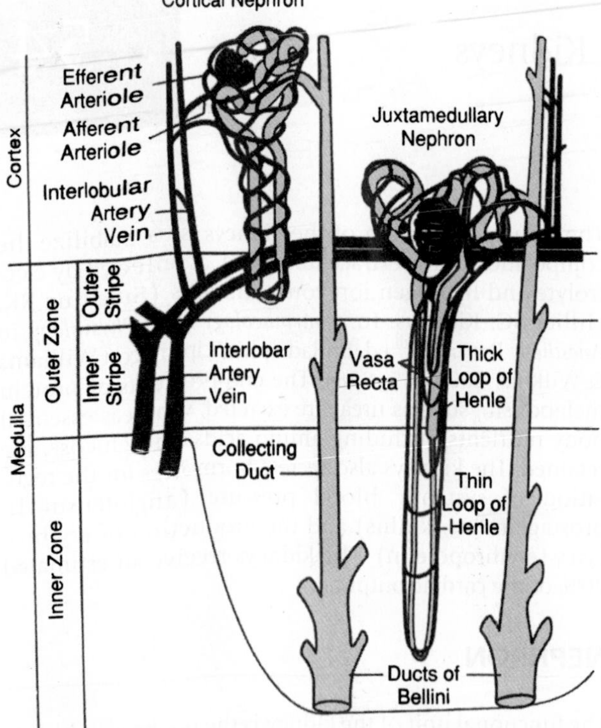

Figure 54-1. Schematic depiction of the nephron and accompanying blood supply. (From Pitts RF. *Physiology of the Kidney and Body Fluids*, 3rd ed. Chicago: Year Book, 1974; with permission.)

Renal Tubule

The components of the renal tubule are the proximal convoluted tubule, the loop of Henle, and the distal convoluted tubule. As the glomerular filtrate travels along the renal tubule, most of its water and varying amounts of solutes are reabsorbed from the renal tubular lumen into peritubular capillaries (Table 54-1). Unwanted metabolic waste products are filtered through glomerular capillaries

TABLE 54-1.

MAGNITUDE AND SITE OF SOLUTE REABSORPTION OR SECRETION IN THE RENAL TUBULES

	Filtered (24 hrs)	Reabsorbed (24 hrs)	Secreted (24 hrs)	Excreted (24 hrs)	Percent Reabsorbed	Location
Water (liters)	180	179		1	99.4	P,L,D,C
Sodium (mEq)	26,000	25,850		150	99.4	P,L,D,C
Potassium (mEq)	600	560	50	90	93.3	P,L,D,C
Chloride (mEq)	18,000	17,850		150	99.2	P,L,D,C
Bicarbonate (mEq)	4,900	4,900		0	10	P,D
Urea (mM)	870	460		410	53	P,L,D,C
Uric acid (mM)	50	49	4	5	98	P
Glucose (mM)	800	800		0	100	P

C, convoluted tubule; D, distal tubule; L, loop of Henle; P, proximal tubule.

but, unlike water and electrolytes, are not reabsorbed as the glomerular filtrate progresses through the renal tubules (see Table 54-1). Ultimately, the urine that is formed is composed mainly of substances filtered through the glomerular capillaries, in addition to small amounts of substances secreted by the renal tubular epithelial cells into the lumens of the renal tubules.

RENAL BLOOD FLOW

The kidneys have an enormous blood supply, receiving 20% to 25% of the cardiac output, despite representing only about 0.5% of the total body weight. Despite this high oxygen delivery via renal blood flow, renal ischemia and acute renal failure are prominent clinical problems, especially in severely injured patients and elderly patients undergoing major vascular surgery. Normally, renal blood flow is approximately 90% to 95% delivered to the renal cortex, with the remainder to the renal medulla.

Influence of Anesthesia and Surgery

All anesthetic drugs, whether inhaled or injected, have the potential to alter renal function by changing systemic blood pressure and cardiac output so that renal blood flow is redistributed away from the outer renal cortex. In this regard, renal ischemia may be prominent despite the absence of systemic hypotension, thus emphasizing that systemic blood pressure may not be a good guide to the adequacy of renal perfusion. Furthermore, intraoperative urine output does not correlate with postoperative changes in renal function as reflected by the plasma creatinine concentrations.

Prostaglandins

Nonsteroidal antiinflammatory drugs that inhibit cyclooxygenase have little or no effect on renal blood flow or glomerular filtration rate in healthy subjects but cause marked decreases in these parameters when the renal circulation is compromised, as by hemorrhage. This emphasizes that vasodilator prostaglandins are important in maintaining renal blood flow and glomerular filtration rate in these circumstances.

Glomerular Capillaries

High pressure in the glomerular capillaries causes them to function in the same manner as the arterial ends of tissue capillaries, with fluid moving continuously out of the glomerular capillaries into Bowman's capsule.

Peritubular Capillaries (Renal Cortex Blood Flow)

Fluid from the renal tubules is absorbed continually into the low-pressure peritubular capillaries (180 liters of fluid is filtered daily through the glomerular capillaries, and all but approximately 1.5 liter is reabsorbed from the renal tubules back into the peritubular capillaries).

Vasa Recta (Renal Medulla Blood Flow)

The function of the renal medulla is to maintain a high osmolarity (produced by solute transport out of the ascending limb of the loop of Henle), to allow the tubular fluid to be concentrated by the osmotic absorption of water from the collecting ducts.

Autoregulation of Renal Blood Flow

Changes in mean arterial pressure between approximately 60 and 160 mm Hg simultaneously autoregulate both renal blood flow and glomerular filtration rate (Fig. 54-2). The concept of autoregulation can be very misleading. For example, when effective circulating volume decreases, a decrease in renal blood flow occurs, regardless of the perfusion pressure and the presence of autoregulation. Thus, underperfusion of the kidneys may

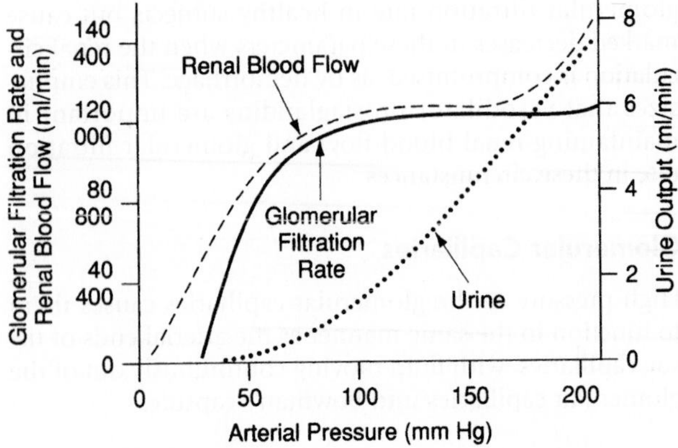

Figure 54-2. Renal blood flow and glomerular filtration rate, but not urine output, are autoregulated between a mean arterial pressure of approximately 60 and 160 mm Hg. (From Guyton AC, Hall JE. *Textbook of Medical Physiology*, 10th ed. Philadelphia: Saunders, 2000; with permission.)

be present, even though mean arterial pressure is in the range for autoregulation of renal blood flow. For this reason, systemic blood pressure may not be a good guide to the adequacy of renal perfusion, especially when vasoconstriction is responsible for maintaining blood pressure in the presence of hypovolemia. Autoregulation of renal blood flow is not abolished during the administration of most anesthetic drugs. Conversely, autoregulation is impaired in severe sepsis, in the presence of acute renal failure, and during cardiopulmonary bypass.

Juxtaglomerular Apparatus

The juxtaglomerular apparatus is the site where the distal renal tubule passes through the angle between renal afferent and efferent arterioles. Juxtaglomerular cells release renin into the circulation, in response to decreased renal blood flow as may accompany hypovolemia, systemic hypotension, renal ischemia, or sympathetic nervous

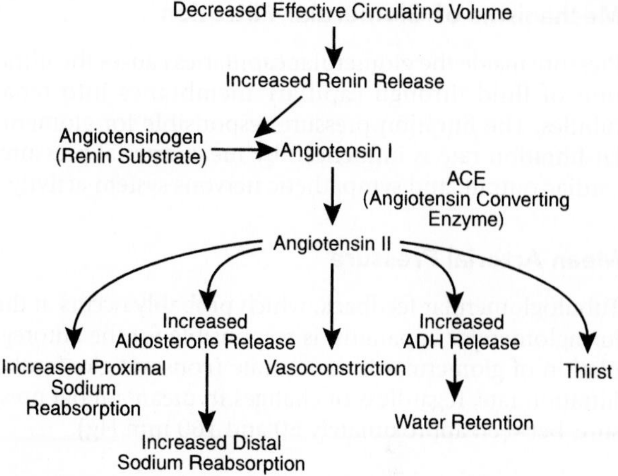

Figure 54-3. The role of the renin-angiotensin system in the maintenance of effective circulating volume. (From Lote CJ, Harper L, Savage COS. Mechanisms of acute renal failure. *Br J Anaesth* 1996;77:82–89; with permission.)

system stimulation (Fig. 54-3). This is an effort by the kidneys to maintain normal renal blood flow and glomerular filtration rate.

GLOMERULAR FILTRATE

Fluid that filters across glomerular capillaries into the renal tubules is designated glomerular filtrate. For all practical purposes, glomerular filtrate is plasma without proteins.

Glomerular Filtration Rate

The glomerular filtration rate is the amount of glomerular filtrate (125 mL/min) formed each minute by all the nephrons. Reabsorption of approximately 99% of this 180 liters of glomerular filtrate occurs during its passage through the renal tubule, resulting in a daily urine output of 1 to 2 liters.

Mechanisms of Glomerular Filtration

Pressure inside the glomerular capillaries causes the filtration of fluid through capillary membranes into renal tubules. The filtration pressure responsible for glomerular filtration rate is influenced by mean arterial pressure, cardiac output, and sympathetic nervous system activity.

Mean Arterial Pressure

Tubuloglomerular feedback, which probably occurs at the juxtaglomerular apparatus, is responsible for the autoregulation of glomerular filtration rate (constant glomerular filtration rate, regardless of changes in mean arterial pressure, between approximately 60 and 160 mm Hg).

Cardiac Output

Because the glomerular filtration rate parallels renal blood flow, it is clear that changes in cardiac output, including those produced by anesthetics, will have an important impact on glomerular filtrate rate.

Sympathetic Nervous System

Excessive sympathetic nervous system stimulation can decrease glomerular blood flow so that urine output decreases to almost zero.

RENAL TUBULAR FUNCTION

Glomerular filtrate flows through renal tubules and collecting ducts, during which time substances are selectively reabsorbed from tubules into peritubular capillaries or secreted into tubules by tubular epithelial cells. The resulting glomerular filtrate entering the renal pelvis is urine. Approximately two-thirds of all reabsorption and secretory processes in renal tubules take place in proximal renal tubules. The major physiologic determinants of the reabsorption of sodium and water are aldosterone, AVP, renal prostaglandins, and atrial natriuretic factor. The energy necessary for the reabsorption of sodium is supplied by the sodium-potassium adenosine triphosphatase (ATPase) system. The proximal convoluted renal tubules have the highest sodium-potassium ATPase activity, and approximately 80% of renal oxygen consumption is used to drive this ATPase enzyme system for sodium reabsorption. Aldosterone promotes the reabsorption of sodium and secretion of hydrogen and potassium in the distal convoluted tubule. More than 99% of the water in the glomerular filtrate is reabsorbed into peritubular capillaries as it passes through renal tubules. Distal renal tubules are almost completely impermeable to water, which is important for controlling the specific gravity of urine. The permeability of the epithelial cells lining the collecting ducts is determined by AVP.

Aquaporins

Aquaporins are protein water channels (tetramers) that facilitate the rapid passage of water across lipid cell membranes at a velocity that exceeds that possible by simple diffusion. Aquaporin-2 is stored in vesicles in the cytoplasm, and vasopressin causes the rapid transcription of these vesicles into the luminal membranes of renal tubular collecting duct cells.

Countercurrent System

The countercurrent system is one in which blood inflow runs parallel and in the opposite direction to outflow. In the kidneys, the U-shaped anatomic arrangement from the peritubular capillaries, known as the vasa recta, to those loops of Henle that extend into the renal medulla make the countercurrent system possible. As a result, the kidneys are able to eliminate solutes with a minimal excretion of water (Fig. 54-4).

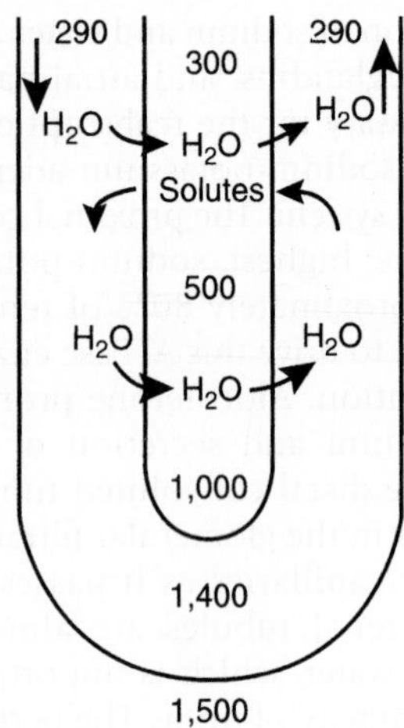

Figure 54-4. Countercurrent exchange of water and solutes in the vasa recta. (From Lote CJ, Harper L, Savage COS. Mechanisms of acute renal failure. *Br J Anaesth* 1996;77:82–89; with permission.)

TUBULAR TRANSPORT MAXIMUM

The tubular transport maximum (Tm) is the maximal amount of a substance that can be actively reabsorbed from the lumens of renal tubules each minute.

REGULATION OF BODY FLUID CHARACTERISTICS

Blood Volume

Blood volume is maintained over a narrow range despite marked daily variations in fluid and solute intake or loss. An increase in blood volume increases cardiac output, which increases blood pressure. Increased systemic blood pressure subsequently leads to renal changes (increased renal blood flow and glomerular filtrate rate) that cause an increased urine output and a return of blood volume to normal. The effects of blood volume on systemic blood pressure, cardiac output, and urine output are slow to develop, requiring several hours to produce a full effect.

Extracellular Fluid Volume

It is not possible to alter blood volume without also simultaneously changing extracellular fluid volume; the extracellular fluid becomes a reservoir for excess fluid that may be administered intravenously during the perioperative period.

Osmolarity

The osmolarity of body fluids is determined almost entirely by the concentration of sodium in the extracellular fluid. The control of sodium ion concentration and, thus, the osmolarity of body fluids is under the influence of the osmoreceptor-AVP mechanism and the thirst reflex.

Osmoreceptor-Arginine Vasopressin Hormone

An increase in the osmolarity of extracellular fluid due to excess sodium ions causes osmoreceptors in the supraoptic nuclei of the hypothalamus to shrink and thereby increase the discharge rate of impulses through the pituitary stalk to the posterior pituitary, where AVP is released. The resulting AVP-induced retention of water dilutes the plasma sodium concentration and returns osmolarity downward toward a normal value.

Thirst Reflex

The most common cause for thirst is an increased sodium concentration in the extracellular fluid. Any change in circulation that leads to the increased production of angiotensin II, such as acute hemorrhage or congestive heart failure, also leads to thirst. Although the sensation of a dry mouth is often associated with the thirst reflex, the blockade of salivary secretions, as by anticholinergic drugs, does not cause humans to drink excessively.

Plasma Concentration of Ions

Potassium

The role of the kidneys in controlling the plasma concentration of potassium is mediated principally by the effects of aldosterone on the renal tubules.

Sodium

Approximately two-thirds of sodium is reabsorbed from the proximal renal tubules, and no more than 10% of the sodium that initially enters the glomerular filtrate is likely to reach the distal renal tubule. In the presence of large amounts of aldosterone, almost all the remaining sodium is reabsorbed, and urinary excretion of sodium approaches zero.

Hydrogen

The kidneys secrete excess hydrogen ions by exchanging a hydrogen ion for a sodium ion, thus acidifying the urine, and by the synthesis of ammonia, which combines with hydrogen to form ammonium.

Calcium

Calcium concentration is controlled principally by the effect of parathyroid hormone on bone reabsorption. A decrease in the plasma concentration of calcium evokes the release of parathyroid hormone, which causes the release of calcium from bone.

Magnesium

Magnesium is reabsorbed by all portions of the renal tubules.

Urea

Urea is the most abundant of the metabolic waste products that must be excreted in urine to prevent an excess accumulation in body fluids.

ATRIAL AND RENAL NATRIURETIC FACTORS

The cardiac atria synthesize, store, and secrete via the coronary sinus an amino acid hormone known as atrial natriuretic peptide (ANP). The renal analog of ANP is renal natriuretic peptide (urodilatin), which is synthesized in renal cortical nephrons.

ACUTE RENAL FAILURE

Acute renal failure is characterized by an abrupt deterioration of renal function, with a decrease in the glomerular filtration rate occurring over a period of hours to days, resulting in the failure of the kidneys to excrete nitrogenous waste products (urea and creatinine) and to maintain fluid and electrolyte homeostasis. Loss of urinary concentrating ability is an early and precise manifestation of acute tubular necrosis, most likely reflecting a failure of the energy-requiring sodium-potassium ATPase pump in the renal tubules.

Classification

Traditionally, acute renal failure is classified as prerenal, intrarenal, or postrenal (Fig. 54-5).

Prerenal Azotemia

Prerenal azotemia denotes a disorder in the systemic circulation that causes renal hypoperfusion. Implicit in this explanation is that a correction of the underlying circulatory disorder (improved cardiac output or repletion of intravascular fluid volume) will restore glomerular filtration. Elderly patients are particularly susceptible to prerenal azotemia because of their predisposition to hypovolemia and high prevalence of renal artery atherosclerosis. Among hospitalized patients, prerenal azotemia is the single most common cause of acute renal failure and is often due to congestive heart failure, hypovolemia,

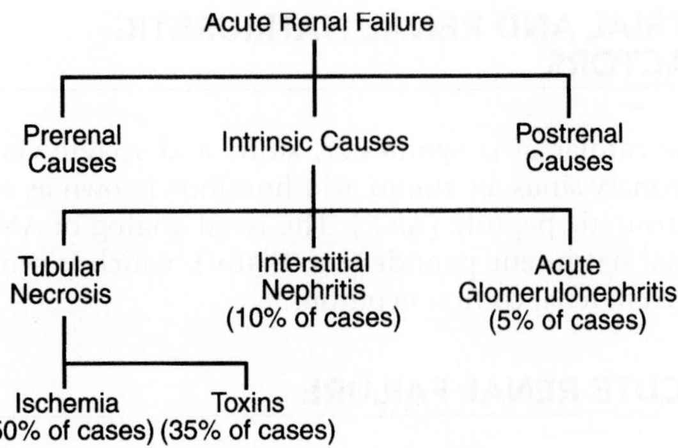

Figure 54-5. Classification of acute renal failure. (From R, Pascual M, Bonventre JV. Acute renal failure. *N Engl J Med* 1996;334:1448–1460; with permission.)

septic shock, or the administration of radiocontrast media, especially in patients with pre-existing renal disease, diabetes, hypovolemia, and concomitant exposure to other nephrotoxins.

Intrinsic Renal Failure

Intrinsic renal failure generally includes renal tubular necrosis, which may be due to ischemia or nephrotoxins. Acute tubular necrosis reflects the destruction of those epithelial cells lining the renal tubules and is most often due to nephrotoxins or renal ischemia, as produced by prolonged decreases in systemic blood pressure and renal blood flow (shock). Acute tubular necrosis due to ischemia of the renal medullary ascending tubular cells is a common cause of acute renal failure in the perioperative period. In this regard, hypoperfusion of the kidneys is the most frequently recognized single insult leading to acute renal failure in the setting of trauma surgery, hemorrhage, or dehydration.

Postrenal Obstructive Nephropathy

Obstructive postrenal failure (renal stones, prostatic hypertrophy, mechanical kinking of catheters) may be a cause of acute renal failure in some patients. Sudden acute oliguria in the perioperative period warrants an evaluation of possible mechanical obstruction to urinary drainage devices.

Oliguric versus Nonoliguric Renal Failure

Acute renal failure may be oliguric (urine output <400 mL/day) or nonoliguric (urine output >400 mL/day). Patients with nonoliguric acute renal failure have a better prognosis than those with oliguric renal failure, probably due to the decreased severity of the causative insult and the fact that many of these patients have drug-associated nephrotoxicity or interstitial nephritis.

Mortality

When acute renal failure occurs in the setting of multiorgan failure, especially in patients with severe hypotension or acute respiratory distress syndrome, mortality rates range from 50% to 80%.

Diagnosis

One of the earliest functional defects seen with renal tubular damage is loss of the ability to concentrate urine (Table 54-2).

TABLE 54-2.
DIFFERENTIAL DIAGNOSIS OF ACUTE RENAL FAILURE

Prerenal Causes	Acute Tubular Necrosis
Urine osmolarity >500 mOsm/liter	Urine osmolarity <350 mOsm/liter
Urinary sodium concentration <20 mEq/liter	Urinary sodium concentration >40 mEq/liter
Fractional excretion of sodium <1%	Fractional excretion of sodium >1%

Treatment

The initial care of patients with acute renal failure is focused on reversing the underlying cause and correcting fluid and electrolyte imbalances (Fig. 54-6). Although restoration of renal blood flow with intravenous volume resuscitation is ineffective in restoring renal function

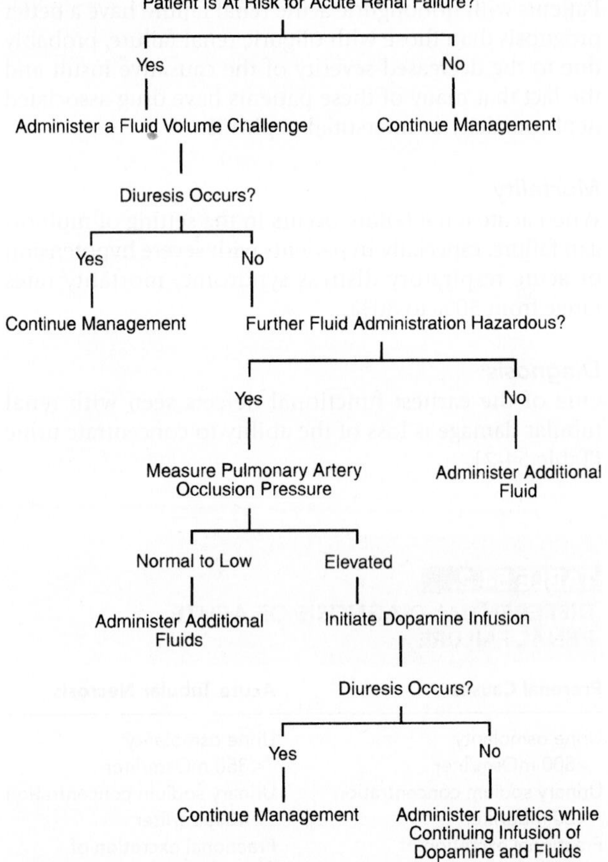

Figure 54-6. Treatment diagram for a patient who develops acute oliguria in the perioperative period.

TABLE 54-3.
CHARACTERISTICS OF PATIENTS AT INCREASED RISK FOR DEVELOPING ACUTE RENAL FAILURE IN THE POSTOPERATIVE PERIOD

Preexisting renal disease
Congestive heart failure
Advanced age
Prolonged renal hypoperfusion
High-risk surgery (abdominal aneurysm resection, cardiopulmonary bypass)
Sepsis
Jaundice

once tubular necrosis is established, volume replacement remains the most effective prophylactic strategy. Aggressive and early treatment of perioperative oliguria is most important for those patients at increased risk for developing acute renal failure (Table 54-3). The occurrence of transient oliguria during elective operations in young patients without preexisting renal disease does not require the same aggressive treatment as does oliguria in elderly patients with preexisting renal disease.

Cytoprotection

Cytoprotection against ischemic reperfusion injury may be provided by calcium channel blockade.

Ischemic Preconditioning

Ischemic preconditioning, in which repeated transient sublethal ischemic events confer resistance to subsequent more severe ischemic insults, occurs in an animal model of acute renal failure and appears to be mediated by adenosine.

CHRONIC RENAL FAILURE

The common denominator present in patients who develop chronic renal failure is a progressive loss of nephron function and decline in glomerular filtration rate (Table 54-4).

TABLE 54-4.
STAGES OF CHRONIC RENAL FAILURE

	Number of Functioning Nephrons (% of Total)	Glomerular Rate Filtration (mL/min)	Signs	Laboratory Changes
Normal	100	125	None	None
Decreased renal reserve	40	50–80	None	None
Renal insufficiency	10–40	12–50	Polyuria, nocturia	Increased BUN and creatinine
Uremia	10	<12	See Table 53-5	See Table 53-5

BUN, blood urea nitrogen.

TABLE 54-5.
MANIFESTATIONS OF CHRONIC RENAL FAILURE

Accumulation of metabolic waste products in blood
Excretion of fixed specific gravity urine
Metabolic acidosis
Hyperkalemia
Anemia (less common with introduction of recombinant erythropoietin)
Platelet dysfunction
Fluid overload and systemic hypertension
Nervous system dysfunction
Osteomalacia

Manifestations of Chronic Renal Failure (Table 54-5)

It has been estimated that 5% of the adult population has preexisting renal disease that may contribute to perioperative morbidity. A comprehensive preoperative evaluation must include a review of renal function tests, keeping in mind that most of these tests are imprecise and insensitive indicators of the degree of renal dysfunction (Table 54-6). Anemia is severe but usually well tolerated, reflecting its slow onset and compensatory increases in tissue blood flow and rightward shift of the oxyhemoglobin dissociation curve in response to acidosis and increased concentrations of 2,3-diphosphoglycerate. Hyperkalemia reflects inability of diseased kidneys to eliminate potassium and has important anesthetic implications, especially with respect to cardiac rhythm and responses at the neuromuscular junction. The accumulation of metabolic waste products in the blood interferes with platelet aggregation, whereas prothrombin time and plasma thromboplastin time usually remain normal. The retention of sodium and water results in fluid overload that may manifest as congestive heart failure and hypertension. Neurologic complications occur in the central

TABLE 54-6.
RENAL FUNCTION TESTS

	Normal Value	Factors that Influence Interpretation
Blood urea nitrogen	8–20 mg/dL	Dehydration Variable protein intake Gastrointestinal bleeding Catabolism
Creatinine	0.5–1.2 mg/dL	Age Skeletal muscle mass Catabolism
Creatinine clearance	120 mL/min	Accurate urine volume measurement

nervous system (confusion or coma), peripheral nervous system (neuropathy), and autonomic nervous system. Dialytic therapy is useful in correcting electrolyte, fluid, and platelet function.

Dialytic Therapy

Indications for initiating dialytic therapy are (a) hyperkalemia and/or acidosis that is not controlled by medical management, and (b) fluid overload that is not responsive to fluid restriction and/or diuretic therapy. Infection remains the main cause of death, despite aggressive dialytic therapy (meticulous aseptic care of intravenous catheters and wounds and avoidance of the use of indwelling urinary catheters are important).

Intermittent Hemodialysis

Hemodialysis is based on the diffusive transport of solute down an osmotic gradient, across a semipermeable membrane. The need to maintain chronic vascular access via a surgically created arteriovenous fistula is a major cause of morbidity in patients with chronic renal failure.

Continuous Hemodialysis

Continuous Hemodialysis is an alternative form of dialysis for critically ill patients with renal failure.

Peritoneal Dialysis

Peritoneal dialysis is effective in patients with acute renal failure associated with hemodynamic instability or when technical support is limited. Surgical placement of an indwelling peritoneal catheter (Tenckhoff catheter) is necessary. Peritonitis is the major complication associated with peritoneal dialysis.

TRANSPORT OF URINE TO THE BLADDER

Urine is transported to the bladder through the ureters, which originate in the pelvis of each kidney. As urine collects in the renal pelvis, the pressure in the pelvis increases and initiates a peristaltic contraction that travels downward along the ureter to force urine toward the bladder. Ureters are well supplied with nerve fibers so that obstruction of a ureter by a stone causes intense reflex constriction and pain. In addition, pain is likely to elicit a sympathetic nervous system reflex (ureterorenal reflex) that causes vasoconstriction of the renal arterioles and a concomitant decrease in urine formation in the kidney served by the obstructed ureter.

55

Liver and Gastrointestinal Tract

LIVER

The liver is the largest organ in the body, weighing approximately 1,500 g and representing 2% of body weight (Stoelting RK, Hillier SC. Liver and gastrointestinal tract. In: *Pharmacology and Physiology in Anesthetic Practice*. 4th ed. Philadelphia, Lippincott Williams & Wilkins, 2006:829–841). Hepatocytes perform diverse and complex functions (Table 55-1).

Anatomy

Blood flows past the hepatocytes via sinusoids from branches of the portal vein and hepatic artery to a central vein (area of contact with plasma is great). Each hepatocyte is also located adjacent to bile canaliculi, which coalesce to form the common hepatic duct. Hepatic lobules are lined by macrophages (derived from circulating monocytes) known as Kupffer's cells, which phagocytize 99% or more of bacteria in the portal venous blood. This is crucial, because the portal venous blood drains the gastrointestinal tract and almost always contains colon bacteria.

Hepatic Blood Flow

The liver receives a dual afferent blood supply from the hepatic artery and portal veins (Fig. 55-1). Total hepatic blood flow is approximately 1,450 mL/min or about 29% of the cardiac output. Of this amount, the portal vein

TABLE 55-1.
FUNCTIONS OF HEPATOCYTES

Absorb nutrients from portal venous blood
Store and release carbohydrates, proteins, and lipids
Excrete bile salts
Synthesize plasma proteins, glucose, cholesterol, and fatty acids
Metabolize exogenous and endogenous compounds

provides 75% of the total flow but only 50% to 55% of the hepatic oxygen supply, because this blood is partially deoxygenated in the preportal organs and tissues (gastrointestinal tract, spleen, pancreas). The hepatic artery provides only 25% of total hepatic blood flow but provides 45% to 50% of the hepatic oxygen requirements.

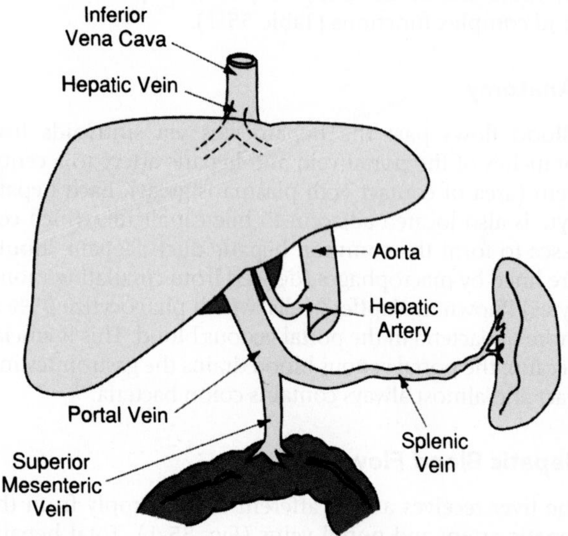

Figure 55-1. Schematic depiction of the dual afferent blood supply to the liver provided by the portal vein and hepatic artery.

Hepatic artery blood flow maintains the nutrition of connective tissues and the walls of bile ducts. For this reason, a loss of hepatic artery blood flow can be fatal because of the ensuing necrosis of vital liver structures. An increase in hepatic oxygen requirements is met by an increase in oxygen extraction rather than a further increase in the already high hepatic blood flow.

Control of Hepatic Blood Flow

Portal vein blood flow is controlled primarily by the arterioles in the preportal splanchnic organs. The fibrotic constriction characteristic of hepatic cirrhosis (most often due to chronic alcohol abuse and hepatitis C) can increase the resistance to portal vein blood flow, as evidenced by portal venous pressures of 20 to 30 mm Hg (portal hypertension). The resulting increased resistance to portal vein blood flow may result in the development of shunts (varices) to allow blood flow to bypass the hepatocytes. Conversely, congestive heart failure and positive pressure ventilation of the lungs impair outflow of blood from the liver because of increased central venous pressure, which is transmitted to hepatic veins. Ascites results when increased portal venous pressures cause the transudation of protein-rich fluid through the outer surface of the liver capsule and gastrointestinal tract into the abdominal cavity. A decrease in portal vein blood flow is accompanied by an increase in hepatic artery blood flow (autoregulation) by as much as 100%. Halothane decreases hepatic oxygen supply to a greater extent than isoflurane, enflurane, desflurane, or sevoflurane when administered in equal potent doses. Surgical stimulation may further decrease hepatic blood flow, independent of the anesthetic drug administered. The greatest decreases in hepatic blood flow occur during intraabdominal operations, presumably due to the mechanical interference of blood flow produced by retraction in the operative area, as well as the release of vasoconstricting substances such as catecholamines.

Reservoir Function

The liver normally contains approximately 500 mL of blood or approximately 10% of the total blood volume. The liver acts as a storage site when blood volume is excessive, as in congestive heart failure, and is capable of supplying extra blood (up to 350 mL) when hypovolemia occurs.

Bile Secretion

Hepatocytes continually form bile (500 mL daily) and then secrete it into bile canaliculi, which empty into progressively larger ducts and ultimately reach the common bile duct. The principal components of bile are bile salts, bilirubin, and cholesterol.

Bile Salts

Bile salts combine with lipids in the duodenum to form water-soluble complexes (micelles) that facilitate the gastrointestinal absorption of fats (triglycerides) and fat-soluble vitamins (vitamin K).

Bilirubin

After approximately 120 days, the cell membranes of erythrocytes rupture, and the released hemoglobin is converted to bilirubin in reticuloendothelial cells (Fig. 55-2).

Jaundice

Jaundice is the yellowish tint of body tissues that accompanies an accumulation of bilirubin in extracellular fluid. Skin color usually begins to change when the plasma concentration of bilirubin increases to approximately three times normal.

Cholesterol

Cholesterol is an important component of cell walls; it is synthesized in tissues from acetate in a reaction catalyzed by β-hydroxy β-methylglutaryl coenzyme A. Cholesterol is transported from the periphery to the liver as high density lipoproteins (HDL).

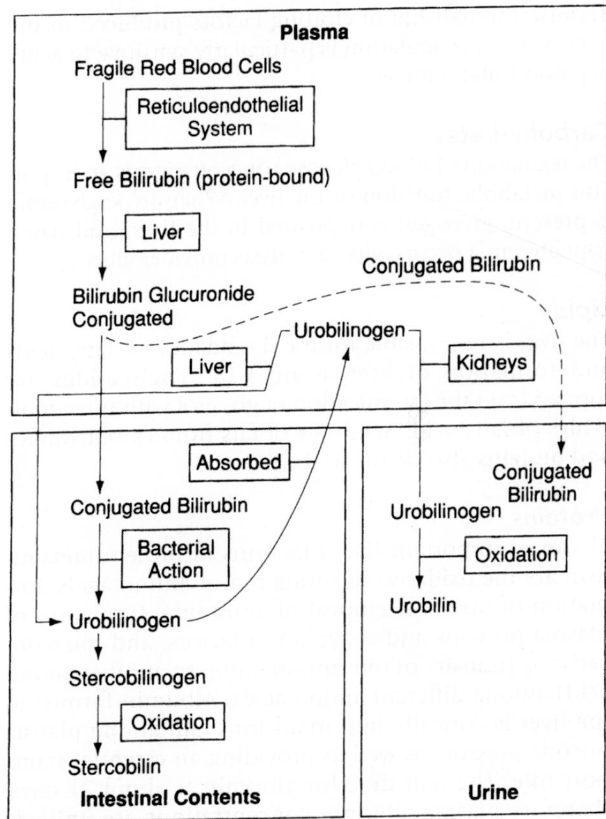

Figure 55-2. Schematic depiction of bilirubin formation and excretion. (From Guyton AC, Hall JE. *Textbook of Medical Physiology*, 10th ed. Philadelphia: Saunders, 2000; with permission.)

Metabolic Functions

The degradation of certain hormones (catecholamines and corticosteroids), as well as drugs, is an important function of the liver. Hepatocytes are the principal site for the synthesis of all the coagulation factors, with the exception of von Willebrand factor and factor VIIIC.

Because the half-life of clotting factors produced in the liver is short, coagulation is particularly sensitive to acute hepatocellular damage.

Carbohydrates

The regulation of blood glucose concentration is an important metabolic function of the liver. When hyperglycemia is present, glycogen is deposited in the liver, and when hypoglycemia occurs, glycogenolysis provides glucose.

Lipids

The liver is responsible for the β-oxidation of fatty acids and formation of acetoacetic acid. Triglycerides are formed from the esterification of glycerol with three molecules of fatty acid. Synthesis of fats from carbohydrates and proteins also occurs in the liver.

Proteins

The most important liver functions in protein metabolism are the oxidative deamination of amino acids, formation of urea for removal of ammonia, formation of plasma proteins and coagulation factors, and interconversions (transfer of one amino group to another amino acid) among different amino acids. Albumin formed in the liver is critically important for maintaining plasma oncotic pressure as well as providing an essential transport role. The half-time for albumin is about 21 days; therefore plasma albumin concentrations are unlikely to be significantly altered in acute hepatic failure.

GASTROINTESTINAL TRACT (FIG. 55-3 AND TABLE 55-2)

Anatomy

The smooth muscle of the gastrointestinal tract is a syncytium, so that electrical signals originating in one smooth muscle fiber are easily propagated from fiber to fiber. Mechanical activity of the gastrointestinal tract is

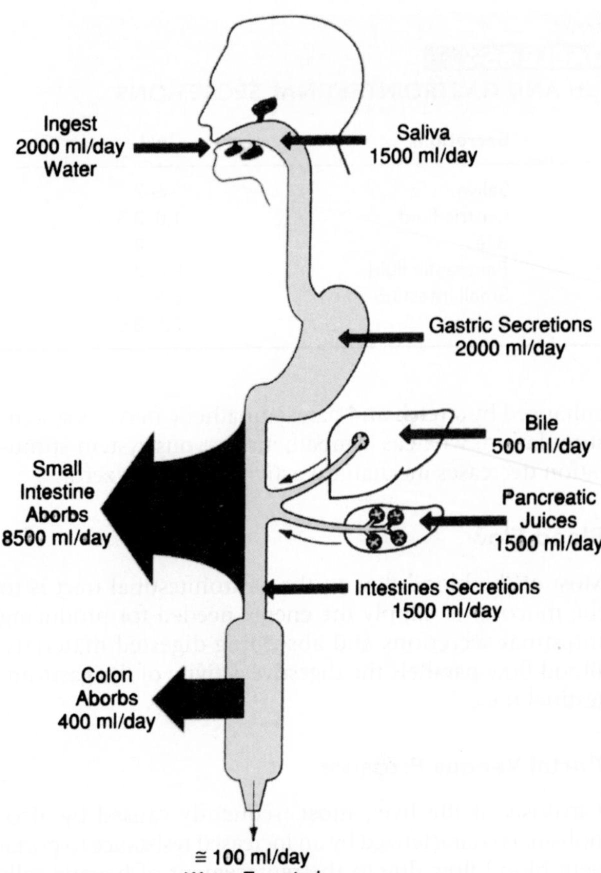

Figure 55-3. Overall fluid balance in the human gastrointestinal tract. Approximately 2 liters of water are ingested each day, and approximately 7 liters of various secretions enter the gastrointestinal tract. Of this 9 liters, about 8.5 liters are absorbed from the small intestine. Approximately 0.5 liter passes to the colon, which normally absorbs 80% to 90% of the water presented to it. (Berne RM, Levy M, Koeppen BM, et al. *Physiology*, 5th ed. St. Louis: Mosby, 2004; with permission.)

TABLE 55-2.
pH AND GASTROINTESTINAL SECRETIONS

Secretions	pH
Saliva	6–7
Gastric fluid	1.0–3.5
Bile	7–8
Pancreatic fluid	8.0–8.3
Small intestine	6.5–7.5
Colon	7.5–8.0

enhanced by stretch and parasympathetic nervous system stimulation, whereas sympathetic nervous system stimulation decreases mechanical activity to almost zero.

Blood Flow

Most of the blood flow to the gastrointestinal tract is to the mucosa, to supply the energy needed for producing intestinal secretions and absorbing digested materials. Blood flow parallels the digestive activity of the gastrointestinal tract.

Portal Venous Pressure

Cirrhosis of the liver, most frequently caused by alcoholism, is characterized by an increased resistance to portal vein blood flow due to the replacement of hepatic cells with fibrous tissue that contracts around the blood vessels. The gradual increase in resistance to portal vein blood flow produced by cirrhosis of the liver causes large collateral vessels to develop between the portal veins and the systemic veins. The most important of these collaterals are from the splenic veins to the esophageal veins. These collaterals may become so large that they protrude into the lumen of the esophagus, producing esophageal varicosities. The esophageal mucosa overlying these varicosities may become eroded, leading to life-threatening hemorrhage. In the absence of the development of adequate collaterals, sustained increases in portal vein pressure may cause protein-containing fluid to escape (ascites) from the surface of the mesentery, gastrointestinal tract, and liver into the peritoneal cavity.

Splenic Circulation

The spleen functions to remove erythrocytes from the circulation.

Innervation

In the absence of sympathetic nervous system or parasympathetic nervous system innervation, the motor and secretory activities of the gastrointestinal tract continue, reflecting the function of the intrinsic nervous system. Impulses from the parasympathetic nervous system increase intrinsic activity, whereas signals from the sympathetic nervous system decrease intrinsic activity.

Motility

The two types of gastrointestinal motility are mixing contractions and propulsive movements characterized as peristalsis. The usual stimulus for peristalsis is distension. Peristalsis is decreased by increased parasympathetic nervous system activity and anticholinergic drugs.

Ileus

Trauma to the intestine or irritation of the peritoneum, as follows abdominal operations, causes adynamic (paralytic) ileus. Peristalsis returns to the small intestine in 6 to 8 hours, but colonic activity may take 2 to 3 days.

Salivary Glands

The principal salivary glands (parotid and submaxillary) produce 0.5 to 1.0 mL/min of saliva (pH of 6 to 7), largely in response to parasympathetic nervous system stimulation.

Esophagus

The upper and lower ends of the esophagus function as sphincters to prevent the entry of air and acidic gastric contents into the esophagus.

Lower Esophageal Sphincter

The intraluminal pressure of the esophagogastric junction is a measure of the strength of the antireflux barrier and is typically quantified with reference to the intragastric pressure (normal <7 mm Hg). The normal lower esophageal sphincter pressure is 10 to 30 mm Hg at end-exhalation. Gastric barrier pressure is calculated as the difference between lower esophageal sphincter pressure and intragastric pressure. This barrier pressure is considered the major mechanism in preventing the reflux of gastric contents into the esophagus. Cricoid pressure decreases lower esophageal sphincter pressure, presumably reflecting the stimulation of mechanoreceptors in the pharynx, created by the external pressure on the cricoid cartilage. General anesthesia decreases lower esophageal sphincter pressure 7 to 14 mm Hg, depending on the degree of skeletal muscle relaxation. Normally, upper esophageal sphincter pressure prevents regurgitation into the pharynx in the awake state. The administration of anesthetic drugs may decrease upper esophageal sphincter pressure even before the loss of consciousness. Despite the decreases in lower esophageal sphincter pressure associated with anesthesia, the incidence of gastroesophageal reflux, as reflected by decreases in esophageal fluid pH, is rare in patients undergoing elective operations.

Gastroesophageal Reflux Disease (GERD)

Transient relaxation of the lower esophageal sphincter, rather than decreased lower esophageal sphincter pressure, is the major mechanism of GERD.

Hiatal Hernia

Hiatal hernia may promote gastroesophageal reflux by trapping gastric acid in the hernia sac, which may then flow backward into the esophagus when the lower esophageal sphincter relaxes during swallowing.

Achalasia

Achalasia reflects a degeneration of neurons in the wall of the esophagus, causing aperistalsis. Dysphagia for both solid foods and liquids is the primary symptom of achalasia. A substantial number of patients complain of heartburn and achalasia; thus achalasia may be confused with GERD.

Esophageal Perforation

Esophageal perforation is a risk of pneumatic dilation therapy for achalasia (a large deflated balloon is passed through the mouth to the lower esophageal sphincter and then rapidly inflated). The endoscopic injection of botulinum toxin into the area of the lower esophageal sphincter blocks the excitatory (acetylcholine-releasing) neurons that contribute to lower esophageal sphincter tone. A patient with achalasia presenting for surgery unrelated to the underlying esophageal motility disorder represents a potential risk for pulmonary aspiration during the perioperative period.

Stomach

The ability of the stomach to secrete hydrogen ions in the form of hydrochloric acid is a hallmark of gastric function.

Gastric Secretions

Total daily gastric secretion is approximately 2 liters with a pH of 1.0 to 3.5. The stomach secretes only a few milliliters of gastric fluid each hour during the periods between digestion. Strong emotional stimulation, such as occurs preoperatively, can increase the interdigestive secretion of highly acidic gastric fluid to >50 mL/hour.

Parietal Cells

Parietal cells secrete an hydrogen ion–containing solution with a pH of approximately 0.8. The secretion of hydrochloric acid depends on the stimulation of receptors in the membrane of parietal cells by histamine, acetylcholine (vagal stimulation), and gastrin. Blockade of receptors with specific antagonist drugs produces effective decreases in acid responses by removing the potentiating effect of the stimulation of these receptors on the responses to other stimuli. Blockade of muscarinic1 receptors is produced by atropine or the more specific anticholinergic pirenzepine. Gastrin receptors can be inhibited by proglumide. Alternatively, the hydrogen-potassium ATPase enzyme system can be inhibited by omeprazole. Pharmacologic manipulation of gastric fluid pH has special implications in the management of patients considered to be at risk for pulmonary aspiration during the perioperative period.

Chief Cells

Pepsinogens secreted by chief cells undergo cleavage to pepsins in the presence of hydrochloric acid. Pepsins are proteolytic enzymes important for the digestion of proteins.

G Cells

Gastrin is secreted by G cells into the circulation, which carries this hormone to responsive receptors in parietal cells to stimulate gastric hydrogen ion secretion.

Gastric Fluid Volume and Rate of Gastric Emptying

The elimination of non-nutrient liquids is an exponential process (volume of liquid emptied per unit of time is directly proportional to the volume present in the stomach), whereas the emptying of solids is a linear process (Fig. 55-4). The emptying of liquids from the stomach begins within 1 minute of ingestion, whereas the emptying

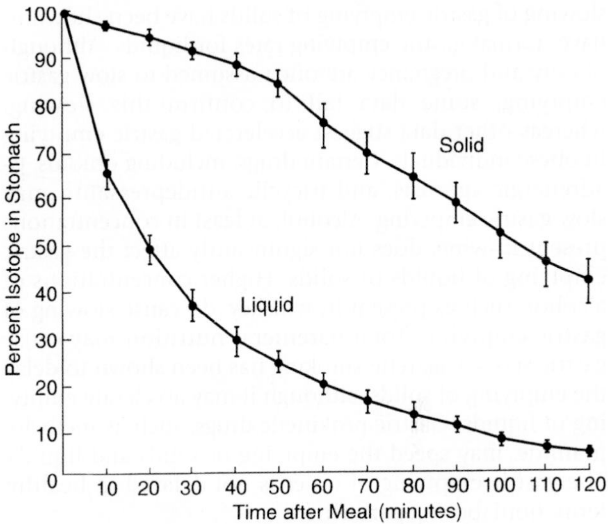

Figure 55-4. Gastric emptying of liquids is exponential, whereas emptying of solids is a linear process. (From Minami H, McCallum RW. The physiology of gastric emptying in humans. *Gastroenterology* 1984;86:1592–1610; with permission.)

of solids typically begins after a lag time of 15 to 137 minutes (median 49 minutes). Clinical manifestations of delayed gastric emptying include anorexia, persistent fullness after meals, abdominal pain, and nausea and vomiting. Emptying of neutral, isoosmolar, and calorically inert solutions is rapid (250 mL of 500 mL of normal saline is emptied in 12 minutes). A small amount of water (up to 150 mL) to facilitate the administration of oral medications shortly before the induction of anesthesia does not produce sustained increases in gastric fluid volume. High lipid and/or caloric content (glucose) slows the emptying of solids from the stomach. Delayed gastric emptying of solids is the most consistent abnormality in diabetics with gastroparesis and is also the most predictably responsive to pharmacologic manipulation. Patients with gastroesophageal reflux and documented slowing of gastric emptying of solids have been shown to have normal gastric-emptying rates for liquids. Although obesity and pregnancy are often assumed to slow gastric emptying, some data fail to confirm this slowing, whereas other data suggest accelerated gastric emptying in obese individuals. Certain drugs, including opioids, β-adrenergic agonists, and tricyclic antidepressants, may slow gastric emptying. Alcohol, at least in concentrations present in wine, does not significantly affect the gastric emptying of liquids or solids. Higher concentrations of alcohol, such as present in whiskey, do cause slowing of gastric emptying. Total parenteral nutrition may cause gastric stasis. Cigarette smoking has been shown to delay the emptying of solids, although it may accelerate emptying of liquids. Gastric prokinetic drugs, such as metoclopramide, may speed the emptying of solids and liquids. The gastric emptying of water is not delayed in healthy, term, nonlaboring parturients.

Gastric Emptying Prior to Elective Surgery

Clear liquids can be administered to adult patients scheduled for elective operations until 2 hours before the induction of anesthesia without increasing gastric fluid volume. It takes 3 to 4 hours for the stomach to empty following a light breakfast (one slice of white bread with butter and jam, 150 mL of coffee without milk or sugar, 150 mL pulp-free orange juice). It is a recommendation that a 6-hour fast should be enforced after a light breakfast.

Opioid-Induced Slowing of Gastric Emptying

Opioid peptides and their receptors are found throughout the gastrointestinal system, with particularly high concentrations in the gastric antrum and proximal duodenum.

Measurement of the Rate of Gastric Emptying

The rate of gastric emptying can be evaluated by a noninvasive electrical bioimpedance method (epigastric impedance method) and indirectly by the acetaminophen absorption technique.

Electrical Bioimpedance Technique

The basis of the bioimpedance technique is that, after the ingestion of fluids with a different conductivity from body tissues, the impedance to an electrical current through the upper abdomen changes.

Acetaminophen Absorption Test

The area under the plasma concentration curve of acetaminophen after oral administration is determined by the rate of gastric emptying, because acetaminophen is not absorbed from the stomach but is rapidly absorbed from the small intestine.

Absorption from the Stomach

The stomach is a poor absorptive area of the gastrointestinal tract because it lacks the villus structure characteristic of absorptive membranes. As a result, only highly lipid-soluble liquids, such as ethanol, and some drugs, such as aspirin, can be absorbed significantly from the stomach.

Vomiting

Vomiting is coordinated by the vomiting center in the medulla, which receives input from multiple sites, including the chemoreceptor trigger zone in the floor of the fourth ventricle, the vestibular apparatus, cortical centers, and the gastrointestinal tract. The blood-brain barrier is poorly developed around the chemoreceptor trigger zone, and emetic substances in the circulation are readily accessible to this site. Serotonin acting at 5-hydroxytryptamine receptors (5-HT3) is an important emetic signal via neural pathways from the gastrointestinal tract ending at the chemoreceptor trigger zone. Pharmacologic antagonism of serotonin emetic signals results in antiemetic effects. The initial manifestation of vomiting often involves nausea, in which gastric peristalsis is reduced or absent, the tone of the upper small intestine is increased, and gastric reflux occurs. Risk factors for postoperative nausea and vomiting include female gender, young age (children), and obesity (perhaps reflecting emetic anesthetic drugs stored in adipose tissue).

Small Intestine

The small intestine is presented with approximately 9 liters of fluid daily (2 liters from the diet and the rest representing gastrointestinal secretions), but only 1 to 2 liters of chyme enters the colon. The small intestine is the site of most of the digestion and absorption of proteins, fats, and carbohydrates (Table 55-3).

Secretions of the Small Intestine

Stimulation of the sympathetic nervous system inhibits the protective mucus-producing function of these glands, which may be one of the factors that causes this area of the gastrointestinal tract to be the most frequent site of peptic ulcer disease.

TABLE 55-3.
SITE OF ABSORPTION

	Duodenum	Jejunum	Ileum	Colon
Glucose	++	+++	++	0
Amino acids	++	+++	++	0
Fatty acids	+++	++	+	0
Bile salts	0	+	+++	0
Water-soluble vitamins	+++	++	0	0
Vitamin B_{12}	0	+	+++	0
Sodium	+++	++	+++	+++
Potassium	0	0	+	++
Hydrogen	0	+	++	++
Chloride	+++	++	+	0
Calcium	+++	++	+	?

Absorption from the Small Intestine

Mucosal folds (valvulae conniventes), microvilli (brush border), and epithelial cells provide an absorptive area of approximately 250 m^2 in the small intestine for nearly all the nutrients and electrolytes, as well as approximately 95% of all the water.

Colon

The functions of the colon are the absorption of water and electrolytes from the chyme and the storage of feces.

Secretion of the Colon

Epithelial cells lining the colon secrete almost exclusively alkaline mucus, which protects the intestinal mucosa against trauma.

Pancreas

Exocrine secretions (approximately 1.5 liters daily) are rich in bicarbonate ions to neutralize duodenal contents and digestive enzymes to initiate breakdown of carbohydrates, proteins, and fats.

Regulation of Pancreatic Secretions

Pancreatic secretions are regulated more by hormonal (secretin) than neural mechanisms.

Skeletal and Smooth Muscle

56

Skeletal muscle is responsible for voluntary actions, whereas smooth muscle and cardiac muscle subserve functions related to the cardiovascular, respiratory, gastrointestinal, and genitourinary systems (Stoelting RK, Hillier SC. Skeletal and smooth muscle. In: *Pharmacology and Physiology in Anesthetic Practice*. 4th ed. Philadelphia, Lippincott Williams & Wilkins, 2006:842–846). Muscle composes 45% to 50% of total body mass, with skeletal muscles accounting for approximately 40% of body mass. The inappropriate activity of smooth muscle is involved in many illnesses including hypertension, atherosclerosis, asthma, and disorders of the gastrointestinal tract.

SKELETAL MUSCLE

Skeletal muscle is made up of individual muscle fibers, each fiber being a single cell. No syncytial bridges exist between cells. Cross striations characteristic of skeletal muscles are due to differences in the refractive indexes of the various parts of the muscle fiber. Each skeletal muscle fiber comprises thousands of fibrils that consist of the contractile proteins known as *myosin, actin, tropomyosin,* and troponin. Myofibrils are suspended inside skeletal muscle fibers in a matrix known as *sarcoplasm*. The sarcoplasm contains mitochondria, enzymes, potassium ions, and extensive endoplasmic reticulum known as the *sarcoplasmic reticulum*. Skeletal muscle has only a limited capacity to form new cells.

Excitation-Contraction Coupling

Excitation-contraction coupling is the process by which the depolarization of the sarcolemma and propagation of an action potential initiates skeletal muscle contraction. An action potential occurs only in response to motor nerve activity and reflects the opening of fast channels in the membrane, allowing rapid inward movement of sodium ions followed by outward movement of potassium ions and depolarization. The action potential is transmitted deep into skeletal muscle to all myofibrils by way of transverse (T) tubules. As action potentials pass down T-tubules, dihydropyridine receptors in the T-tubules undergo conformational changes that result in the opening of sarcoplasmic calcium channels (ryanodine receptors), which in turn causes the release of calcium ions from the sarcoplasmic reticulum into the immediate vicinity of all myofibrils. Calcium ions bind to troponin, thus abolishing the inhibitory effect of troponin on the interaction between myosin and actin. As a result, the head of a myosin molecule links to an actin molecule (cross-bridge), producing movement of myosin on actin, which is repeated in serial fashion to produce a contraction of the muscle fiber. The immediate source of chemical energy for contraction is provided by adenosine triphosphate (ATP). Each interaction of myosin with actin results in the hydrolysis of ATP. The amount of ATP present in a skeletal muscle fiber is sufficient to maintain full contraction for <1 s. This emphasizes the importance of rephosphorylation of ADP to form ATP. Shortly after releasing calcium, the sarcoplasmic reticulum begins to reaccumulate this ion by an active transport process (calcium pump). Once the calcium concentration in the sarcoplasm has been lowered sufficiently, cross-bridging between myosin and actin ceases, and the skeletal muscle relaxes. Failure of the calcium ion pump results in sustained skeletal muscle contraction and marked increases in heat production, leading to malignant hyperthermia.

Neuromuscular Junction

The neuromuscular junction is the site at which presynaptic motor nerve endings meet the postsynaptic membranes of skeletal muscles (motor end plates). Acetylcholine is synthesized in the cytoplasm of the nerve terminal and stored in synaptic vesicles. A nerve impulse arriving at the nerve ending causes the release of approximately 60 vesicles, each containing an estimated 10,000 molecules of acetylcholine. In the absence of calcium, or in the presence of excess magnesium ions, the release of acetylcholine is greatly decreased. Acetylcholine diffuses across the synaptic cleft to excite skeletal muscles, but within 1 ms, the neurotransmitter is hydrolyzed by acetylcholinesterase enzyme (true cholinesterase) in the folds of the sarcolemma.

Mechanism of Acetylcholine Effects

Nicotinic acetylcholine receptors comprise five subunits, arranged in a nearly symmetric fashion, that extend through the cell membrane (see Chapter 8). The binding of two acetylcholine molecules (one molecule at each α-subunit) causes a conformation change in the receptor so that sodium enters into the interior of the cell. As a result, the resting transmembrane potential increases in this local area of the motor end-plate, creating a local action potential known as the *end-plate potential*. The threshold potential at which skeletal muscle fibers are stimulated to contract is approximately 50 mV.

Altered Responses to Acetylcholine

Nondepolarizing neuromuscular-blocking drugs compete with acetylcholine at α-subunits of the receptor and thus prevent changes in the permeability of skeletal muscle membranes (see Chapter 8). As a result, an end-plate potential does not occur, and neuromuscular transmission is effectively prevented. Anticholinesterase drugs inhibit acetylcholinesterase enzyme, allowing an accumulation of acetylcholine at receptors and the subsequent displacement of nondepolarizing neuromuscular-blocking drugs from the α-subunits (see Chapter 9).

Blood Flow

Skeletal muscle blood flow can increase more than 20 times (a greater increase than in any other tissue of the body) during strenuous exercise. Among inhaled anesthetics, isoflurane is a potent vasodilator, producing marked increases in skeletal muscle blood flow.

Innervation

Skeletal muscles are innervated by large myelinated α-motor neurons that originate from cell bodies in the ventral (anterior) horns of the spinal cord (Fig. 56-1) The nerve axon exits via the ventral root and reaches the muscle through a mixed peripheral nerve. Motor nerves branch in the skeletal muscle, with each nerve terminal innervating a single muscle cell.

Denervation Hypersensitivity

Denervation of skeletal muscle causes atrophy of the involved muscle and the development of abnormal excitability of the skeletal muscle to its neurotransmitter, acetylcholine.

SMOOTH MUSCLE

Smooth muscle is distinguished anatomically from skeletal and cardiac muscle because it lacks visible cross-striations (actin and myosin are not arranged in regular arrays). Calcium ions are released from the sarcoplasmic reticulum into the myoplasm when stimulatory neurotransmitters, hormones, or drugs bind to receptors on the sarcolemma. Calcium ion channels on the sarcoplasmic reticulum of smooth muscles includes ryanodine receptors (similar to those present in skeletal muscles) and inositol 1,4,5-triphosphate (IP3)-gated calcium ion

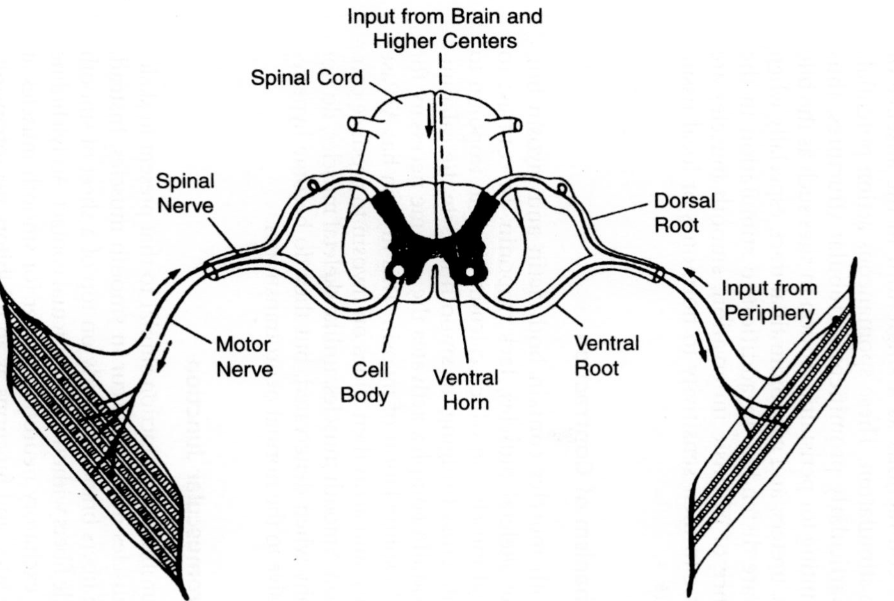

Figure 56-1. Schematic depiction of skeletal muscle innervation. (From Berne et al., *Physiology*, 5th ed. St. Louis: Mosby, 2004; with permission.)

channels. Visceral smooth muscle is characterized by cell membranes that contact adjacent cell membranes, forming a functional syncytium that often undergoes spontaneous contractions as a single unit in the absence of nerve stimulation. These spontaneous action potentials are particularly prominent in tubular structures, thus accounting for peristaltic motion in sites such as the bile ducts, ureters, and gastrointestinal tract, especially when they are distended. In addition to stimulation in the absence of extrinsic innervation, smooth muscles are unique in their sensitivity to hormones or local tissue factors.

Mechanism of Contraction

Smooth muscles contain both actin and myosin but, unlike skeletal muscles, lack troponin. In contrast to skeletal muscles, in which calcium binds to troponin to initiate cross-bridging, in smooth muscle the calcium-calmodulin complex activates the enzyme necessary for the phosphorylation of myosin. This myosin has ATPase activity, and actin then slides on myosin to produce contraction. Smooth muscles, unlike skeletal muscles, do not atrophy when denervated, but they do become hyperresponsive to the normal neurotransmitter.

Neuromuscular Junction

A neuromuscular junction similar to that present in skeletal muscles does not occur in smooth muscles. Instead, nerve fibers branch diffusely on top of a sheet of smooth muscle fibers without making actual contact. Acetylcholine is an excitatory neurotransmitter for smooth muscles at some sites, and functions as an inhibitory neurotransmitter at other sites. Norepinephrine exerts the reverse effect of acetylcholine.

Uterus

Uterine smooth muscle is characterized by a high degree of spontaneous electrical and contractile activity (unlike the heart, no pacemaker exists). The availability of calcium ions greatly influences the response of uterine smooth muscle to physiologic and pharmacologic stimulation or inhibition. α-Excitatory and β-inhibitory receptors are also present in the myometrium.

Erythrocytes and Leukocytes

57

ERYTHROCYTES

Erythrocytes (red blood cells, RBCs) are the most abundant of all cells in the body (25 trillion of the estimated total 75 trillion cells), and they have an irreplaceable role in the delivery of oxygen to tissues (Stoelting RK, Hillier SC. Erythrocytes and leukocytes, In: *Pharmacology and Physiology in Anesthetic Practice.* 4th ed. Philadelphia, Lippincott Williams & Wilkins, 2006:847–856). In addition to transporting hemoglobin, RBCs contain large amounts of carbonic anhydrase. This enzyme speeds the reaction between carbon dioxide and water, making it possible to transport carbon dioxide from tissues to the lungs for elimination. Hemoglobin in RBCs is an excellent acid–base buffer, providing approximately 70% of the buffering power of whole blood.

Anatomy

RBCs are biconcave disks with a mean diameter of 8 μ. The average number of RBCs in each milliliter of plasma, and thus the hemoglobin concentration and hematocrit, varies with the individual, gender, and barometric pressure (Table 57-1). Each gram of hemoglobin is capable of combining with 1.34 mL of oxygen.

Bone Marrow

In the adult, RBCs, platelets, and many of the leukocytes are formed in bone marrow. When the bone marrow produces

TABLE 57-1.
ERYTHROCYTES IN THE PLASMA

	Contents
Erythrocytes (mL)	
Male	$4.3–5.9 \times 10^6$
Female	$3.5–5.5 \times 10^6$
Hematocrit (%)	
Male	39–55
Female	36–48
Hemoglobin (g/dL)	
Male	13.9–16.3
Female	12.0–15.0

RBCs at a rapid rate, many of the cells are released into the blood before they are mature. Overall, the bone marrow is one of the largest organs of the body, approaching the size and weight of the liver.

Control of Production

The total mass of RBCs in the circulation is regulated within narrow limits so that the number of cells is optimal to provide tissue oxygenation without an excessive number that would adversely increase viscosity of blood and decrease tissue blood flow. Any event that causes the amount of oxygen transported to tissues to decrease, as in anemia, chronic pulmonary disease, or cardiac failure, will stimulate the production of RBCs by the bone marrow.

Erythropoietin

Erythropoietin is a glycoprotein synthesized in response to arterial hypoxemia, and it stimulates RBC production in the bone marrow. When arterial hypoxemia is corrected, erythropoietin production decreases to zero almost immediately. The absence of kidneys removes the source of renal erythropoietic factor, which results in anemia. Therapy with recombinant human erythropoietin is an alternative to blood transfusion, if the clinical condition of the patient permits sufficient time for stimulation of erythropoiesis to correct anemia. Four weekly subcutaneous doses of erythropoietin are usually sufficient to produce a reticulocyte response.

Vitamins Necessary for Formation

Vitamin B_{12} (cyanocobalamin) is necessary for the synthesis of DNA. Lack of this vitamin results in the failure of nuclear maturation and division, which is particularly evident in rapidly proliferating cells such as RBCs. Many months of impaired vitamin B_{12} absorption are necessary before maturation failure macrocytic anemia manifests.

Destruction

RBCs normally circulate an average of 120 days after leaving the bone marrow. Hemoglobin released from ruptured RBCs is rapidly phagocytized by reticuloendothelial cells.

BLOOD GROUPS

Genetically determined antigens (agglutinogens) are present on the cell membranes of RBCs (most antigenic are the A, B, and Rh agglutinogens).

ABO Antigen System (Table 57-2)

In the absence of the A or B antigen, the opposite antibody (agglutinin) is present in the circulation (see Table 57-2).

TABLE 57-2.
ABO ANTIGEN SYSTEM

Blood Type	Incidence (%)	Genotype	Antigens (Agglutinogens)	Antibodies (Agglutinins)
O	47	OO		anti-A, anti-B
A	41	OA,AA	A	anti-B
B	9	OB,BB	B	anti-A
AB	3	AB	A,B	

Blood Typing

Blood typing is the in vitro mixing of a drop of the patient's blood with plasma containing antibodies against the A or B antigen. *Cross-matching* is the procedure that determines the compatibility of the patient's blood with the donor's RBCs and plasma.

Rh Blood Types

Six common types of Rh antigens exist—designated C, D, E, c, d, and e—and they are collectively known as the Rh factor. An individual who is Rh-negative develops anti-Rh antibodies only when exposed to RBCs containing the C, D, or E antigens. An Rh-negative mother typically becomes sensitized to the Rh-positive factor in her child during the first few days after delivery, when degenerating products of the placenta release Rh-positive antigens into the maternal circulation. If these Rh antigens are destroyed at this time, before an anti-Rh antibody response occurs, the mother will not become sensitized for subsequent pregnancies. This goal is achieved by injecting antibodies [Rh (D) immune globulin] against the antigen before it can evoke the formation of antibodies.

Hemolytic Transfusion Reactions

The transfusion of ABO type blood that is different from that of the recipient results in agglutination of the transfused RBCs by antibodies present in the plasma of the recipient. In addition to agglutination, this antigen–antibody interaction may result in the immediate hemolysis of the transfused RBCs. When the rate of hemolysis is rapid, the plasma concentration of hemoglobin may exceed the binding capacity of haptoglobin, and free hemoglobin continues to circulate. Acute renal failure often accompanies a severe transfusion reaction.

LEUKOCYTES (TABLE 57-3)

Normally, each milliliter of blood contains 4,000 to 11,000 leukocytes, the most numerous being neutrophils.

TABLE 57-3.
CLASSIFICATION OF LEUKOCYTES

	Cells per mL of Plasma (Range)	% of Total (Range)
Granulocytes		
Neutrophils	3,000–6,000	55–65
Eosinophils	0–300	1–3
Basophils	0–100	0–1
Monocytes/macrophages	300–500	3–6
Lymphocytes	1,500–3,500	25–35
Total leukocytes	4,000–11,000	

Granulocytes and monocytes are formed from stem cells in the bone marrow. After birth, some lymphocytes are formed in bone marrow, but most are produced in the thymus, lymph nodes, and spleen, from precursor cells that came originally from the bone marrow.

Neutrophils

Neutrophils are the most numerous leukocytes in the blood, representing approximately 60% of the circulating leukocytes. These cells seek out, ingest, and kill bacteria (phagocytosis) and thus represent the body's first line of defense against bacterial infection. A marked increase (up to fivefold) in the number of circulating neutrophils (leukocytosis) occurs within a few hours after bacterial infection or onset of inflammation. Intense exercise lasting only 1 minute can cause the number of circulating neutrophils to increase threefold (physiologic neutrophilia).

Eosinophils

Eosinophils account for approximately 20% of circulating leukocytes. After release from the bone marrow into the circulation, most eosinophils migrate within 30 minutes into extravascular tissues where they survive 8 to 12 days. Eosinophils show a special propensity to collect at sites of antigen–antibody reactions in tissues, most likely in response to a chemotactic stimulus.

Basophils

Basophils in the blood are similar to mast cells in tissues in that both types of cells contain histamine and heparin. Degranulation of these cells occurs when immunoglobulin E (IgE) selectively attaches to the membranes of previously sensitized basophils or mast cells. The subsequent release of histamine and perhaps other chemical mediators is responsible for the manifestations of allergic reactions.

Tryptase

Tryptase is a neutral protease that is stored in the granules of mast cells present in tissues. Mast cell degranulation results in increased plasma concentrations of tryptase, as evidence of anaphylaxis. Increased plasma concentrations of histamine, as evidence of basophil and/or mast cell degranulation, are difficult to measure accurately because the half-life of histamine in plasma is brief.

Monocytes

Monocytes enter the circulation from the bone marrow but, after approximately 24 hours, migrate into tissues to become macrophages. These macrophages, like neutrophils, contain peroxidase and lysosomal enzymes and are actively phagocytic. Macrophages constitute the reticuloendothelial system.

Kupffer's Cells

Kupffer's cells line the hepatic sinuses and serve as a filtration system to remove bacteria that have entered the portal blood from the gastrointestinal tract.

Reticulum Cells

Reticulum cells phagocytize foreign particles as they pass through lymph nodes.

Alveolar Macrophages

Alveolar macrophages are present in alveolar walls and can phagocytize invading organisms that are inhaled. Macrophages often form a giant cell capsule around carbon particles.

Histiocytes

Histiocytes phagocytize invading organisms that gain access when the skin is broken.

Cytokines

Cytokines are synthesized by activated macrophages and lymphocytes and act as hormone-like molecules to regulate immune responses (Table 57-4). These proteins act as secondary messengers and induce the synthesis and expression of specific adhesion molecules on endothelial cells and leukocytes that promote the attachment and transmigration of leukocytes (chemoattractants and leukocyte activators). The term *interleukin* emphasizes that these proteins facilitate communication between/among (inter) leukocytes (leukin). Overall, interleukins are considered to be a group of regulatory proteins that act to control many aspects of the immune and inflammatory response. Interleukin-6 is the principal cytokine released after surgery. Cytokines tend to be paracrine (act on nearby cells) or autocrine (act on the same cell), rather than endocrine (secreted into the circulation to act on distant cells).

Lymphocytes

Lymphocytes cells play a prominent role in immunity.

Agranulocytosis

Agranulocytosis is the acute cessation of leukocyte production by the bone marrow (due to nuclear radiation, drugs). Usually, sufficient stem cells (hemocytoblasts) remain after injury to allow the recovery of bone marrow function if fatal infection is prevented by appropriate antibiotic therapy.

TABLE 57-4.
EXAMPLES OF CYTOKINES AND THEIR CLINICAL RELEVANCE

Cytokine	Cellular Sources	Clinical Effects	Clinical Impact
Interleukin-1	Macrophages	Activation of T cells and macrophages Promotion of inflammation	Implicated in the pathogenesis of septic shock, rheumatoid arthritis and atherosclerosis
Interleukin-2	Type 1 helper T cells	Activation of lymphocytes, macrophages	Used to induce lymphokine- and activated killer cells Used in the treatment of renal-cell carcinoma
Interleukin-4	Type 2 helper T cells	Activation of lymphocytes Activation of monocytes	Stimulates IgE production (allergy)
Interleukin-5	Type 2 helper T cells	Differentiation of eosinophils	Monoclonal antibody against Interleukin-5

TABLE 57-4.
(continued)

Cytokine	Cellular Sources	Clinical Effects	Clinical Impact
Interleukin-6	Type 2 helper T cells	Activation of lymphocytes Differentiation of B cells Production of acute-phase proteins	Acts as an autocrine growth factor
Interleukin-8	T cells and macrophages	Chemotaxis of neutrophils, basophils, and T cells	Increased in diseases accompanied by neutrophilia
Interleukin-11	Bone marrow stromal cells	Production of acute-phase proteins	Decrease chemotherapy-induced thrombocytopenia
Interleukin-12	Macrophages and B cells	Production of interferon	Adjuvant for vaccines

Bacterial Destruction

Leukocytes participate in the destruction of bacteria by the processes of diapedesis, chemotaxis, and phagocytosis. Opsonization also makes bacteria susceptible to phagocytosis.

Diapedesis

Neutrophils and monocytes can squeeze through pores in blood vessels through diapedesis.

Chemotaxis

Chemotaxis is the phenomenon by which different chemical substances in tissues cause neutrophils and monocytes to move either toward or away from the chemical. Chemotaxis is effective up to 100 μm away from an inflamed tissue. Because almost no tissue is more than 30 to 50 μm away from a capillary, the chemotactic signal can rapidly attract large numbers of leukocytes to the inflamed area. Chemotaxis may be inhibited by inhaled anesthetics.

Opsonization

Opsonization is the coating of bacteria by immunoglobulin G (IgG) and complement proteins (opsonins), thus making the microorganisms susceptible to phagocytosis.

Phagocytosis

On approaching a particle to be phagocytized, the neutrophil projects pseudopodia around the particle. Most natural substances of the body, including neutrophils and monocytes, have electronegative surfaces. Conversely, necrotic tissues and foreign particles often are electropositive and thus are attracted to phagocytes.

INFLAMMATION

Inflammation is a series of sequential changes that occur in tissues in response to injury. Soon after inflammation begins, the inflamed area is invaded by neutrophils and macrophages.

IMMUNITY

Immunity is the ability to resist all types of organisms or toxins that could damage tissues or organs. Cell-mediated immunity and humoral immunity are the two types of immune defense systems designed to protect the body against organisms or toxins that cause tissue damage (Fig. 57-1) . The principal defense against bacterial infection is provided by humoral immunity, due to circulating antibodies in the γ-globulin fraction of plasma proteins. Cellular immunity is responsible for delayed allergic reactions, the rejection of foreign tissue, and the destruction of early cancer cells. Cellular immunity also serves as a major defense against infections caused by viruses, fungi, and bacteria such as *Mycobacterium tuberculosis*. Short-term anesthesia has not been shown to adversely impact the immune system, although high doses of anesthetics (as used for long-term sedation) may reach tissue concentrations sufficient to cause a suppression of cellular immune mechanisms.

B Lymphocytes and T Lymphocytes

Those lymphocytes responsible for humoral immunity are designated B lymphocytes and those responsible for cellular immunity are T lymphocytes (see Fig. 57-1). Morphologically, B lymphocytes and T lymphocytes are indistinguishable. B lymphocytes differentiate into memory B cells and plasma cells. Plasma cells are the source of γ-globulin antibodies responsible for humoral immunity. T lymphocytes are categorized as helper/inducer T cells, suppressor T cells, cytotoxic T cells, and memory T cells. Helper/inducer T cells and suppressor T cells are involved in the regulation of antibody production by B lymphocyte derivatives, and cytotoxic T cells destroy foreign cells, as represented by organ transplants. Helper/inducer T cells may be designated T4 cells because they often have on their surface a glycoprotein marker called T4; cytotoxic and suppressor T cells may be designated T8 cells

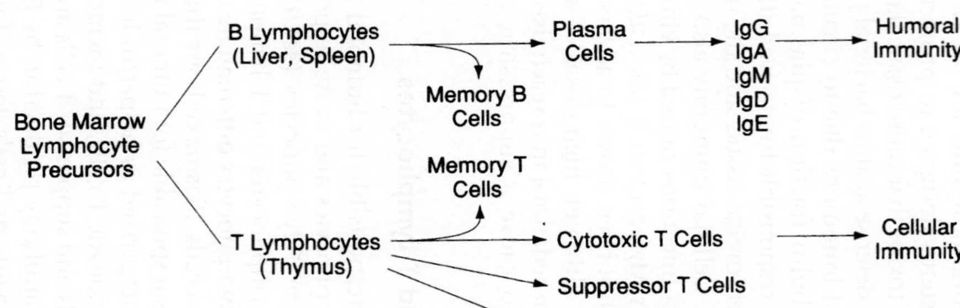

Figure 57-1. Schematic depiction of the immune system.

for a similar reason. The human immunodeficiency virus (HIV) specifically attacks helper/inducer T lymphocytes (T4 cells), causing eventual loss of immune function and death from cancer or infections due to normally nonpathogenic bacteria.

Antigens

Antigens are foreign proteins or chemicals that evoke the production of antibodies. The critical event in the initiation of the complex immune process that leads to the destruction of foreign pathogens or self-antigens is antigen-induced activation, proliferation, and differentiation of T lymphocytes.

Antibodies

The entry of antigens into lymphoid tissues causes clones of B lymphocytes to form plasma cells capable of producing γ-globulin antibodies specific for activity against that antigen (primary response). Some B lymphocytes, however, remain dormant in the lymphoid tissue, functioning as B memory cells. Subsequent exposure to the antigen causes these memory cells to participate in an exaggerated antibody response (secondary response), when compared with the primary response. The increased intensity and duration of the secondary response is the reason why vaccination is often achieved by injection of the antigen in multiple small doses several weeks apart.

Structure

Plasma cells form γ-globulin antibodies, which are grouped into five classes of immunoglobulins: IgG, IgA, IgM, IgD, and IgE (Table 57-5).

Mechanism of Action

Antibodies act by (a) direct effects on the antigen, (b) activation of the complement system, or (c) initiation of an anaphylactic reaction.

TABLE 57-5.
PROPERTIES OF IMMUNOGLOBULINS

	IgG	IgA	IgM	IgD	IgE
Location	Plasma Amniotic fluid	Plasma Saliva Tears	Plasma	Plasma	Plasma
Plasma concentration (mg/dL)	600–1,500	85–380	50–400	<15	0.01–0.03
Plasma half-time	21–23	6	5	2–8	1–5
Function					
Complement activation	+	–	+	–	–
Degranulation of mast cells	–	–	–	–	+
Bacterial lysis	+	–	+	–	–
Opsonization	+	?	–	–	–
Agglutination	+	+	+	–	–
Virus inactivation	+	+	+	–	–

Complement System

Complement is a system of enzyme precursors that are normally present in the plasma in an inactive form. Complement activation proceeds in a sequential fashion, comparable to the blood coagulation cascade. Protamine and heparin-protamine complexes can activate the complement cascade.

Anaphylactic Reaction

An anaphylactic reaction occurs when an antigen attaches to IgE antibodies on the cell membranes of circulating basophils or tissue mast cells. This antigen–antibody interaction changes the permeability of the cell membrane, leading to degranulation and the release of chemical mediators (histamine, leukotrienes, prostaglandins) into the circulation. These chemical mediators are responsible for the symptoms (hypotension, bronchoconstriction, edema) of an anaphylactic reaction. In some highly sensitized individuals, the degranulation resulting from the antigen–antibody interaction may be so explosive that life-threatening hypotension or bronchoconstriction occurs. Less explosive reactions are characterized by urticaria, in which an antigen enters the skin and evokes the local release of histamine. Hay fever results when the antigen–antibody reaction occurs in the nose, in contrast to asthma, in which the reaction occurs in the bronchioles of the lungs.

TISSUE TYPING

Tissue typing is possible in much the same way that blood is typed. The most important antigens that cause the rejection of transplanted tissue are the human leukocyte antigens (HLAs). HLAs are also present on the cell membranes of leukocytes. As a result, tissue typing can be accomplished by determining the types of antigens on the recipient's lymphocyte membranes.

58

Hemostasis and Blood Coagulation

Blood consists of components derived from many different sources, including the bone marrow, vascular endothelium, and reticuloendothelial system (Stoelting RK, Hillier SC. Hemostasis and blood coagulation. In: *Pharmacology and Physiology in Anesthetic Practice.* 4th ed. Philadelphia, Lippincott Williams & Wilkins, 2006:857–860). Under normal circumstances, the blood remains a liquid system, permitting the flow and delivery of vital nutrients to tissues. When vascular injury occurs, however, components of this liquid coagulate in a complex cascade of reactions involving multiple enzymes and inhibitor systems designed to transform blood into a solid clot, localized to the site of vascular injury.

HEMOSTATIC MECHANISM

The hemostatic response involves three processes characterized as (a) primary hemostasis, (b) coagulation, and (c) fibrinolysis.

Primary Hemostasis (Platelet Plug)

Primary hemostasis takes place within seconds of vascular endothelial injury and is characterized by the formation of a platelet plug. Aspirin inhibits the platelet release reaction and subsequent aggregation by irreversibly acetylating cyclooxygenase. Primary hemostasis is controlled by the balance between thromboxane A2 and prostacyclin. The platelet plug mechanism is important for closing the minute breaks in small blood vessels that occur hundreds of times daily. When the number of platelets is decreased, small hemorrhagic areas appear under the skin and internally.

Vascular Spasm

In addition to the steps that initiate the formation of a platelet plug, the wall of the cut blood vessel immediately contracts, which serves to decrease blood loss from the damaged vessel. This contraction results from neural reflexes initiated by pain impulses from the traumatized vessel and the release of vasoconstricting substances, such as serotonin, from platelets. Vascular spasm is most intense in severely traumatized or crushed blood vessels. The sharply cut or transected blood vessel, as occurs during surgery, undergoes less vascular spasm, and blood loss is decreased less.

Megakaryocytes

Megakaryocytes are giant cells in the bone marrow from which cytoplasmic fragments are pinched off and extruded into the circulation as nuclear platelets. Approximately 150,000 to 350,000 platelets normally are present in each milliliter of blood, with an average life span of 8 to 12 days.

Clot Formation

The fundamental reaction in blood clotting is the conversion of fibrinogen to fibrin by the action of activated thrombin. Activator substances from the traumatized vascular wall and platelets initiate this process within 15 to 20 s, and after 3 to 6 minutes, the cut end of a blood vessel is filled with clot. If whole blood is allowed to clot, and the clot is removed, the remaining fluid is serum. Serum is thus plasma with factors I, II, V, and VII removed.

Growth of Fibrous Tissue

The invasion of a blood clot by fibroblasts causes the formation of connective tissue throughout the clot.

Coagulation

Coagulation takes place in three essential steps (Fig. 58-1). The coagulation process is closely intertwined with primary hemostasis and fibrinolysis.

Clotting Factors

More than 50 different substances that promote (procoagulants) or inhibit (anticoagulants) coagulation have been identified in blood and tissues (Table 58-1). Normally, anticoagulants (antithrombin III, protein C, protein S) predominate, and blood does not coagulate. When a blood vessel is transected or damaged, the activity of the procoagulants in the area of the damage becomes

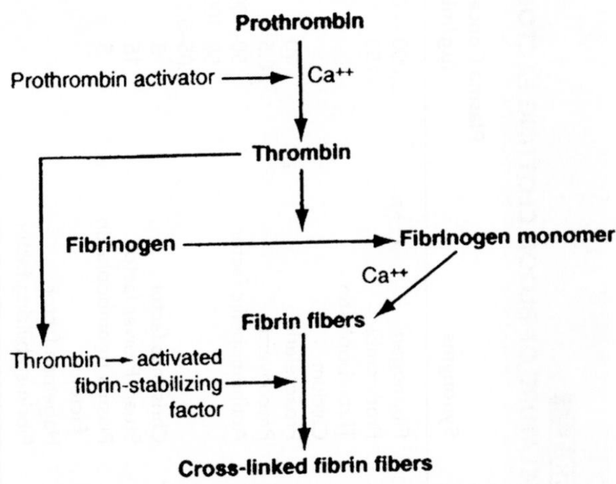

Figure 58-1. Pathway for conversion of prothrombin to thrombin and polymerization of fibrinogen from fibrin fibers (From Guyton AC, Hall JE. *Textbook of Medical Physiology*, 10th ed. Philadelphia: Saunders, 2000; with permission.)

TABLE 58-1.

NOMENCLATURE OF BLOOD CLOTTING FACTORS

Factor	Synonyms	Plasma Concentration (μg/mL)	Half-Time (hrs)	Stability in Stored Whole Blood
I	Fibrinogen	2,000–4,000	95–120	No change
II	Prothrombin	150	65–90	No change
III	Thromboplastin			
IV	Calcium			
V	Proaccelerin	10	15–24	Labile
VII	Proconvertin	0.5	4–6	No change
VIII	Antihemophilic factor	50–100	10–12	Labile
VIII:vWF		50–100		
VIII:C		0.05–0.10		
IX	Christmas factor	3	18–30	No change
X	Stuart-Prower factor	15	40–60	No change
XI	Plasma thromboplastin factor	5	45–60	Labile
XII	Hageman factor			
XIII	Fibrin-stabilizing factor			

predominant, and clot formation occurs. During the process of coagulation, a portion of the protein procoagulant molecule is cleaved and the "activated clotting factor" is designated by lowercase "a" after the Roman numeral of the factor. Most of the coagulation proteins are synthesized in the liver, with the exception of von Willebrand (vWF) factor VIII, which is synthesized by endothelial cells and megakaryocytes. Continued clot formation occurs only where blood is not flowing, because the flow of blood dilutes thrombin and other procoagulants released during the clotting process. Within a few minutes after the clot is formed, it begins to contract, and it typically expresses most of its fluid after 30 to 60 minutes. Platelets are necessary for this clot retraction to occur. Failure of clot retraction is an indication that the number of circulating platelets is inadequate.

Pathway for Coagulation

Coagulation is triggered by exposure of blood to "tissue factor" that is extrinsic to blood (tissue factor pathway of coagulation).

Tissue Factor Pathway of Coagulation

Coagulation is initiated when damage to blood vessels exposes tissue factor (thromboplastin) to circulating factor VII. Prothrombin, as well as factors VII, IX, and X, depends on the presence of vitamin K for synthesis in the liver. Lack of vitamin K resulting from the absence of bile salts or the presence of severe liver disease may prevent normal prothrombin formation. Failure of the liver to synthesize prothrombin leads to a decrease in its plasma concentration below normal levels in 24 hours.

Endogenous Anticoagulants

Antithrombin III is a circulating substance that binds to thrombin, thus preventing its conversion to fibrin. The binding of antithrombin III to thrombin is greatly facilitated by heparin. Protein C is a circulating substance that inhibits the activity of factors VIII:C and V. Protein S enhances the effect of protein C. An increased incidence of thrombosis occurs in patients with deficient amounts of antithrombin III, protein C, or protein S. Heparin is not an effective anticoagulant when administered to patients with deficient antithrombin III levels.

Drotrecogin-α

Drotrecogin-α (activated) is a recombinant form of human activated protein C that is indicated for the reduction of mortality in adult patients with sepsis associated with acute organ dysfunction.

Impact of Progressive Blood Loss

It is likely that stress, tissue trauma with release of tissue thromboplastin, and increases in the plasma concentrations of catecholamines offset any hypocoagulable tendency resulting from hemodilution and loss of coagulation factors during progressive blood loss. These offsetting factors are probably responsible for the increase in coagulability seen in many surgical patients experiencing moderate to massive blood loss.

Fibrinolysis

Fibrinolysis leads to the dissolution of fibrin clots and restores normal blood flow through blood vessels. Plasmin is formed in response to thrombin and tissue plasminogen activator, leading to the lysis of fibrin clots and production of fibrin split products. The therapeutic use of plasminogen activators is in the dissolution of intravascular clots by plasmin without a major effect on circulating fibrinogen. The excess activity of plasmin causes the destruction of clotting factors I, II, V, VIII, and XII. As a result, the lysis of clots may also be associated with hypocoagulability of the blood.

THROMBOEMBOLISM

An embolus is a fragment of the thrombus that breaks off and travels in the blood until it lodges at a site of vascular narrowing. For this reason, an embolus originating in an artery usually occludes a more distal and smaller artery. Conversely, an embolus originating in a vein commonly lodges in the lungs and causes pulmonary vascular obstruction. Thromboembolism is likely to occur in the presence of (a) any condition that causes a roughened endothelial vessel wall, such as arteriosclerosis, infection, or trauma, and (b) a slowing of blood flow. Slow or sluggish blood flow means activated clotting factors are less diluted and carried away slowly, thus increasing the likelihood of localized clotting. Vascular stasis in leg veins associated with pregnancy or postoperative immobility is a common precipitating event for the formation of a venous thrombus and subsequent pulmonary embolism.

DISSEMINATED INTRAVASCULAR COAGULATION

Disseminated intravascular coagulation reflects the entrance of substances into the circulation that cause an elaboration of thrombin, leading to widespread thrombosis in small blood vessels. Hypofibrinogenemia occurs when fibrinogen is consumed in the formation of these thrombi. Other clotting factors along with platelets may also be consumed.

Metabolism of Nutrients

59

Metabolism refers to all the chemical and energy transformations that occur in the body (Stoelting RK, Hillier SC. Metabolism of nutrients. In: *Pharmacology and Physiology in Anesthetic Practice.* 4th ed. Philadelphia, Lippincott Williams & Wilkins, 2006:857–860). The oxidation of nutrients (carbohydrates, fats, and proteins) results in the production of carbon dioxide, water, and high-energy phosphate bonds (adenosine triphosphate [ATP]) necessary for life processes (Fig. 59-1). ATP from the metabolism of nutrients is necessary to provide energy for the transport of ions across cell membranes and thus to maintain the distribution of these ions, which is necessary for propagation of nerve impulses. In addition to its function in energy transfer, ATP is also the precursor of cyclic adenosine monophosphate (cAMP).

CARBOHYDRATE METABOLISM

At least 99% of all the energy derived from carbohydrates is used to form ATP in the cells.

Glycogen

After entering cells, glucose can be used immediately for the release of energy to cells or it can be stored as a polymer of glucose known as glycogen. The ability to form glycogen makes it possible to store substantial quantities

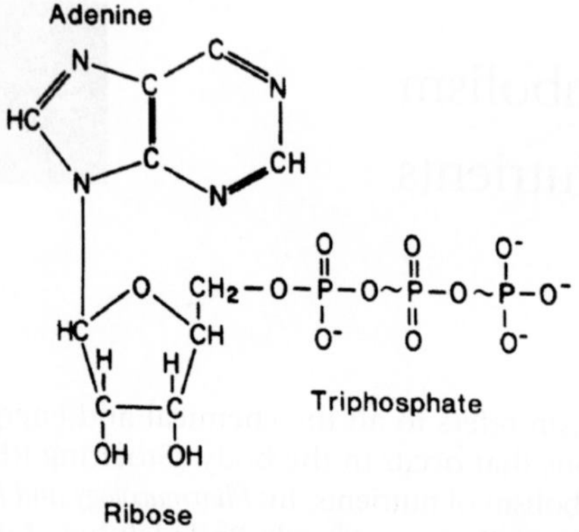

Adenine

Triphosphate

Ribose

Figure 59-1. Metabolism of nutrients in cells is directed toward the ultimate synthesis of adenosine triphosphate (ATP). Energy necessary for physiologic processes and chemical reactions is derived from the high energy phosphate bonds of ATP.

of carbohydrates without significantly altering the osmotic pressure of intracellular fluids.

Gluconeogenesis

Gluconeogenesis is the formation of glucose from amino acids and the glycerol portion of fat. This process occurs when body stores of carbohydrates decrease below normal levels. Gluconeogenesis is stimulated by hypoglycemia.

Energy Release from Glucose

Glucose is progressively broken down, and the resulting energy is used to form ATP. The most important means by which energy is released from the glucose molecule is by glycolysis and the subsequent oxidation of the end-products of glycolysis.

Anaerobic Glycolysis

In the absence of adequate amounts of oxygen, a small amount of energy can be released to cells by anaerobic glycolysis because the conversion of glucose to pyruvate does not require oxygen.

LIPID METABOLISM

Lipids include phospholipids, triglycerides, and cholesterol. The basic lipid moiety of phospholipids and triglycerides is fatty acids. Fatty acids are long-chain hydrocarbon organic acids that, when bound to albumin, are known as free fatty acids. Phospholipids include lecithins, cephalins, and sphingomyelins, which are formed principally in the liver and are important in the formation of myelin and cell membranes. Triglycerides, after absorption from the gastrointestinal tract, are transported in the lymph and then, by way of the thoracic duct, into the circulation in droplets known as *chylomicrons*. Triglycerides are used in the body mainly to provide energy for metabolic processes similar to those fueled by carbohydrates. Cholesterol does not contain fatty acids, but its sterol nucleus is synthesized from degradation products of fatty acid molecules, thus giving it many of the physical and chemical properties characteristic of lipids (Fig. 59-2). Lipoproteins are synthesized principally in the liver and are mixtures of phospholipids, triglycerides, cholesterol, and proteins (Table 59-1). The presumed function of lipoproteins is to provide a mechanism of transport for lipids throughout the body. Lipoproteins are classified according to their density, which is inversely proportional to their lipid content.

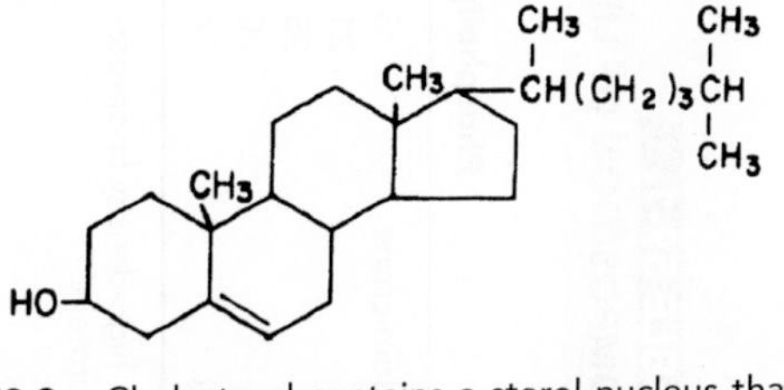

Figure 59-2. Cholesterol contains a sterol nucleus that is synthesized from the degradation products of fatty acid molecules.

TABLE 59-1.
COMPOSITION OF LIPIDS IN THE PLASMA

	Phospholipid (%)	Triglyceride (%)	Free Cholesterol (%)	Cholesterol Esters (%)	Protein (%)	Density
Chylomicrons	3	90	2	3	2	0.94
LDL	21	6	7	46	20	1.019–1.063
HDL	25	5	4	16	50	1.063–1.21
IDL	20	40	5	25	10	1.006–1.019
VLDL	17	55	4	18	8	0.94–1.006

HDL, high-density lipoprotein; IDL, intermediate-density lipoprotein; LDL, low-density lipoprotein; VLDL, very-low-density lipoprotein.

In the liver, low density lipoproteins (LDLs) are taken up by receptor-mediated endocytosis. An intrinsic feedback control system increases the endogenous production of cholesterol when exogenous intake is decreased, explaining the relatively modest lowering effect on plasma cholesterol concentrations produced by low-cholesterol diets. Statins, drugs that selectively inhibit HMG-CoA and effectively lower plasma LDL cholesterol concentrations, seem to provide protection against acute cardiac events, perhaps reflecting antiinflammatory effects. In the absence of adequate carbohydrate metabolism (starvation or uncontrolled diabetes mellitus), large quantities of acetoacetic acid, β-hydroxybutyric acid, and acetone accumulate in the blood to produce ketosis, because almost all the energy of the body must come from the metabolism of lipids. In contrast to glycogen, large amounts of lipids can be stored in adipose tissue and in the liver. A major function of adipose tissue is to store triglycerides until they are needed for energy.

PROTEIN METABOLISM

Approximately 75% of the solid constituents of the body are proteins (Table 59-2). All proteins are composed of the same 20 amino acids, and several of these must be

TABLE 59-2.
TYPES OF PROTEINS

Globular	Fibrous	Conjugated
Albumin	Collagen	Mucoprotein
Globulin	Elastic fibers	Structural components of cells
Fibrinogen	Keratin	
Hemoglobin	Actin	
Enzymes	Myosin	
Nucleoproteins		

TABLE 59-3.
AMINO ACIDS

Essential	Nonessential
Arginine	Alanine
Histidine	Asparagine
Isoleucine	Aspartic acid
Leucine	Cysteine
Lysine	Glutamic acid
Methionine	Glutamine
Phenylalanine	Glycine
Threonine	Proline
Tryptophan	Serine
Valine	Tyrosine

supplied in the diet because they cannot be formed endogenously (essential amino acids) (Table 59-3). In proteins, amino acids are connected into long chains by peptide linkages. The type of protein formed by the cell is genetically determined. In proximal renal tubules, amino acids that have entered the glomerular filtrate are actively transported back into the blood.

Storage of Amino Acids

Immediately after entry into cells, amino acids are conjugated under the influence of intracellular enzymes into cellular proteins. These proteins can be rapidly decomposed again into amino acids and transported out of cells into blood to maintain optimal plasma amino acid concentrations. Cancer cells are prolific users of amino acids, and, simultaneously, the proteins of other tissues become markedly depleted.

Plasma Proteins

Plasma proteins are represented by (a) albumin, which provides colloid osmotic pressure; (b) globulins necessary for natural and acquired immunity; and (c) fibrinogen, which polymerizes into long fibrin threads during the coagulation of blood. Essentially, all plasma albumin and fibrinogen and 60% to 80% of the globulins are formed in the liver. The remainder of the globulins are formed in lymphoid tissues and other cells of the reticuloendothelial system.

Albumin

Albumin is the most abundant plasma protein and is principally responsible for maintaining plasma osmotic pressure. In addition, albumin is important as a transporter of plasma-bound substances, often including exogenously administered drugs. The normal daily synthesis of albumin is about 10 g, and the half-life for this protein may be as long as 22 days. Therefore, serum albumin concentrations may not be noticeably decreased in early states of acute hepatic failure.

Coagulation Factors

Hepatocytes are the site of synthesis of all protein coagulation factors, with the exception of von Willebrand factor and factor VIII:C. Coagulation may be rapidly impaired by acute liver failure, reflecting the short plasma half-life of certain coagulation factors (factor VII, 100 to 300 minutes).

Use of Proteins for Energy

After cells contain a maximal amount of protein, any additional amino acids are either deaminated (oxidative deamination) to keto acids that can enter the citric acid cycle to become energy or are stored as fat. Deamination of surplus amino acids may also be coupled with the transfer of an amino acid group from one amino acid to another amino acid (transamination.) Ammonia resulting from transamination is converted to urea in the liver for excretion by the kidneys (acute hepatic failure manifests by an accumulation of toxic concentrations of ammonia). The conversion of amino acids to glucose or glycogen is gluconeogenesis, and the conversion of amino acids into fatty acids is ketogenesis. Carbohydrates and lipids spare protein stores because they are used in preference to proteins for energy.

EFFECT OF STRESS ON METABOLISM

Stress increases the secretion of cortisol, catecholamines, and glucagon resulting in increased endogenous glucose production (hepatic gluconeogenesis) and hyperglycemia (provides glucose to cells involved in wound healing and inflammatory responses). Increased lipolysis reflects stress-induced β-stimulation. A predictable response to stress is the catabolism of proteins in skeletal muscles.

OBESITY

Given the importance of energy stores to individual survival and reproductive capacity, the ability to conserve energy in the form of adipose tissue would at one time have conferred a survival advantage. For this reason, human genes that favor energy intake and storage are presumed to be present, although not yet identified. The combination of easy access to calorically dense foods and a sedentary lifestyle has made the metabolic consequences of these presumed genes maladaptive (Table 59-4). Obesity is associated with a three- to fourfold increase in the risk of ischemic heart disease, stroke, and diabetes mellitus compared with the general population. The increased risk for morbidity and mortality extend beyond measurements of body mass index and fat distribution, as reflected by the diagnosis of *Metabolic Syndrome* (syndrome X, insulin-resistance syndrome) (Table 59-5). The risk of anesthesia may be increased in morbidly obese patients, reflecting mechanical (airway, positioning, ventilation) and comorbid conditions (diabetes mellitus, systemic hypertension).

TABLE 59-4.
DRUGS COMMONLY ASSOCIATED WITH WEIGHT GAIN

Classification	Drug	Alternative Drug
Antidepressants	Tricyclic antidepressants	Selective serotonin reuptake inhibitors
	Monoamine oxidase inhibitors	
Antidiabetics	Insulin	Metformin, acarbose
	Sulfonylureas	
	Thiazolidinediones	
Antiepileptics	Gabapentin	Lamotrigine
	Valproic acid	
	Topiramate	
Antipsychotics	Clozapine	Haloperidol
Steroids	Glucocorticoids	

TABLE 59-5.
CRITERIA FOR DIAGNOSIS OF METABOLIC SYNDROME (ANY THREE OF THE FOLLOWING CHARACTERISTICS)

Characteristic	Specific Finding
Waist circumference	Males >102 cm (40 inches) Females >88 cm (35 inches)
Blood glucose concentration (fasting)	>110 mg/dL
Increased systemic blood pressure	Systolic >130 mm Hg Diastolic >85 mm Hg
Serum triglyceride concentration	>150 mg/dL
High density lipoprotein cholesterol concentration	Males <40 mg/dL Females <50 mg/dL

Pharmacologic Treatment

Phentermine is an appetite suppressant that is utilized for short-term therapy intended to induce weight loss. In the past, this drug was frequently used in combination with fenfluramine (no longer clinically available). Long-term pharmacologic therapy intended to induce weight loss utilizes sibutramine or orlistat. Side effects of sibutramine include cardiovascular stimulation (important to monitor blood pressure and heart rate), and this drug is not recommended in patients with untreated systemic hypertension or coronary artery disease. Orlistat inhibits lipases in the gastrointestinal lumen, thus antagonizing triglyceride hydrolysis and decreasing fat absorption by about 30%. Because orlistat is not absorbed, its ability to cause weight loss likely reflects the resulting low-fat diet and lower caloric intake.

Physiology of the Newborn and Elderly

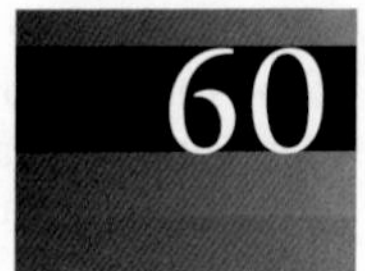

The physiology of both the neonatal and the elderly patient can be characterized by decreased functional reserve (Stoelting RK, Hillier SC. Physiology of the newborn and elderly. In: *Pharmacology and Physiology in Anesthetic Practice.* 4th ed. Philadelphia, Lippincott Williams & Wilkins, 2006:869–879). Additional demands and the coexisting diseases commonly encountered in the perioperative period may place a significant burden on organ systems that already have little functional reserve.

NEONATAL PHYSIOLOGY

The relatively high metabolic rate of the neonate (oxygen consumption is approximately 6 mL per kg per minute versus 3 mL per kg per minute in the adult) is the crucial determinant of cardiopulmonary function.

Neonatal Cardiovascular Physiology

The fetal circulation is characterized by high pulmonary vascular resistance, low systemic vascular resistance (placenta), and right to left shunting via the foramen ovale and ductus arteriosus.

Aeration of Lungs at Birth

The aeration of the lungs at birth causes a rapid decline in pulmonary vascular resistance and an increase in pulmonary blood flow. Increasing blood return to the heart via the pulmonary veins raises the pressure of the left atrium above that of the right atrium, causing a functional closure of the foramen ovale. The functional closure of the ductus arteriosus is, in part, mediated by an increase in arterial oxygen partial pressure and is complete within the first 10 to 15 hours.

Foramen Ovale and Ductus Arteriosus

Because the foramen ovale and ductus arteriosus are only functionally closed in the neonatal period, the neonatal circulation is able to revert readily to the fetal pattern, particularly in response to the physiologic stresses occasionally encountered in the perioperative period (hypoxemia, hypercarbia, acidosis).

Right-to-Left Shunting

Right-to-left shunting, by causing arterial hypoxemia, causes a further increase in pulmonary vascular resistance, thus creating a vicious circle.

Neonatal Myocardium

The neonatal myocardium contains immature contractile elements and is less compliant than the adult myocardium; therefore, only a limited increase in cardiac output is to be gained from aggressive volume loading in the normovolemic newborn.

Cardiac Output

Because contractile reserve is limited, neonatal cardiac output is exquisitely heart-rate dependent.

To meet the elevated metabolic demand, neonatal cardiac output relative to body weight is twice that of the adult. This is achieved by a relatively rapid heart rate (140 beats per minute), because stroke volume cannot be significantly increased.

Baroreflex Activity

Because neonatal baroreflex activity is impaired, the response to hemorrhage produces little increase in heart rate or change in total peripheral resistance. Thus, even a modest (10%) reduction in blood volume will cause a

15% to 30% decrease in mean blood pressure in the newborn infant.

Hematocrit

The marginal cardiovascular reserve of the neonate and the leftward shift of the fetal hemoglobin dissociation curve are the rationale underlying the recommendation that the hematocrit be maintained at 30% or higher.

Respiratory Physiology of the Newborn

The respiratory system of a term neonate at birth is immature, and postnatal development continues through early childhood.

Alveolar Maturation

Complete alveolar maturation does not occur until 8 to 10 years of age (the ratio of alveolar surface area to body surface area is one-third that of the adult). At birth, the infant possesses approximately one-tenth of the adult population of alveoli (neonatal alveolar minute ventilation is twice that of the adult).

Increasing respiratory rate, rather than tidal volume, is the most efficient means to increase alveolar ventilation in the newborn.

Lungs

The neonatal lung has a greater tendency to collapse, and the infant is obliged to utilize active mechanisms to maintain normal lung volumes (Table 60-1).

Functional Reserve Capacity

Neonatal functional reserve capacity (FRC) may decrease significantly during anesthesia, particularly during periodic breathing and apnea. The combination of increased oxygen consumption and a reduced FRC means that apnea and hypoventilation are associated with marked and rapid desaturation.

TABLE 60-1.
ACTIVE MECHANISMS USED BY NEONATES TO MAINTAIN LUNG VOLUME*

Rapid respiratory rate—early termination of expiration
Intercostal muscle activity in expiration—stabilizes compliant chest wall
Expiration against partially closed glottis—retards expiratory flow

*Significantly attenuated by general anesthesia.

Hypoxic Response

The impaired neonatal ventilatory responses to hypoxia and hypercarbia are contributing factors to the development of life-threatening apnea and hypoventilation in the postoperative period.

Neonatal Thermoregulation

The neonate tends to become hypothermic during general anesthesia much more rapidly than the adult, because of a relatively large surface area, thinner layer of insulating subcutaneous fat, and a limited capability for thermogenesis.

TABLE 60-2.
FACTORS THAT ENHANCE HEAT LOSS IN PEDIATRIC PATIENTS DURING ANESTHESIA AND SURGERY

Decrease in thermoregulatory threshold
Low ambient temperatures in operating room
Preparation of the skin with cold solutions
Infusion of cold solutions
Anesthesia-induced vasodilation
High flow nonrebreathing anesthesia systems

TABLE 60-3.
INTERVENTIONS THAT PREVENT HEAT LOSS IN PEDIATRIC PATIENTS DURING ANESTHESIA AND SURGERY

Increase ambient temperature in operating room (28–30°C)
Radiant heat lamps
Wrapping the extremities
Use nonvolatile warmed solutions for skin preparation
Administration of warmed intravenous fluids and blood products
Warmed and humidified inhaled gases
Forced air warming devices

Heat Loss (Table 60-2)

Intraoperative hypothermia will markedly delay emergence from anesthesia. Several interventions may prevent heat loss in pediatric patients during anesthesia and surgery (Table 60-3).

Neonatal Fluid, Electrolyte, and Renal Physiology (Table 60-4)

The neonate is at risk for overhydration, dehydration, metabolic acidosis, and hyponatremia, necessitating meticulous attention to intraoperative fluid therapy.

TABLE 60-4.
CHARACTERISTICS OF NEONATAL FLUID, ELECTROLYTE, AND RENAL PHYSIOLOGY

Increased total body water
Increased extracellular fluid volume
Increased water turnover rate
Reduced glomerular filtration rate
Obligate sodium losers

Neonates have decreased glycogen stores and are prone to hypoglycemia after relatively brief periods of starvation (risk for hypoglycemia and the need for supplemental glucose is an essential element of the intraoperative fluid plan).

Neonatal Neurophysiology

The neural connections required for the transmission and perception of pain are functional by the 24th week of gestation. Failure to provide analgesia for neonatal pain causes up-regulation of the nociceptive pathways in the dorsal horn of the spinal cord.

Preterm Infant Pathology

Periventricular-intraventricular hemorrhage occurs in 40% to 50% of premature infants. Preterm infants are also at risk for the retinopathy of prematurity (prematurity is the primary etiologic factor).

THE PHYSIOLOGY OF THE ELDERLY

Aging and the Cardiovascular System

The decline in cardiac function that occurs with aging in the healthy individual appears to be related in part to decreasing functional demand. Indeed, when exercise and conditioning are maintained into the later decades, the decline in cardiovascular function is markedly attenuated.

Heart

Increases in cardiac output in response to severe exertion are attenuated by approximately 20% to 30% in the elderly, principally because the heart rate response to severe exercise is diminished.

Loss of the atrial "kick," such as during atrial fibrillation, is particularly poorly tolerated.

Diastolic dysfunction is a major contributor to cardiovascular disease in the elderly population and is exacerbated by several coexisting diseases (Table 60-5).

TABLE 60-5.
COMMONLY ENCOUNTERED DISEASES OF THE ELDERLY ASSOCIATED WITH DIASTOLIC DYSFUNCTION

Systemic hypertension
Coronary artery disease
Cardiomyopathy
Aortic stenosis
Atrial fibrillation
Diabetes
Chronic renal disease

Dyspnea in the elderly may indicate congestive heart failure and/or pulmonary disease.

Large Vessels

Structural changes in the large vessels are an important element of the aging process and contribute significantly to the age-related changes in the heart (pulse wave is reflected back from the peripheral circulation and augments systolic pressure). Both systolic pressure and pulse pressure are increased, and left ventricular afterload is elevated.

Endothelial Function

Endothelial function is important for the regulation of vasomotor responses, coagulation, fibrinolysis, immunomodulation, and vascular growth and proliferation. Age-related endothelial dysfunction can be characterized as a decrease in the ability of the endothelium to dilate blood vessels in response to physiologic and pharmacologic stimuli.

Conduction System

The proportion of pacemaker cells decreases from 50% in late childhood to less than 10% at 75 years, thus contributing to an increased incidence of first- and second-degree heart block, sick sinus syndrome, and atrial fibrillation in the elderly.

Autonomic and Integrated Cardiovascular Responses

Aging is associated with increased norepinephrine entry into the circulation and deficient catecholamine reuptake at nerve ending, yet the cardiovascular response to increased adrenergic stimulation is attenuated by down-regulation of post-receptor signaling, decreased receptor density, and reduced contractile response of the myocardium.

β-Agonists

The response to exogenously administered β-agonists, such as isoproterenol, is similarly attenuated.

Orthostatic Hypotension

Orthostatic hypotension is common in the elderly and is associated with syncope, falls, and cognitive decline.

Anesthetic and Ischemic Preconditioning in the Aging Heart

Anesthetic preconditioning may be markedly attenuated in the elderly, and the utility of preconditioning strategies in this age group is uncertain.

Aging and the Respiratory System (Tables 60-6 and 60-7)

Respiratory System Mechanics and Architecture

Aging is associated with a loss of lung elasticity that is responsible for a decrease in lung recoil, thus making the lung more distensible.

Lung Volumes and Capacities (Table 60-8)

Expiratory Flow

A progressive decline occurs in FEV_1 and functional vital capacity (FVC) with age that is independent of smoking or environmental exposure.

TABLE 60-6.
INTRINSIC AND EXTRINSIC EVENTS THAT INFLUENCE THE RESPIRATORY SYSTEM DURING AGING

Intrinsic to the Aging Process	Environmental, Behavioral, and Disease Related
Decreased bronchiolar caliber	Industrial and environmental pollution
Decreased alveolar surface area	Smoking
Increased lung collagen content	General deconditioning
Decreased lung elastin content	Coexisting disease
Kyphoscoliosis	
Increased thoracic cage rigidity	
Decreased diaphragmatic strength	

Diffusing Capacity and Alveolar to Arterial Oxygen Gradient

Gas-exchange efficiency declines with aging as a result of increasing intrapulmonary shunting and decreasing lung-diffusing capacity. The result is a linear decline in resting

TABLE 60-7.
FUNCTIONAL CONSEQUENCES OF THE INTRINSIC AND EXTRINSIC EVENTS THAT INFLUENCE THE RESPIRATORY SYSTEM DURING AGING

Decrease in lung elastic recoil
Increase in lung compliance
Decrease in oxygen diffusing capacity
Premature airway closure causing V/Q mismatch and increased alveolar-to-arterial oxygen gradient
Small airway closure and gas trapping
Decreased expiratory flow rates

TABLE 60-8.
CHANGES IN LUNG VOLUMES AND CAPACITIES WITH AGING

Increase	Decrease	No Change
Residual volume Functional residual capacity Closing capacity (airway closure may occur during tidal breathing)	Vital capacity	Total lung capacity

supine PaO_2 between early adulthood and 65 years of age (~ 0.5 mm Hg per year).

V/Q Mismatch
Small airway closure causes V/Q mismatch and shunting.

Shunting
Cardiac output is often decreased in the elderly, to the extent that mixed venous oxygen tension is decreased (modest amounts of shunting may produce a significant decrease in PaO_2).

Upper Airway Protective Reflexes

Cough effectiveness is reduced in the elderly because of diminished reflex sensitivity and impaired muscle function (increased incidence of aspiration pneumonia).

Control of Breathing, Chemoreceptors, and Integrated Responses

Increases in heart rate and minute ventilation in response to elevations in $PaCO_2$ or decreases in PaO_2 are markedly attenuated in the elderly. These responses are further attenuated by the administration of opioids and sedative/hypnotic drugs. Thus, the elderly are at particular risk from life-threatening respiratory depression in the perioperative period.

Exercise Capacity

Exercise capacity in the elderly may be limited by both decreased cardiovascular and respiratory reserve.

Sleep Disordered Breathing

The incidence of sleep disordered breathing increases with age, especially in men.

Thermoregulation in the Elderly

Resting Core Temperature (Table 60-9)

Response to Cold Stress (Table 60-10)

The attenuated cold-stress responses of the elderly are further diminished by general and regional anesthesia. Perioperative hypothermia is very likely in the elderly patient, unless active measures are taken to maintain normothermia.

Response to Heat Stress (Table 60-10)

The response to heat stress may be markedly attenuated in the elderly, and this places a significant burden on the cardiovascular system.

Gastrointestinal Function in the Elderly

Liver (Table 60-11)

TABLE 60-9.
FACTORS ASSOCIATED WITH REDUCED RESTING CORE TEMPERATURES IN THE ELDERLY

Neurologic disease
Diabetes
Low body weight
Lack of self-sufficiency
Consumption of less than two meals per day
Smoking
Alcohol consumption

TABLE 60-10.
FACTORS RESPONSIBLE FOR ATTENUATED THERMAL STRESS RESPONSES IN THE ELDERLY

Heat Stress Response	Cold Stress Response
Reduced sweat gland output	Loss of muscle mass
Reduced ability to increase cutaneous blood flow	Reduced ability for cutaneous vasoconstriction
Reduced ability to increase cardiac output	
Less redistribution of cardiac output from core to peripheral circulations	

Gastro-Esophageal Physiology

Gastric emptying of solid material appears to be relatively normal in the healthy elderly population.

Gastro-Esophageal Reflux Disease

Gastro-esophageal reflux disease (GERD) is more frequent in the elderly (Table 60-12).

Several medications that are commonly prescribed in the elderly population predispose to GERD by decreasing lower esophageal sphincter tone (Table 60-13).

TABLE 60-11.
CHANGES RELATED TO AGING THAT MANIFEST AT THE LIVER

Decreased liver mass and hepatic blood flow (decreased first pass metabolism)
Preservation of hepatocellular function
Possible decreased albumin production (related to nutrition)
Increased α-1-acid glycoprotein concentrations
Possible decreased production of plasma cholinesterase

TABLE 60-12.
FACTORS PREDISPOSING TO THE INCREASED INCIDENCE OF GASTROESOPHAGEAL REFLUX DISEASE IN THE ELDERLY

Increased prevalence of sliding hiatal hernia
Shortened intra-abdominal segment of the lower esophageal sphincter
Impaired clearance of refluxed acid
Use of medications that reduce lower esophageal sphincter pressure
Decreased esophageal peristalsis pressure

TABLE 60-13.
MEDICATIONS COMMONLY ADMINISTERED IN THE ELDERLY THAT REDUCE LOWER ESOPHAGEAL SPHINCTER TONE AND PREDISPOSE TO GASTROESOPHAGEAL REFLUX

Anticholinergics
Antidepressants
Nitrates
Calcium channel blockers
Theophylline

TABLE 60-14.
CHANGES IN RENAL FUNCTION IN THE ELDERLY

Decreased cortical nephron population
Reduction in renal mass
Decreased glomerular filtration rate (serum creatinine unchanged due to decreased skeletal muscle mass)
Decreased renal blood flow

TABLE 60-15.
FACTORS THOUGHT TO BE RESPONSIBLE FOR THE SIGNIFICANT DECREASE IN LEAN MUSCLE MASS THAT OCCURS WITH AGING

Decreased motor neuron innervation
Decreased physical activity
Endocrine shift towards catabolism (reduced insulin-like-growth factor-1 secretion)
Decreased androgen (testosterone and estrogen) secretion
Decreased total caloric intake
Decreased protein consumption and protein synthesis
Inflammatory mediators and cytokines (Interleukins 1 and 6, tumor necrosis factor)

Renal Function in the Elderly (Table 60-14)

Muscle Mass and Aging

Aging is associated with a significant decline in neuromuscular performance (sarcopenia) (Table 60-15). Diminished muscle mass has significant implications for the elderly patient during the perioperative period (Table 60-16).

Neurophysiology of Aging (Table 60-17)

TABLE 60-16.
PERIOPERATIVE FUNCTIONAL CONSEQUENCES OF THE LOSS OF MUSCLE MASS THAT TYPICALLY ACCOMPANIES AGING

Impaired postoperative mobilization and ambulation
Reduced cough effectiveness
Reduced shivering thermogenesis
Altered drug disposition
Reduced neuromuscular functional reserve
Prolonged recovery and hospitalization

TABLE 60-17. NEUROPHYSIOLOGICAL MANIFESTATIONS OF AGING
Decreased sensitivity to benzodiazepines and opioids
Decreased MAC for volatile anesthetics
Postoperative delirium
Cognitive impairment
Hyperacute neuroendocrine response to stress (may cause dendritic atrophy)

Drug Index

Note: Page numbers followed by f indicate figures; page numbers followed by t indicate tables

Subject Index

Note: Page numbers followed by f indicate figures; page numbers followed by t indicate tables

B

P

T

W

Z